Textbook of SARS-CoV-2 and COVID-19

Textbook of SARS-CoV-2 and COVID-19

Epidemiology, Pathophysiology, Immunology, Clinical Manifestations, Treatment, Complications, and Preventive Measures

Edited by

Subramani Mani, MBBS, PhD

Independent Research Consultant
Former Associate Professor, Department of Medicine
University of New Mexico School of Medicine
Albuquerque, New Mexico
Former Assistant Professor, Department of Biomedical
Informatics, Vanderbilt University,
Franklin, Tennessee

Jörn-Hendrik Weitkamp, MD

Professor of Pediatrics
Monroe Carrell Jr. Children's Hospital
Vanderbilt University Medical Center,
Nashville, Tennessee

Elsevier

1600 John F. Kennedy Blvd.
Ste 1800
Philadelphia, PA 19103-2899

TEXTBOOK OF SARS-COV-2 AND COVID-19:   ISBN: 978-0-323-87539-4
EPIDEMIOLOGY, PATHOPHYSIOLOGY, IMMUNOLOGY, CLINICAL MANIFESTATIONS,
TREATMENT, COMPLICATIONS, AND PREVENTIVE MEASURES

Senior Content Development Manager: Somodatta Roy Choudhury
Senior Content Strategist: Charlotta Kryhl
Senior Content Development Specialist: Shilpa
Publishing Services Manager: Shereen Jameel
Project Manager: Vishnu T. Jiji
Senior Designer: Amy Buxton

Printed in India
Last digit is the print number: 9 8 7 6 5 4 3 2 1

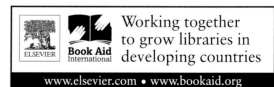

We dedicate this book to all the survivors and victims of SARS-CoV-2 and COVID-19, the frontline workers in the fight against the pandemic, all health care personnel, health policy employees, and scientists engaged in the struggle to control and neutralize the virus.

—Subramani Mani and Jörn-Hendrik Weitkamp

I dedicate this book fondly to my alma mater, Medical College, Trivandrum, India, where I first observed the rays of light illuminate the workings of the human body in health and disease and absorbed the foundations of the science and art of clinical medicine.

And to my high school, the Attakulangara Government Central High School, Trivandrum, which opened my eyes and ears to the magical mysteries of science, where giant canopy trees cover its lawns, woodpeckers and owls tease you playfully, and butterflies flutter colorfully and carelessly, nature in all its furious and enchanting avatars of torrential rain, scorching sun, cool breeze, drizzle, and rainbow provides the perfect natural background for the lessons of the teachers, setting an ideal environment for minds to open, develop, and broaden.

And to the Medical Service Center, India, founded by my friends and colleagues, which provides volunteer medical services during natural disasters, including the COVID-19 pandemic.

To my professor, Dr. P.P. Joseph, MBBS, MRCP, a doyen of clinical medicine who had the patience to respond to all my clinical questions and train me.

And to Dr. V. Venugopal, MBBS, a loving friend, a great doctor, and a fighter for social justice.

—Subramani Mani

I dedicate this book to my parents Anita and Fritz, who have supported me during all steps of life; my coach, critic, and loving wife Asli; and my wonderful children Alara, Selin, and Alp.

—Jörn-Hendrik Weitkamp

Contributors

Jamie Aranda, MD, FAAEM, FACEP
Assistant Professor of Emergency
    Medicine,
Department of Emergency
    Medicine,
Medical College of Wisconsin,
    Milwaukee, Wisconsin

Goundappa K. Balasubramani, PhD
Research Associate Professor,
Department of Epidemiology,
School of Public Health,
University of Pittsburgh,
Pittsburgh, Pennsylvania

Ritu Banerjee, MD, PhD
Professor, Department
    of Pediatrics,
 Vanderbilt University Medical
    Center,
Nashville, Tennessee

Behin Barahimi, MD
Associate Professor,
Department of Ophthalmology
    and Visual Sciences,
Vanderbilt Eye Institute,
Nashville, Tennessee

Laura A. Binari, MD
Transplant Nephrology Fellow,
    Division of Nephrology,
Department of Medicine,
Vanderbilt University Medical
    Center,
Nashville, Tennessee

David M. Brooks, MD
Clinical Fellow,
Division of Neonatology,
Department of Pediatrics,
Vanderbilt University Medical
    Center,
Nashville, Tennessee

Anna Burgner, MD, MEHP
Assistant Professor,
Division of Nephrology,
Department of Medicine,
Vanderbilt University Medical
    Center,
Nashville, Tennessee

Alexander De Castro-Abeger, MD
Pediatric Ophthalmology and
    Strabismus Fellow,
Vanderbilt Eye Institute,
Nashville, Tennessee

Matthew Chinn, MD, FAEMS
Assistant Professor,
Department of Emergency
    Medicine,
Medical College of Wisconsin,
    Milwaukee, Wisconsin

Amparo de la Peña, PhD
Vice President of Pharmacometric
    Services, Simulations Plus,
    Cognigen division
Senior Research Advisor and
Asset Manager,
Chorus, Eli Lilly,
Indianapolis, Indiana

Ally Esch, DO
Emergency Medicine Resident,
Medical College of Wisconsin,
Milwaukee, Wisconsin

Mark E. Garcia, MD
Assistant Professor of Medicine,
Division of Cardiology,
University of New Mexico School
    of Medicine,
Albuquerque, New Mexico

Ben Geoffrey A.S., PhD
Bioinformatician,
Srivathi AI,
Bangalore, India

Pravin George, DO
Director,
Critical Care Medical Informatics,
INOVA Health System,
Assistant Professor of Neurology,
Case Western University School
    of Medicine,
Cleveland, Ohio

Karen E. Gilcs, MD, MS
Psychiatry Resident,
Department of Psychiatry and
    Behavioral Sciences,
Emory University School of
    Medicine,
Atlanta, Georgia

Aarthi Goverdhan, PhD
Senior Scientist,
Qiagen,
Redwood City, California

Daniel Griffin, MD, PhD
Instructor in Clinical Medicine,
Columbia University,
New York, New York

Sylvia Groth, MD
Assistant Professor,
Department of Ophthalmology
    and Visual Sciences,
Vanderbilt Eye Institute,
Nashville, Tennessee

Madihah Hepburn, MD
Neurocritical Care Attending,
Dept of Stroke & Neurosciences,
Summa Health System,
Akron, Ohio

Nancy Jacobson, MD
Assistant Professor of Emergency
    Medicine,
Department of Emergency
    Medicine,
Medical College of Wisconsin,
Wisconsin, Milwaukee

Sarah Kim, PhD
Assistant Professor,
Department of Pharmaceutics,
College of Pharmacy,
University of Florida,
Orlando, Florida

Charles A. Knirsch, MD, MPH
Vice President,
Clinical Research and
    Development, Pfizer,
New York, New York

Srinivasan Krishnaswami, PhD
Independent Consultant for
  Chemical Technologies,
Sravathi Advance Process
  Technologies Private Limited,
Bangalore, India

Sriram Krishnaswami, PhD
Vice President,
Medicine Team Leader,
Global Product Development
  Oncology, Pfizer,
Groton, Connecticut

Pooja Lal, MD
Gastroenterology and Hepatology
  Fellow,
Vanderbilt University Medical
  Center,
Nashville, Tennessee

Susan M. Lopata, MD
Assistant Professor,
Division of Neonatology,
Department of Pediatrics,
Vanderbilt University Medical
  Center,
Nashville, Tennessee

Subramani Mani, MBBS, PhD
Independent Research Consultant,
Former Associate Professor,
Department of Medicine,
University of New Mexico School
  of Medicine,
Albuquerque, New Mexico
Former Assistant Professor,
Department of Biomedical
  Informatics,
Vanderbilt University,
Franklin, Tennessee

Natalie N. McCall, MD
Assistant Professor,
Division of Nephrology,
Department of Medicine,
Vanderbilt University Medical
  Center,
Nashville, Tennessee

William M. McDonald, MD
Professor and Chair,
Department of Psychiatry and
  Behavioral Sciences,
Emory University School of
  Medicine,
Atlanta, Georgia

**Sujatha S. Menon, M Pharm,
MS Pharm, PhD**
Senior Director,
Clinical Pharmacology (I&I),
Global Product Development
  Pfizer,
Groton, Connecticut

Cullen P. Moran, MD
Ophthalmology Resident,
Vanderbilt Eye Institute,
Nashville, Tennessee

Sivakumar Nagaraju, MD
Pulmonary and Critical Care
  Physician,
Lovelace Medical Group,
Albuquerque, New Mexico

Christopher Newey, DO, MS, FNCS
Assistant Professor of Neurology,
  Cleveland Clinic Lerner College
  of Medicine
Staff Physician, Cerebrovascular
  and Epilepsy Centers,
  Cleveland Clinic
Medical Director, NSICU Cleveland
  Clinic Akron General,
Akron, Ohio

Mary Patricia Nowalk, PhD, RDN
Professor, Department of Family
  Medicine,
University of Pittsburgh, School
  of Medicine,
Pittsburgh, Pennsylvania

Dhyanesh A. Patel, MD
Assistant Professor of Medicine,
Division of Gastroenterology,
Hepatology, and Nutrition,
Department of Medicine,
Vanderbilt University Medical
  Center,
Nashville, Tennessee

Amelie Pham, MD
Clinical Fellow,
Division of Maternal-Fetal Medicine,
Department of Obsterics and
  Gynecology,
Vanderbilt University Medical
  Center,
Nashville, Tennessee

**Krishna Ramakrishnamenon Prasad,
MD**
Past Medical Director,
Emergency Medicine Department,
Aurora Medical Center,
Summit, Wisconsin

**Sathishkumar Ramalingam, MD,
FACP, FHM**
Assistant Professor,
Burrell College of Osteopathic
  Medicine,
Department of Hospital medicine,
Lovelace Medical Center,
Albuquerque, New Mexico

John C. Ray, MD, MBA
Assistant Professor,
Department of Emergency Medicine,
Medical College of Wisconsin,
Senior Medical Director,
Froedtert Emergency Department,
Milwaukee, Wisconsin

Mythily Srinivasan, MDS, PhD
Associate Professor,
Indiana University School
  of Dentistry,
Indiana University–Purdue
  University,
Indianapolis, Indiana

Amit K. Srivastava, PhD
Senior Director,
Vaccines Medical and Scientific
  Affairs, Pfizer,
Cambridge, Massachusetts

Jennifer L. Thompson, MD
Associate Professor,
Division of Maternal-Fetal Medicine,
Department of Obstetrics and
  Gynecology,
Vanderbilt University Medical
  Center,
Nashville, Tennessee

Thankam Thyvalikakath, MDS, DMD, PhD
Professor and Director Dental
  Informatics Core,
Indiana University School
  of Dentistry,
Indiana University–Purdue
  University,
Indianapolis, Indiana

Michael F. Vaezi, MD, PhD
Professor, Division of
  Gastroenterology, Hepatology,
  and Nutrition, Department of
  Medicine, Vanderbilt
  University Medical Center,
  Nashville, Tennessee

Andreas Wack, PhD
Principal Group Leader,
Immunoregulation Lab,
The Francis Crick Institute,
  London, United Kingdom

Robert S. Wallis, MD, FIDSA, FRCPE
Chief Science Officer, Aurum
Institute, Johannesburg, South
  Africa
Professor (Adjunct) Vanderbilt
  and Case Western Reserve
  Universities

Charles B. Nemeroff, MD, PhD
Professor and Chair,
Department of Psychiatry and
  Behavioral Sciences,
Dell Medical School, The University
  of Texas at Austin,
Austin, Texas

Jörn-Hendrik Weitkamp, MD
Professor of Pediatrics, Monroe
  Carrell Jr. Children's Hospital,
Vanderbilt University Medical
  Center,
Nashville, Tennessee

Acknowledgments

First and foremost, we are greatly indebted to all the chapter contributors who made this book possible. Without their dedicated and diligent efforts in putting together each chapter in a timely manner we could not have taken it to press with an accelerated timeline. In particular, SM would like to thank Dr. Prasad and Dr. Krishnaswami (Pfizer) for suggesting colleagues as prospective authors and then motivating them to be part of this endeavor.

Robin Carter, Charlotta Kryhl, and Patricia Geary of Elsevier enthusiastically facilitated a quick review of our book proposal while patiently answering our innumerable queries. Once the decision was made to proceed, Shilpa, Vishnu and Baljinder Kaur from Elsevier took over the formidable task of going through all the submitted chapters and taking it to production, satisfying the publisher's stringent requirements and guidelines in a time-sensitive manner.

SM specifically would like to recall with gratitude the innumerable discussions with Dr. Prasad, Dr. Krishnaswami, and Shanthi regarding the scope, content, and direction of the book in the early stages of the proposal development. SM also feels indebted to Dr. Krishnaswami and Shanthi for their valuable feedback on the earlier drafts of chapters he coauthored.

Subramani Mani, MBBS, PhD
Jörn-Hendrik Weitkamp, MD

The SARS-CoV-2 pandemic has entered its third year. The novel corona virus continues to evolve and adapt, extending its reach across all the six continents and sparing no single country along its many trajectories of spread. From Alpha through the currently raging Omicron variant, the virus has spawned a number of versions of varying infectivity and virulence generating multiple waves and surges along the way. As of January 2022, the number of people who have tested positive for the virus exceeds 300 million, with more than 5 million deaths globally.

In spite of national and international efforts, not always well-coordinated, to prevent, contain, mitigate, and control the spread of the virus and the development of effective vaccines, antiviral agents, and other therapeutics during the pandemic, there is no clear end in sight at the time of this writing. However, there are certain signs of optimism emanating from the limited progress humanity has made in its fight against the virus and COVID-19, the disease it causes.

During this period, tens of thousands of articles have delved into various aspects of the virus and disease, and many articles have been published in scientific journals, along with the extensive coverage of the pandemic in the popular media. All of these have contributed to the creation of a broad awareness of the problem and the significant challenges everyone is facing. However, critical details of the science of SARS-CoV-2 and COVID-19 remain scattered and sometimes even submerged among the mounds of these publications, which are accumulating at a pace that makes it virtually impossible for students, trainees, health care providers, researchers, and health policy makers to keep up with important and relevant developments in a timely manner. Public health agencies, professional societies, and journal portals have tried to alleviate the problem by developing and maintaining guidelines and putting together article collections and document clusters catering to different sections of readers.

Our goal in putting together this textbook on SARS-CoV-2 and COVID-19 has been to collate, distill, synthesize, abstract, and organize in one place the advancing but scattered knowledge spread throughout the published literature related to the novel corona virus and disease. This posed a challenge as the pandemic itself was evolving; our solution was to focus on the basics, maintain an appropriate balance of breadth and depth while limiting the temporal scope of the effort to the first 18 months of the pandemic to keep our endeavor manageable and timebound. We have been fortunate to put together a high-quality team of physicians and scientists for this task, and their dedicated effort in crafting the individual chapters has been commendable. We as editors feel confident that the authors have succeeded immensely in overcoming the challenges of abstracting relevant knowledge from the copious published literature on the epidemiology, biology, pathophysiology, clinical manifestations, and management of COVID-19.

During the early days of the pandemic when there was a lot of confusion, fear, and misinformation and the science of SARS-CoV-2 and COVID-19 was gradually emerging, Dr. Rajeevan P.P., the secretary of the Kerala state (SM's home state in India) chapter of the Breakthrough Science Society (BSS), a grassroots organization based in India with a mission of fighting superstition and inculcating scientific thought in society, invited SM to give a Zoom talk on the emerging pandemic. Then, over the summer of 2020, when the race for the development of vaccines for COVID-19 was accelerating, generating interest and enthusiasm on the one hand while also stirring up controversies, SM gave a second talk on vaccine basics and the COVID-19 vaccine race. The talks were well received, and the idea of abstracting relevant knowledge from the glut of publications related to SARS-CoV-2 and COVID-19, which was making it hard for various stakeholders to keep up with the essential science behind the pandemic, was born. After making a short list of potential chapter authors, SM quickly reached out to HW at Vanderbilt, with whom he had collaborated on research while SM was at Vanderbilt, for a chapter contribution. We then started discussing the details of the book proposal, and it soon became clear that we would be coediting the proposed textbook. HW put forward a list of potential chapter authors from Vanderbilt University Medical Center. SM then reached out to Dr. Krishnaswami, a senior scientist at Pfizer, and Dr. Prasad, an emergency physician SM knew from his medical school days at Trivandrum Medical College (Kerala, India), and put together a long list of prospective authors. After convincing ourselves of the feasibility of the project based on the enthusiastic response we received, we drafted a formal book proposal over the next couple of weeks and submitted it to Elsevier.

It was pandemic time, and we had set ourselves up to edit a book on the virus and the disease responsible for the pandemic. Moreover, as the pandemic was evolving, we had to compress the submission and editing timeline and expedite the process to maintain time sensitivity. Despite immense challenges, including personal setbacks and tragedies many authors faced—losing a loved one, being hospitalized with COVID-19, personal and family health setbacks, getting injured in a car accident, etc.—the authors did a magnificent job of surmounting the obstacles and delivered the promised manuscripts on time and keeping the publication schedule on track.

The textbook has been developed with comprehensiveness and scientific rigor in mind, addressing both the breadth and depth requirements. The book covers the biology, epidemiology, pathogenesis, immunology, clinical features, current treatment, and prevention strategies, including a few special topics related to the virus (SARS-CoV-2) and the disease (COVID-19). The book has been organized into four parts: (1) basics, 4 chapters; (2) clinical, 8 chapters; (3) pediatrics, 2 chapters; and (4) special topics, 4 chapters, for a total of 18 chapters. To achieve our goal, we recruited contributors with diverse backgrounds, training, expertise, and scholarship to undertake this important scholarly task. The various contributors are drawn from the pool of practicing physicians from different disciplines, physician scientists, and applied research scientists. All of the authors are involved in treating COVID-19 patients and/or pursuing clinical investigations, applied research, or data analytics and literature reviews pertaining to SARS-CoV-2 and COVID-19.

The book is expected to serve the needs of medical students, advanced nursing students, graduate students in biological sciences and the schools of public health, physicians undergoing residencies and fellowship training in medical specialties, other health care trainees, practicing physicians, health care researchers, and possibly public health policy makers. It also should be of value to a section of the public seeking in-depth knowledge of SARS-CoV-2 and COVID-19 that is ravaging the lives of many people, including their friends and family members.

Medical students, nursing students, and graduate students pursuing advanced degrees in biology and public health need textbooks that cover a disease or a set of related clinical conditions in a comprehensive manner while providing sufficient bibliographic material as citations for them to explore further when needed. The textbook provides sufficient bibliographic references after each chapter for more in-depth study. Each specific chapter is expected to provide a solid foundation on the topic with pointers to relevant original published sources.

Physicians undergoing residencies and fellowship training would like to look up material that will help answer clinical questions at the point of care, and the e-book version could fulfill such a need. The bibliography will enable them to understand material at greater depth for detailed clinical reports or for research papers if they are pursuing clinical research projects. Individual chapters synthesize the state of the art in scientific literature to help provide a starting point for those pursuing advanced degrees or training.

Similarly, for other health care trainees, practicing physicians, health care researchers, and public health policy makers, the book can serve as a source of quick reference to answer questions that arise during their workday. In addition, for the inquisitive section of the public, many of the chapters would provide useful information in sufficient detail to answer their questions and address their concerns regarding the pandemic. The following is a short introduction to each of the included chapters.

In Chapter 1, Drs. Balasubramani and Nowalk present the epidemiology of SARS-CoV-2 and COVID-19. The authors take us on a tour of the important countries on the flight path of the virus during the first wave of the pandemic, discussing the morbidity and mortality and contrasting the damage caused with the mitigation and control measures adopted by the respective countries.

In Chapter 2, Dr. Goverdhan delves into the detailed molecular structure of the virus and the clever mechanisms used by the pathogen to enter human host cells to start the infection. The article also covers the principles of diagnostic tests available to detect infection by the virus.

In Chapter 3, Drs. Knirsch, Wallis, Srivastava, and Wack take us on a *tour de force* of the various types of immune mechanisms triggered by the novel corona virus in the host. The authors also discuss in detail the immunopathology of mild to severe versions of COVID-19.

In Chapter 4, Drs. Mani and Griffin provide a big-picture view of the manifestations of COVID-19 in various organs and systems, starting with the respiratory system. The authors also cover the important comorbidities that make individuals susceptible to severe disease and present some of the observed racial and ethnic disparities in susceptibility to the virus.

In Chapter 5, Drs. Nagaraju, Ramalingam, and Mani discuss in detail the pathophysiology of acute respiratory distress syndrome and the different manifestations of COVID-19 lung injury. The authors address the management of various complications resulting from COVID-19 lung injury, illustrating their narrative with three representative case reports highlighting severe COVID-19.

In Chapter 6, Drs. Mani and Garcia describe the spectrum of varied cardiovascular manifestations and explore the four pathophysiological mechanisms leading to cardiac injury—the renin angiotensin system, direct viral infection of the myocardium, cytokine-mediated cardiac injury, and COVID-19–associated thrombosis. The authors then discuss the complications of cardiac injury and their management highlighted by three case reports.

In Chapter 7, Drs. Hepburn, Newey, and George present the various neurological manifestations and discuss in detail the resulting complications after SARS-CoV-2 infection. The authors also include two case reports from their practice to illustrate many of the significant clinical findings.

In Chapter 8, Drs. Srinivasan and Thyvalikakath describe the oral cavity manifestations of COVID-19 and the postulated mechanisms underlying these pathological conditions. The chapter also discusses salivary diagnostics for virus detection and for understanding the transmission characteristics of the SARS-CoV-2. The authors also address the challenges faced by dental offices and practices in pandemic times.

In Chapter 9, Drs. Lal, Patel, and Vaezi illustrate the pathophysiology and clinical manifestations of SARS-CoV-2 for the gastrointestinal system. They discuss the impact of SARS-CoV-2 on gut microbiota and review the implications of COVID-19 in patients with inflammatory bowel disease, chronic liver disease, and pancreatic disorders.

In Chapter 10, Drs. Binari, McCall, and Burgner deliberate the multifactorial pathogenesis of acute kidney injury (AKI) in patients with COVID-19. They describe cellular mechanisms and propose treatment options. They further discuss populations specifically vulnerable to sequelae from SARS-CoV-2 infection, such as patients with end-stage kidney disease (ESKD) and kidney transplant patients.

In Chapter 11, Drs. Barahimi, Moran, De Castro-Abeger, and Groth describe the ophthalmic manifestations of COVID-19, including the anterior segment of the eye, the orbit, eyelids, retina, microvasculature, and uvea, as well as neuroophthalmologic manifestations and specific considerations for pediatric populations.

In Chapter 12, Drs. Giles, Nemeroff, and McDonald report on neuropsychiatric symptoms of COVID-19. Although depression, anxiety, mania, delirium, catatonia, and psychosis have been well documented during acute infection, many patients continue to experience psychiatric symptoms after recovering from the acute infection, and others have developed new symptoms such as posttraumatic stress and psychosis.

In Chapter 13, Drs. Pham, Brooks, Lopata, Thompson, and Weitkamp describe the impact of maternal SARS-CoV-2 infection on the fetus and newborn. The chapter includes a history of perinatal coronavirus infections, implication of SARS-CoV-2 infection for the pregnant mother, manifestations of the virus in the placenta, management suggestions during pregnancy, and consequences of maternal COVID-19 for the fetus and newborn.

In Chapter 14, Dr. Banerjee discusses how the COVID-19 pandemic has affected children and adolescents. The chapter includes epidemiology, pathogenesis, clinical manifestations, and treatment options, as well as the effect of reduced physical activity, social isolation, stress, and disruptions in income, food, and other determinants of health. The chapter has sections on the multisystem inflammatory syndrome in children (MIS-C) and specific consequences of SARS-CoV-2 infection in immunocompromised children.

In Chapter 15, Drs. Ray, Chinn, Aranda, Jacobson, Esch, and Prasad highlight the challenges faced by emergency medicine as a specialty in providing needed care to COVID-19 and non–COVID-19 patients reporting to the emergency department. The chapter addresses in detail the workup and management of COVID-19 patients in the emergency medicine setting.

In Chapter 16, Drs. Krishnaswami, de la Peña, Kim, and Menon discuss in detail the evolving scenario of therapeutics available for the management of COVID-19 patients. The authors also lay out the different pharmacological strategies based on clinical efficacy and safety and discuss approaches to making informed decisions when multiple therapeutic options become available.

In Chapter 17, Drs. Krishnaswami and Geoffrey illustrate our current understanding of the function and structure of the SARS CoV-2 proteome and the proteins currently targeted for treatment of COVID-19. Additionally, the chapter covers interactions of viral proteins with host proteins, identification of new protein targets, known virus variants, and an overview of currently known and emerging therapeutic solutions.

In Chapter 18, Drs. Mani and Griffin provide a basic understanding of the science of vaccines and then go into the details of the development and deployment of the leading COVID-19 vaccines. Specifically, the chapter provides descriptions of vaccine target selection and postulated mechanisms of action of the mRNA vaccines shown to be effective in preventing COVID-19.

The pandemic continues to evolve, and along with it the science and practice of understanding both the virus and disease are also advancing. We are aware that future editions of the textbook incorporating the new developments would be required to keep up with the scientific progress and provide updates. We consider this first edition as a worthy starting point.

Subramani Mani, MBBS, PhD
Jörn-Hendrik Weitkamp, MD

Contents

The Basics: Epidemiology, Biology, Pathogenesis, Immunology, and Natural History

CHAPTER

1 Epidemiology of SARS-CoV-2 and COVID-19

Goundappa K. Balasubramani, PhD, and Mary Patricia Nowalk, PhD, RDN

OUTLINE

The severe acute respiratory syndrome coronavirus-2 (SARS-CoV-2) causes a highly contagious disease called *COronaVIrus Disease* 2019 (COVID-19). The virus was first reported in Wuhan city, Hubei Province of China in December 2019; in less than 3 months it spread globally and was declared a global pandemic by the World Health Organization (WHO) on March 11, 2020.[1] By March 24, 2020, the novel SARS-CoV-2 had been observed in all seven continents and in 222 countries and territories, with 163,788,738 confirmed cases and a mortality rate of 2.1%.

Symptoms of SARS-CoV-2 infection include fever or chills, cough, shortness of breath, fatigue, muscle or body aches, headache, loss of taste or smell, sore throat, congestion or runny nose, nausea or vomiting, and diarrhea.[2] Severe cases often develop pneumonia, acute respiratory distress syndrome (ARDS), and multiple organ failure.[3]

Less than 2 weeks after the Wuhan Municipal Health Commission announced the detection of the first cases of coronavirus-associated pneumonia, the WHO issued comprehensive technical guidance on how to detect, test, and manage potential cases based on available information. The first official confirmed novel coronavirus case outside of Wuhan was recorded in Thailand on January 13, 2020, and the United States reported its first case on January 21, 2020.[4] Approximately 3 weeks later, on February 11, 2020, the WHO announced that the disease caused by the novel coronavirus would be named COVID-19. Within 5 days, significant transmission of SARS-CoV-2 and increasing cases of COVID-19 were reported in Iran, Italy, and Spain, and the first cases were reported on the African continent on February 25, 2020.

By March 7, 2020, the total number of confirmed COVID-19 cases worldwide had reached over 100,000. The WHO, alarmed at the rapidity of spread and severity of disease, issued a statement calling for "action to stop, contain, control, delay, and reduce the impact of the virus at every opportunity,"[5] and on March 11, 2020, the WHO announced that COVID-19 was officially a "pandemic." One month later, on April 4, 2020, infections had mushroomed 10-fold to over 1 million cases of COVID-19 worldwide.

The virus has spread in stages known as surges or waves because of their episodic increase in cases, peak, sometimes a plateau, and gradual decline. These waves of viral transmission can be isolated and studied to reveal the details of the spread during these specific periods and determine any precipitating events or related factors. A study conducted with COVID-19 patients before January 20, 2020 found that the average incubation period for the disease was 5.2 days (95% confidence interval [CI], 4.1–7.0) and the 95th percentile was 12.5 days; the number of individuals likely to be infected by each case (the R_0) was estimated to be 2.2.[6] A later review found R_0 values ranging from 1.4 to 4.6, with a mean of 3.28.[7] The epidemic doubling time was 7.4 days; however, doubling time will vary with the intensity of the mitigation efforts.[8]

The COVID-19 pandemic has been characterized by several waves that differ in size and intensity across countries and continents. A wave is over when the number of new cases per day declines and then plateaus.

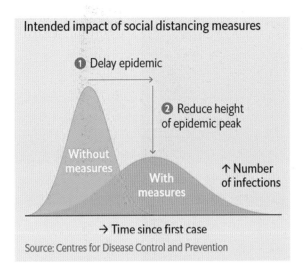

Intended impact of social distancing measures

❶ Delay epidemic

❷ Reduce height of epidemic peak

Without measures

With measures

↑ Number of infections

→ Time since first case

Source: Centres for Disease Control and Prevention

Fig. 1.1 Without mitigation efforts to limit the spread of the SARS-CoV-2, the epidemic curve showing the number of infections over time is expected to be steep *(blue),* with the potential to overwhelm health care systems. By practicing social distancing to limit person-to-person contact, the rate of new infections should be slower *(tan),* thus "flattening the curve." (Flattening the curve. 2020, The Economist 434 [9183]. Copyright from Rights Link/The Economist Group Limited; Order Number: 5084401039568, June 08, 2021.)

"Flattening the curve" is a phrase that was commonly used in the early months of the pandemic, when efforts were focused on preventing transmission because health care facilities were in jeopardy of being unable to care for all cases. Flattening the curve means reducing transmission so that the number of daily new cases[9] is reduced and maintained over a longer period. Locales that observed strict social distancing and other mitigation efforts typically observed flattening of their first wave of the pandemic (Fig. 1.1).

In March 2020, Italy, Iran, and New York City were the hardest-hit regions, with daily cases peaking at 6557 new cases per day in Italy, 3186 cases day in Iran, and 21,000 new cases per day in New York City. In April 2020, COVID-19 cases started to spike in Brazil, and by mid-May COVID-19 cases were surging in India. At the same time, several countries, including Spain, Iran, Italy, Denmark, Israel, Germany, New Zealand, and Thailand, began to ease their lockdown restrictions because of reduction in cases. The total number of cases surpassed 5 million globally on May 21, 2020, a number that had doubled to 10 million by the end of June 2020. Globally, COVID-19 deaths had surpassed half a million people by June 28, 2020, according to the Reuters tally, but doubled to over 1 million on September 18, 2020,[10] 191 days after the WHO declared the novel coronavirus outbreak a global pandemic.

In October 2020, the United States entered its third surge of coronavirus cases, the beginning of its deadliest phase yet. The United States accounted for the highest number of cases and deaths in the world at this point, and globally cases surpassed 50 million by early November 2020.

As of May 18, 2021, over 163 million people had tested positive for COVID-19 and over 3.3 million people had died from the disease across the globe. To date, the three countries most affected by COVID-19 infections are the United States (confirmed cases 32,356,034 and 1.8% mortality), India (confirmed cases 23,702,832 and 1.1% mortality), and Brazil (confirmed cases 15,209,990 and 2.8% mortality).[11] Since March 2020, the overall case fatality rate (CFR) was reported to be around 2.1%; as of May 17, 2021, the CFR has decreased to 0.87%[12] (Fig. 1.2).

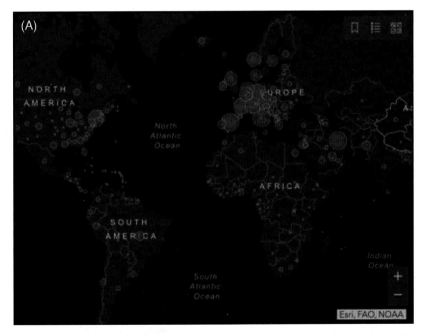

Fig. 1.2 Chronology of the Coronavirus Pandemic. March 2020, 1.2A; May 2020, 1.2B; December 2020, 1.2C; June 2021, 1.2D. (Dong E, Du H, Gardner L. An interactive web-based dashboard to track COVID-19 in real time. *Lancet Infect Dis.* 20(5):533-534. doi:10.1016/S1473-3099(20)30120-1.)

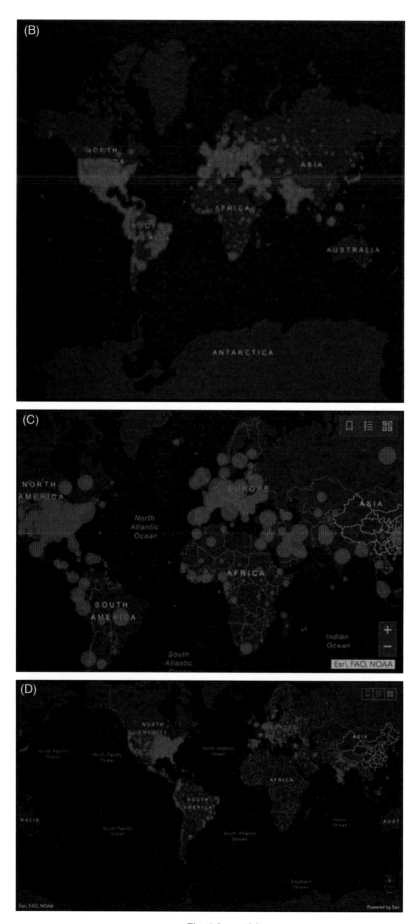

Fig. 1.2 cont'd

The most significant factor in controlling the pandemic has been the introduction of COVID-19 vaccines. The COVAX Facility, a system designed to equitably distribute COVID-19 vaccines worldwide, was developed as testing of COVID-19 vaccine candidates was ongoing. By July 15, 2020, the COVAX Facility had been accepted by over 150 countries, representing over 60% of the world's population. Pfizer/BioNtech's COVID-19 vaccine was authorized for use in the United Kingdom on December 2, 2020, and the US Food and Drug Administration (FDA) issued emergency use authorization (EUA) for the Pfizer/BioNtech vaccine on December 11, 2020, and EUA for Moderna's COVID-19 vaccine on December 18, 2020. Immediately after approval for use, these vaccines were being administered to health care workers and other priority groups. At the end of February 2021, the one-dose Johnson & Johnson vaccine was given EUA by the FDA. As of this writing, individuals as young as 5 years old may receive a COVID-19 vaccine in the United States. Early reports find high vaccine effectiveness for the COVID-19 two-dose vaccines.[13]

Because of the propensity of viruses to mutate, new coronavirus variants are already emerging. Currently six coronavirus variants that are causing significant numbers of symptomatic infections have been identified and are variants of interest or variants of concern.[14] The B.1.1.7 variant was first detected in the United Kingdom but has since been reported in the United States (December 2020). The B.1.351 variant was initially detected in South Africa in December 2020 and was identified in the United States at the end of January 2021. The P.1 variant was first detected in travelers from Brazil at an airport in Japan in early January 2021 and found to be circulating in the United States later that month. The B.1.427 and B.1.429 variants were first identified in California in February 2021 and were classified as variants of concern in March 2021. The B.1.617 variants were first detected in December 2020 in the state of Maharashtra, India. They are currently listed as variants of interest. These variants are concerning because of evidence that they may be more contagious, more virulent, less susceptible to treatment, and/or capable of causing reinfections.

In the following sections, the epidemiology of COVID-19 is presented by continent, starting from its occurrence in Asia. Within each continent, selected countries are discussed as examples of different approaches to mitigation and control of the SARS-CoV-2, especially those with high morbidity and mortality rates. The second part of the chapter deals with risk factors for COVID-19.

Asia

China

The first cases of novel coronavirus (SARS-CoV-2)–infected pneumonia occurred in Wuhan, Hubei Province, China, in December 2019.[6] Morbidity was low; 55% of the patients who developed symptoms before the end of December 2019 were related to exposure at Wuhan's Huanan Wholesale Seafood Market. The first stage of epidemic transmission was primarily a local outbreak among people with a direct contact history at the seafood market. In the second phase, interpersonal and cluster transmission occurred in multiple communities and families in Wuhan in early January. This was the community dissemination stage of the epidemic. During the second half of January, in particular after the January 25, 2020 celebration of the Chinese New Year, there was a remarkable increase in the number of infected patients in affected cities outside Hubei Province. These cases were attributed to population movement in anticipation of the New Year.

An interim report by an independent panel commissioned by the WHO[15,16] found the initial Chinese response to the new disease to be inadequate. In response, China imposed a city-wide, strictly enforced lockdown of Wuhan that shocked the rest of the world. Nearly 11 million people were quarantined, and face masks and social distancing were mandatory. Hundreds of field hospitals were erected within days to deal with overwhelming cases of COVID-19. Despite the Wuhan lockdown, COVID-19 outbreaks occurred in other major Chinese cities such as Beijing and Shanghai. These were quickly controlled using the same immediate lockdowns and swift mass testing. Entry into China was managed by introducing new restrictions and quarantine control. Although considered to be harsh, these measures eventually proved effective in mitigating the spread of the virus. From January 3, 2020 to May 21, 2021, there have been 105,647 confirmed cases of COVID-19, with 4861 deaths reported to the WHO.[17]

Japan

The first SARS-CoV-2 infection was confirmed in Japan on January 16, 2020, in a person who had returned from Wuhan, China. Multiple cases of COVID-19 were identified by the end of February 2020 throughout Japan. A second outbreak of infection occurred in Japan around mid-March 2020. However, the level of testing for SARS-CoV-2 conducted in Japan during the two initial outbreaks of COVID-19 was lower than in other countries.[18] The total number of cases of COVID-19 reported in Japan is 97,074, with one of the lowest COVID-19 death rates per capita (1.356 deaths/100,000 population).

Vietnam

Between the first case being reported on January 23, 2020 and August 13, 2020, Vietnam had 911 confirmed cases with 21 fatalities (2% case fatality rate). In response, the Vietnamese government took draconian measures to curb the infection rate, including social distancing, locking down businesses, suspending entry of all foreigners from March 2020 until further notice, and closing the border between Vietnam and Cambodia. These measures were effective, and Vietnam reported 6314 confirmed cases and 46 deaths as of May 21, 2021.[19,20] However, from May 12, 2021 onward, community transmission cases have been reported from Bac Giang, Hung Yen, Hai Duong, Dien Bien, and Hanoi.

Vietnam reported its first case of the coronavirus variant from the United Kingdom on January 2, 2021 and has reinstituted closures of businesses such as movie theaters and sidewalk cafes, schools, and public transportation and banned inbound flights from the United Kingdom and South Africa.

Taiwan

Taiwan had been spared the worst of the pandemic by containing the spread of COVID-19 among its population of 24 million without a complete lockdown. The island recorded 1128 cases and 12 deaths by the end of April 2021. Most of these cases had been imported from travelers. Although Taiwan is currently experiencing a surge, reporting more than 6761 cases and 59 deaths as of May 27, 2021, these numbers are significantly smaller than those in most countries and territories worldwide.[20]

The newest outbreak, causing over 200 daily cases in the week of May 17, 2021, is thought to have started because authorities had relaxed quarantine requirements for airline crew members in mid-April 2021. New social-distancing rules limiting social gatherings, closing some businesses, and tightening border restrictions have been implemented.[21]

India

The first case of COVID-19 in India was reported on January 30, 2020 in an Indian student evacuated from Wuhan, and the first death was reported on March 12, 2020.[22,23] By August 2020, India had reported several million cases, with more cases among younger people than has been reported in higher-income countries. Deaths were concentrated in 50- to 64-year-olds.[22]

India's COVID-19 cases started to decline in September 2020, after peaking near 100,000 daily infections. After a plateau, cases began to rise again in March 2021, and the current peak is more than double the previous one, the severity of which has been described by comparison with the previous one, "the second wave has made the last one look like a ripple in a bathtub."[24] This surge has been attributed to a combination of factors, including the emergence of highly infectious SARS-CoV-2 variants (coronavirus variant B.1.617 was first detected in India in February 2021), a rise in unrestricted social interactions, and low vaccine coverage.

In addition, inadequate resources and measures to combat the spread of COVID-19 have caused India to be considered the epicenter of the global COVID-19 pandemic. India now represents 50% of COVID-19 cases and 30% of deaths globally.[25] From January 3, 2020 to May 21, 2021, there have been 26,031,991 confirmed cases of COVID-19 and 291,331 deaths in India.[26]

Nepal

The surge in cases in India caused a critical upsurge in cases in Nepal, with which it shares a border. The cumulative cases in this country of 29 million are more than 513,000, with more than 6300 deaths as of May 23, 2021.[21] The surging 9300 daily COVID-19 cases are overloading Nepal's fragile health care system, and the country faces severe shortages of medical supplies and vaccines.[21] Thus the pandemic easily crosses borders.

Russia

Russia is among the four countries with the highest number of confirmed COVID-19 cases as of May 11, 2020.[27] The COVID-19 cases in Russia started later than in many neighboring European countries. Russia acted early to reduce importation of the virus by implementing quarantine for passengers arriving from China (January 23, 2020), closure of the land border with China (January 31, 2020), cancellation of most incoming flights from China (February 1, 2020), restrictions on the entrance of non-Russian citizens from China (February 4), and restrictions on access from Iran and South Korea in late February 2020.[28-30] In the Russian Federation, from January 3, 2020 to May 21, 2021, there have been 4,983,845 confirmed cases of COVID-19, with 117,739 deaths, reported to the WHO.[31]

Iran

Iran was among the first countries to experience large numbers of COVID-19 cases, but the rate of infection slowed after December 2020[32] as a result of containment measures such as movement restrictions and business closures across the country. After averaging 14,000 daily new cases, after December 1, 2020, the average daily new COVID-19 cases declined 50% to 6000 to 7000 and fatalities declined by approximately 50% and hospitalizations by 40%.[33] Overall, the pandemic has caused 2,865,864 cases and claimed 79,219 lives in Iran.[32]

Europe

France reported the first recognized case of COVID-19 in Europe on January 24, 2020, and within 6 weeks, all 27 countries of the European Union reported cases. Italy was the epicenter for cases early in the pandemic, reporting 62% of cases in Europe during the first week of March 2020. Italian cases and deaths were concentrated in the northern regions of Veneto and Lombardy during the latter part of February, likely as a result of environmental conditions there (see later section). On March 13, 2020, the WHO declared Europe the epicenter of the COVID-19 pandemic with more reported cases and deaths than the rest of the world combined.[34] In a historic move, on March 17, 2020, the European Union closed all its external borders to prevent further spread of the virus.[35] However, SARS-CoV-2 continued to spread quickly throughout the region, so that by the first week of April, Spain reported 21%, Italy 20%, Germany 15%, and France 11% of cases in Europe.

Differences across European countries can be attributed to a number of factors, including differences in population density, population size, the rapidity with which national governments imposed restrictions on movement of residents, availability of personal protective equipment (PPE) and sanitation supplies, and the restrictiveness of and adherence to stay-at-home and quarantine orders. Countries with fewer deaths locked down earlier, had shorter epidemics that peaked earlier, and had smaller populations.[36]

Sweden, for example, stood out among European countries by not imposing restrictions on movement, masking requirements, or crowd sizes and instead relying on herd immunity to contain the epidemic. In addition, testing, contact tracing, source identification, and reporting were limited and considered inadequate.[37] The effect was that Sweden's cases and deaths (>1 million cases and >14,000 deaths) are higher than those of other Scandinavian countries (Norway 120,000 cases and 781 deaths; Finland 91,000 cases and 929 deaths[38]) as of May 21, 2021. The United Kingdom has experienced three waves of the pandemic and has reported 4.458 million cases and 127,710 deaths.[39] The first nonclinical trial dose of the Pfizer/BioNTech COVID-19 vaccine was given December 8, 2020 in the United Kingdom, and vaccination began in earnest. Around the same time, a new variant of SARS-CoV-2, B.1.1.7,[40] was beginning to spread, initiating the third surge of cases and the implementation of renewed travel and social distancing restrictions.

As of May 21, 2021,[41] the European Union reported 51,599,270 cases and 1,093,462 deaths; the countries reporting the most deaths were France (5.568 million cases, 108,314 deaths), Italy (4.183 million cases, 125,028 deaths[42]), and Germany (3.64 million cases, 87,667 deaths[43]).

Americas

United States

The SARS-CoV-2 virus was introduced into the United States in January and February 2020 by travelers returning from China's Hubei Province, where the virus was first recognized, and subsequently spread to their household contacts.[44] No connection with international travel was found among cases by late February. Early in the pandemic, cases were concentrated on the East and West Coasts. Gatherings of persons from different locations, followed by return to their home communities, played a significant role in the early US spread of COVID-19. Over 3 weeks in late February to early March, the number of US COVID-19 cases increased more than 1000-fold. By mid-March, transmission had become widespread, and by April 21, a total of 793,669 confirmed COVID-19 cases had been reported in the United States, the majority resulting from widespread community transmission. Schuchat et al.[44] report that four factors contributed to the speed with which the virus spread in the United States. Those factors include:

1. Continued importation of the virus by travelers infected elsewhere (e.g., on cruise ships or in countries experiencing outbreaks). Restrictions on international travel did not occur until March 11, 2020, when the US President banned all travel from 26 European countries and declared a national emergency on March 13, 2020.[45]
2. Amplification of spread in local communities and across states occurred as a result of unrestricted attendance at professional and social events.
3. Rapid spread occurred in facilities housing people in close proximity such as long-term care facilities and high-density urban areas, with the added importation to these areas by high levels of daily ingress and egress.
4. Limited testing and contact tracing caused challenges in virus detection, concurrent circulation with influenza and influenza and pneumonia hospitalizations caused failure to recognize COVID-19 symptoms and infectivity, and cryptic transmission occurred from persons who were asymptomatic or presymptomatic.

During March 2020, national, state, and local governments, public health agencies, businesses, and schools began to implement mitigation strategies, issuing stay-at-home orders, virtual learning, organized case detection, contact tracing, and quarantine, but the response was uncoordinated and inconsistent. Thus different parts of the United States experienced varying levels of COVID-19 activity.[46]

By June 9, 2020, New York State had the highest number of cases (>379,000) reported in the United States, with over half of these cases in New York City. At the same time, Washington state reported 24,354 cases and 1176 deaths and California was in a state of emergency, with 133,489 cases and 4697 deaths. By contrast, states in the Midwest reported lower cases and deaths at the same time: Kansas 10,972 cases and 238 deaths,[47] Arkansas 10,327 cases and 172 deaths,[48] and Wisconsin 21,308 cases and 661 deaths.[49] Nationally,

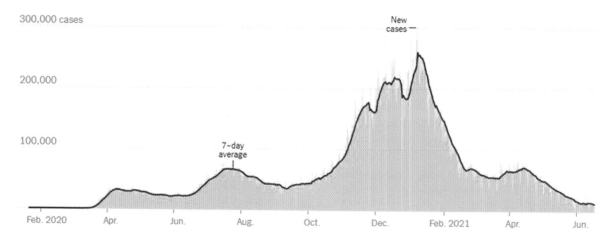

Fig. 1.3 Epidemic Curve of COVID-19 Cases in the United States: February 2020 to June 2021. *Yellow lines* represent reporting anomalies. (From US Trend-Reported Cases. Coronavirus in the U.S.: Latest Map and Case Count." The *New York Times.* June 18, 2021. Copyright obtained from PARS International, License Agreement REF # 000095571 dated June 18, 2021.)

there were 1,933,560 reported cases with 110,220 deaths from COVID-19.

As the summer of 2020 began, PPE and sanitizing supplies became more widely available so that all people could access masks to prevent the spread of the virus. More information about how the virus spread was available, mass testing centers and testing protocols were in place, temporary intensive care units (ICUs) were opened in many hospitals, and more ventilators were becoming available. Despite promulgation through social media of ineffective and sometimes dangerous remedies for COVID-19,[50] better treatments for COVID-19 cases were being developed and testing of vaccine candidates had begun.[51] Although much of the United States had managed to flatten the curve, approximately 3 weeks after the Memorial Day holiday on May 30, 2020, cases began to surge again. This second wave of COVID-19 occurred in much of the United States because of lax adherence to social distancing protocols and family gatherings that included individuals from outside the household, the region, and state as the 7-day moving average doubled from 21,518 cases on June 1, 2020 to 43,767 cases on July 1, 2020.[52]

After the summer wave, cases began to plateau through the fall when students stayed home from school and learned virtually, and most sports, entertainment, political gatherings, concerts, and other events that draw large groups of people continued to be curtailed. In addition, masking and social distancing had become commonplace and were being enforced in retail and other establishments.

In early winter, states that had seen little COVID-19 disease experienced surges. For example, Georgia on December 1, 2020 had 4261 new cases, which increased to 8371 new cases by December 31, 2020.[53] During the second week of December (December 11) the Pfizer/BioNTech COVID-19 vaccine received EUA and was

recommended by the Advisory Committee on Immunization Practices (ACIP) for individuals 16 years and older.[54] A week later (December 18), the Moderna COVID-19 vaccines received EUA,[55] and on December 19, 2020, the ACIP recommended its use in persons 18 years and older.[56] Because of limited initial supplies, health care workers and residents of long-term care facilities were prioritized to receive the vaccine.[54] Later, non–health care frontline essential workers and adults 75 years and older became eligible for vaccination; thereafter adults 65 years and older and younger adults ages 16 to 64 years with high-risk conditions became eligible.[57] Initially, the rollout of vaccinations was slow and demand was high. At the end of February, a third vaccine (Janssen) became available[58] and over the next several weeks, supplies and logistics for vaccinating large numbers of people were in place. Soon thereafter, children as young as 12 years of age were also given authorization by the regulatory agencies to be vaccinated.[59] By May 20, 2021, 125,453,423 million Americans had received at least one dose of a COVID-19 vaccine.[60] In response, COVID-19 cases began to decline, and restrictions on masking and social distancing were relaxed.[61] Schools and businesses began to reopen, and capacity for indoor gatherings was increased in many places (Fig. 1.3).

Canada

In Canada, the first few cases were reported on January 28, 2020, and the first death was reported on March 9, 2020.[48] As of May 18, 2021, there have been roughly 1,338,141 reported cases and 25,018 deaths related to COVID-19 in Canada. The highest number of cases were seen in highly populated provinces, such as Ontario, with 513,102 confirmed cases and 8506 deaths, and Quebec, with 364,396 confirmed cases and 11,050 deaths. Ontario and Quebec reported the most cases (65.5%) and deaths (78.1%).[62]

As observed in other developed countries, there was an increased risk of more severe outcomes for Canadians aged 65 and older with compromised immune systems or underlying medical conditions.[63] However, Canada's mitigation plan and considerable investment in research and development[64] have led to dramatic successes in reducing the spread of COVID-19.[65] These plans included significant cooperation among national and local governmental agencies with the preservation of local control over mitigation strategies to fit local circumstances and appropriate funding to support individuals, businesses, and local governments. Of the 13 jurisdictions reporting updates, no new deaths were reported in 6 provinces and territories in the previous 24 hours as of May 19, 2021, with 4.1% of the 33,754,111 tested identified as positive for COVID-19.[62]

Mexico

The first case of COVID-19 detected in Mexico was on February 27, 2020. On April 30, 2020, 64 days after this first diagnosis, the number of patients had increased exponentially, reaching 19,224 confirmed cases and 1859 (9.67%) deaths.[66] Cases of COVID-19 in Mexico were predominantly caused by community-based transmission, and the majority of cases of COVID-19 were located in Mexico City. Of 12,656 confirmed cases, most infected individuals were between the ages of 30 and 59 years (65.9%), with a mean age of 46 years. There was a higher incidence rate in men (58%) than in women (42%). Patients who died had one or more comorbidities, in particular, hypertension (46%), diabetes (39%), and obesity (30%). There have been 2,385,512 cases in Mexico and 220,746 deaths as of May 19, 2021.

Haiti

Among countries of the Western Hemisphere, Haiti has been spared the worst of the COVID-19 pandemic. With 13,906 cases and 288 deaths[67] as of May 25, 2021, Haiti has one of the lowest death rates from COVID-19 in the world.[68] This Caribbean nation often struggles with high rates of infectious diseases, yet has a COVID-19 death rate of 22 per million, compared with the United States at 1800 per million, and parts of Europe that are nearing 3000 per million.

Haiti's success has not been attributed to innovative interventions or strict adherence to masking, social distancing, and quarantine. Rather, it is likely due to Haiti's demographic distribution. Haiti is a young country, with an average age of 23 years. Although a significant number of people were infected by the virus in the summer of 2020, most showed no symptoms. In fact, Haiti closed its COVID-19 units in the fall of 2020 because of a lack of patients. According to Dr. Jacqueline Gautier, Director of the St. Damien Pediatric Hospital, "COVID-19 hasn't become a daily concern for most Haitians." A surge such as that seen in India may occur in Haiti given the capricious nature of the disease and the fact that Haiti has refused COVID-19 vaccines supplied through the COVAX program.

Latin America

Nearly 6 weeks after the first reported cases in the United States (March 10, 2020), Panama became the second country in Latin America and the first Central American country to have a confirmed coronavirus-related death, in an individual who had traveled to Spain and returned infected. On March 11, 2020, Honduras reported its first two cases of COVID-19 involving two women who had traveled to Europe.

According to the Pan American Health Organization, three factors accounted for most of the spread of COVID-19 into and within the Americas: importation, community transmission, and outbreaks in enclosed areas such as nursing homes. Brazil has had the highest number of confirmed cases (15,812,055) with 441,691 deaths as of May 21, 2021.[69,70] São Paulo is the largest city in South America and receives the greatest proportion of international flights in Brazil. Cities in Brazil are densely populated, with large numbers of poor people, indigenous people, and people living in close quarters.[71] Cases and deaths were relatively low in Brazil until its first peak began in June 2020, with a second surge that began in January 2021. In an editorial published in May 2021, Hallal and Victoria[72] argue that Brazil's current devastating COVID-19 crisis in which Brazil accounts for 12% of all COVID-19 cases and more than a quarter of deaths,[73] despite having 2.7% of the world's population, is due to several factors. They include denial of science and consequent failure to implement social distancing, lockdowns, masking, and other mitigation strategies; denial of the value of vaccines and consequent failure to procure vaccines, especially those with the highest efficacy; and the practice of sending infected patients, particularly those infected with the new P.1 variant, to hospitals in other cities in because of overcrowded conditions in the area where patients live, contributing to the spread of more highly transmissible infections.

In the last few weeks of May 2021, Argentina had reported record-breaking numbers of daily cases (39,000/day up from 5000/day in March 2021) and deaths (744/day up from 112/day in March 2021).[21] More than 3.5 million cases and more than 74,000 deaths were reported as of May 23, 2021. In response, the government of Argentina has implemented strict containment measures, including closing schools and nonessential businesses and banning social, religious, and sporting events until the end of May 2021. Argentina has the second highest COVID-19 burden, with

3,191,097 cases and 68,311 deaths; followed by Colombia with 3,031,726 cases and 78,771 deaths; Peru with 1,897,000 cases and 66,770 deaths; Panama with 368,368 cases and 6282 deaths; Honduras with 222,228 cases and 5789 deaths; and Costa Rica with 273,714 cases and 3456 deaths as of May 12, 2021. In total, there were more than 21,390,349 cases of COVID-19 reported in South America as of May 18, 2021.[41]

Africa

The African continent was the last and least affected by the COVID-19 pandemic to date.[74] The African continent confirmed its first case of COVID-19 in Egypt on February 14, 2020. In sub-Saharan Africa, the first case was reported in Nigeria on February 27, 2020.[75,76] Most of the initial cases of COVID-19 in Africa were imported from Europe and the United States rather than from the original COVID-19 epicenter, China.[77] Africa's first wave of the pandemic peaked in July 2020, when the mean daily number of new cases was 18,273.

Reporting for African countries in five regional groupings indicates Central (9 countries, 121.2 thousand cases, 2000 deaths); Western (15 countries, 444.3 thousand cases, 5600 deaths); Eastern (14 countries, 6.8 million tests, 468.5 thousand cases, 8500 deaths), Northern (7 countries, 1.2 million cases, 35,200 deaths); and Southern (10 countries, 1.9 million cases, 59,300 deaths). The most-affected countries are South Africa (1,538,961 cases, 3.4% mortality) and Egypt (52,251 cases, 7.2% mortality).

As of December 31, 2020, 40 African countries had experienced or were experiencing a more severe second wave of the pandemic, with the continent reporting a mean of 23,790 daily new cases.[78] As of May 19, 2021, there were 2,763,421 COVID-19 cases and 65,602 deaths, accounting for 3.4% of worldwide cases and 3.6% of deaths and surpassing those figures from the early months of the global pandemic.[79] This wave was in part due to new virus variants that emerged in South Africa. Since peaking in mid-January 2021, overall cases and deaths have trended downward; however, countries throughout the African region continue to report sustained transmission and increases in some areas, highlighting the importance of examining multiple epidemiological variables at the regional and country levels over time.[78] As of May 2, 2021, the African region reported over 42,000 new cases,[80] a 15% decrease, and 1000 new deaths, a 13% decrease compared with the previous week. The highest numbers of new cases were reported from South Africa (3% decrease), Ethiopia (34% decrease), and Cameroon (8% increase). The highest numbers of new deaths were reported from South Africa (32% decrease), Ethiopia (12% decrease), and Kenya (1% increase).

Several factors have significantly affected the epidemiology of COVID-19 in the African continent,[81,82] including (1) late arrival of the pandemic; (2) weak diagnostics, such as inadequate COVID-19 testing (as of December 31, 2020, 17 countries reported test-to-case ratios less than the recommended 10–30:1); (3) lack of essential medical supplies; and (4) a largely susceptible population (18 countries reported CFRs greater than the global CFR of 2.2%). The true epidemiology of COVID-19 in the African continent and the actual number of cases remain unknown because of inadequate testing capacity. Furthermore, 48 countries had five or more stringent public health and social measures in place by April 15, 2020; this number had decreased to 36 as of December 31, 2020, despite an increase in cases in the preceding month.

Cases and mortality in Africa are likely to be affected by the presence of other diseases. The Infectious Disease Vulnerability Index (IDVI, 2016) pointed out that of 25 countries most vulnerable to infectious diseases, 22 are in the African region. The WHO Africa estimates that 26 million people infected with human immunodeficiency virus (HIV), 2.5 million with tuberculosis, 71 million with hepatitis B or C, and 213 million with malaria live in Africa.[83–86] Moreover, noncommunicable diseases, such as cardiovascular diseases, cancers, chronic respiratory diseases, and diabetes, that affect the ability to fight infectious diseases increase the burden of COVID-19 in Africa.[87,88]

Oceania

Australia

The first case of novel coronavirus in Australia (nCoV-19) was reported in Victoria on January 25, 2020, with an additional three cases confirmed in New South Wales later that day.[89] A total of 12 cases of nCoV-19 infection were notified up until February 1, 2020. All 12 cases reported a travel history to China, especially to Wuhan, Hubei Province. On March 16, 2020, the Australian Ministry of Health declared a public health emergency.

Mitigation measures were imposed by the third week of March 2020 that included (1) a ban on nonessential indoor gatherings of 100 people or more, (2) considering only essential travel, (3) strict visitor rules for aged care facilities, (4) social distancing of 1.5 m, and (5) allowing student nurses to work in situations that assisted with pandemic response. By March 24, 2020, Tasmania, Northern Territory, South Australia, Western Australia, and Queensland announced closed borders and travel restrictions.[89] In addition, by the end of March 2020, South Australia, Western Australia, New South Wales, Tasmania, Northern Territory, Australian Capital Territory, Victoria, and Queensland had all announced, cumulatively, billions of dollars' worth of economic stimulus and support packages.

Australia continues to report low numbers of COVID-19 cases; in the 2 weeks reporting from April 26 to May 9, 2021, the daily average number of cases was 12. As of May 23, 2021, the total number of cases was 30,011, with 910 deaths reported. Reported cases have been higher among males than females in all age groups older than 30 years.

New Zealand

New Zealand's rapid and immediate response to the COVID-19 pandemic has resulted in extremely low rates of infection and death. Working together with local public health officials, the New Zealand government invested a considerable amount of money in a "go hard, go early" strategy to combat the spread of the virus. Prevention policies were implemented by local infectious disease experts that were individually applied to each clinic or hospital department, with an emphasis on coordination and communication.[90] The "hard-and-early" strategy was effective because New Zealand adopted a set of nonpharmaceutical interventions to stop the spread of COVID-19 and governments supplied resources such as personnel, PPE, laboratory supplies, etc. as they were requested. As other high-income countries have reported an increasing number of cases since August, 2020, New Zealand is one of the few countries globally with low COVID-19 cases and deaths, reporting 2313 confirmed cases with 29 deaths since March 2020.[91]

Australia's and New Zealand's successes prove that a robust public health response focused on vigilant testing, well-functioning surveillance systems, and strict adherence to quarantine that are both enforced and supported by government, are the key to fighting a pandemic.[92,93]

Risk Factors for COVID-19

As the pandemic swept across the world, the general public, public health officials, and governmental agencies watched in trepidation as SARS-CoV-2 arrived in each locality and cases began to surge. Tracking of cases was initiated to elucidate the population subgroups at greatest risk for infection, severe disease, and death. Many of the epidemiological studies were based on population-level factors and data. These studies were meant to inform systems to prepare for a surge in cases and allocate resources to the areas of greatest need. In the United States and elsewhere, PPE and sanitation supplies were in short supply and government officials were initially reluctant to impose sheltering in place orders and other restrictions on people's movement. All of these factors contributed to unequal risk from a virus to which the entire population was naïve and should have been equally vulnerable.

In December, 2020, Woolf et al.[94] published an editorial declaring COVID-19 as the leading cause of death in the United States, surpassing both heart disease and malignant neoplasms. This conclusion was based on COVID-19 deaths through October 2020, before the predicted 2020–2021 winter surge, which ultimately occurred, surpassing even the first spring 2020 surge.[95] Provisional mortality data for 2020 named COVID-19 the third leading cause of death, with an overall 15.9% increase in age-adjusted mortality.[96]

Early reports of risk factors for severe disease and death were older age, male sex, and presence of one or more chronic diseases, including diabetes, obesity, cardiovascular disease, and chronic lung disease.[97-99] Other chapters are devoted to the relationships of COVID-19 and these chronic diseases.

Sex

Differences in COVID susceptibility and mortality between males and females have been noted. Early reports from China suggested higher rates of COVID-19 cases among males (1.27:1 male-to-female ratio),[100] as well as COVID-19 deaths.[97] Studies from Korea[101] and the United States[102] showed higher numbers of cases among females, whereas other studies showed no sex-based differences.[103] Studies in the United States reported higher odds of severe outcomes and mortality associated with male sex.[102,104] These findings were later confirmed in which males were more frequently hospitalized, admitted to the ICU, intubated, and prescribed vasopressors.[105] These varied findings may be due to differences in sample sizes, inclusion criteria, and methodology. Large studies, including data from multiple countries have confirmed that there are male and female differences in both COVID-19 cases and deaths. Importantly, sex-based differences in COVID-19 cases are age dependent, with confirmed cases higher among females in younger ages (10–50 years) and among males at ages younger than 10 and older than 50 years.[106] On the other hand, case fatality rates for COVID-19 across 38 countries were significantly higher for males (7.3; 95% CI, 5.4–9.2) compared with females (4.4; 95% CI, 3.4–5.5; $P < .001$).[107] Moreover, the risk for death for males increases with increasing age. Among nursing home patients, risk for mortality was significantly higher for males than females.[108]

Many reasons, both biological and nonbiological, have been posited to explain these differences. For example, females have been shown to have stronger cell-mediated and humoral immune responses to viral and other microbial infections.[103,109] These differences are thought to be related to the sex hormone milieu—estrogen is immune enhancing and testosterone is immune suppressive.[109,110] Fig. 1.4 illustrates the potential role of hormonal and humoral factors proposed for the observed sex-based differences in susceptibility to SARS-CoV-2. Additionally, females have longer life expectancy and lower mortality from coronary heart

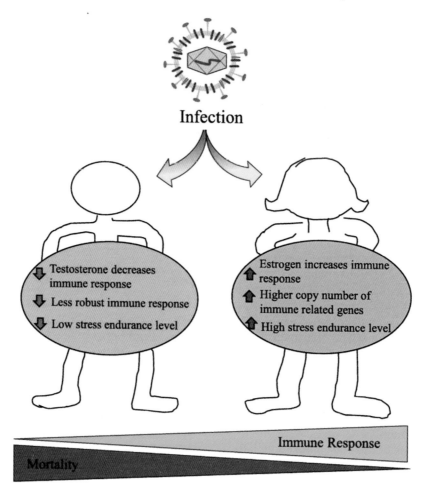

Fig. 1.4 Sex-based differences in mortality may be explained by higher levels of estrogen in females, greater numbers of immune-related genes on the X chromosome, and females' higher stress endurance levels. (Reproduced with permission. Pradhan A, Olsson PE. Sex differences in severity and mortality from COVID-19: are males more vulnerable? *Biol Sex Differ.* 2020 Sep 18;11(1):53. doi:10.1186/s13293-020-00330-7. PMID: 32948238; PMCID: PMC7498997.)

disease and other chronic diseases, all of which are related to COVID-19 mortality.[102] Some have attributed sex differences in COVID-19 mortality to social differences such as the higher frequency of male smokers, less health care–seeking behavior among males,[107] and higher exposure to environmental toxins[111] among males, because more females stay home to care for children[103] (see Fig. 1.4).

Age

The oldest members of the US population have been disproportionately affected by COVID-19, with 80.1% of deaths occurring in those aged 65 years and older, compared with 17.3% for 45 to 64 years and 2.6% for those younger than 45 years.[95] In a review of age-related morbidity and mortality of COVID-19, Kang and Jung[112] summarize clear evidence of an exponential increase in COVID-19 deaths with increasing age. Although this pattern does not differ from the mortality risks from many chronic diseases, Kang and Jung note that mortality related to COVID-19 does not display the U-shaped curve (with highest mortality among the youngest and

oldest individuals) typical of other respiratory viruses such as influenza.

However, the pattern of age-based cases of COVID-19 varies across countries. For example, Natale et al.[113] reported relative illness ratios (RIRs) that account for the proportion of COVID-19 cases for a given age group among all cases in relation to that age group's proportion of the entire population. (That is, for any given age group, a RIR >1 indicates that the age group has a higher proportion of cases compared with other age groups.) Although RIRs generally increased from the youngest to older age groups, two European countries, Spain and Italy, showed sharper increases in RIR for groups older than 60 to 65 years, whereas two Asian countries, China and Korea, had RIRs much lower for those age groups.[113] These geographic differences may be attributed to the stage of the pandemic and the resultant differences in testing at the time of the study (i.e., the initial surge in cases in China occurred weeks before similar surges were observed in Italy, Iran, and US coastal cities). Moreover, China and Korea began to test asymptomatic and symptomatic individuals sooner than the United States and Europe, where the shortage of testing capability resulted in testing being reserved for symptomatic or more severe cases to more effectively isolate and treat these cases. Detection of asymptomatic cases may vary across age groups and could result in different RIRs.

Differences in COVID-19 incidence by age also have been attributed to differences in exposure. Children's exposure to infections usually occurs in daycare settings, schools, and within the home from infected family members. As the pandemic began, these nonhome sites were closed and families sheltered at home, thus significantly reducing children's exposure to the virus. A systematic literature review reported that children and adolescents have lower susceptibility to SARS-CoV-2 than adults, and children younger than 10 to 14 years appear to be less susceptible to SARS-CoV-2 than older children and adults (20 years and older).[114] In one reviewed study, children (under 20 years of age) had pooled odds ratio (OR) of being an infected contact of 0.56 (95% CI, 0.37–0.85) compared with adults. COVID-19 is generally a mild disease in children, including infants. However, a small proportion develop severe disease requiring ICU admission and prolonged ventilation, although fatal outcomes are rare.

On the other end of the age spectrum, a significant number of older individuals in the United States reside in communal living facilities, including residential care communities and nursing homes (2015–16 estimates of 2.16 million) with over 1.2 million direct caregivers (nursing and social work).[115] Although these facilities limited visitors, they could not eliminate interactions among residents and staff, leading to rapid spread of infection in long-term care facilities.

Older individuals are more vulnerable to infectious diseases because of reduced ability to mount a robust immune response to the infectious agent and chronic subclinical systemic inflammation.[116] Moreover, the presence of other chronic conditions such as chronic lung or heart disease may make these systems less resilient to infection. Conversely, children infrequently have comorbidities, may be less susceptible to infection, and/or may be less likely to develop severe symptoms. In absence of chronic high-risk conditions, children may be less likely to be tested and diagnosed, resulting in underestimation of true incidence. Based on this evidence, Kang and Jung[112] surmised that susceptibility to *infection* is likely similar across age groups, but susceptibility to *symptomatic infection* seems to increase with age.

Long-Term Care Facilities

Among older individuals, nursing home residents have experienced especially high mortality related to COVID-19, in part because of close living quarters, underlying health conditions, and the need for close, hands-on care. In a review of studies from Australia, Europe, and the United States, the percentage of total COVID-19 deaths ranged from 18.6% to 67% in April and May of 2020 to 26.6% to 78.2% in August 2020.[117] Nursing home staff in six states also experienced significant increases in cases even after mitigation measures were in place.[118] COVID-19 spread in long-term care facilities can be attributed to three types of factors: facility, staff, and patient factors.

Facility Factors

Facility characteristics associated with the probability of having at least one COVID-19 case in unadjusted analyses include larger size, nonchain status, urban location, and larger percentage of African-American residents. Percentage of Medicaid patients, five-star rating for quality, prior infection violation, and ownership (chain, government owned, etc.) were not related to COVID-19 cases. A facility's number of cases was directly related to larger size and for-profit status.[119] Other studies that used multivariate logistic regression to control for other factors confirmed that higher quality rating was related to lower COVID-19 cases[120] and deaths.[121] For-profit status and larger size were related to higher COVID-19 cases and deaths,[121] as were percent of racial/ethnic minority patients[120] and percent of non-White residents.[121] In contrast, increased percentage of Medicaid patients was related to an increased number of COVID-19 cases[120] and deaths.[122] One multistate study of nursing homes found that larger size and the prevalence of SARS-CoV-2 in the county where the facility was located were significantly related to higher numbers of COVID-19 cases.[123] In a study of New York, New Jersey, and Connecticut nursing homes, the highest probability of having six or more COVID-19 deaths was found in larger nursing facilities, those with higher occupancy rates, and for-profit homes.[122] A study from Canada compared long-term care homes in two provinces, Ontario and British Columbia. It found that factors related to the long-term care system of British Columbia that had been established before the pandemic resulted in an environment that was more resilient and better prepared to protect its residents from coronavirus than was the case in Ontario. Whereas Ontario experienced a resident infection rate of 7.6% and mortality rate of 2.3%, British Columbia's infection rate was 1.7% and mortality rate was 0.6%. The differences in COVID-19 cases were attributed to pre-pandemic increased funding for long-term care (additional $19/resident per day), fewer shared rooms (24% vs. 63%), more not-for-profit ownership (66% vs. 42%), and more frequent comprehensive inspections.[124] Resident COVID-19 case fatality rates were slightly higher in British Columbia (33.5%) than in Ontario (30.5%), suggesting that facility factors may determine infection rates, although patient factors likely contributed to mortality.

Staffing Factors

Some of the factors related to high nursing home rates are staff members working while contagious, inadequate training of staff, part-time staff working in multiple sites, shortage of PPE such as masks and gloves, and limited testing for infection among both staff and residents.[125] Li et al.[120] reported that a 20-minute increase per resident per day in registered nurse staffing time was associated with a 22% reduction in COVID-19 cases and 26% reduction in COVID-19 deaths. This finding was confirmed in a multistate study in which facilities with more than 100 beds in which increased direct care hours per patient-day was associated with a 4.8% decrement in probability of having six or more COVID-19 deaths.[122] Liu et al.[124] reported that the extra funding to British Columbia nursing homes was used for staff salaries and contributed to lower COVID-19 cases in residents.

Patient Factors

Studies have also examined nursing home patient factors that are related to the risk for COVID-19. One study of New York, New Jersey, and Connecticut nursing homes reported higher probability of having six or more COVID-19 deaths in nursing facilities whose patients had higher activities of daily living (ADL) scores, that is, required greater assistance with activities of daily living.[122] Increased incidence of neurological pathological conditions—especially dementia, which is frequently accompanied by lower physical functioning—have been reported to increase the risk for COVID.[125] In a study of mortality within 30 days among COVID-19 cases living in nursing homes in the United States, odds of death were 46% higher for residents 80 to 84 years compared with residents 75 to 79 years old; women had odds of death 31% lower than for men; residents with diabetes were 21% more likely to die and those with chronic kidney disease were 33% more likely to die than residents without these conditions. The odds of death were doubled (OR, 2.09; 95% CI, 1.68–2.59) for those with moderate cognitive impairment and nearly tripled (OR, 2.79; 95% CI, 2.14–3.66) for those with severe cognitive impairment compared with residents without cognitive impairment, while the odds of death were 49% and 64% higher for those with moderate and severe physical impairment, respectively.[126] In contrast to the facility factor of percent of residents who are non-White or a racial or ethnic minority predicting higher risk for COVID-19, personal racial category did not affect risk for death from COVID-19 in this study. A study in an Italian nursing home confirmed that increased COVID-19 mortality was related to male sex, older age, and greater physical impairment.[108]

By virtue of their diminished physical and cognitive capacities, nursing home residents are at greater risk for all-cause mortality. However, several factors—the communal living situation (often without isolation areas), insufficient testing of residents and staff, the need for close-contact care, limited supply of PPE, and exposure to staff who may be inadequately trained or working in multiple facilities—has placed nursing home residents at highest risk for COVID-19 infection and subsequently death.

Race/Ethnicity

The US death toll from COVID-19 indicates that 61% of deaths were among Whites, 19% among Hispanics, 15% among Blacks, 4% among Asians, and 1.2% among American Indian/Native American/Native Alaskans and Pacific Islanders[95]; however, these numbers do not tell the whole story.

The Kaiser Family Foundation compared the proportion of COVID-19 cases among racial/ethnic groups with their relative proportions in each state's population. As of April 30, 2021, 15 states had higher percentages of cases among Blacks, 33 states had higher percentages of cases among Hispanics, and 2 states had higher percentages of cases among Asians than their respective proportions of their state's population.[127]

California was one of the first states to report COVID-19 cases (January 26, 2020).[128,129] A study that used county-level data and tracked the racial distribution of COVID-19 cases over the first 175 days of the pandemic found rapidly changing geospatial distribution of the disease. After the first 50 days, the case distribution resembled the distribution of Asian Americans; whereas 125 days later, the distribution of COVID-19 cases was more similar to the geospatial distribution of African Americans in California. Predominantly White communities consistently bore less COVID-19 burden.[130]

Numerous other reports have highlighted the unequal burden of COVID-19 on communities of color. A study in Chicago found that Black residents, who represented 31% of the population, accounted for 42% of COVID-19 deaths, whereas the opposite was true for neighborhoods with higher percentages of Asian and White residents.[111] Millett et al.,[131] examined county-level characteristics of the entire United States and similarly reported that counties with higher proportions of Black residents (>13%) had higher risk ratios for COVID-19 infection (1.24; 95% CI, 117–1.33) and COVID-19 deaths (1.18; 95% CI, 1.07–1.40) than counties with lower proportions of Black residents after controlling for potential confounders such as age, poverty, and comorbidities. Furthermore, this study found that the 20% of counties determined to have high proportions of Black residents accounted for 52% of COVID-19 cases and 58% of COVID-19 deaths. Another national study of US counties used percentages of Black and other racial/ethnic groups as a continuous variable and confirmed the higher infection risk ratio for Blacks as 1.03

(95% CI, 1.02–1.04) when controlling for demographic and socioeconomic variables.[132]

In a regional study of New York counties, Black race was not associated with COVID-19 prevalence when accounting for poverty rates.[133] In a more granular study of New York City using zip codes, a relatively small number of zip code areas accounted for the highest rates of COVID-19 infections. In multivariable models that accounted for chronic lung and heart disease, age, housing density, and proportion of African-American residents, the likelihood of COVID-19 infection as measured by incidence density ratio was 2.29 for Black race and 1.5 for age older than 65 years.[134] In studies focused on individual risk factors for severe outcomes of COVID-19, Black race was associated with risk for mechanical ventilation (adjusted hazard ratio, 1.52; 95% CI, 1.25–1.85)[104] but not with mortality.[102,104]

An ecological study was performed to examine risk for COVID-19 infection and death among Latinos across the United States using a proportion of 17.8% or more Latino to designate high Latino population. The findings were not uniform across the United States. In counties in the Northeast and Midwest, COVID-19 infections were related to higher proportions of Latino residents after adjusting for sociodemographic characteristics such as age and language spoken at home, comorbidities, and factors such as housing densities. COVID-19 deaths were only related to proportion of Latino residents in the Midwest.[135] Notably, these disparities were not observed in the South, which has a higher proportion of Back individuals who have been disproportionately affected by COVID-19 and a higher proportion of undocumented immigrants who do not tend to use health care services.[135] Strully et al.[132] reported higher COVID-19 cases associated with larger county immigrant populations (infection risk ratio [IRR], 1.09; 95% CI, 1.07–1.12), and with residents from Central America (IRR, 1.13; 95% CI, 1.07–1.20).[132] Individual-level data from a study in Rhode Island indicated that the risk ratio for COVID-19 infection for the Hispanic/Latino population was 4.97 (95% CI, 2.59–9.53) compared with non-Hispanic Whites and 2.61 (95% CI, 1.7–4.0) compared with Blacks.[136]

Racial/ethnic differences in COVID-19 incidence and mortality are not limited to the United States, nor to majority minority ethnic groups. Indigenous and native peoples such as Native Americans, who represent small percentages of the world's populations, have been disproportionately affected by COVID-19. For example, Native Americans in New Mexico comprise 11% of the population, yet as of April 2021, they represent 15.8% of cases and 27.7% of COVID-19 deaths. By comparison, Whites make up 81.9% of the population, 17.8% of cases, and 29.9% of deaths. However, the age-adjusted mortality rate for Native Americans/Alaskan Indians was 651.3/100,000 compared with 79.2/100,000 population for Whites.[137]

Reports from the United Kingdom show similar disparities in COVID-19 mortality among various ethnic and racial minority groups, including Black African, Black Caribbean, and South Asians from Bangladesh and Pakistan.[138,139] In Brazil, less than 10% of the population is Black and 47.7% is White.[140] In a study as of August 2020, using a database of over 3 million COVID-19 cases, the COVID-19 incidence rate was higher among Whites (1038.7/100,000) than Blacks (713.6/100,000), but the case fatality rate among Whites was 3.2% compared with 4.9% among Blacks, for a relative risk (RR) of 1.5 (95% CI, 1.46–1.54).[141]

Sociodemographic and Economic Factors

Numerous attempts have been made to explain the racial and ethnic disparities in COVID burden. It was established early in the pandemic that those with pre-existing comorbid conditions, older age, and smoking were at higher risk for death from COVID-19.[98] Given that in the United States, Black and Hispanic individuals have higher rates of obesity, diabetes, chronic heart disease, chronic lung disease, and hypertension, it followed that these communities of color would be more severely affected by the coronavirus. Significantly higher COVID-19 cases have been reported in areas with more African American residents even when adjusting for presence of comorbidities, such as heart disease, and environmental factors.[134] Other research has demonstrated that factors including social determinants of health are at play.

Several of the studies cited earlier also examined environmental and social determinants of risk for COVID-19. Oronce et al.,[142] compared the state-level Gini index, a measure of income inequality, to COVID cases and deaths. A higher Gini index represents more income inequality. In unadjusted analyses, greater income inequality was significantly correlated with COVID-19 cases and deaths. However, when adjusting for potential confounders, such as age, sex, race/ethnicity, level of poverty, etc., income was no longer associated with cases, but states with higher Gini indexes had more COVID-19 deaths than states with lower Gini indexes. Each unit change in Gini index resulted in 27.2% more deaths.[142] Similarly, the social vulnerability index, which measures a community's resilience using socioeconomic status (SES), minority status and language, housing and transportation, and household composition and disability, was assigned to counties across the United States and compared with COVID-19 burden. When overall vulnerability domains were combined, risk for COVID-19 infection was 63% higher (RR, 1.63; 95% CI, 1.49–1.78) and risk for COVID-19 death was 73% higher (RR, 1.73; 95% CI,

1.55–1.93) for residents of the most vulnerable counties. When individual domains were examined, significantly higher RRs for COVID-19 infection and death were associated with increased vulnerability in the SES (poverty, unemployment), housing and transportation (crowded housing, access to a personal vehicle), and minority status and language (non–English speaking) domains.[143]

One study looked at changes in mobility as measured by New York subway ridership as well as measures of socioeconomic disadvantage such as median income, work in essential services, race/ethnicity, health insurance status, and education level. This study reported that ridership on the subway was significantly related to engaging in "essential" work when adjusting for other measures of SES. Increased mobility or less ability to socially distance by staying home, using non-public transportation, or even leaving the city, as well as lower median income, working in essential services, being non-White and/or Hispanic, not having health insurance, and having a high school education or less were significantly related to higher risk for COVID-19 disease.[144] Another study in New York confirmed evidence that neighborhoods with larger percentages of Black and Hispanic residents had higher rates of both COVID-19 cases and deaths, but the factor most related to increased cases was the proportion of essential workers. This factor was not related to the number of COVID deaths among majority Black communities.[145] A national study of county characteristics associated with COVID-19 burden reported an association with lack of health insurance with a population-attributable burden for cases of 3.3% in counties with a lower proportion of Black residents compared with 4.2% for counties with a higher proportion of Black residents.[131]

A study of neighborhood characteristics associated with COVID-19 mortality in Chicago found significant relationships between the percentage of White versus non-White residents. That is, majority-minority neighborhoods recorded the highest death rates, with notably higher rates among Whites in those neighborhoods than in those with higher percentages of White residents. Moreover, the neighborhoods with more "barriers to social distancing," such as fewer households with broadband Internet, fewer residents with college education, more residents without health insurance, had higher COVID-19 mortality.[111] However, when death rates were analyzed by race/ethnic group, most neighborhood characteristics were no longer significantly related in Hispanic individuals, and all became insignificant among Black individuals; the neighborhood characteristics, however, remained significant among Whites. That is, neighborhood characteristics had a greater effect on risk for death among Whites than among racial/ethnic minorities. McClure et al.[147] argue that occupational settings drive racial/ethnic disparities in

COVID-19 burden. For example, Black, Hispanic, and undocumented immigrant workers are overrepresented in industries such as construction, meat packing, agricultural production, health care and nursing homes, and grocery store chains.[146] They argue that these populations have had less access to PPE, have fewer chances to work from home, work in close proximity without the ability to socially distance, work shifts, rely on public transportation, work multiple jobs, or do not have access to sick time, all of which put them at a disadvantage for preventing COVID-19 infection and transmission.[147]

International studies have shown increased levels of COVID-19 burden associated with lower income (Peru),[148] overcrowded housing (England),[138] lower SES (Korea),[149] income inequality (Brazil),[150] health care access (Brazil),[151] and socioeconomic factors such as place of residence and occupation (England and Wales).[139]

As Bambra et al.[152] point out, disadvantaged communities, many of which are majority ethnic and/or racial minority, have higher rates of chronic diseases such as hypertension; diabetes; chronic cardiovascular, respiratory, liver, and renal diseases; obesity; smoking; and cancer. Many of these diseases are related to higher risk for COVID-19 infection and result from adverse working conditions associated with lower pay/lower skill jobs. Marginalized populations live in segregated communities with concentrated poverty, increased exposure to air and water pollution, low-quality housing and reduced access to health care services,[152] leading to well-documented health disparities.[153]

Thus, as Demenech et al.[150] summarized, socioeconomically disadvantaged people are at increased risk of COVID-19 burden because of (1) differential exposure to the virus from crowding on public transportation, in homes, and at work; (2) differential susceptibility because of low food/nutritional quality or quantity, increased stress, inadequate access to health care, and occupation-related risks; or (3) differential consequences to exposure such as fewer options for prevention and treatment. When combined with higher risk for chronic diseases, these social determinants of health have created increased risk and burden of COVID-19 among racial and ethnic minorities and other disadvantaged populations.

Air Pollution

After the initial onset of the pandemic in China, Italy was one of the hardest hit countries, especially the Po Valley region of northern Italy.[154] Beijing, China and the Po Valley are known for their high levels of industrial pollution that includes fine particulate matter and the noxious gases nitrogen dioxide (NO_2), carbon monoxide, ozone, and sulfur dioxide. The propensity of this region to air inversions, which trap air and prevent

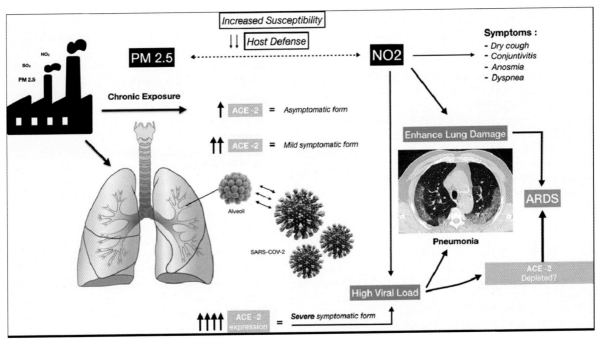

Fig. 1.5 Severe lung disease may be induced by the combined effect of small particulate matter (*PM* 2.5) and nitrogen dioxide (*NO₂*). Chronic exposure to PM 2.5 is thought to cause overexpression of angiotensin-converting enzyme-2 (*ACE-2*), facilitating viral entry into cells and depleting ACE-2 stores. Increased NO₂ is associated with increased inflammatory response and cellular damage. The combination of high viral load and ACE-2 depletion exacerbates lung injury. *ARDS,* Acute respiratory distress syndrome. (Frontera A, Cianfanelli L, Vlachos K, Landoni G, Cremona G. Severe air pollution links to higher mortality in COVID-19 patients: The "double-hit" hypothesis. *J Infect.* Aug 2020;81(2):255-259. doi:10.1016/j.jinf.2020.05.031.)

air exchange, causes longer exposure to air pollution. Three studies used ecological data to map concentrations of pollutants over specific regions, including China and Europe. One study found that concentrations of particulate matter were highest both in Beijing and northern Italy and were related to excess COVID-19 burden. The authors speculated that the fine particulate matter causes the virus to be suspended in air longer than it would in air without such pollution, thus potentially increasing one's exposure to the virus.[155] Fig. 1.5 illustrates the pathophysiological mechanisms postulated to explain the roles of fine particulate matter and NO₂ in causing ARDS, a hallmark of severe lung disease in COVID-19. Another study mapped NO₂ levels over northern Italy, Spain, and parts of surrounding countries during January and February 2020, reporting the highest number of deaths in the five regions with the highest concentrations of NO₂.[156] The author attributed the effect to chronic exposure to NO₂ causing lung inflammation that rendered the lungs less able to withstand infection by the coronavirus. A third, Italian study reported significant correlations between fine particulate matter levels and COVID-19 cases and severe outcomes (ICU admission, death).[155] These authors speculated that chronic exposure to fine particulate matter caused overexpression of angiotensin-converting enzyme-2 (ACE-2), allowing for easier penetration of the virus into lung cells. An ecological study conducted in the United States using county-level data for fine particulate matter and COVID-19 deaths found that an increase of 1 μg/m³ was associated with an 8% (95% CI, 2%–15%) increase in COVID-19 mortality.[157]

Conclusion

A global pandemic offers a vast array of opportunities to study the epidemiology of a disease caused by a newly emerged virus. This overview presents what is currently known after 18 months since the identification of SARS-CoV-2 and the declaration of the pandemic. New knowledge about the virus characteristics, treatment modalities, and risk factors for disease and death is being acquired daily. Despite our understanding of effective mitigation techniques and the availability of highly effective vaccines, cases of COVID-19 continue to accumulate and the death toll grows. As communities begin to reopen and new virus variants emerge, the epidemiology of COVID-19 will continue to evolve and thus its true patterns of infection, spread, risk, morbidity, and mortality will not be fully known until the pandemic has abated.

REFERENCES

1. Du Toit A. Outbreak of a novel coronavirus. *Nat Rev Microbiol.* Mar 2020;18(3):123. doi:10.1038/s41579-020-0332-0.
2. Centers for Disease Control and Prevention (CDC). Symptoms of COVID-19 (Last Updated Feb 22, 2021, Accessed May 27, 2021). Centers for Disease Control and Prevention (CDC). Accessed 05/20/2021, https://www.cdc.gov/coronavirus/2019-ncov/symptoms-testing/symptoms.html.

3. Zhou F, Yu T, Du R, et al. Clinical course and risk factors for mortality of adult inpatients with COVID-19 in Wuhan, China: a retrospective cohort study. *Lancet.* Mar 28 2020;395(10229):1054–1062. doi:10.1016/S0140-6736(20)30566-3.

4. World Health Organization. Novel Coronavirus (2019-nCoV): situation report, 3. 2020. 2020-01-23. https://apps.who.int/iris/handle/10665/330762.

5. World Health Organization (WHO). WHO statement on cases of COVID-19 surpassing 100 000 (Last Updated Mar 7, 2020, Accessed May 21, 2021). World Health Organization (WHO). https://www.who.int/news/item/07-03-2020-who-statement-on-cases-of-covid-19-surpassing-100-000.

6. Li Q, Guan X, Wu P, et al. Early transmission dynamics in Wuhan, China, of novel coronavirus-infected pneumonia. *N Engl J Med.* Mar 26 2020;382(13):1199–1207. doi:10.1056/NEJMoa2001316.

7. Liu Y, Gayle AA, Wilder-Smith A, Rocklöv J. The reproductive number of COVID-19 is higher compared to SARS coronavirus. *J Travel Med.* Mar 13 2020;27(2):taaa021. doi:10.1093/jtm/taaa021.

8. Lurie MN, Silva J, Yorlets RR, Tao J, Chan PA. Coronavirus disease 2019 epidemic doubling time in the United States before and during stay-at-home restrictions. *J Infect Dis.* 2020;222(10):1601–1606. doi:10.1093/infdis/jiaa491.

9. Johns Hopkins University & Medicine - Coronavirus Resource Center. New COVID-19 Cases Worldwide - Have Countries Flattened the Curve? (Last Updated and Accessed May 28, 2021). https://coronavirus.jhu.edu/data/new-cases.

10. Higgins-Dunn N. The coronavirus has now killed more than 1 million people and upended the global economy in less than nine months (Last Updated and Accessed May 28, 2021). CNBC. https://www.cnbc.com/2020/09/28/the-coronavirus-has-killed-more-than-1-million-people-and-upended-the-global-economy.html.

11. Johns Hopkins University & Medicine - Coronavirus Resource Center. Mortality Analyses - How does Mortality differ across Countries? (Last Updated and Accessed May 28, 2021). https://coronavirus.jhu.edu/data/mortality.

12. Ministry of Health and Family Welfare. Dr. Harsh Vardhan reviews Public Health Response to COVID-19 and Progress of Vaccination with 9 States/UTs (Last Updated May 21, 2021, Accessed May 28, 2021). Press Information Bureau (PIB). https://pib.gov.in/PressReleaseIframePage.aspx?PRID=1720679.

13. Centers for Disease Control and Prevention (CDC). Effectiveness of Pfizer-BioNTech and Moderna Vaccines Against COVID-19 Among Hospitalized Adults Aged ≥65 Years — United States, January–March 2021 (Posted Apr 28, 2021, Last Accessed May 28, 2021). Centers for Disease Control and Prevention (CDC). Updated 04/28/2021. Accessed 5/28/2021, https://www.cdc.gov/mmwr/volumes/70/wr/mm7018e1.htm?s_cid=mm7018e1_w.

14. Centers for Disease Control and Prevention (CDC). About Variants of the Virus that Causes COVID-19 (Last Updated April 2, 2021). Centers for Disease Control and Prevention (CDC). Accessed 05/20/2021, https://www.cdc.gov/coronavirus/2019-ncov/transmission/variant.html.

15. Independent Panel for Pandemic Preparedness and Response (for the WHO Executive Board). The Independent Panel for Pandemic Preparedness and Response - Second report on progress (Last Updated Jan 15, 2021, Accessed May 21, 2021). The Independent Panel for Pandemic Preparedness and Response. https://theindependentpanel.org/wp-content/uploads/2021/01/Independent-Panel_Second-Report-on-Progress_Final-15-Jan-2021.pdf.

16. Nebehay S. Independent pandemic review panel critical of China, WHO delays (Last Updated Jan 18, 2021, Accessed May 28, 2021). Reuters. https://www.reuters.com/article/us-health-coronavirus-who-panel/independent-pandemic-review-panel-critical-of-china-who-delays-idUSKBN29N1V1.

17. Worldometers. China Coronavirus Cases (Last Updated May 21, 2021). Worldometers. Accessed 05/21/21, https://www.worldometers.info/coronavirus/country/china.

18. Sekizuka T, Itokawa K, Hashino M, et al. A genome epidemiological study of SARS-CoV-2 introduction into Japan. *mSphere.* Nov 11 2020;5(6). doi:10.1128/mSphere.00786-20.

19. Dezan Shira & Associates V. Vietnam Business Operations and the Coronavirus: Updates (Last Updated and Accessed May 23, 2021). https://www.vietnam-briefing.com/news/vietnam-business-operations-and-the-coronavirus-updates.html/.

20. Worldometers. Coronavirus Cases (Last Updated and Accessed May 21, 2021). Worldometers. Accessed 05/21/21, https://www.worldometers.info/coronavirus/?fbclid=IwAR19og-43nWLhrj3zfKmxPl5_mXk7LSHvCNN26PvKXsCiK-FEASChMEVJo5qM.

21. Yen Nee Lee. *India isn't the only one. Covid cases are rising at record levels in these places too*: CNBC; May 25, 2021. https://www.cnbc.com/2021/05/25/covid-argentina-nepal-and-others-see-cases-rising-rapidly-like-india.html, https://www.cnbc.com/2021/05/25/covid-argentina-nepal-and-others-see-cases-rising-rapidly-like-india.html.

22. Laxminarayan R, Wahl B, Dudala SR, et al. Epidemiology and transmission dynamics of COVID-19 in two Indian states. *Science.* Nov 6 2020;370(6517):691–697. doi:10.1126/science.abd7672.

23. Laxminarayan R, Jameel S, Sarkar S. India's battle against COVID-19: progress and challenges. *Amer J Trop Med Hygiene.* 07 Oct. 2020;103(4):1343–1347. doi:10.4269/ajtmh.20-0992.

24. Mallapaty S. India's massive COVID surge puzzles scientists. *Nature.* Apr 2021;592(7856):667–668. doi:10.1038/d41586-021-01059-y.

25. McKenzie S. What we know about the Covid-19 variant first found in India (Last Updated May 17, 2021, Accessed May 26, 2021). CNN. https://www.cnn.com/2021/05/17/health/variant-india-explained-coronavirus-intl-cmd/index.html.

26. Worldometers. India Coronavirus Cases (Last Updated May 21, 2021). Worldometers. Accessed 05/21/21, https://www.worldometers.info/coronavirus/country/india/.

27. Worldometers. Reported Cases and Deaths by Country or Territory (Last Updated and Accessed May 11, 2021). Updated 05/11/2021. Accessed 05/11/2021, https://www.worldometers.info/coronavirus/#countries.

28. The Moscow Times. Russia Closes Far East Border Over Coronavirus (Last Updated Jan 30, 2020, Accessed May 21, 2021). The Moscow Times. https://www.themoscowtimes.com/2020/01/30/russia-closes-far-east-border-over-coronavirus-a69100.

29. TASS Russian News Agency. Russia restricts air travel with China from February 1 due to coronavirus (Updated Feb 1, 2020, Accessed May 21, 2021). https://tass.com/economy/1115335.

30. Government R. A number of decisions have been taken to prevent the entry into Russia of coronavirus infection from the territory of the People's Republic of China. (Last Updated Feb 1, 2020, Accessed May 21, 2021). government.ru. http://government.ru/docs/38900/.

31. Worldometers. Russia Coronavirus Cases (Last Updated May 21, 2021). Worldometers. Accessed 05/21/21, https://www.worldometers.info/coronavirus/country/russia.

32. Worldometers. Iran Coronavirus Cases (Last Updated and Accessed May 28, 2021). Worldometers. Accessed 05/28/21, https://www.worldometers.info/coronavirus/country/iran/.

33. The United Refugee Agency - UNHCR. COVID-19 response in the Islamic Republic of Iran (Updated Dec 2020, Last Accessed May 26, 2021). https://reliefweb.int/sites/relief-web.int/files/resources/UNHCR%20Iran%20COVID%20response%20Dec%202020.pdf.

34. World Health Organization. 2020. WHO Director-General's opening remarks at the media briefing on COVID-19. [assessed 2020 April 18]. https://www.who.int/dg/speeches/detail/who-director-general-s-opening-remarks-at-the-mission-briefing-on-covid-19-13-march.

35. European Commission. COVID-19: Temporary Restriction on Non-Essential Travel to the EU COM(2020) 115 final. March 16, 2020. https://ec.europa.eu/info/sites/default/files/communication-travel-on-the-eu.pdf.

36. Dye C, Cheng RCH, Dagpunar JS, Williams BG. The scale and dynamics of COVID-19 epidemics across. *Europe. R Soc Open Sci.* Nov 2020;7(11):201726. doi:10.1098/rsos.201726.

37. Claeson M, Hanson S. COVID-19 and the Swedish enigma. *Lancet.* Jan 23 2021;397(10271):259–261. doi:10.1016/S0140-6736(20)32750-1.

38. European Centre for Disease Prevention and Control (ECDC). COVID-19 situation update for the EU/EEA (Last Updated May 21, 2021). European Centre for Disease Prevention and Control. Accessed 5/21/21, https://www.ecdc.europa.eu/en/cases-2019-ncov-eueea.

39. Worldometers. United Kingdom Coronavirus Cases (Last Updated May 21, 2021). Worldometers. Accessed 05/21/21, https://www.worldometers.info/coronavirus/country/uk/.

40. Wise J. Covid-19: New coronavirus variant is identified in UK. *BMJ.* 2020;371:m4857. doi:10.1136/bmj.m4857.

41. European Centre for Disease Prevention and Control (ECDC). COVID-19 situation update worldwide (Last Updated May 18, 2021). European Centre for Disease Prevention and Control. Accessed 5/19/21, https://www.ecdc.europa.eu/en/geographical-distribution-2019-ncov-cases.

42. Worldometers. Italy Coronavirus Cases (Last Updated May 21, 2021). Worldometers. Accessed 05/21/21, https://www.worldometers.info/coronavirus/country/italy.

43. Worldometers. Germany Coronavirus Cases (Last Updated May 21, 2021). Worldometers. Accessed 05/21/21, https://www.worldometers.info/coronavirus/country/germany.

44. Schuchat A, Team CC-R. Public health response to the initiation and spread of pandemic COVID-19 in the United States, February 24-April 21, 2020. *MMWR Morb Mortal Wkly Rep.* May 8 2020;69(18):551–556. doi:10.15585/mmwr.mm6918e2.

45. Neilson S, Woodward A. A comprehensive timeline of the coronavirus pandemic at 1 year, from China's first case to the present (Published and Last Updated Dec 24, 2020). The Insider. https://www.businessinsider.com/coronavirus-pandemic-timeline-history-major-events-2020-3. Accessed 5/21/2021.

46. Sanyaolu A, Okorie C, Hosein Z, et al. Global pandemicity of COVID-19: situation report as of June 9, 2020. *Infect Dis (Auckl).* 2021;14:1178633721991260. doi:10.1177/1178633721991260.

47. Kansas Department of Health and Environment. COVID-19 Cases in Kansas (Last Updated May 19, 2021). Kansas Department of Health and Environment. https://www.coronavirus.kdheks.gov/160/COVID-19-in-Kansas.

48. Worldometers. Canada Coronavirus Cases (Last Updated May 21, 2021). Worldometers. Accessed 05/20/21, https://www.worldometers.info/coronavirus/country/canada/https://www.worldometers.info/coronavirus/country/canada/.

49. Wisconsin Department of Health Services. COVID-19: Wisconsin Cases (Last Updated May 20, 2021). Wisconsin Department of Health Services. Accessed 05/19/21, https://www.dhs.wisconsin.gov/covid-19/cases.htm.

50. Pazzanese C. Battling the 'pandemic of misinformation' (May 8, 2020). The Harvard Gazette Updated 5/8/2020. https://news.harvard.edu/gazette/story/2020/05/social-media-used-to-spread-create-covid-19-falsehoods/.

51. Irfan U. The case for ending the Covid-19 pandemic with mass testing (April 13, 2020). Vox.com. Updated 05/19/2021. https://www.vox.com/2020/4/13/21215133/coronavirus-testing-covid-19-tests-screening.

52. Centers for Disease Control and Prevention (CDC). COVID Data Tracker (Updated Daily, Accessed May 19, 2021). Centers for Disease Control and Prevention (CDC). Accessed 5/19/21, https://covid.cdc.gov/covid-data-tracker/#datatracker-home.

53. Johns Hopkins University & Medicine - Coronavirus Resource Center. America is reopening but have we flattened the curve? See trends in confirmed cases for all 50 states - Georgia (Last updated May 21, 2021). Johns Hopkins University & Medicine. Accessed 05/21/21, https://coronavirus.jhu.edu/data/new-cases-50-states/georgia.

54. Centers for Disease Control and Prevention (CDC). The Advisory Committee on Immunization Practices' Interim Recommendation for Use of Pfizer-BioNTech COVID-19 Vaccine — United States, December 2020 (Published Dec 18, 2020, Last Accessed May 21, 2021). Centers for Disease Control and Prevention (CDC). Updated 12/18/2020. Accessed 5/21/2021, https://www.cdc.gov/mmwr/volumes/69/wr/mm6950e2.htm.

55. Coronavirus (COVID-19) Update: FDA Authorizes Pfizer-BioNTech COVID-19 Vaccine for Emergency Use in Adolescents in Another Important Action in Fight Against Pandemic (Press Release May 10, 2021). May 10, 2021, https://www.fda.gov/news-events/press-announcements/coronavirus-covid-19-update-fda-authorizes-pfizer-biontech-covid-19-vaccine-emergency-use.

56. Centers for Disease Control and Prevention (CDC). The Advisory Committee on Immunization Practices' Interim Recommendation for Use of Moderna COVID-19 Vaccine — United States, December 2020 (Published Jan 1, 2021, Last Accessed May 21, 2021). Centers for Disease Control and Prevention (CDC). Updated 01/01/2021. Accessed 5/21/2021, https://www.cdc.gov/mmwr/volumes/69/wr/mm695152e1.htm.

57. Centers for Disease Control and Prevention (CDC). The Advisory Committee on Immunization Practices' Updated Interim Recommendation for Allocation of COVID-19 Vaccine — United States, December 2020 (Published Jan 1, 2021, Last

Accessed May 21, 2021). Centers for Disease Control and Prevention (CDC). Updated 01/01/2021. Accessed 5/21/2021, https://www.cdc.gov/mmwr/volumes/69/wr/mm695152e2.htm.

58. National Institutes of Health (NIH). Statement from NIH and BARDA on the FDA Emergency Use Authorization of the Janssen COVID-19 Vaccine (News Release Feb 27, 2021). National Institutes of Health (NIH). Accessed 05/21/21, https://www.nih.gov/news-events/news-releases/statement-nih-barda-fda-emergency-use-authorization-janssen-covid-19-vaccine.

59. Centers for Disease Control and Prevention (CDC). The Advisory Committee on Immunization Practices' Interim Recommendation for Use of Pfizer-BioNTech COVID-19 Vaccine in Adolescents Aged 12–15 Years — United States, May 2021 (Published May 14, 2021, Last Accessed May 21, 2021). Centers for Disease Control and Prevention (CDC). Updated 05/14/2021. Accessed 5/21/2021, https://www.cdc.gov/mmwr/volumes/70/wr/mm7020e1.htm.

60. Centers for Disease Control and Prevention (CDC). COVID-19 Vaccinations in the United States (Updated Daily, Accessed May 20, 2021). https://covid.cdc.gov/covid-data-tracker/#-vaccinations.

61. Centers for Disease Control and Prevention (CDC). When You've Been Fully Vaccinated - How to Protect Yourself and Others (Updated May 16, 2021). Centers for Disease Control and Prevention (CDC). Updated 5/16/21. Accessed 05/17/21, https://www.cdc.gov/coronavirus/2019-ncov/vaccines/fully-vaccinated.html.

62. Government of Canada. COVID-19 daily epidemiology update (Last Updated May 26, 2021, Accessed May 26, 2021). https://health-infobase.canada.ca/covid-19/epidemiological-summary-covid-19-cases.html?measure=tested&stat=num&measure=tested&stat=num.

63. Fisman DN, Bogoch I, Lapointe-Shaw L, McCready J, Tuite AR. Risk factors associated with mortality among residents with coronavirus disease 2019 (COVID-19) in long-term care facilities in Ontario, Canada. *JAMA Netw Open.* Jul 1 2020;3(7):e2015957. doi:10.1001/jamanetworkopen.2020.15957.

64. Canadian Institutes of Health Research. Government of Canada funds 49 additional COVID-19 research projects – Details of the funded projects (Last Updated Aug 8, 2020, Accessed May 26, 2021). Government of Canada. Updated 8/8/2020. Accessed 05/26/2021, https://www.canada.ca/en/institutes-health-research/news/2020/03/government-of-canada-funds-49-additional-covid-19-research-projects-details-of-the-funded-projects.html.

65. The Organisation for Economic Co-operation and Development (OECD). The territorial impact of COVID-19: Managing the crisis across levels of government (Last Updated Nov 10, 2020. Accessed May 25, 2021). OECD. Updated 11/10/2020. Accessed 5/25/2021, https://www.oecd.org/coronavirus/policy-responses/theterritorial-impact-of-covid-19-managing-the-crisis-across-levels-of-government-d3e314e1/.

66. Suarez V, Suarez Quezada M, Oros Ruiz S, Ronquillo De Jesus E. Epidemiology of COVID-19 in Mexico: from the 27th of February to the 30th of April 2020. *Rev Clin Esp (Barc).* Nov 2020;220(8):463–471. Epidemiologia de COVID-19 en Mexico: del 27 de febrero al 30 de abril de 2020. doi:10.1016/j.rce.2020.05.007.

67. Worldometers. Haiti Coronavirus Cases (Updated Daily, Accessed May 25, 2021). Worldometers. Accessed 05/25/21, https://www.worldometers.info/coronavirus/country/haiti/.

68. NPR. One Of The World's Poorest Countries Has One Of The World's Lowest COVID Death Rates (May 4, 2021, Accessed May 25, 2021). NPR. https://www.npr.org/sections/goatsandsoda/2021/05/04/992544022/one-of-the-worlds-poorest-countries-has-one-of-the-worlds-lowest-covid-death-rat.

69. Statista. Number of deaths due to the novel coronavirus (COVID-19) in Latin America and the Caribbean by country (Last Updated May 2021). Accessed 05/19/21, https://www.statista.com/statistics/1103965/latin-america-caribbean-coronavirus-deaths/.

70. World Health Organization (WHO). COVID-19 Statistics - Brazil (last Updated May 14, 2021). World Health Organization (WHO). Accessed 05/21/21, https://covid19.who.int/region/amro/country/br.

71. Hallal PC, Hartwig FP, Horta BL, et al. SARS-CoV-2 antibody prevalence in Brazil: results from two successive nationwide serological household surveys. *Lancet Glob Health.* Nov 2020;8(11):e1390–e1398. doi:10.1016/S2214-109X(20)30387-9.

72. Hallal PC, Victora CG. Overcoming Brazil's monumental COVID-19 failure: an urgent call to action. Nature Medicine. 2021/05/06 2021;doi:10.1038/s41591-021-01353-2.

73. World Health Organization (WHO). COVID-19 WHO Coronavirus (COVID-19) Dashboard (last Updated May 21, 2021). World Health Organization (WHO). Accessed 05/21/21, https://covid19.who.int.

74. Fox B. The last continent to face up COVID-19, Africa 'needs to wake up' (Published Mar 20, 2020. Updated May 13, 2020). Euractiv.com. Updated May 21, 2021. https://www.euractiv.com/section/botswana/news/the-last-continent-to-face-up-covid-19-africa-needs-to-wake-up/.

75. World Health Organization (WHO). COVID-19 cases top 10 000 in Africa(last Updated April 7, 2020). World Health Organization (WHO). Accessed 05/21/21, https://www.afro.who.int/news/covid-19-cases-top-10-000-africa.

76. Nigeria Centre for Disease Control. First Case of Corona Virus Disease confirmed in Nigeria (Last Updated Feb 28, 2020, Accessed May 21, 2021). Nigeria Centre for Disease Control. Updated 2/28/20. Accessed 5/21/21, https://ncdc.gov.ng/news/227/first-case-of-corona-virus-disease-confirmed-in-nigeria.

77. MacLean R. Africa Braces for Coronavirus, but Slowly (Published Mar 17, 2020, Updated Jun 29, 2020, Accessed May 21, 2021). The New York Times. doi:https://www.nytimes.com/2020/03/17/world/africa/coronavirus-africa-burkina-faso.html.

78. Salyer SJ, Maeda J, Sembuche S, et al. The first and second waves of the COVID-19 pandemic in Africa: a cross-sectional study. *Lancet.* Apr 3 2021;397(10281):1265–1275. doi:10.1016/S0140-6736(21)00632-2.

79. African Union - Africa Centres for Disease Control and Prevention. COVID 19 Vaccine Perceptions: A 15 country study (Updated Mar 10, 2021, Accessed May 21, 2021). https://africacdc.org/download/covid-19-vaccine-perceptions-a-15-country-study/.

80. World Health Organization (WHO). Weekly epidemiological update on COVID-19 - 4 May 2021 (Accessed May 21, 2021). World Health Organization (WHO). Accessed 05/21/21, https://www.who.int/publications/m/item/weekly-epidemiological-update-on-covid-19-4-may-2021.

81. Kaseje N. Why Sub-Saharan Africa needs a unique response to COVID-19 (Published Mar 30, 2020, Accessed May 21, 2021). Mar 30, 2020.

82. African Center for Strategic Studies. Mapping Risk Factors for the Spread of COVID-19 in Africa (Published Apr 3, 2020, Updated May 13, 2020, Accessed May 21, 2021). African Center for Strategic Studies. https://africacenter.org/spotlight/mapping-risk-factors-spread-covid-19-africa/.

83. World Health Organization (WHO). World AIDS Day 2019 (Accessed May 21, 2021). World Health Organization (WHO). Accessed 05/21/21, https://www.who.int/campaigns/world-aids-day/2019.

84. World Health Organization (WHO). World Hepatitis Day 2019 (Accessed May 21, 2021). World Health Organization (WHO). Accessed 05/21/21, https://www.who.int/campaigns/world-hepatitis-day/2019.

85. World Health Organization (WHO). World Tuberculosis Day 2019 (Accessed May 21, 2021). World Health Organization (WHO). Accessed 05/21/21, https://www.who.int/campaigns/world-tb-day/2019.

86. World Health Organization (WHO). World malaria report 2019 (Updated Dec 4, 2019, Accessed May 21, 2021). World Health Organization (WHO). Accessed 05/21/21, https://www.who.int/publications/i/item/9789241565721.

87. Mudie K, Jin MM, Tan, et al. Non-communicable diseases in sub-Saharan Africa: a scoping review of large cohort studies. *J Glob Health*. Dec 2019;9(2):020409. doi:10.7189/jogh.09.020409.

88. World Health Organization (WHO). Global status report on noncommunicable diseases 2010 (Cited Apr 17, 2020, Accessed May 21, 2021). World Health Organization (WHO). https://www.who.int/nmh/publications/ncd_report_full_en.pdf.

89. Storen R, Corrigan N. *COVID-19: a chronology of state and territory government announcements up until 30 June 2020*: Parliament of Australia - Department of Parliamentary Services; 2020. Research Paper Series, 2020-2110/22/2020https://parlinfo.aph.gov.au/parlInfo/download/library/prspub/7614514/upload_binary/7614514.pdf. Accessed 05/21/21. https://www.aph.gov.au/About_Parliament/Parliamentary_Departments/Parliamentary_Library/pubs/rp/rp2021/Chronologies/COVID-19StateTerritoryGovernmentAnnouncements#_ftn1.

90. Melinek MD J. Culture Shock: Why New Zealand's Response to COVID-19 Worked - A first-hand account from a doctor from the U.S. who lives in New Zealand (Nov 24, 2020, Last Accessed May 24, 2021). https://www.medpagetoday.com/blogs/working-stiff/89867.

91. World Health Organization (WHO). World Health Emergency Dashboard - New Zealand (Accessed and Last Updated May 26, 2021). World Health Organization (WHO). https://covid19.who.int/region/wpro/country/nz.

92. Robert A. Lessons from New Zealand's COVID-19 outbreak response. *Lancet Public Health*. Nov 2020;5(11):e569–e570. doi:10.1016/S2468-2667(20)30237-1.

93. Australian Government - Department of Health. Coronavirus (COVID-19) current situation and case numbers (Last Updated May 17, 2021, Accessed May 18, 2021). Australian Government - Department of Health. https://www.health.gov.au/news/health-alerts/novel-coronavirus-2019-ncov-health-alert/coronavirus-covid-19-current-situation-and-case-numbers.

94. Woolf SH, Chapman DA, Lee JH. COVID-19 as the leading cause of death in the United States. *JAMA*. Jan 12 2021;325(2):123–124. doi:10.1001/jama.2020.24865.

95. Statistics CfDCaPC-NCfH. COVID-19 Mortality Overview - Provisional Death Counts for Coronavirus Disease 2019 (COVID-19). Page last reviewed April 23, 2021. Centers for Disease Control and Prevention (CDC). Updated 04/23/2021. Accessed 04/25/2021, https://www.cdc.gov/nchs/covid19/mortality-overview.htm.

96. Ahmad FB, Cisewski JA, Miniño A, et al. Provisional Mortality Data — United States, 2020 (MMWR Morb Mortal Wkly Rep 03/31/2021;70:519–522). Updated 3/31/2021. Accessed 04/25/2021, 4/25/2021. https://www.cdc.gov/mmwr/volumes/70/wr/mm7014e1.htm.

97. Huang C, Wang Y, Li X, et al. Clinical features of patients infected with 2019 novel coronavirus in Wuhan, China. *Lancet*. Feb 15 2020;395(10223):497–506. doi:10.1016/S0140-6736(20)30183-5.

98. Zheng Z, Peng F, Xu B, et al. Risk factors of critical & mortal COVID-19 cases: A systematic literature review and meta-analysis. *J Infect*. Aug 2020;81(2):e16–e25. doi:10.1016/j.jinf.2020.04.021.

99. CDC COVID-19 Response Team. Preliminary Estimates of the Prevalence of Selected Underlying Health Conditions Among Patients with Coronavirus Disease 2019 - United States, February 12-March 28, 2020. PMC7119513 Journal Editors form for disclosure of potential conflicts of interest. No potential conflicts of interest were disclosed., Updated Apr 3. Accessed 13, 69. https://www.cdc.gov/nchs/covid19/mortality-overview.htm.

100. Qi C, Zhu YC, Li CY, et al. Epidemiological characteristics and spatial-temporal analysis of COVID-19 in Shandong Province. *China. Epidemiol Infect*. Jul 6 2020;148:e141. doi:10.1017/S095026882000151X.

101. Korean Society of Infectious DKorean Society of Pediatric Infectious DKorean Society of E. Report on the Epidemiological Features of Coronavirus Disease 2019 (COVID-19) Outbreak in the Republic of Korea from January 19 to March 2, 2020. *J Korean Med Sci*. Mar. 16. 2020;35(10):e112. doi:10.3346/jkms.2020.35.e112.

102. Suleyman G, Fadel RA, Malette KM, et al. Clinical characteristics and morbidity associated with coronavirus disease 2019 in a series of patients in metropolitan Detroit. *JAMA Netw Open*. Jun 1 2020;3(6):e2012270. doi:10.1001/jamanetworkopen.2020.12270.

103. Kopel J, Perisetti A, Roghani A, Aziz M, Gajendran M, Goyal H. Racial and gender-based differences in COVID-19. *Front Public Health*. 2020;8:418. doi:10.3389/fpubh.2020.00418.

104. Ioannou GN, Locke E, Green P, et al. Risk factors for hospitalization, mechanical ventilation, or death among 10131 US veterans with SARS-CoV-2 infection. *JAMA Netw Open*. Sep 1 2020;3(9):e2022310. doi:10.1001/jamanetworkopen.2020.22310.

105. Gomez JMD, Du-Fay-de-Lavallaz JM, Fugar S, et al. Sex differences in COVID-19 hospitalization and mortality. *J Womens Health (Larchmt)*. May 2021;30(5):646–653. doi:10.1089/jwh.2020.8948.

106. Piemonti L, Scavini M. Gender and Age Effects on the Rates of Infection and Deaths in Individuals with Confirmed SARS-CoV-2 Infection in Six European Countries. TheLancet.com (ePub ahead of print) 04/28/2020.

107. Scully EP, Haverfield J, Ursin RL, Tannenbaum C, Klein SL. Considering how biological sex impacts immune responses and COVID-19 outcomes. *Nat Rev Immunol*. Jul 2020;20(7):442–447. doi:10.1038/s41577-020-0348-8.

108. Cangiano B, Fatti LM, Danesi L, et al. Mortality in an Italian nursing home during COVID-19 pandemic: correlation with gender, age, ADL, vitamin D supplementation, and limitations of the diagnostic tests. *Aging (Albany NY)*. Dec 22 2020;12(24):24522–24534. doi:10.18632/aging.202307.

109. Pradhan A, Olsson PE. Sex differences in severity and mortality from COVID-19: are males more vulnerable? *Biol Sex Differ*. Sep 18 2020;11(1):53. doi:10.1186/s13293-020-00330-7.

110. Strope JD, Chau CH, Figg WD. Are sex discordant outcomes in COVID-19 related to sex hormones? *Semin Oncol*. Oct 2020;47(5):335–340. doi:10.1053/j.seminoncol.2020.06.002.

111. Scannell Bryan M, Sun J, Jagai J, et al. Coronavirus disease 2019 (COVID-19) mortality and neighborhood characteristics in Chicago. *Ann Epidemiol*. Apr 2021;56:47–54, e5. doi:10.1016/j.annepidem.2020.10.011.

112. Kang SJ, Jung SI. Age-related morbidity and mortality among patients with COVID-19. *Infect Chemother*. Jun 2020;52(2):154–164. doi:10.3947/ic.2020.52.2.154.

113. Natale F, Ghio D, Tarchi D, Goujon A, Conte A. Natale, F.,Ghio, D., Tarchi, D., Goujon, A., Conte, A. COVID-19 Cases and Case Fatality Rate by age (published May 4, 2020). European Commission. Updated 05/04/2020. Accessed 04/25/2021, https://knowledge4policy.ec.europa.eu/publication/covid-19-cases-case-fatality-rate-age_en.

114. Viner RM, Mytton OT, Bonell C, et al. Susceptibility to SARS-CoV-2 infection among children and adolescents compared with adults: a systematic review and meta-analysis. *JAMA Pediatr*. Feb 1 2021;175(2):143–156. doi:10.1001/jamapediatrics.2020.4573.

115. U.S. DEPARTMENT OF HEALTH AND HUMAN SERVICES; Centers for Disease Control and Prevention; National Center for Health Statistics. National Center for Health Statistics - Vital and Health Statistics. Long-term Care Providers and Services Users in the United States, 2015–2016. Series 3, Number 43 (DHHS Publication No. 2019–1427). National Center for Health Statistics - Vital and Health Statistics Updated February 2019. Series 3, Number 43 (DHHS Publication No. 2019–1427). https://www.cdc.gov/nchs/data/series/sr_03/sr03_43-508.pdf.

116. Gruver AL, Hudson LL, Sempowski GD. Immunosenescence of ageing. *J Pathol*. Jan 2007;211(2):144–156. doi:10.1002/path.2104.

117. Thompson DC, Barbu MG, Beiu C, et al. The impact of COVID-19 pandemic on long-term care facilities worldwide: an overview on international issues. *Biomed Res Int*. 2020;2020:8870249. doi:10.1155/2020/8870249.

118. Konetzka RT, Gorges RJ. Nothing much has changed: COVID-19 nursing home cases and deaths follow fall surges. *J Am Geriatr Soc*. Jan 2021;69(1):46–47. doi:10.1111/jgs.16951.

119. Abrams HR, Loomer L, Gandhi A, Grabowski DC. Characteristics of U.S. nursing homes with COVID-19 cases. *J Am Geriatr Soc*. Aug 2020;68(8):1653–1656. doi:10.1111/jgs.16661.

120. Li Y, Temkin-Greener H, Shan G, Cai X. COVID-19 infections and deaths among Connecticut nursing home residents: facility correlates. *J Am Geriatr Soc*. Sep 2020;68(9):1899–1906. doi:10.1111/jgs.16689.

121. He M, Li Y, Fang F. Is there a link between nursing home reported quality and COVID-19 cases? Evidence from California skilled nursing facilities. *J Am Med Dir Assoc*. Jul 2020;21(7):905–908. doi:10.1016/j.jamda.2020.06.016.

122. Unruh MA, Yun H, Zhang Y, Braun RT, Jung HY. Nursing home characteristics associated with COVID-19 deaths in Connecticut, New Jersey, and New York. *J Am Med Dir Assoc*. Jul 2020;21(7):1001–1003. doi:10.1016/j.jamda.2020.06.019

123. White EM, Kosar CM, Feifer RA, et al. Variation in SARS-CoV-2 prevalence in U.S. skilled nursing facilities. *J Am Geriatr Soc*. Oct 2020;68(10):2167–2173. doi:10.1111/jgs.16752.

124. Liu M, Maxwell CJ, Armstrong P, et al. COVID-19 in long-term care homes in Ontario and British Columbia. *CMAJ*. Nov 23 2020;192(47):E1540–E1546. doi:10.1503/cmaj.201860.

125. Surveillance of COVID-19 at longterm care facilities in the EU/EE (Published May 19, 2020). European Centre for Disease Prevention and Control (ECDC). https://www.ecdc.europa.eu/sites/default/files/documents/covid-19-long-term-care-facilities-surveillance-guidance.pdf.

126. Panagiotou OA, Kosar CM, White EM, et al. Risk factors associated with all-cause 30-day mortality in nursing home residents with COVID-19. *JAMA Intern Med*. Apr 1 2021;181(4):439–448. doi:10.1001/jamainternmed.2020.7968.

127. KFF - State Health Facts. COVID-19 Cases by Race/Ethnicity (Last Updated May 3, 2021). KFF - State Health Facts. Updated 5/3/21. Accessed 4/25/21, https://www.kff.org/other/state-indicator/covid-19-cases-by-race-ethnicity/?currentTimeframe=0&sortModel=%7B%22colId%22:%22Location%22,%22sort%22:%22asc%22%7D.

128. Worldometers. First 20 cases in the United States (Last Updated May 20,2021). Updated 05/20/2021. Accessed 05/20/2021, https://www.worldometers.info/coronavirus/country/us/#first-cases.

129. Centers for Disease Control and Prevention (CDC). CDC confirms additional cases of 2019 Novel Coronavirus in United States (Last Updated January 26, 2020). Centers for Disease Control and Prevention (CDC). Updated 01/26/21. Accessed 05/20/2021, https://www.cdc.gov/media/releases/2020/s0126-coronavirus-new-cases.html.

130. Cuomo RE. Shift in racial communities impacted by COVID-19 in California. *J Epidemiol Community Health*. Oct 16 2020. doi:10.1136/jech-2020-215148.

131. Millett GA, Jones AT, Benkeser D, et al. Assessing differential impacts of COVID-19 on black communities. *Ann Epidemiol*. Jul 2020;47:37–44. doi:10.1016/j.annepidem.2020.05.003.

132. Strully K, Yang TC, Liu H. Regional variation in COVID-19 disparities: connections with immigrant and Latinx communities in U.S. counties. *Ann Epidemiol*. Jan 2021;53:56–62, e2. doi:10.1016/j.annepidem.2020.08.016.

133. Takagi H, Kuno T, Yokoyama Y, et al. Ethnicity/race and economics in COVID-19: meta-regression of data from counties in the New York metropolitan area. *Journal of Epidemiology and Community Health*. 2021;75(2):205–206. doi:10.1136/jech-2020-214820.

134. DiMaggio C, Klein M, Berry C, Frangos S. Black/African American Communities are at highest risk of COVID-19: spatial modeling of New York City ZIP Code-level testing results. *Ann Epidemiol.* Nov 2020;51:7–13. doi:10.1016/j.annepidem.2020.08.012.

135. Rodriguez-Diaz CE, Guilamo-Ramos V, Mena L, et al. Risk for COVID-19 infection and death among Latinos in the United States: examining heterogeneity in transmission dynamics. *Ann Epidemiol.* Dec 2020;52:46–53, e2. doi:10.1016/j.annepidem.2020.07.007.

136. Weng CH, Saal A, McGuire DC, Chan PA. Persistently high SARS-CoV-2 positivity rate and incidence for Hispanic/Latinos during state reopening in an urban setting: a retrospective cohort study. *Epidemiol Infect.* Jan 18 2021;149:e25. doi:10.1017/S0950268821000133.

137. New Mexico Health Department. NEW MEXICO COVID-19 MORTALITY UPDATE (Last Updated May 03, 2021). Accessed 04/25/21, https://cv.nmhealth.org/wp-content/uploads/2021/05/COVID-19-Mortality-Rates-Public-Report_05.03.2021.pdf.

138. Daras K, Alexiou A, Rose TC, Buchan I, Taylor-Robinson D, Barr B. How does vulnerability to COVID-19 vary between communities in England? Developing a Small Area Vulnerability Index (SAVI). *J Epidemiol Community Health.* Feb 4 2021. doi:10.1136/jech-2020-215227.

139. Office for National Statistics. Latest data and analysis on coronavirus (COVID-19) in the UK and its effect on the economy and society (Accessed April 25, 2021). Accessed 04/25/2021, https://www.ons.gov.uk/peoplepopulationandcommunity/healthandsocialcare/conditionsanddiseases.

140. BBC News. Brazil 2010 census shows changing race balance (Last Updated 11/17/2011). BBC News. Accessed 04/25/21, https://www.bbc.com/news/world-latin-america-15766840.

141. Martins-Filho PR, Araujo BCL, Sposato KB, Araujo AAS, Quintans-Junior LJ, Santos VS. Racial disparities in COVID-19-related deaths in Brazil: black lives matter? *J Epidemiol.* Mar 5 2021;31(3):239–240. doi:10.2188/jea.JE20200589.

142. Oronce CIA, Scannell CA, Kawachi I, Tsugawa Y. Association between state-level income inequality and COVID-19 cases and mortality in the USA. *J Gen Intern Med.* Sep 2020;35(9):2791–2793. doi:10.1007/s11606-020-05971-3.

143. Khazanchi R, Beiter ER, Gondi S, Beckman AL, Bilinski A, Ganguli I. County-level association of social vulnerability with COVID-19 cases and deaths in the USA. *J Gen Intern Med.* Sep 2020;35(9):2784–2787. doi:10.1007/s11606-020-05882-3.

144. Sy KTL, Martinez ME, Rader B, White LF. Socioeconomic disparities in subway use and COVID-19 outcomes in New York City. *medRxiv.* May 30 2020. doi:10.1101/2020.05.28.20115949.

145. Phuong Do D, Frank R. Unequal burdens: assessing the determinants of elevated COVID-19 case and death rates in New York City's racial/ethnic minority neighbourhoods.

Journal of Epidemiology and Community Health. 2021;75(4):321–326. doi:10.1136/jech-2020-215280.

146. Rho HJ, Brown H, Fremstad S. A Basic Demographic Profile of Workers in Frontline Industries (Last Updated April 2020, Accessed May 21, 2021). Center for Economic and Policy Research (CEPR). https://cepr.net/wp-content/uploads/2020/04/2020-04-Frontline-Workers.pdf.

147. McClure ES, Vasudevan P, Bailey Z, Patel S, Robinson WR. Racial capitalism within public health: how occupational settings drive COVID-19 disparities. *Am J Epidemiol.* Nov 2 2020;189(11):1244–1253. doi:10.1093/aje/kwaa126.

148. Renteria ER, Cespedes P, Cerna K, et al. Epidemiologic patterns of COVID-19 incidence in the province of Lima. *Ann Epidemiol.* Feb 2021;54:27–28. doi:10.1016/j.annepidem.2020.09.018.

149. Jeong HE, Lee J, Shin HJ, Shin JY. Socioeconomic disparities in Korea by health insurance type during the COVID-19 pandemic: a nationwide study. *Epidemiol Health.* 2021;43:e2021007. doi:10.4178/epih.e2021007.

150. Demenech LM, Dumith SC, Vieira M, Neiva-Silva L. Income inequality and risk of infection and death by COVID-19 in Brazil. *Rev Bras Epidemiol.* 2020;23:e200095. Desigualdade economica e risco de infeccao e morte por COVID-19 no Brasil doi:10.1590/1980-549720200095.

151. Thome B, Rezende LFM, Schveitzer MC, Monteiro CN, Goldbaum M. Differences in the prevalence of risk factors for severe COVID-19 across regions of Sao Paulo City. *Rev Bras Epidemiol.* 2020;23:e200087. doi:10.1590/1980-549720200087.

152. Bambra C, Riordan R, Ford J, Matthews F. The COVID-19 pandemic and health inequalities. *J Epidemiol Community Health.* Nov 2020;74(11):964–968. doi:10.1136/jech-2020-214401.

153. Williams DR, Collins C. Racial residential segregation: a fundamental cause of racial disparities in health. *Public Health Rep.* Sep-Oct 2001;116(5):404–416. doi:10.1093/phr/116.5.404.

154. Goumenou M, Sarigiannis D, Tsatsakis A, et al. COVID19 in Northern Italy: An integrative overview of factors possibly influencing the sharp increase of the outbreak (Review). *Mol Med Rep.* Jul 2020;22(1):20–32. doi:10.3892/mmr.2020.11079.

155. Frontera A, Cianfanelli L, Vlachos K, Landoni G, Cremona G. Severe air pollution links to higher mortality in COVID-19 patients: the "double-hit" hypothesis. *J Infect.* Aug 2020;81(2):255–259. doi:10.1016/j.jinf.2020.05.031.

156. Ogen Y. Assessing nitrogen dioxide (NO_2) levels as a contributing factor to coronavirus (COVID-19) fatality. *Sci Total Environ.* Jul 15 2020;726:138605. doi:10.1016/j.scitotenv.2020.138605.

157. Wu X, Nethery RC, Sabath BM, Braun D, Dominici F. Exposure to air pollution and COVID-19 mortality in the United States: a nationwide cross-sectional study. *medRxiv.* Apr 7 2020. doi:10.1101/2020.04.05.20054502.

SARS-CoV-2: Structure, Pathogenesis, and Diagnosis

Aarthi Goverdhan, PhD

OUTLINE

SARS-CoV-2 and Coronaviruses

Evolutionary Origins

In the last two decades, three coronaviruses have caused outbreaks of varying scales, with the pandemic caused by severe acute respiratory syndrome coronavirus 2 (SARS-CoV-2) representing the most recent threat to human health at a global level. Aside from severe acute respiratory syndrome coronavirus (SARS-CoV) and Middle East respiratory syndrome coronavirus (MERS-CoV), which were responsible for the first two outbreaks of the 21st century, only four other coronaviruses that cause relatively mild disease in humans have been discovered: HCoV-229E, HCoV-NL63, HCoV-OC43, and HCoV-HKU1.[1,2] The SARS, MERS, and COVID-19 outbreaks have demonstrated that zoonotic coronaviruses can successfully cross species barriers to infect humans and cause a high level of pathogenicity and mortality.

SARS-CoV-2 belongs to the order Nidovirales, family Coronaviridae, subfamily Coronavirinae, and genus Betacoronavirus. Within the genus Betacoronavirus, four distinct lineages are assigned: HCoV-OC43 and HCoV-HKU1 belong to lineage A, SARS-CoV and SARS-CoV-2 belong to lineage B, and MERS-CoV belongs to lineage C.[3] SARS-CoV-2 is further classified under the subgenus Sarbecovirus.[4,5] SARS-CoV and MERS-CoV both originated in bats, palm civets acted as the intermediate host for SARS-CoV, and camels served as the intermediate host for MERS-CoV.[6-8] The genome of SARS-CoV-2 shares 80% sequence identity with SARS-CoV and presents a high degree of sequence identity to the genomes of bat coronaviruses RaTG13 and RmYN02.[9,10] The high level of similarity to bat-derived coronaviruses suggests that SARS-CoV-2 must have also originated in bats.[4,9] Although sarbecoviruses are known to undergo frequent recombination, assessment of the SARS-CoV-2 genome revealed no evidence to suggest that it originated from a recent recombination event. Early studies characterizing SARS-CoV-2 reported that it uses the same human receptor as SARS-CoV, angiotensin-converting enzyme-2 (ACE2), to enter and infect host cells. In contrast, MERS-CoV uses a receptor called dipeptidyl peptidase 4 (DPP4).[7] Interestingly, SARS-CoV-2 possesses a polybasic cleavage site insertion (PRRA sequence) in the spike protein at the junction of the S1 and S2 subunits, which resembles a sequence that is present in MERS-CoV but absent in SARS-CoV and RaTG13.[11] This sequence was identified as a putative furin cleavage site that may be acted upon by the proprotein convertase furin during viral egress.

The discovery of a coronavirus similar to SARS-CoV-2, pangolin CoV, in Malayan pangolins showing clinical signs of infection drove the suspicion that pangolins may serve as the intermediate host for SARS-CoV-2.[12] The receptor-binding domain (RBD) in the spike protein of pangolin-CoV was almost identical to that of SARS-CoV-2, but pangolin-CoV lacked the furin cleavage site found in SARS-CoV-2.[13] Moreover, many bat-derived coronaviruses, such as RmYN02, have been reported to contain a similar insertion in spike protein at the S1/S2 junction, suggesting that SARS-CoV-2 likely

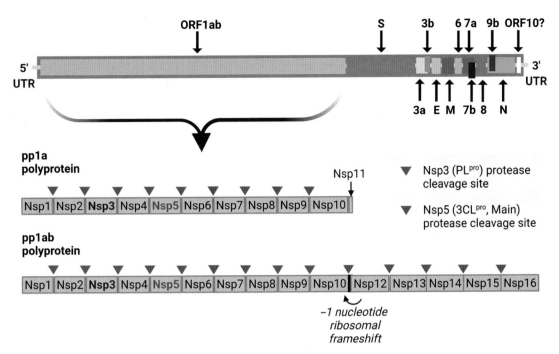

Fig. 2.1 SARS-CoV-2 Genome. In addition to the 5′ and 3′ untranslated regions *(UTR)*, the SARS-CoV-2 genome contains coding regions for structural proteins spike protein *(S)*, envelope protein *(E)*, membrane protein *(M)*, and nucleocapsid protein *(N)*, and many open reading frames (ORF1ab, ORF3a, ORF3b, ORF6, ORF7a, ORF7b, ORF8, ORF9b, and ORF10). ORF9b is an alternative reading frame located within the *N* gene. ORF10 may not generate a functional protein in SARS-CoV-2. ORF1ab makes up more than 60% of the genome, and produces two polyproteins: pp1ab and pp1a, which are proteolytically cleaved by nonstructural protein 5 (Nsp5) and Nsp3 to yield the full set of nonstructural proteins. Nsp1-11 is generated through cleavage of the pp1a polyprotein, whereas Nsp1-10 and Nsp12-16 are generated through cleavage of the pp1ab polyprotein. The pp1ab polyprotein is produced from ORF1ab by a ribosomal frameshifting event involving a (–1) nucleotide shift during translation.

originated from multiple recombination events that occurred within viruses inhabiting bats and other species. With the accumulating evidence, it appears unlikely that pangolins acted as intermediate hosts facilitating SARS-CoV-2 spillover to humans.[13,14] Although the involvement of an intermediate host cannot be ruled out, it has been suggested that SARS-CoV-2 may have spilled over directly from bats to humans without requiring an intermediate host.[15] The origin and cross-species transmission of SARS-CoV-2 is still under investigation and remains a subject of debate.

Structure, Genome, and Proteome

The positive-sense single-stranded RNA genome of SARS-CoV-2 extends to 29,891 nucleotides and encodes 9860 amino acids.[16] In addition to the flanking 5′ and 3′ untranslated regions (UTRs), the SARS-CoV-2 genome includes coding regions for the structural proteins spike glycoprotein (S), envelope protein (E), membrane glycoprotein (M), and nucleocapsid protein (N), and several open reading frames (ORF1ab, ORF3a, ORF3b, ORF6, ORF7a, ORF7b, ORF8, ORF9b, and ORF10) that code for accessory structural and nonstructural proteins (Fig. 2.1).[64]

The first electron micrographs of SARS-CoV-2 revealed virus particles described as spherical with some pleomorphism and distinctive spikes that created the appearance of a solar corona.[17] Coronavirus particles consist of an outer lipid bilayer envelope inserted with the spike, membrane, and envelope structural proteins. The inner core contains a helical nucleocapsid structure that is formed by the association of nucleocapsid phosphoproteins with the viral genomic RNA (Fig. 2.2).

Structural Proteins

Spike Protein

The spike glycoprotein (S) is a structural protein that is critical for binding to the ACE2 receptor on host cells and facilitating cell entry.[18] The S protein is embedded into the outer lipid bilayer envelope in a uniform distribution and extends out from the virion surface, producing the defining "corona"-like appearance.[19] The SARS-CoV-2 S protein is a densely glycosylated homotrimeric class I fusion protein that is divided into two subunits, S1 and S2, which are separated by a multibasic furin protease cleavage site.[20] The S1 subunit forms a globular head that binds to the host cell receptor, and the S2 subunit facilitates viral membrane fusion with the host cell membrane.[21] The S1 subunit is composed of an amino- or N-terminal domain (NTD) and a

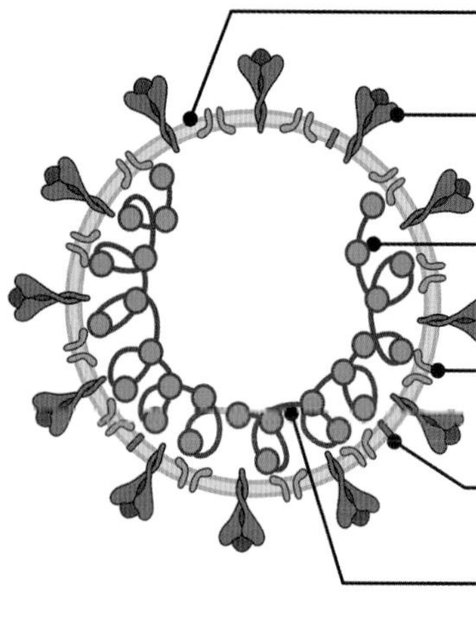

Outer lipid bilayer envelope

Spike (S) protein

Nucleocapsid (N) protein

Membrane (M) protein

Envelope (E) protein

Viral genomic RNA

Fig. 2.2 Viral Structure. Coronavirus particles consist of an outer lipid bilayer envelope that is studded with the spike (S), membrane (M), and envelope (E) structural proteins. The spike protein protrudes out from the viral envelope, giving the appearance of a solar corona. The inner core of the virion consists of a helical nucleocapsid structure formed by the association of nucleocapsid (N) phosphoproteins with viral genomic RNA.

carboxy- or C-terminal domain (CTD). The S1 subunit CTD functions as the RBD that binds to the human ACE2 (hACE2) receptor.[18,22]

The S protein exists in a metastable prefusion conformation. On binding to the host cell receptor, it undergoes a significant structural transformation to enable fusion of the viral membrane with the host cell membrane.[23] The furin cleavage site (RRXR motif) at the S1/S2 junction is proteolytically cleaved, leading to the separation of S1 from S2; however, the two subunits remain noncovalently bound to each other.[19,24] After S1/S2 cleavage and engagement of the RBD with the host cell ACE2 receptor, another cleavage site (S2′) in the S2 subunit is exposed, and this site also must be cleaved by proteases to release the fusion peptide, which is essential for membrane fusion and viral infectivity.[25] Receptor binding destabilizes the prefusion trimer, resulting in the shedding of the S1 subunit and transition of the S2 subunit to a stable postfusion conformation.

To engage the host cell receptor, the RBD in the S1 subunit undergoes hinge-like structural movements that either expose or hide the residues involved in receptor recognition. The accessible state is referred to as the "open" or "up" conformation, and the inaccessible state is referred to as the "closed" or "down" conformation (Fig. 2.3). The RBD consists of a core and a receptor binding motif (RBM), with the latter directly mediating contacts with the ACE2 receptor. Various studies have reported either equivalent or higher binding affinity of the SARS-CoV-2 RBD for ACE2, compared with its counterpart in SARS-CoV.[18,22–24,26]

Envelope Protein

The envelope glycoprotein (E) in SARS-CoV-2 is an integral membrane protein of only 75 amino acids in length.[27] Envelope proteins are viroporins, which are generally described as virally encoded small proteins that can form pores in the membranes of host cell organelles and modulate ion channel activity, among other functions.[28] In lipid bilayers that mimic the endoplasmic reticulum–Golgi intermediate compartment (ERGIC)

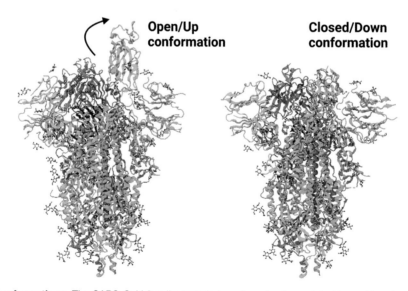

Open/Up conformation

Closed/Down conformation

Fig. 2.3 Spike Protein Conformations. The SARS-CoV-2 spike protein is a densely glycosylated homotrimeric class I fusion protein that is divided into two subunits: S1 and S2, with S1 binding to the angiotensin-converting enzyme-2 *(ACE2)* receptor on host cells, and S2 mediating membrane fusion. To bind to the ACE2 receptor, the receptor binding domain (RBD) in the S1 subunit undergoes hinge-like movements that either expose ("open" or "up" conformation) or hide ("closed" or "down" conformation) the residues that mediate receptor recognition. Protein data bank (PDB) structure IDs: 6VXX and 6VYB. (From Walls AC, Park YJ, Tortorici MA, et al. Structure, function, and antigenicity of the SARS-CoV-2 spike glycoprotein. *Cell.* 2020;181[2]:281-292.e286. https://doi.org/10.1016/j.cell.2020.02.058)

membrane, the SARS-CoV-2 E protein transmembrane domain forms a five-helix bundle that surrounds a narrow pore, a homopentameric cation channel.[27] The elucidated N-terminal lumen/C-terminal cytoplasmic membrane topology of SARS-CoV-2 E is conducive to the conduction of Ca^{2+} ions out of the ERGIC lumen, a role that may link the E protein to host inflammasome activation based on similar topology and involvement of the SARS-CoV E protein in this process.[27,29–31] Examination of E protein from other coronaviruses indicates that the protein is abundantly expressed in infected cells, but only a small proportion of the protein is incorporated into the virion envelope. The larger proportion is localized at sites of intracellular trafficking, such as the endoplasmic reticulum (ER), Golgi, and ERGIC membranes. At these sites, the E protein plays a role in virion assembly and budding.[28]

Membrane Protein

The most abundant protein in coronaviruses, the Membrane protein (M), is a transmembrane glycoprotein that plays a role in delineation of the viral envelope shape and size. The M protein acts as a scaffold to regulate virion assembly by binding to other viral structural proteins at the site of budding and bringing them together to form the viral envelope.[28] The M protein is functionally dimeric and may be able to associate with other M dimers to form a matrix-like layer. The M protein network possesses intrinsic membrane-bending properties, but its interactions with the S protein, E protein, and N protein–viral RNA complexes are important for effective membrane curvature and has an impact on virion size.[32,33] The M protein interacts with the spike protein to facilitate its retention in the ERGIC/Golgi complex.[28] The M protein can adopt two conformations; the elongated conformer of M protein plays a role in spike incorporation into new virions.[32] The structural properties of this conformer facilitate the formation of a rigid and convex viral envelope. The C-terminal domain of the M protein further interacts with and stabilizes the internal core and N protein–RNA complexes that make up the nucleocapsid, to promote completion of virion assembly.[34] Expression of the M, S, and E proteins is minimally required for the production of SARS-CoV-2 noninfectious virus-like particles.[35]

Nucleocapsid Protein

The Nucleocapsid (N) protein is a multivalent RNA-binding protein, the primary role of which is to package the 30-kb-long genomic RNA compactly into viral ribonucleoprotein (vRNP) complexes that can be accommodated into the approximately 80-nm-diameter viral lumen.[36] The N protein self-associates and naturally exists in a dimeric state, although it can also form oligomers, a property that is likely important for the formation of vRNPs.[37] The protein consists of two globular domains, the NTD and the CTD, with the NTD containing RNA-binding sites that may interact with the viral genomic RNA packaging signal and the CTD forming a dimer with an RNA-binding groove to aid in vRNP assembly. The NTD and CTD are separated by a central, highly conserved, intrinsically disordered region containing a serine arginine (SR)–rich sequence with multiple phosphorylation sites that are targeted by cytoplasmic kinases to regulate the function of the N protein. The N protein also includes N-terminal and C-terminal intrinsically disordered regions; the latter and the CTD are both involved in M protein binding to anchor the vRNP complex to the inner surface of the viral envelope.[38]

Structural analysis of SARS-CoV-2 viruses by cryo-electron tomography revealed that vRNPs associated with the viral envelope were stacked into cylindrical or helical filament-like assemblies.[33] Efficient packing of the virus particles by N proteins could be accomplished through a "beads on a string" formation with viral RNA linking neighboring vRNPs. Another study determined that the vRNPs in SARS-CoV-2 existed in different arrangements based on the shape of the virions.[36] In spherical virions, there was a higher incidence of membrane-proximal vRNPs packed internally against the envelope in a "hexon" formation. In ellipsoidal virions, membrane-free vRNPs were arranged like pyramids or in "tetrahedron" formations. However, in both arrangements, neighboring vRNPs were equally spaced apart, and in situ projection suggests that tetrahedrons might be able to assemble into hexons. Therefore the vRNP triangle presents a durable building block that can withstand environmental and mechanical stresses and allows for the adoption of various arrangements within the virion.[36]

Accessory Proteins
ORF3a

SARS-CoV-2 ORF3a encodes a viroporin that shares 73% sequence identity with SARS-CoV ORF3a.[39–41] ORF3a has been demonstrated to play a role in blocking autophagy and conferring viral escape from lysosomal destruction, a function reported to be unique to SARS-CoV-2 ORF3a and not observed in its SARS-CoV counterpart.[42,43] Additionally, ORF3a is involved in inflammasome activation, pyroptosis, and apoptosis induction.[39,41,44]

ORF3b

Because of the presence of premature stop codons, ORF3b is a short protein that is 22 amino acids in length, with no homology to its SARS-CoV counterpart, which is 154 amino acids long and known to function as an interferon (IFN) antagonist. As a result of the completely different sequences, SARS-CoV-2 ORF3b was originally predicted to lack any similarity in function to SARS-CoV ORF3b. However, this novel short protein has been demonstrated to be a potent IFN antagonist that can suppress type I IFN (IFN-I) induction even more effectively than SARS-CoV ORF3b.[45] SARS-CoV-2–related viruses found in bats and pangolins encode a similar truncated ORF3b with IFN antagonist activity. The C-terminal region of SARS-CoV ORF3b contains a nuclear localization signal (NLS) that is lacking in SARS-CoV-2 ORF3b. Truncation of the C-terminus of SARS-CoV ORF3b enhances its IFN antagonist activity, suggesting that the NLS may impair its ability to block the nuclear translocation of IRF3, a transcription factor that induces IFN-β (*IFNB1*) expression.

ORF6

SARS-CoV-2 ORF6 shares only 66% sequence similarity with its counterpart in SARS-CoV, and this variation in sequence mainly occurs at the C-terminus.[46] SARS-CoV ORF6 plays a key role in antagonizing IFN signaling, and its C-terminal tail is critical for this function. Despite the differences in sequence, SARS-CoV-2 ORF6 displays an equivalent ability to antagonize IFN signaling by blocking nuclear translocation of the transcription factors IRF3, STAT1, and STAT2.[46,47] By directly interacting with NUP98-RAE1 in the nuclear pore complex by its CTD, SARS-CoV-2 ORF6 has been reported to interfere with the docking of the karyopherin/importin complex.[47] ORF6 also interacts with karyopherin α2 (*KPNA2*), presenting an alternative mechanism that could disrupt nuclear translocation of proteins involved in IFN signaling.[48]

ORF7a

Similar to its SARS-CoV ortholog, SARS-CoV-2 ORF7a is a transmembrane protein of 121 amino acids, including an immunoglobulin-like (Ig-like) ectodomain and a hydrophobic transmembrane domain. The Ig-like domain is typically found in proteins that mediate cell adhesion or protein protein binding. The Ig-like domain in SARS-CoV-2 ORF7a mediates interactions with CD14+ monocytes.[49] Although SARS-CoV-2 ORF7a is structurally similar to SARS-CoV ORF7a, the latter does not interact efficiently with CD14+ monocytes. Additionally, ORF7a plays a role in blocking type I IFN (IFN-I) signaling through inhibition of STAT2 phosphorylation, which consequently blocks nuclear translocation of STAT1.[48,50] SARS-CoV-2 ORF7a also antagonizes restriction of viral replication by bone marrow stromal antigen (BST-2), which acts as a potent inhibitor of viral egress.[51]

ORF7b

The ORF7b protein in SARS-CoV-2 is 43 amino acids long, with approximately 60% sequence similarity to SARS-CoV.[52] The protein contains a transmembrane domain with a putative leucine zipper that may promote multimerization. SARS-CoV-2 ORF7b has been shown to play a role in the attenuation of IFN-I signaling by suppressing STAT1/STAT2 phosphorylation, a step that is essential for their functional activation.[48]

ORF8

ORF8 encodes a 121–amino acid accessory protein displaying less than 20% sequence identity to its counterpart in SARS-CoV. ORF8 contains a predicted Ig domain.[53] The structure of SARS-CoV-2 ORF8 as revealed by X-ray crystallography describes a core that is similar to ORF7a, with the additional presence of two dimerization interfaces.[54] ORF8 is likely to be a secreted protein because ORF8 antibodies represent one of the major markers of SARS-CoV-2 infection.[55,56] ORF8 plays a putative role in modulating the host antiviral immune response and has been reported to downregulate major histocompatibility complex (MHC) expression.[57] ORF8 protein also directly interacts with the interleukin-17 (IL-17) receptor A (*IL17RA*) and activates signaling through the IL-17 pathway, leading to nuclear factor-kappa B (NF-κB) activation and proinflammatory cytokine secretion.[58,59]

ORF9b

ORF9b is an alternative ORF within the nucleocapsid (*N*) gene. In infected cells, SARS-CoV-2 RNA activates IFN signaling through the RIG-I-MAVS–dependent pathway. Like its ortholog in SARS-CoV, ORF9b protein localizes to the mitochondrial membrane and suppresses IFN-I signaling by blocking MAVS activation.[58,60] ORF9b additionally blocks IFN production by inhibiting NF-κB activation.[61]

ORF10

As the final ORF located at the 3′ end of the SARS-CoV-2 genome, ORF10 may code for a putative protein of 38 amino acids containing an alpha-helical region.[62] It does not share sequence similarity with known proteins from SARS-CoV. Through exogenous expression of ORF10, a study reported that the protein could interact with members of a cullin-2 RING E3 ligase complex, specifically with ZYG11B, leading to the hypothesis that ORF10 may be able to hijack the function of ubiquitin ligase complexes.[62] Another study confirmed the interaction with ZYG11B, but unearthed no evidence to indicate that ORF10 could regulate the function of the E3 ligase complex or that this interaction may have any impact on viral processes.[63] The annotation of ORF10 as an ORF in the SARS-CoV-2 genome has been called into question by studies noting the challenge of detecting subgenomic reads for its transcript, indicating that such a protein may not be produced by the virus.[64–67]

Nonstructural Proteins

ORF1ab

The original Wuhan publication lists ORF1a and ORF1b as separate genes, whereas the NCBI reference sequence (NC_045512.2) combines them under ORF1ab.[68,69] Located near the 5′ terminus, ORF1ab spans two-thirds of the genome and encodes the overlapping polyproteins pp1a and pp1ab. The pp1ab polyprotein is generated through a programmed ribosomal frameshifting event.[70] Proteolytic cleavage of the polyproteins by its gene products, the nonstructural protein 5 (Nsp5) and Nsp3 proteases, yields 11 and 15 nonstructural proteins from pp1a and pp1ab respectively (see Fig. 2.1). Nonstructural proteins play a variety of roles in the viral replication and transcription complex (RTC), including RNA synthesis, processing, and proofreading (Table 2.1).

Sequencing and Variants

Genome sequences of SARS-CoV-2 strains detected around the world have been deposited in the GISAID repository, providing a valuable resource for tracking temporal and geographic variations in sequence over the course of the pandemic.[71] The first SARS-CoV-2 sequences derived from patients in Wuhan were almost identical to each other, indicating a recent and common origin for the virus.[5,9,17,72]

In general, RNA viruses have higher mutation rates compared with DNA viruses, because RNA-dependent RNA polymerases typically lack proofreading mechanisms that limit the incorporation of mutations into the viral genome. However, coronaviruses and a few other related RNA viruses of the order Nidovirales represent an exception and demonstrate lower mutation rates compared with other RNA viruses.[73] For reference, the SARS-CoV-2 genome has been reported to accumulate mutations at a rate that is half the mutation rate of influenza and one-quarter the mutation rate of human immunodeficiency virus.[74] This difference may be attributed to the function of the Nsp14 exoribonuclease in SARS-CoV-2, a proofreading enzyme that is essential for the maintenance of viral genome integrity in coronaviruses.[75] Although mutations in the SARS-CoV-2 genome are expected to occur, most mutations are likely to be neutral or mildly deleterious, and only a minority are likely to confer any fitness advantage to the virus. Nevertheless, monitoring sequence variations in the viral genome, with a focus on mutations in proteins that may have an impact on the behavior of the virus and affect infectivity, transmissibility, pathogenicity, and antigenicity, is integral to the effort of containing the pandemic.

Deletions involving ORF7a, ORF7b, and ORF8 constituted the early emergent variants, detected in the January to February 2020 time frame.[76,77] The most common variant was a deletion of 382 nucleotides that truncated ORF7b and deleted most of ORF8, including the transcription regulatory sequence.[76] A 29-nucleotide deletion in ORF8 that was associated with reduced virulence had previously been detected in SARS-CoV strains at the mid-to-late phase of the SARS epidemic.[78] However, the impact of such deletions on infectivity and pathogenicity could not be evaluated because the SARS epidemic came to a natural end. Evaluation of the 382-nucleotide deletion variant in SARS-CoV-2 indicated that the virus retained its replicative fitness, but the deletion may have altered the immune-evasive function of ORF8, resulting in an enhanced immune response to the virus.[76] This variant was linked to milder disease severity and a reduction in the systemic release of proinflammatory cytokines.[79] Consistent with these observations, the 382-nucleotide deletion variant was not detected in patient samples beyond March 2020.[79]

Mutations emerging in the S1 subunit of the spike protein are of special interest because of the critical role of this domain in host cell receptor binding and recognition by neutralizing antibodies (Fig. 2.4). The NTD is targeted by antibodies that specifically recognize epitopes in this region; epitope binning of a large number of NTD-specific monoclonal antibodies (mAbs) revealed multiple antigenic sites.[80] However, one particular site that included residues 14-20, 140-158, and 245-264 was recognized by all known NTD-specific antibodies and aptly named an "NTD supersite." Beyond the NTD, the RBD in the S1 subunit is immunodominant and represents the primary target of neutralizing antibodies. Therefore mutations in this region can contribute to immune escape.[81] However, mutations emerging in the RBD must not be significantly damaging to hACE2 binding and virus entry into host cells. Outside of the RBD and the NTD, other mutations in the S1 subunit of spike protein may also impact SARS-CoV-2 infectivity and transmissibility.

In March 2020, a variant strain of SARS-CoV-2 that harbored a D614G (23403A > G) substitution in the S1 subunit of the spike protein spread rapidly to become the predominant strain worldwide.[82–84] By June 2020, this strain, represented by clade "G" (also called clade A2a or type VI), and its offspring "GH" and "GR," grew to become the most common clades, representing 74% to 78% of all sequenced SARS-CoV-2 genomes.[82,83] Studies functionally characterizing the D614G mutation demonstrated increased infectivity of viruses harboring this mutation when tested using both pseudotyped viruses and isogenic recombinant SARS-CoV-2.[82,85–88] Enhanced viral replication was observed in primary

Table 2.1 SARS-CoV-2 Nonstructural Proteins[a]

Protein	Function
Nsp1 (virulence factor)	Nsp1 suppresses host gene expression by blocking cellular mRNA nuclear export and shutting down translation of mRNA.[162–164]
Nsp2	In SARS-CoV, Nsp2 interacts with host cell proteins such as prohibitin 1 and prohibitin 2 and may be involved in the disruption of host cellular processes.[230,231]
Nsp3 (papain-like cysteine protease, Pl[pro])	Nsp3, the largest Nsp, is a transmembrane protein containing multiple functional domains including a Mac1 domain with mono-ADP-ribosyl hydrolase activity.[171,172] Through its protease activity, Nsp3 cleaves sites in the pp1a and pp1ab polyproteins to yield Nsps. Nsp3 can also remove ubiquitin (Ub) and the Ub-like protein modifier interferon stimulated gene 15 (ISG15) from cellular proteins. SARS-CoV-2 Nsp3 has a preference for mono-Ub and ISG15 over K48-linked and K63-liked polyUb.[169,232] SARS-CoV Nsp3 plays an important role in viral RNA replication by recruiting N protein to the RTC and promotes formation of double-membrane vesicles that house viral replication complexes.
Nsp4	Nsp4 is a transmembrane glycoprotein. Interactions of Nsp4 with Nsp3 and Nsp6 drive the formation of double-membrane vesicles for viral replication.[233]
Nsp5 (3C-like protease, 3CL[pro]; main protease, M[pro])	Nsp5, the viral chymotrypsin-like cysteine protease enzyme or main protease, performs proteolytic processing of most of the cleavage sites in the pp1a and pp1ab polyproteins to generate the component Nsps. Because of its critical role in the generation of viral Nsp proteins, Nsp5 is indispensable for virion production.[234]
Nsp6	Nsp6 is a transmembrane protein that is involved in double-membrane vesicle formation and interacts with Nsp4.[233] It also plays a role in autophagosome formation and maturation.[235,236]
Nsp7	Nsp7 forms the primase complex together with Nsp8, and acts as an accessory subunit of the RNA-dependent RNA polymerase complex. The primase complex performs de novo initiation and primer extension. Nsp7 plays a crucial role in RNA binding by the Nsp7-Nsp8-Nsp12 complex.[155,237]
Nsp8	Nsp8 possesses RNA-dependent RNA polymerase activity.[238] Nsp8 demonstrates de novo initiation and primer extension activity during RNA synthesis, and forms a complex with Nsp7. Primase activity lies in the N-terminal of Nsp8 and requires the formation of large oligomeric complexes to bring the active site residues into proximity.[237]
Nsp9	Nsp9 is a dimeric RNA-binding protein with a preference for single-stranded nucleic acids. Nsp9 is essential for replication.[239,240]
Nsp10	Nsp10 is an essential cofactor for Nsp14 and Nsp16, forming a part of the exonuclease and RNA-capping subcomplex. Nsp10 can bind to single- and double-stranded RNA and DNA.[241,242]
Nsp11	Nsp11 is a short peptide with unknown function that forms the final Nsp in the pp1a polyprotein. In pp1ab, the N-terminal sequence of Nsp11 lies between the Nsp10/11 junction and the ORF1ab frameshift site, and becomes the N-terminal part of Nsp12.[243]
Nsp12 (RdRp)	Nsp12 is the main RNA-dependent RNA polymerase (RdRp) that performs viral RNA synthesis. During viral RNA replication, RdRp forms a complex with Nsp7, Nsp8, and proteins involved in proofreading and capping.[155]
Nsp13	Nsp13 is a helicase and RNA-5′-triphosphatase. Nsp13 helicase activity is stimulated by binding to Nsp12. Nsp13 unwinds double-stranded DNA and RNA in a 5′–3′ direction, a function that is involved in genomic RNA synthesis by the polymerase complex.[242] Additionally, Nsp13 may facilitate proofreading by stimulating backtracking by the viral replication and transcription complex.[244]
Nsp14	Nsp14 is a bifunctional enzyme with 3′–5′ exoribonuclease activity and N7-guanine methyltransferase activities involved in maintaining replication fidelity and performing 5′-RNA capping respectively. It forms a part of the exonuclease and capping subcomplex, which associates with the Nsp7-Nsp8-Nsp12 polymerase complex.[155]
Nsp15	Nsp15 is a uridine-specific endoribonuclease that preferentially cleaves RNA on the 3′ side of uridines. Nsp15 may be involved in immune evasion by viral RNA processing. Polyuridine tracts at the 5′-end of negative-strand viral RNA intermediates can provoke an IFN response. Through its nuclease activity, Nsp15 may prevent activation of host antiviral sensors by regulating the length of the polyuridine tails and cleaving other sites within the viral RNA to limit the formation of double-stranded RNA (dsRNA) intermediates.[245]
Nsp16	Nsp16 is a 2′-O-methyltransferase that functions as an integral component of the RNA capping machinery. Nsp16 methylates the 5′ cap of viral RNA to mimic human mRNA and prevent viral recognition by the sensor MDA5 in the host cell. Nsp16 was shown to be indispensable for coronavirus replication in cell culture.[241]

[a]The functions of nonstructural proteins Nsp1-16 are summarized. This information is based on recently published research about their functions in SARS-CoV-2 or based on knowledge about the functions of their SARS-CoV counterparts.

ADP, Adenosine diphosphate; *IFN,* interferon; *MDA5,* melanoma differentiation–associated 5; *mRNA,* messenger ribonucleic acid; *Nsp,* nonstructural proteins; *RTC,* replication and transmission complex.

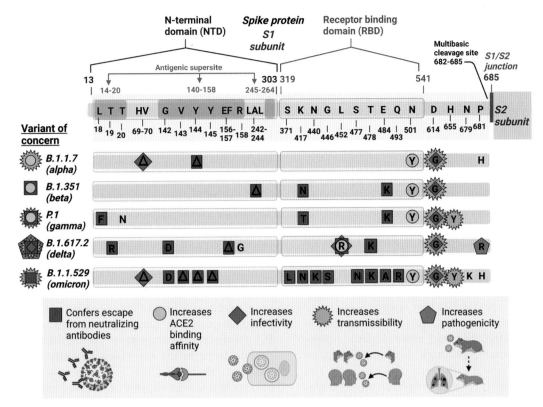

Fig. 2.4 Notable Mutations Detected in S1 Subunit of Spike Protein in Variants of Concern. As of February 2022, five SARS-CoV-2 sequence variants were designated as variants of concern (VOC). The N-terminal domain (NTD) ranging from amino acids 13-303 is the target of many neutralizing antibodies. Notable mutations in this region include deletions affecting amino acids L18-T20, H69-V70, D142G, V143-Y145, E156-F157, R158G, and L242-L244. The receptor binding domain (RBD) ranging from amino acids 319-541 is involved in angiotensin-converting enzyme-2 (ACE2) receptor binding and is also a major target of neutralizing antibodies. Mutations in this region that are found in multiple VOCs include K417N/T, T478K, E484K/A, N501Y, D614G, H655Y, and P681R/H These mutations may confer immune escape, increase ACE2 binding affinity, or increase infectivity, transmissibility, or pathogenicity. Based on the information available at present, the alpha variant possesses increased transmissibility and a slight increase in ACE2 receptor binding affinity. The beta variant demonstrates higher ACE2 binding affinity and notably increases resistance to neutralizing antibodies. The gamma variant is associated with increased transmissibility, an increase in ACE2 binding affinity that is comparable to the beta variant, and resistance to certain monoclonal antibodies but not polyclonal sera. The delta variant is associated with enhanced transmissibility, infectivity, pathogenicity, and immune escape. Early reports suggest that the omicron variant is associated with increased transmissibility and resistance to neutralizing antibodies.

human airway epithelial cells, including bronchial and nasal airway epithelial cell cultures.[21,85,86] This was consistent with reports that the D614G mutation was associated with higher viral loads in the upper respiratory tract of patients.[82,85,89] There was no indication of increased pathogenicity in animal models, which agreed with the observed lack of association of the D614G variant with altered mortality or clinical severity.[21,82,89] Hamster and ferret models are useful tools to study SARS-CoV-2 transmission because of their susceptibility to infection and the similarity of the disease developed by the animals to the pan-respiratory moderate to severe COVID-19 and upper respiratory tract–localized mild infection observed in humans, respectively.[21] In hamster and ferret models of SARS-CoV-2 infection, the D614G mutation–harboring virus demonstrated increased transmissibility.[21,86] D614G was further shown to enhance viral entry into hACE2–expressing cells.[19,87,90] At the structural level, D614G disrupted a critical inter-protomer contact and shifted S protein conformation toward the "open" or "up" ACE2 binding–competent state to promote membrane fusion with target cells.[20,87,91] Studies using pseudotyped viruses suggested that D614G could affect S protein processing and shedding or increase functional S protein incorporation into virions.[19,20,92] However, experiments performed using isogenic viruses expressing additional SARS-CoV-2 structural proteins did not corroborate these effects on S protein processing and incorporation.[85–87] Viruses that harbored the D614G mutation were as susceptible to neutralization by antibodies and perhaps even slightly more susceptible.[19,87,90]

Since the beginning of the pandemic, various SARS-CoV-2 strains have emerged in different parts of the world. As of February 2022, the World Health Organization (WHO) has categorized five strains as variants of concern—strains B.1.1.7, B.1351, P.1, B.1.617.2, and B.1.1.529.

The B.1.1.7 variant (also known as 501Y.V1; WHO label: alpha) that first emerged in the United Kingdom harbors 17 nonsynonymous mutations, including the D614G mutation and 8 additional mutations in the spike protein: ΔH69-V70, ΔY144, N501Y, A570D, P681H, T716I, S982A, and D1118H.[93] Preliminary evidence suggests that this variant may possess increased transmissibility and may be associated with an increased risk for mortality.[94–100] The only mutation localized to the RBD, N501Y, has been reported to increase hACE2 binding affinity, which likely signifies an increase in the ACE2 binding affinity of the B.1.1.7 variant over the original strain.[101,102] Although mice normally demonstrate poor susceptibility to SARS-CoV-2 infection because of suboptimal recognition of the mouse ACE2 receptor, the N501Y mutation facilitates adaptation and successful infection by SARS-CoV-2 in a mouse model; therefore N501Y may enhance cross-species transmission.[103,104] However, there is no evidence to indicate that the N501Y mutation increases infectivity of the virus in the context of hACE2–expressing cells.[105] The P681H mutation is located adjacent to the furin cleavage site (RRAR) that spans amino acids 682-685. To a limited extent, the P681H mutation enhances spike protein cleavage and fusogenic potential of the alpha variant, although this mutation alone does not increase virion infectivity in vitro.[246,248] The ΔH69-V70 deletion increases infectivity, enhances incorporation of cleaved spike protein into virions, and accelerates syncytium formation.[108,109,249] The ΔY144 deletion is located within the NTD supersite and confers resistance to NTD-specific monoclonal antibodies.[110] Overall, the B.1.1.7 variant is less sensitive to some monoclonal antibodies, but in general remains susceptible to neutralizing antibodies.[93,111] The combination of spike mutations in this variant may be associated with a modest, if any, reduction in vaccine efficacy.[111–113]

B.1.351 is a variant of concern that also harbors the N501Y mutation found in the B.1.1.7 strain. The B.1.351 variant (also known as 501Y.V2; WHO label: beta), which was first detected in South Africa, harbors eight lineage-defining mutations in the spike protein, including the D614G mutation: D80A, D215G, ΔL242-L244, K417N, E484K, N501Y, and A701V.[114] This variant shows no apparent difference in infectivity but greatly enhances immune escape by conferring resistance to neutralization by mAbs and convalescent and vaccine-elicited polyclonal sera; this observation has raised much concern in the international community.[105,115–118] Additionally, because of the combination of mutations in the RBD, the B.1.351 variant is reported to possess increased ACE2 binding affinity, higher than that of B.1.1.7.[118] Multiple studies have shown that the E484K mutation confers resistance to neutralizing antibodies.[115,119–123] In addition, deep mutational scanning in yeast indicates that E484K might slightly increase ACE2 binding affinity.[102] Mutations at K417, including K417N and K417T, occur in multiple variants of interest, and have been identified as escape mutations that can cause resistance to monoclonal neutralizing antibodies.[120,122,124]

Beyond the established effects of the RBD mutations E484K, K417N, and N501Y, the deletion of residues 243-244 also has been shown to cause resistance to NTD-specific neutralizing antibodies.[108]

The P.1 variant (also known as 501Y.V3; WHO label: gamma) which was first detected in Brazil, includes 10 new nonsynonymous mutations in the spike protein besides the D614G mutation: L18F, T20N, P26S, D138Y, R190S, K417T, E484K, N501Y, H655Y, and T1027I.[125–127] The P.1 strain shares the triplet combination of mutations found in the B.1.351 variant—K417X, E484K, and N501Y—indicating convergent molecular adaptation.[127] The H655Y mutation has been shown to enhance transmissibility in a hamster model of SARS-CoV-2 infection.[246] The L18F mutation in the antigenic supersite reduces neutralization by NTD mAbs.[110] Overall, the P.1 variant is estimated to possess higher transmissibility and demonstrates an increase in ACE2 binding affinity to an extent similar to that of B.1351. As a result of the presence of nearly identical mutations in the RBD, the P.1 strain also demonstrates a significant degree of escape from mAbs targeting the RBD, in a manner similar to that of B.1351. However, unlike B.1351, the P.1 strain does not show a substantial reduction in neutralization by polyclonal sera, suggesting that it is unlikely to affect vaccine efficacy.[128]

The B.1.617.2 variant (WHO label: delta) that was first detected in India is reported to contain multiple conserved changes in the spike protein, including the D614G mutation: T19R, T95I, G142D, ΔE156-F157, R158G, L452R, T478K, P681R, and D950N.[129] The P681R mutation has been linked to increased spike protein cleavage, enhanced spike protein fusogenicity and syncytium formation, and increased pathogenicity of the delta variant.[250,251] Analysis of sequences deposited in GISAID revealed that L452R emerged independently in various strains in the December 2020 to February 2021 time frame.[131] The L452R mutation increases ACE2 binding affinity, enhances entry into cells coexpressing ACE2 and TMPRSS2, increases pseudovirus infectivity against human airway lung organoids, and may increase viral replication.[132,133] The L452R mutation additionally confers escape from neutralization by mAbs and polyclonal human immune sera, and evades antigen recognition by human leukocyte antigen (HLA)–restricted cellular immunity.[80,122,133] The T470-T478 loop is a critical determinant of spike RBD recognition by the ACE2 receptor.[134] The T478K mutation is yet to be extensively characterized, but was found to be enriched upon exposure to weak neutralizing antibodies.[129] Another substitution mutation at the same position, T478I, confers resistance to neutralizing mAbs and polyclonal human immune sera, and the T478S mutation has been demonstrated to increase ACE2 binding.[135,136] The ΔE156-F157 and G142D mutations are located within the same NTD supersite as the ΔY144 mutation and may evade recognition by

NTD-specific antibodies.[80] In August 2021, B.1.617.2 strain became the dominant strain in the United States and in much of the world. This strain has been reported to possess increased transmissibility and establish much higher viral loads in patients, hinting at enhanced replicative potential and infectivity.[137,138] Additionally, B.1617.2 can escape neutralization by antibodies that target both RBD and non-RBD epitopes. Although the existing vaccines remain effective against B.1.617.2, their efficacy may be reduced.[139,140]

The B.1.1.529 variant (WHO label: omicron) was identified in Botswana and South Africa in November 2021. Within a few weeks, the omicron variant spread rapidly across the globe and became the predominant source of new Covid-19 cases. B.1.1.529 contains over 30 non-synonymous mutations in spike protein. It shares many mutations in spike protein with other variants of concern, including – ΔH69-70, T95I, G142D, K417N, T478K, N501Y, D614G, H655Y, and P681H; additionally, the E484A and Δ143-145 mutations are similar to previously observed mutations that confer escape from neutralizing antibodies.[253,254] B.1.1.529 also contains an insertion mutation (ins214EPE), a small deletion mutation (ΔN211), and several novel mutations – A67V, L212I, G339D, S371L, S373P, S375F, N440K, G446S, S477N, Q493R, G496S, Q498R, Y505H, T547K, N679K, N764K, D796Y, N856K, Q954H, N969K, and L981F. Many of the mutations affecting the RBD and the NTD are expected to cause resistance to neutralizing antibodies.[135,248,253,262] The omicron variant escapes neutralization by convalescent sera from patients previously infected with other SARS-CoV-2 variants and with the two-dose series of mRNA vaccines; however, booster doses are reported to reinstate protection against this variant.[255–257,259,260] Various studies have reported that the RBD of the omicron variant either possesses increased or similar ACE2 binding affinity compared to the original Wuhan strain.[253,255,258,263] Preliminary evidence suggests that the omicron variant is highly transmissible.[264] Unlike the delta variant, the omicron variant does not efficiently infect the lungs but replicates successfully in the bronchus and in the upper respiratory tract.[248,264] This may be linked to the route of host cell entry employed by the omicron variant; preliminary studies indicate that omicron uses the cathepsin-mediated endosomal route of cell entry instead of TMPRSS2-dependent membrane fusion.[248,265] Despite the presence of mutations such as P681H and H655Y which have been shown to increase S protein cleavage, the omicron variant displays reduced fusogenic potential and decreased syncytia formation compared to other variants.[246,248] In addition to its inability to effectively infect lung cells, this may contribute to the attenuation in pathogenicity reported for the omicron variant. However, further investigations are necessary to fully characterize the omicron variant. While much research has been performed to evaluate the effect of individual mutations observed in spike protein, it is important to keep in mind that the properties of a SARS-CoV-2 variant are dictated by the sum total of mutational effects on Spike protein, and additionally by mutations in other structural, accessory, and nonstructural proteins that have not yet been characterized. To end the pandemic, it is essential to continue monitoring the emergence of new variants and investigate their impact on receptor binding, host cell entry, infectivity, transmissibility, pathogenicity, escape from neutralizing antibodies, and detection by diagnostic tests.

Mechanisms of SARS-CoV-2 Pathogenesis

Receptor Binding and Entry Into Host Cells

Early studies characterizing the SARS-CoV-2 virus revealed that ACE2 is the host cell receptor exploited by the virus for cell entry.[9,141] ACE2 is an integral transmembrane protein that functions as a carboxypeptidase and plays an important role in the regulation of blood pressure.[142] The spike protein, which binds to the peptidase domain of ACE2, contains two sites that have to be cleaved to unleash the full infectivity of the virus, a process referred to as S protein "priming." The S1/S2 junction of SARS-CoV-2 contains a furin cleavage site, which is the first site to be cleaved by host cell proteases. Spike protein cleavage may be carried out in producer cells by furins or furin-like enzymes during trafficking in the secretory pathway or by cathepsins in the late endosome or endolysosome of target cells. Alternatively, cleavage may occur at the target cell surface before viral entry, by transmembrane serine proteases such as TMPRSS2. After S1/S2 cleavage, a second cleavage site becomes exposed, the S2′ site. Cleavage at this site is necessary for liberating the S2 fusion peptide and initiating viral membrane fusion with the host cell membrane.

The furin cleavage site is reported to be an important determinant of viral transmission in ferret models of SARS-CoV-2 infection.[25] Using lentiviral pseudotypes and a cell culture–adapted SARS-CoV-2 virus with an S1/S2 deletion, the polybasic furin cleavage site has been shown to confer a selective advantage to SARS-CoV-2 in lung cells and primary human airway epithelial cells. This selective advantage depends on the expression of the cell surface protease TMPRSS2, which has been demonstrated to be essential for SARS-CoV-2 S protein priming and viral entry into lung cells.[141,143,144]

The presence of the polybasic cleavage site in the spike protein provides a unique advantage to SARS-CoV-2 by increasing susceptibility to furin-mediated cleavage in the producer cells.[145] The resulting virions with pre-cleaved spike proteins demonstrate enhanced entry into TMPRSS2-expressing cells in the human airway and lungs. Furin-dependent cleavage of the poly-basic site potentiates the infectivity of the virions by promoting the processing of spike in the producer cell and making the S2′ cleavage site accessible to TMPRSS2 at the receiver cell surface. TMPRSS2 cleaves the spike protein at S2′ and promotes early entry at or in the vicinity of the cell surface, rather than late entry through the endosome, which is characteristic of cathepsin-dependent cleavage.[25] By reducing reliance on low pH–dependent and cathepsin-mediated cleavage in the late endosomes, the polybasic furin cleavage site confers escape from restriction by innate immune antiviral proteins belonging to the IFN-induced transmembrane protein family (IFITM), which localize to the late endosomes and prevent the entry of double-enveloped viruses.[25,146] Alteration of the furin cleavage site ablates processing by furin and promotes the incorporation of uncleaved spike protein into virions.[24,143] Loss of this site is associated with a reduced replication rate and attenuated infection in both hamster and K18-hACE2 transgenic mouse models of SARS-CoV-2 pathogenesis.[143,147] Additionally, mutation of the SARS-CoV-2 furin cleavage site eliminates cell–cell fusion, which is a mechanism by which viruses can spread from infected cells to neighboring cells.[143] This is mediated by spike protein from newly formed virions which are released to the cell surface. At the surface, spike protein binds ACE2 to promote fusion with neighboring cells, a phenomenon that is characterized by the formation of large multinucleate cells or syncytia.[261] TMPRSS2 enhances virion infectivity by increasing syncytia formation. Unlike the effect observed with loss of the cleavage site, loss of furin alone does not eliminate cell–cell fusion or infectivity if TMPRSS2 is expressed by the acceptor cell.[148] Therefore, although the polybasic cleavage site is essential for both infectivity and fusogenic activity, cleavage at this site is not exclusively mediated by furin.

The proprotein convertase furin is a type I transmembrane protein that is widely expressed in various cells and tissues. Furin is ubiquitously expressed; thus the expression levels and distribution of ACE2 and TMPRSS2 across various tissues and organs is the factor that likely dictates SARS-CoV-2 organotropism. In general, ACE2 is expressed at lower levels compared with TMPRSS2, but ACE2 and TMPRSS2 are detected in both the nasal and bronchial epithelium. ACE2 is expressed in multiple epithelial cell types throughout the airway, including alveolar epithelial type II (AT2) cells, which play a central role in SARS-CoV-2 pathogenesis.[149,150] TMPRSS2 presents a broader distribution and higher expression across various tissue types, suggesting that ACE2 expression may be the limiting factor for initial SARS-CoV-2 infection and tropism. TMPRSS2 is expressed only in a subset of cells expressing ACE2, indicating that the virus may use cathepsins or other proteases for S protein priming in certain cell types. ACE2+, TMPRSS2+ cells in the nasal and airway passages are mostly secretory

goblet and multiciliated cells, whereas those in the lungs are AT2 cells.[149,151]

Replication and Assembly

Upon membrane fusion or endocytic entry, viral genomic RNA is released by uncoating and translated by the host cell protein translation machinery. The polyproteins pp1a and pp1ab are proteolytically cleaved by their own component proteins Nsp3 (PL^{pro}) and Nsp5 (3CL^{pro}, main protease) to generate the full series of viral nonstructural proteins (Nsp1-16). Most of the Nsps are involved in the formation of the viral RTC and function to create a cellular environment that is conducive for viral RNA synthesis, virion assembly, and infection.

Positive-sense viral genomic RNA is used as a template to generate full-length negative-sense copies for replication, and subgenomic negative-sense RNAs to produce the nested set of subgenomic mRNAs (sgmRNAs).[65,152] The cytosol of coronavirus-infected cells, such as those infected with SARS-CoV-2, contain a high density of double-membrane vesicles derived from the ER. These double-membrane vesicles constitute the sites of viral genomic RNA replication and subgenomic mRNA transcription, providing a protective and resource-rich environment away from disruptive host cell factors, with dsRNA replication intermediates segregated in the interior.[33,153] The viral nonstructural proteins Nsp3, Nsp4, and Nsp6 are implicated in the formation of double-membrane vesicles and in anchoring of the RTC to the vesicular membrane.[154] The RTC includes multiple viral nonstructural proteins, with the core polymerase complex formed by Nsp12, Nsp7, and Nsp8.

Nsp12, the main RdRp, possesses low RNA polymerization activity on its own. However, the primase complex proteins Nsp7 and Nsp8 greatly stimulate its catalytic activity by promoting RNA binding.[155] The SARS-CoV-2 core polymerase complex is formed by the Nsp12 subunit bound to an Nsp7-Nsp8 heterodimer, with an additional Nsp8 subunit bound at a different site.[156–159] Nsp12 extensively interacts with RNA through the phosphate-ribose backbone, implying sequence-independent binding. The holoenzyme for viral replication includes other Nsp proteins to incorporate proofreading and capping functions, such as the Nsp13 RNA 5′-triphosphatase with helicase activity, and the Nsp10-Nsp14-Nsp16 exonuclease and capping subcomplex.

Double-membrane vesicles housing the RTC contain membrane-spanning molecular complexes formed by Nsp3 that connect the interior of the vesicle with the cytosol.[160] These pores are expected to act as a conduit for the exit of viral sgmRNA and genomic RNA products to sites of translation and encapsidation by N protein, respectively. N protein is translated in the cytoplasm and encapsidates nascent genomic RNA to form the nucleocapsid. Viral structural proteins (S, E, and M) are

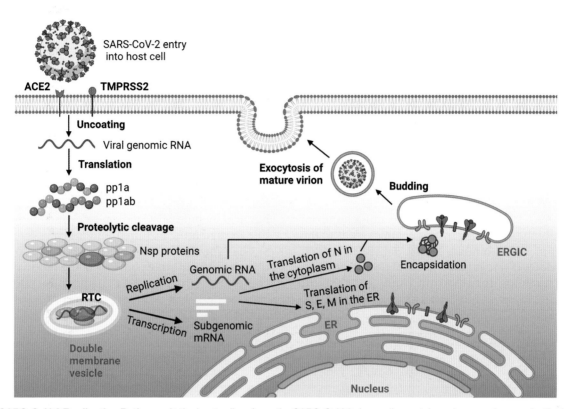

Fig. 2.5 SARS-CoV-2 Replication Pathway. At the host cell surface, the SARS-CoV-2 virus spike protein undergoes cleavage by the transmembrane protease TMPRSS2 and engages the angiotensin-converting enzyme-2 (ACE2) receptor. After cell entry, uncoating releases the viral genomic RNA. Translation of ORF1ab generates polyproteins pp1a and pp1ab through a ribosomal frameshifting event. These polyproteins are subsequently cleaved by their own gene products, the proteases nonstructural protein-5 (Nsp5) and Nsp3, to yield 16 SARS-CoV-2 Nsps. The cytosol of cells infected by SARS-CoV-2 harbor high densities of double-membrane vesicles derived from the endoplasmic reticulum (ER). These double-membrane vesicles house the viral replication and transcription complex (RTC), which consists of at least Nsp12 (RNA-dependent RNA polymerase [RdRp]), Nsp7, and Nsp8, which make up the minimal polymerase unit, but likely also includes other Nsps responsible for proofreading and processing. Viral subgenomic mRNAs for spike (S), envelope (E), and membrane (M) are translated in the ER and the proteins are trafficked to the ER-Golgi intermediate compartment (ERGIC). The subgenomic mRNA for Nucleocapsid (N) is translated in the cytosol. The newly synthesized viral genomic RNA interacts with the N protein and undergoes encapsidation to form the viral nucleocapsid. In the endoplasmic reticulum–Golgi intermediate compartment (ERGIC), virion assembly involves interaction of the S, E, and M proteins with the nucleocapsid, followed by budding into smooth-walled vesicles, which subsequently transport the virions to the cell surface and release them outside the cell through exocytosis.

translated in the ER and transported to the ERGIC, the main site of coronavirus assembly. Interaction with encapsidated genomic RNA in the ERGIC induces budding into the lumen of secretory vesicles, which ultimately fuse with the plasma membrane, releasing the virions from the infected cell by exocytosis.[161] The viral replication process is illustrated in Fig. 2.5.

Disruption of Host Cellular Processes and Defenses

Coronaviruses hijack the host cell machinery and resources to produce viral proteins and replicate. To do this, CoVs must first block protein synthesis of host cellular mRNA.

Nsp1, the "host shutoff factor," which plays a multifaceted role in the suppression of host protein synthesis by coronaviruses, undergoes rapid proteolytic release from the polyprotein. SARS-CoV-2 Nsp1 inhibits the nuclear export of cellular mRNAs by interacting with the host mRNA export receptor heterodimer NXF1-NXT1.[162] Through its C-terminal, Nsp1 binds to the 40S ribosomal subunit and occludes the mRNA entry tunnel, thereby suppressing host cellular mRNA translation.[163–165] Beyond Nsp1, Nsp8 and Nsp9 bind to the signal recognition particle to disrupt host cell protein trafficking, whereas Nsp16 binds to the mRNA recognition domains of U1 and U2 splicing RNAs and affects mRNA splicing at a global level.[166] By disrupting the production of host proteins, including those involved in IFN-I signaling, these nonstructural proteins blunt the host cell innate immune response and antiviral defense mechanisms.

IFN-I and IFN-III induction upon SARS-CoV-2 infection plays a critical role in the innate defense mechanism by limiting viral replication.[167] Type I IFNs (IFN-α and IFN-β) are widely expressed, whereas type III IFN (IFN-λ) responses are mainly restricted to mucosal surfaces. SARS-CoV-2 viral replication has been reported to induce a delayed IFN response in lung epithelial cells. Pathogen-associated molecular patterns (PAMPs), including dsRNA intermediates produced during viral replication, can be recognized by pattern recognition receptors (PRRs) such as retinoic acid–inducible gene I (RIG-I), melanoma differentiation–associated 5 (MDA5), and Toll-like receptor 3 (TLR3). In SARS-CoV-2–infected lung epithelial cells, MDA5 and laboratory of genetics and physiology 2 (LGP2) protein were primarily involved in the IFN response, with MDA5 acting as the main viral dsRNA sensor.[167] MDA5 triggers formation of the mitochondrial antiviral-signaling protein (MAVS) signaling complex consisting of proteins MAVS-TRAF3-TRAF6-TOM70 on the mitochondrial outer membrane. Signaling by this complex leads to the activation of TANK-binding kinase 1 (TBK1), which phosphorylates IFN regulatory factor 3 (IRF3), promoting its nuclear localization and subsequent

transcriptional activation of IFN-β. IRF3, IRF5, and NF-κB drive IFN-β and IFN-λ induction in lung epithelial cells infected with SARS-CoV-2.[167] Secreted IFN-β and IFN-λ bind to and activate their respective receptors on infected cells and neighboring cells, which leads to phosphorylation and heterodimerization of STAT1-STAT2.[168] The STAT1-STAT2 heterodimer recruits IRF9 to form ISGF3, which then translocates to the nucleus. ISGF3 binds to IFN-stimulated response elements (ISRE) in the promoters of hundreds of genes with antiviral functions, called IFN-stimulated genes (ISGs) =, and induces their expression. Proteins encoded by ISGs not only induce strong antiviral innate immune responses but also include MHC molecules, which play a critical role in regulating acquired immunity.

The type II interferon, IFN-γ, signals through a distinct pathway in which binding of the IFN to its receptor complex induces STAT1 phosphorylation and

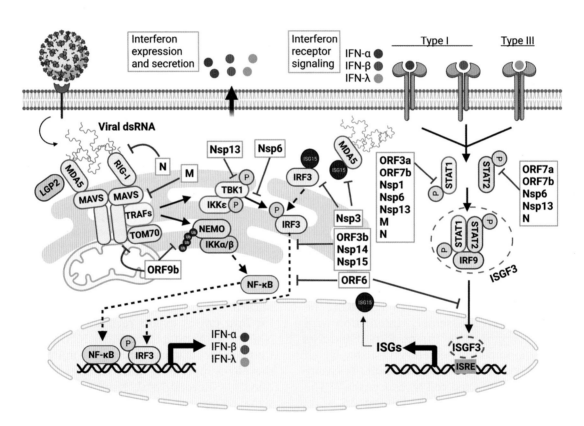

Fig. 2.6 Antagonism of Interferon Signaling by SARS-CoV-2 Proteins. Retinoic acid–inducible gene I (RIG-I) and melanoma differentiation–associated 5 (MDA5) are pattern recognition receptors that are activated on recognition of viral dsRNA in the cytoplasm of infected cells. This prompts oligomerization of RIG-I or MDA5 and promotes its association with the adaptor protein mitochondrial antiviral signaling protein (MAVS) through their respective caspase activation and recruitment domain (CARD) domains. LGP2 is a viral RNA sensor that lacks a CARD domain and therefore lacks the ability to activate downstream signaling, but it is known to potentiate signaling downstream of MDA5 by promoting MDA5-RNA interactions. The interaction between RIG-I/MDA5 and MAVS induces the formation of signaling complexes that include TOM70, TRAF3/6, and other signaling molecules. Activation of IKKε/TBK1 and IKKα/IKKβ/NEMO result in the activation of interferon regulating factor-3 (IRF3) and nuclear factor-kappa B (NF-κB), respectively, which translocate to the nucleus and transcriptionally activate the production of type I (IFN-α, β) and type III (IFN-λ) interferons, which are then secreted by the infected cell. The secreted IFN ligands bind to and activate their cognate receptor complexes on the surfaces of the infected cells and neighboring noninfected cells. This subsequently results in the phosphorylation and activation of STAT1 and STAT2, which heterodimerize and bind to the transcription factor IRF9 to form a complex called ISGF3. This complex translocates to the nucleus, where it binds to response elements (ISRE) in the promoters of IFN stimulated genes (ISG) and activates their transcription. SARS-CoV-2 proteins antagonize IFN signaling at various stages, resulting in the blockade of IFN production and suppression of ISG expression. Additionally, Nsp3 may actively remove ISG15 from proteins like MDA5 and IRF3 to attenuate IFN signaling.

homodimerization to produce the IFN-g activated factor (GAF). GAF translocates to the nucleus and activates genes that contain gamma-activated sequence (GAS) promoter elements. Through these different types of IFNs, STAT1 can activate different sets of ISGs.[168] Importantly, the genes activated by the STAT1-STAT2 heterodimer regulate the innate immune response on viral RNA sensing, whereas the genes activated by the STAT1 homodimer induce proinflammatory responses and promote macrophage activation.

Coronaviruses have evolved complex mechanisms to escape viral recognition and suppress the IFN response. In addition to forming double-membrane vesicles to shield dsRNA intermediates that can be recognized by cytosolic PRRs, viral mRNA is "capped" by Nsp14 and Nsp16 and modified by Nsp15 to prevent recognition by PRRs. Capping of viral RNA at the 5′ end consists of an N-methylated guanosine triphosphate and a C2′-O-methyl-ribosyladenine and serves to disguise viral RNA to resemble human mRNA. It also ensures efficient translation by the cellular machinery and stabilizes the RNA.

The de-ISGylation and de–adenosine diphosphate (ADP)–ribosylation activities of Nsp3 play a role in the evasion of innate immunity. ISGylation is a posttranslational modification similar to ubiquitination in which ISG15, a small protein that is highly induced by IFN-I, is conjugated to target proteins and modulates their functions. Interestingly, SARS-CoV-2 Nsp3 preferentially cleaves ISG15, whereas its SARS-CoV counterpart preferentially cleaves polyubiquitin chains.[169] MDA5-mediated viral RNA sensing depends on the ISGylation of its caspase activation and recruitment domain (CARD), which promotes its oligomerization. By actively performing de-ISGylation, Nsp3 antagonizes MDA5 activation.[170] Additionally, Nsp3 cleaves ISG15 from IRF3, which leads to decreased phosphorylation and reduced nuclear translocation of IRF3.[169] By mimicking host cell sensing of viral nucleic acids through treatment with poly(I:C) which normally induces IFN-β expression, expression of SARS-CoV-2 Nsp3 was observed to decrease the activation of the *IFNB1* promoter more effectively compared with SARS-CoV Nsp3. SARS-CoV-2 Nsp3 also contains a Mac1 domain, which can remove mono-ADP ribose modifications generated by PARP14 on host cell protein substrates.[171,172] These modifications are involved in the IFN response, and their removal alters STAT1 regulation and hinders IFN production.[173] Mutation of the Mac1 domain in SARS-CoV Nsp3 induced IFN production and resulted in attenuated infection in a mouse model.[174] Therefore, through these different mechanisms, SARS-CoV-2 Nsp3 is expected to play a key role in attenuating the IFN-I response.

Several other SARS-CoV-2 proteins also antagonize IFN signaling at various levels by inhibiting IRF3 nuclear translocation, by blocking STAT1/STAT2 phosphorylation and nuclear translocation and by suppressing ISG transcription (Fig. 2.6). Nsp13 binds to and blocks TBK1 phosphorylation, and Nsp6 binds to TBK1 and inhibits IRF3 phosphorylation.[48] ORF6 inhibits both STAT1 and IRF3 nuclear translocation, whereas ORF3b, Nsp14, and Nsp15 block IRF3 nuclear translocation.[45,46,175] Nsp6, Nsp13, and ORF7b suppress STAT1/STAT2 phosphorylation. Nsp1, ORF3a, and M protein inhibit STAT1 phosphorylation, whereas ORF7a inhibits STAT2 phosphorylation. SARS-CoV-2 N protein can suppress IFN-b induction by two mechanisms: by interacting directly with RIG-I through its DExD/H-box helicase domain, which is responsible for viral RNA sensing, and by binding and inhibiting STAT1/STAT2 phosphorylation and nuclear translocation.[176,177] ORF9b protein localizes to the mitochondrial membrane to suppress IFN-I signaling by associating with the substrate-binding site of TOM70, which is involved in the activation of MAVS.[58,60] Additionally, during SARS-CoV-2 infection in primary human pulmonary alveolar epithelial cells, ORF9b has been shown to accumulate and antagonize IFN signaling by interrupting the K63-linked polyubiquitination of NF-κB essential modulator (NEMO) protein, consequently inhibiting canonical IKKα/β-NEMO-NF-κB signaling and blocking IFN production.[61] SARS-CoV-2 M protein functions as an IFN antagonist by directly interacting with MAVS and preventing the formation of the RIG-I/MDA5-MAVS-TRAF3-TBK1 signaling complexes.[178,179]

In addition to the IFN response, human cells have evolved mechanisms to clear pathogens through autophagy and lysosomal destruction. Late endosome-localized SARS-CoV-2 ORF3a facilitates the evasion of this host cell defense mechanism by inhibiting the fusion of autophagosomes with lysosomes. It performs this function by directly interacting with and sequestering the HOPS complex protein VPS39, thereby preventing the assembly of the STX17-SNAP29-VAMP8 SNARE complex.[42,43] ORF3a expression also impairs lysosome function.

The BST-2 is an inhibitory ISG that has been shown to restrict the release of many viruses that undergo budding either at the ERGIC or at the plasma membrane. It performs this function by tethering the virions to the intracellular membrane or cell surface. BST-2 has been reported to antagonize late-stage SARS-CoV-2 viral replication and egress, as evidenced by a decrease in the release of viral-like particles in the presence of BST-2. However, SARS-CoV-2 ORF7a directly interacts with BST-2 in the perinuclear region and antagonizes its restrictive function.[51]

Through these various mechanisms, SARS-CoV-2 proteins evade host cell defenses and disrupt cellular processes to carry out viral replication and propagate.

Cell Death, Inflammation, and Immune Response

The host's ability to mount an effective and timely innate immune response is crucial for blockade of viral replication and determines the clinical outcome of viral infection. In the absence of a successful innate immune response, the virus can replicate to high titers and provoke an excessive proinflammatory reaction. A cytokine storm is marked by heightened production of proinflammatory cytokines and immune cell hyperactivation, which can lead to extensive organ damage.[180] Acute respiratory distress syndrome (ARDS), which is observed in severe cases of COVID-19, may be driven by a cytokine storm.[181,182]

Studies on SARS-CoV-2 differ in their conclusion regarding the timing, extent, and duration of the IFN-I response elicited by infection, with many studies reporting delayed and impaired IFN-I and IFN-III responses, as detected by low levels of IFN-α, IFN-β, and IFN-λ in the serum of patients with severe or critical COVID-19. This is associated with increased viral loads and high amounts of chemokines and proinflammatory cytokines.[183–186] Reportedly, IFN responses were induced in some critically ill patients at a late stage, whereas proinflammatory cytokines such as tumor necrosis factor (TNF), IL-6, and IL-8 were persistently produced at an early stage during infection and preceded the IFN response.[185]

However, other studies indicate that the IFN-I response is intact in COVID-19 patients. Single-cell RNA sequencing in patients with severe COVID-19 has shown that the IFN-I response occurs along with TNF-induced and IL-1β–induced inflammation in peripheral blood mononuclear cells (PBMCs), suggesting that the increased inflammation that is observed early on in severe disease may be driven by IFN-I signaling.[187] This observation has been corroborated using cell culture and ferret models of SARS-CoV-2 infection.[184] In a mouse model of SARS-CoV-2 infection, IFN-I signaling induced ISG expression and recruitment of proinflammatory cells in the lung, but did not restrain viral replication, suggesting that even when IFN-I signaling is activated, it may not effectively suppress SARS-CoV-2 viral replication.[188] In this study, the authors observed an acute inflammatory immune response marked by the infiltration of monocytes, macrophages, neutrophils, activated T cells (CD4+ and CD8+), and natural killer (NK) cells. Likewise, high levels of proinflammatory monocyte-derived macrophages have been observed in the bronchoalveolar lavage fluid of patients with severe COVID-19, in contrast to healthy individuals and patients with mild disease.[189] In a hamster model of SARS-CoV-2 infection, IFN signaling by STAT2 activation controlled viral dissemination but elicited strong inflammatory responses in the lungs with neutrophil infiltration and edema, leading to lung damage. Hamsters with STAT2 ablation (STAT2–/–) were observed

to develop less pronounced lung pathological conditions, supporting the hypothesis that IFN signaling may be partially responsible for the hyperinflammatory response in patients with severe disease.[190]

Severe cases of COVID-19 are not just associated with higher serum levels of proinflammatory cytokines and chemokines, but analyses of postmortem lung tissues in fatal cases have also detected extensive lung damage.[191,192] The NLRP3 (NOD-, LRR- and pyrin domain-containing protein 3) inflammasome is a protein complex that is important for the antiviral response. Inflammasome sensors such as NLRP3 can recognize PAMPs and cellular damage on viral infection, leading to the cleavage and activation of caspase-1, IL-1β, and IL-18. However, hyperactivation of the inflammasome can cause pathological injury to organs. In a mouse model of SARS-CoV infection, ion channel activity of the E protein was shown to promote inflammasome activation; inflammasome-derived IL-1β, in addition to TNF and IL-6, induced a phenotype resembling ARDS, with extensive lung damage and edema, ultimately resulting in a fatal outcome.[193] In patients with moderate and severe COVID-19, activated NLRP3 inflammasomes were detected in PBMCs and in tissues from fatal cases.[191] Higher levels of IL-18 and Casp1p20 (active caspase-1) in the serum of patients were linked to disease severity and poor outcomes.

Although cell death is an important mechanism for clearing pathogens, inflammatory cell death can also result in severe inflammation and organ damage. Pyroptosis is a form of inflammatory cell death induced by inflammasome hyperactivation.[187] It is caused by gasdermin-mediated pore formation in the plasma membrane, which leads to cellular swelling and lysis (Fig. 2.7). Gasdermins are strategically expressed by immune cells and epithelial cells at mucosal and skin barriers. The release of IL-1β and IL-18 on pyroptosis recruits immune cells to the site of infection to facilitate pathogen clearance. SARS-CoV-2 has been reported to induce pyroptosis in the monocytes and macrophages of COVID-19 patients.[44,194] In patients with severe COVID-19, lung tissues displayed infiltration of monocytes, neutrophils, and plasma cells, with infiltrating proinflammatory macrophages demonstrating high expression of IL-1β, IL-18, and IL-6. SARS-CoV-2 ORF7a may contribute to the recruitment of monocytes to infected lungs. The Ig-like domain in SARS-CoV-2 ORF7a strongly interacts with CD14+ monocytes in peripheral blood and acts as an immunomodulatory factor that triggers an inflammatory response.[49]

Infiltrating macrophages in the lung tissue of COVID-19 patients also display characteristics of edema, which is associated with pyroptosis. SARS-CoV-2 ORF3a protein may play a role in macrophage pyroptosis and promote the cytokine storm by stimulating the expression of IL-1β, IL-18, and IL-6, and activating the NLRP3 inflammasome.[41,44] SARS-CoV ORF3a protein has also

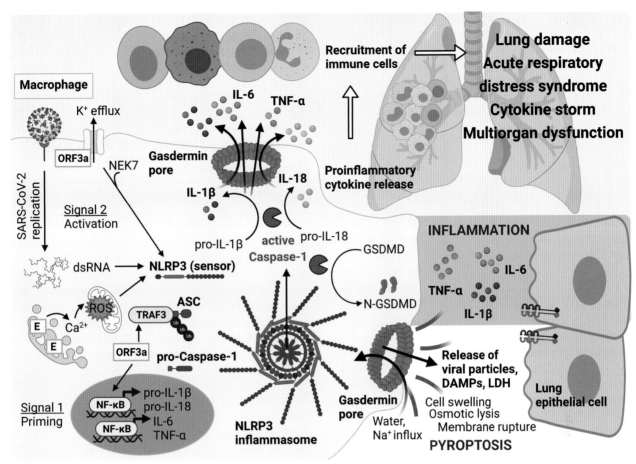

Fig. 2.7 SARS-CoV-2–Induced Pyroptotic Cell Death of Macrophages and the Impact of Hyperinflammation and Immune Cell Recruitment. SARS-CoV-2 infection has been linked to an inflammatory form of cell death called pyroptosis in pulmonary macrophages derived from infiltrating inflammatory monocytes. The NLRP3 inflammasome is a large supramolecular complex composed of a sensor (NLRP3), adaptor (ASC), and effector (pro-Caspase-1). NLRP3 inflammasome activation typically requires two signals: a priming signal and an activation signal. The priming signal leads to the transcriptional upregulation of inflammasome components and induces posttranslational modifications of NLRP3 that regulate its activation. The SARS-CoV-2 viroporin ORF3a may play a role in the priming step and additionally induce the expression of other cytokines such as interleukin-6 *(IL-6)* through nuclear factor-kappa B (NF-κB) activation. The second signal is activation of the NLRP3 sensor, which can be mediated by various stimuli such as sensing of viral dsRNA or K⁺ efflux from the cell. SARS-CoV-2 ORF3a may induce K⁺ efflux by acting as an ion channel in the plasma membrane, which results in NEK7-NLRP3 association and activation of the NLRP3 inflammasome. SARS-CoV E protein is known to act as an ion channel in the endoplasmic reticulum (ER)/Golgi membrane and promote Ca²⁺ leakage into the cytoplasm, which causes mitochondrial damage and results in the production of reactive oxygen species (ROS) and release of oxidized mtDNA, both of which can act as a second signal for inflammasome activation. Once NLRP3 is activated, it passes on this signal to ASC, which oligomerizes and associates with pro-caspase-1 through its caspase activation and recruitment domain (CARD) domain, promoting the formation of the NLRP3 inflammasome. By bringing multiple pro-caspase-1 molecules in close proximity to each other, ASC promotes autoproteolysis of pro-caspase-1 to produce active Caspase-1. SARS-CoV ORF3a promotes K63-linked polyubiquitination of ASC by TRAF3, which also promotes inflammasome formation. Active caspase-1 promotes pyroptosis by cleaving the inactive precursors pro-IL1β and pro-IL-18 to generate active IL-1β and IL-18. Additionally, caspase-1 processes gasdermin-D (GSDMD) to release the N-terminal fragments (N-GSDMD) that form the characteristic gasdermin pore in the cell membrane—the final step in the execution of pyroptosis. IL-1β and IL-18 are secreted through these pores; Na⁺ and water influx through the pores causes cell swelling, membrane rupture and lysis, releasing the contents of the cell, including DAMPs such as adenosine triphosphate (ATP), viral RNA, viral particles, and lactate dehydrogenase (LDH) which serves as a marker of cell damage and death. Pyroptotic macrophages may secrete proinflammatory cytokines such as IL-6 and tumor necrosis factor (TNF-α). The release of cytokines and cellular contents attract more immune cells to the site of infection, resulting in a hyperinflammatory milieu that induces further damage to lung cells, precipitating acute respiratory distress syndrome. In the process, proinflammatory cytokines and viral particles are released into circulation, which can lead to the proliferation of the inflammatory response with systemic effects on other organs, eventually causing multiorgan dysfunction.

been reported to activate the inflammasome through two mechanisms: by inducing K63-linked ubiquitination of apoptosis-associated speck-like protein containing a CARD (ASC) by TRAF3 and by promoting K⁺ efflux from the cell. Interestingly, the SARS-CoV-2 ORF3a protein can also induce apoptotic cell death through the extrinsic pathway, which depends on caspase-8 cleavage and activation.[39] Under certain conditions, initiators and mediators of apoptosis, such as caspase-8 and caspase-3, have been reported to induce a lytic form of cell death.[195] SARS-CoV-2 infection activates caspase-8, resulting in cell apoptosis and the secretion of inflammatory cytokines through the necroptosis pathway in lung epithelial cells.[196] These hallmarks were also observed in an hACE2–transgenic mouse model of SARS-CoV-2 infection. Additionally, analysis of lung sections from patients with fatal COVID-19 revealed apoptosis, necroptosis, necrotic cell debris, inflammatory cell infiltration, and pulmonary interstitial fibrosis, which is a marker of immune pathogenesis. Through caspase-8 activation, SARS-CoV-2 not only induced cell death but also triggered massive inflammatory responses contributing to the lung damage observed in COVID-19 patients with critical disease.

Recognition of PAMPs by PRRs, in combination with inflammatory cytokine signaling, can induce a process called PANoptosis, a unique form of inflammatory cell death. This process is regulated by the PANoptosome, which provides a combined platform for the induction of inflammasome-mediated pyroptosis, apoptosis, and necrosis.[195,197] Among all the cytokines that are released by cells during SARS-CoV-2 infection, a study tied TNF-α and IFN-γ specifically to caspase-8/FADD–mediated PANoptosis, driving a cytokine storm similar to that observed with severe COVID-19 disease and sepsis.[198] Mice treated with a combination of TNF-α and IFN-γ demonstrated signs of cytokine shock with extensive inflammation and lung damage. On SARS-CoV-2 infection, neutralizing antibodies against TNF-α and IFN-γ, or PANoptosis inhibitors, were able to protect the mice from mortality.

Interestingly, SARS-CoV-2 ORF8 has been reported to downregulate MHC-I in host cells.[57] In ORF8-expressing cells, MHC-I molecules are selectively targeted for lysosomal degradation by an autophagy-dependent mechanism. As a result, cytotoxic T lymphocytes do not efficiently eliminate ORF8-expressing cells.

Because ACE2 and TMPRSS2 are expressed in multiple organs other than the lungs, it is unclear if SARS-CoV-2 causes extensive organ damage as a result of direct infection of cells, or if this damage is inflicted by the dysregulated immune response and hyperinflammatory response. Based on the current knowledge, it seems that both mechanisms may contribute to the multiorgan dysfunction observed with SARS-CoV-2 infection, although the dysregulated immune and hyperinflammatory responses likely induce more systemic effects throughout the human body. It must be noted that some studies disagree with the universal relevance of cytokine storms to severe COVID-19 infections, based on the observation that only a subset of severe COVID-19 cases are reported to manifest with the features of cytokine storm and that levels of inflammatory cytokines detected in the circulation of most patients with severe COVID-19 are lower than the levels observed with influenza infection or ARDS.[199,200] It is possible that there are other mechanisms that significantly contribute to the devastating effects of SARS-CoV-2 infection in the other severe cases. SARS-CoV-2 may affect the normal physiological function of ACE2 by binding to it, promoting its internalization from the cell surface and downregulating its expression, which could have far-reaching consequences because ACE2

plays an important role in counterbalancing the vasoconstrictive, procoagulant, and proinflammatory effects of ACE-induced angiotensin II.[201–203] Further investigations are necessary to pinpoint the common underlying factors in severe cases of COVID-19 that distinguish them from mild infections.

Testing for Present and Past Infection

Diagnostic Tests

Many of the symptoms associated with COVID-19 overlap with symptoms caused by other respiratory pathogens. To confirm infection by SARS-CoV-2, the presence of viral nucleic acids or antigens matching the virus must be detected using molecular biology techniques. An alternative method is to detect the presence of antibodies against viral proteins. However, thus far, the specificity and sensitivity of antibody tests are not considered ideal for diagnostic purposes. Here, we outline the most commonly used techniques for determination of present and past infection by SARS-CoV-2.

Polymerase Chain Reaction–based Tests

Because of their high specificity and sensitivity, nucleic acid amplification tests (NAATs) based on real-time reverse transcription quantitative polymerase chain reaction (RT-qPCR) are the gold-standard tests for detecting SARS-CoV-2 infection. For initial diagnostic testing, the Centers for Disease Control and Prevention (CDC) recommends collecting an upper respiratory tract sample from the patient; however, under certain conditions, lower respiratory tract samples such as sputum, bronchoalveolar lavage fluid, or tracheal aspirates also may be used.[204] Nasopharyngeal or oropharyngeal specimens are collected using sterile swabs, typically within a week after the patient has started exhibiting symptoms, when high viral loads are present in the upper respiratory tract.[205,206] After collecting the specimen, which contains cells infected with the virus and free viral particles, the first step is to perform RNA extraction. Next, purified viral RNA is converted to complementary DNA (cDNA) in a reverse transcription (RT) reaction. The cDNA is then amplified by Taq polymerase in a quantitative and fluorescence-based PCR reaction using primers that are specific to regions of the SARS-CoV-2 viral genome.[207] The number of replication cycles required to generate a fluorescent signal are denoted by the cycle threshold (Ct) value. A lower Ct value is representative of higher viral loads, with a Ct value less than 40 reported as a positive test result.[205] Primers from RT-PCR kits developed by various clinical laboratories and diagnostic companies may differ with respect to the regions in the SARS-CoV-2 genome that they target. To avoid false negatives, primers should target sequences that display minimal variability across strains, focusing on regions that are less likely to undergo mutation. The most common targets for SARS-CoV-2 detection are sequences within N, Nsp12 (ORF1ab), E, and S. From sample collection to receiving the final results, the total turnaround time for diagnostic RT-qPCR tests may vary, ranging from a few hours to a few days. This presents the most significant disadvantage of relying on RT-qPCR tests for early detection and ensuring that infected individuals do not come into contact with others before the test results become available. More recently, saliva-based RT-qPCR tests for SARS-CoV-2 detection have also become available. Although the performance of such tests must be confirmed in larger studies, preliminary reports have demonstrated sensitivity and specificity comparable to nasopharyngeal swab nucleic acid amplification tests, making them a convenient option for tests allowing at-home sample collection.[208,209]

Antigen Tests

As the name indicates, rapid antigen tests have the advantage of generating faster results, facilitating point-of-care testing. However, they are not as sensitive as RT-qPCR tests. Antigen tests are immunoassays that evaluate the presence of a specific SARS-CoV-2 viral antigen in patient samples, using lateral flow or enzyme-linked immunosorbent assay (ELISA). If using nasopharyngeal swabs, specimens are immersed in buffer to extract the viral proteins and then applied to the device, which contains immobilized antibodies against the viral antigen. Saliva-based antigen tests are also available. If the viral antigen is present in the patient sample, a visually detectable signal is produced, typically in under 30 minutes.[207] A positive result indicates current infection. The viral antigens detected in these tests are expressed only when the virus is in its active replicative state, and therefore the antigen test must be done during the early acute phase of infection, when the viral load is high in the respiratory tract. The N protein is the most frequently used target for antigen testing, although studies have also shown that specific antibodies against the spike protein also could be used in antigen testing.[210–213] An alert has been issued by the US Food and Drug Administration (FDA) about false-positive results obtained from certain antigen tests, cautioning that this may occur in populations with low prevalence of infection.[214]

Emerging Diagnostics
RT-LAMP–based Tests

As an alternative to RT-qPCR–based tests, reverse transcription loop-mediated isothermal amplification (RT-LAMP) tests are NAATs that are performed by incubation at a constant temperature, which simplifies the workflow and provides scalability.[215] This approach could be useful in small community settings that lack the necessary resources and equipment to perform RT-qPCR tests. RT-LAMP reactions use a DNA polymerase with

tolerance for elevated temperatures. RNA is added to a reaction containing a reverse transcriptase, a DNA polymerase, and oligonucleotides for each; this sample is incubated at a constant temperature for 20 to 60 minutes to allow cDNA production and amplification. The primers typically target the N gene or ORF1ab. Finally, to detect cDNA production, a colorimetric approach may be used, in which a pH indicator causes a color change with accumulating DNA levels. Validation of RT-LAMP assays for detecting SARS-CoV-2 have indicated that the assays possess high sensitivity and specificity. However, the colorimetric RT-LAMP assay was observed to be more effective for detecting positivity in individuals with medium to high viral loads and did not perform as efficiently with low viral loads, revealing an important limitation to keep in mind.

CRISPR-Cas12/13–based Tests
The clustered regularly interspaced short palindromic repeats (CRISPR-Cas) system is a widely used tool for genome editing. Originally derived from bacterial adaptive immune systems, the Cas12 and Cas13 RNA-guided enzymes can directly target and cleave single- and double-stranded DNA or single-stranded RNA (ssRNA), respectively. Cas13 forms a nuclease-inactive ribonucleoprotein complex together with a CRISPR RNA (crRNA) containing a programmable spacer sequence. When the complex binds to its complementary target RNA, Cas13 is activated and cleaves the target nucleic acids in addition to indiscriminately cleaving any other ssRNA in solution.[216,217] For diagnostic testing, the crRNAs can be designed to target different genomic regions of SARS-CoV-2, such as the N gene, E gene, or ORF1ab. Target RNA binding and cleavage mediated by Cas13 then can be detected through colorimetric or fluorescent methods to produce a test result. CRISPR-Cas12–based tests function similarly but use DNA substrates.[218] Rapid CRISPR-Cas13a–based assays without preamplification steps have facilitated the development of at-home tests that can be self-administered with a nasal swab.[216] Saliva-based tests based on CRISPR-Cas12a activity also have been reported, offering a convenient option that maintains high sensitivity.[219] CRISPR-based tests provide quick results, facilitate point-of-care testing, and may be able to augment the gold-standard PCR tests.

Antibody Tests

Serological testing is important for monitoring infection rates in populations and also can be used for diagnosing infection in certain cases, but the CDC does not recommend using it to diagnose acute SARS-CoV-2 infection.[220] Antibody tests can be used in combination with the gold-standard RT-PCR test to improve detection in individuals with asymptomatic disease or in those with mild COVID-19 who are uncertain about the timeline of symptom onset. The combined sensitivity of RT-PCR and IgM ELISA targeting the nucleocapsid antigen is reported to be much higher, with the former producing higher positivity within the first week of symptom onset, whereas the latter can produce positive results after the first week.[205] IgM and IgG antibody tests based on ELISA are reported to be more than 95% specific for diagnosing COVID-19 infection. For antibody testing, lateral flow devices, ELISA, or chemiluminescent immunoassay (CIA) methods may be used with patient serum, plasma, or blood. On infection by SARS-CoV-2, the human body mounts an immune response and produces antibodies against specific viral antigens, such as the abundantly expressed nucleocapsid protein and the spike protein. Antibodies against the spike protein target the S1 protein subunit and the RBD.[221–224] IgM and IgG antibodies can be detected within the first week after symptom onset, but higher levels may be observed in the second or third week. IgM and IgG seroconversion occurred in all patients within a 4-week time frame after symptom onset.[206,225,226] IgM levels gradually drop beyond the 2-week time point and eventually reach basal levels, whereas IgG antibodies remain at high levels and persist for several months after infection.[224,227] Individuals with severe COVID-19 may mount a more pronounced antibody response with higher antibody titers and persistence, whereas seroreversion has been reported in patients with mild COVID-19.[223] Detection of IgG antibodies in patient-derived serum or saliva can provide an idea about the incidence of past infection and can also inform about present infection if detected together with IgM.[228,229] Because of its highly immunogenic nature, the N protein constitutes an effective antigen for designing antibody tests with high sensitivity, and the S protein can be leveraged to design antibody tests with improved specificity. IgG antibodies to the SARS-CoV-2 RBD have been observed to strongly correlate with anti-S neutralizing antibody titers, which could be useful for estimating protection against future infection in unvaccinated individuals.[224] However, these tests are not recommended for assessing protection after receiving the vaccine.[220] Antibody cross-reactivity with SARS-CoV and other coronaviruses may also occur, and therefore antibody tests must be well validated before use and caution must be observed while interpreting results.

Conclusion

In contrast to the SARS-CoV and MERS-CoV outbreaks that were locally contained and self-limiting, the pandemic driven by the emergence of the SARS-CoV-2 virus has posed a challenge to the entire world and caused significant loss of life. The transmission characteristics of SARS-CoV-2 compared with its predecessors have transformed it into a formidable foe. Although the

mechanisms are yet to be clearly defined, we know that the virus can successfully evade the host innate immune response and replicate to high viral loads in the respiratory tract, inducing hyperinflammatory responses and extensive organ damage. The battle is not over yet, with the virus constantly evolving and new variants being discovered in different parts of the world, many of which contain mutations conferring variable degrees of immune escape and enhancing cell entry to further promote virus infectivity. Globally, countries are engaged in a race to vaccinate their population, while the scientific community attempts to stay one step ahead to ensure that vaccines remain effective against newly evolving variants. The vast literature on SARS-CoV-2 and COVID-19 based on the high-quality scientific research performed in various countries provides an invaluable resource to understand coronavirus pathogenesis and its devastating effects on the human host. Hopefully, this will enable us to contain the current pandemic and prevent similar outbreaks in the future.

Acknowledgments

All the figures in this chapter were created with BioRender.com. Fig. 2.2 was adapted from "Human Coronavirus Structure" by BioRender.com (2021); retrieved from https://app.biorender.com/biorender-templates.

REFERENCES

1. Walsh EE, Shin JH, Falsey AR. Clinical impact of human coronaviruses 229E and OC43 infection in diverse adult populations. *J Infect Dis.* 2013;208(10):1634–1642. https://doi.org/10.1093/infdis/jit393.
2. Gaunt ER, Hardie A, Claas EC, et al. Epidemiology and clinical presentations of the four human coronaviruses 229E, HKU1, NL63, and OC43 detected over 3 years using a novel multiplex real-time PCR method. *J Clin Microbiol.* 2010;48(8):2940–2947. https://doi.org/10.1128/jcm.00636-10.
3. Fung TS, Liu DX. Human coronavirus: host-pathogen interaction. *Annu Rev Microbiol.* 2019;73:529–557. https://doi.org/10.1146/annurev-micro-020518-115759.
4. Boni MF, Lemey P, Jiang X, et al. Evolutionary origins of the SARS-CoV-2 sarbecovirus lineage responsible for the COVID-19 pandemic. *Nat Microbiol.* 2020;5(11):1408–1417. https://doi.org/10.1038/s41564-020-0771-4.
5. Lu R, Zhao X, Li J, et al. Genomic characterisation and epidemiology of 2019 novel coronavirus: implications for virus origins and receptor binding. *Lancet.* 2020;395(10224):565–574. https://doi.org/10.1016/s0140-6736(20)30251-8.
6. Zhong NS, Zheng BJ, Li YM, et al. Epidemiology and cause of severe acute respiratory syndrome (SARS) in Guangdong, People's Republic of China, in February, 2003. *Lancet.* 2003;362(9393):1353–1358. https://doi.org/10.1016/s0140-6736(03)14630-2.
7. Cui J, Li F, Shi ZL. Origin and evolution of pathogenic coronaviruses. *Nat Rev Microbiol.* 2019;17(3):181–192. https://doi.org/10.1038/s41579-018-0118-9.

8. Guan Y, Zheng BJ, He YQ, et al. Isolation and characterization of viruses related to the SARS coronavirus from animals in southern China. *Science*. 2003;302(5643):276–278. https://doi.org/10.1126/science.1087139.

9. Zhou P, Yang XL, Wang XG, et al. A pneumonia outbreak associated with a new coronavirus of probable bat origin. *Nature*. 2020;579(7798):270–273. https://doi.org/10.1038/s41586-020-2012-7.

10. Zhou H, Chen X, Hu T, et al. A novel bat coronavirus closely related to SARS-CoV-2 contains natural insertions at the S1/S2 cleavage site of the spike protein. *Curr Biol*. 2020;30(11):2196–2203. e2193. https://doi.org/10.1016/j.cub.2020.05.023.

11. Zhang T, Wu Q, Zhang Z. Probable Pangolin Origin of SARS-CoV-2 Associated with the COVID-19 Outbreak. *Curr Biol*. 2020;30(7):1346–1351. e1342. https://doi.org/10.1016/j.cub.2020.03.022.

12. Xiao K, Zhai J, Feng Y, et al. Isolation of SARS-CoV-2-related coronavirus from Malayan pangolins. *Nature*. 2020;583(7815):286–289. https://doi.org/10.1038/s41586-020-2313-x.

13. Liu P, Jiang JZ, Wan XF, et al. Are pangolins the intermediate host of the 2019 novel coronavirus (SARS-CoV-2)? *PLoS Pathog*. 2020;16(5):e1008421. https://doi.org/10.1371/journal.ppat.1008421.

14. Frutos R, Serra-Cobo J, Chen T, et al. COVID-19: Time to exonerate the pangolin from the transmission of SARS-CoV-2 to humans. *Infect Genet Evol*. 2020;84:104493. https://doi.org/10.1016/j.meegid.2020.104493.

15. MacLean OA, Lytras S, Weaver S, et al. Natural selection in the evolution of SARS-CoV-2 in bats created a generalist virus and highly capable human pathogen. *PLoS Biol*. 2021;19(3):e3001115. https://doi.org/10.1371/journal.pbio.3001115.

16. Chan JF, Kok KH, Zhu Z, et al. Genomic characterization of the 2019 novel human-pathogenic coronavirus isolated from a patient with atypical pneumonia after visiting Wuhan. *Emerg Microbes Infect*. 2020;9(1):221–236. https://doi.org/10.1080/22221751.2020.1719902.

17. Zhu N, Zhang D, Wang W, et al. A Novel Coronavirus from Patients with Pneumonia in China, 2019. *N Engl J Med*. 2020;382(8):727–733. https://doi.org/10.1056/NEJMoa2001017.

18. Shang J, Ye G, Shi K, et al. Structural basis of receptor recognition by SARS-CoV-2. *Nature*. 2020;581(7807):221–224. https://doi.org/10.1038/s41586-020-2179-y.

19. Zhang L, Jackson CB, Mou H, et al. SARS-CoV-2 spike-protein D614G mutation increases virion spike density and infectivity. *Nat Commun*. 2020;11(1):6013. https://doi.org/10.1038/s41467-020-19808-4.

20. Gobeil SM, Janowska K, McDowell S, et al. D614G mutation alters SARS-CoV-2 spike conformation and enhances protease cleavage at the S1/S2 junction. *Cell Rep*. 2021;34(2):108630. https://doi.org/10.1016/j.celrep.2020.108630.

21. Zhou B, Thao TTN, Hoffmann D, et al. SARS-CoV-2 spike D614G change enhances replication and transmission. *Nature*. 2021;592(7852):122–127. https://doi.org/10.1038/s41586-021-03361-1.

22. Wang Q, Zhang Y, Wu L, et al. Structural and functional basis of SARS-CoV-2 entry by using human ACE2. *Cell*. 2020;181(4):894–904. e899. https://doi.org/10.1016/j.cell.2020.03.045.

23. Wrapp D, Wang N, Corbett KS, et al. Cryo-EM structure of the 2019-nCoV spike in the prefusion conformation. *Science*. 2020;367(6483):1260–1263. https://doi.org/10.1126/science.abb2507.

24. Walls AC, Park YJ, Tortorici MA, et al. Structure, function, and antigenicity of the SARS-CoV-2 spike glycoprotein. *Cell*. 2020;181(2):281–292.e286. https://doi.org/10.1016/j.cell.2020.02.058.

25. Peacock TP, Goldhill DH, Zhou J, et al. The furin cleavage site in the SARS-CoV-2 spike protein is required for transmission in ferrets. *Nat Microbiol*. 2021. https://doi.org/10.1038/s41564-021-00908-w.

26. Lan J, Ge J, Yu J, et al. Structure of the SARS-CoV-2 spike receptor-binding domain bound to the ACE2 receptor. *Nature*. 2020;581(7807):215–220. https://doi.org/10.1038/s41586-020-2180-5.

27. Mandala VS, McKay MJ, Shcherbakov AA, et al. Structure and drug binding of the SARS-CoV-2 envelope protein transmembrane domain in lipid bilayers. *Nat Struct Mol Biol*. 2020;27(12):1202–1208. https://doi.org/10.1038/s41594-020-00536-8.

28. Schoeman D, Fielding BC. Coronavirus envelope protein: current knowledge. *Virol J*. 2019;16(1):69. https://doi.org/10.1186/s12985-019-1182-0.

29. Duart G, García-Murria MJ, Grau B, et al. SARS-CoV-2 envelope protein topology in eukaryotic membranes. *Open Biol*. 2020;10(9):200209. https://doi.org/10.1098/rsob.200209.

30. Nieto-Torres JL, Dediego ML, Alvarez E, et al. Subcellular location and topology of severe acute respiratory syndrome coronavirus envelope protein. *Virology*. 2011;415(2):69–82. https://doi.org/10.1016/j.virol.2011.03.029.

31. Nieto-Torres JL, Verdiá-Báguena C, Jimenez-Guardeño JM, et al. Severe acute respiratory syndrome coronavirus E protein transports calcium ions and activates the NLRP3 inflammasome. *Virology*. 2015;485:330–339. https://doi.org/10.1016/j.virol.2015.08.010.

32. Neuman BW, Kiss G, Kunding AH, et al. A structural analysis of M protein in coronavirus assembly and morphology. *J Struct Biol*. 2011;174(1):11–22. https://doi.org/10.1016/j.jsb.2010.11.021.

33. Klein S, Cortese M, Winter SL, et al. SARS-CoV-2 structure and replication characterized by in situ cryo-electron tomography. *Nat Commun*. 2020;11(1):5885. https://doi.org/10.1038/s41467-020-19619-7.

34. Siu YL, Teoh KT, Lo J, et al. The M, E, and N structural proteins of the severe acute respiratory syndrome coronavirus are required for efficient assembly, trafficking, and release of virus-like particles. *J Virol*. 2008;82(22):11318–11330. https://doi.org/10.1128/jvi.01052-08.

35. Swann H, Sharma A, Preece B, et al. Minimal system for assembly of SARS-CoV-2 virus like particles. *Sci Rep*. 2020;10(1):21877. https://doi.org/10.1038/s41598-020-78656-w.

36. Yao H, Song Y, Chen Y, et al. Molecular Architecture of the SARS-CoV-2 Virus. *Cell*. 2020;183(3):730–738. e713. https://doi.org/10.1016/j.cell.2020.09.018.

37. Carlson CR, Asfaha JB, Ghent CM, et al. Phosphoregulation of Phase Separation by the SARS-CoV-2 N Protein Suggests a Biophysical Basis for its Dual Functions. *Mol Cell*. 2020;80(6):1092–1103.e1094. https://doi.org/10.1016/j.molcel.2020.11.025.

38. Lu S, Ye Q, Singh D, et al. The SARS-CoV-2 nucleocapsid phosphoprotein forms mutually exclusive condensates with RNA and the membrane-associated M protein. *Nat Commun.* 2021;12(1):502. https://doi.org/10.1038/s41467-020-20768-y.

39. Ren Y, Shu T, Wu D, et al. The ORF3a protein of SARS-CoV-2 induces apoptosis in cells. *Cell Mol Immunol.* 2020;17(8):881–883. https://doi.org/10.1038/s41423-020-0485-9.

40. Issa E, Merhi G, Panossian B, et al. SARS-CoV-2 and ORF3a: Nonsynonymous Mutations, Functional Domains, and Viral Pathogenesis. *mSystems.* 2020;5(3). https://doi.org/10.1128/mSystems.00266-20.

41. Xu H, Akinyemi IA, Chitre SA, et al. SARS-CoV-2 viroporin encoded by ORF3a triggers the NLRP3 inflammatory pathway. *Virology.* 2022; 568:13–22. https://doi.org/10.1016/j.virol.2022.01.003.

42. Miao G, Zhao H, Li Y, et al. ORF3a of the COVID-19 virus SARS-CoV-2 blocks HOPS complex-mediated assembly of the SNARE complex required for autolysosome formation. *Dev Cell.* 2021;56(4):427–442.e425. https://doi.org/10.1016/j.devcel.2020.12.010.

43. Zhang Y, Sun H, Pei R, et al. The SARS-CoV-2 protein ORF3a inhibits fusion of autophagosomes with lysosomes. *Cell Discov.* 2021;7(1):31. https://doi.org/10.1038/s41421-021-00268-z.

44. Zhang J, Wu H, Yao X, et al. Pyroptotic macrophages stimulate the SARS-CoV-2-associated cytokine storm. *Cell Mol Immunol.* 2021;18(5):1305–1307. https://doi.org/10.1038/s41423-021-00665-0.

45. Konno Y, Kimura I, Uriu K, et al. SARS-CoV-2 ORF3b Is a Potent Interferon Antagonist Whose Activity Is Increased by a Naturally Occurring Elongation Variant. *Cell Rep.* 2020;32(12):108185. https://doi.org/10.1016/j.celrep.2020.108185.

46. Lei X, Dong X, Ma R, et al. Activation and evasion of type I interferon responses by SARS-CoV-2. *Nat Commun.* 2020;11(1):3810. https://doi.org/10.1038/s41467-020-17665-9.

47. Miorin L, Kehrer T, Sanchez-Aparicio MT, et al. SARS-CoV-2 Orf6 hijacks Nup98 to block STAT nuclear import and antagonize interferon signaling. *Proc Natl Acad Sci U S A.* 2020;117(45):28344–28354. https://doi.org/10.1073/pnas.2016650117.

48. Xia H, Cao Z, Xie X, et al. Evasion of Type I Interferon by SARS-CoV-2. *Cell Rep.* 2020;33(1):108234. https://doi.org/10.1016/j.celrep.2020.108234.

49. Zhou Z, Huang C, Zhou Z, et al. Structural insight reveals SARS-CoV-2 ORF7a as an immunomodulating factor for human CD14(+) monocytes. *iScience.* 2021;24(3):102187. https://doi.org/10.1016/j.isci.2021.102187.

50. Cao Z, Xia H, Rajsbaum R, et al. Ubiquitination of SARS-CoV-2 ORF7a promotes antagonism of interferon response. *Cell Mol Immunol.* 2021;18(3):746–748. https://doi.org/10.1038/s41423-020-00603-6.

51. Martin-Sancho L, Lewinski MK, Pache L, et al. Functional landscape of SARS-CoV-2 cellular restriction. *Mol Cell.* 2021. https://doi.org/10.1016/j.molcel.2021.04.008.

52. Fogeron M-L, Montserret R, Zehnder J, et al. SARS-CoV-2 ORF7b: is a bat virus protein homologue a major cause of COVID-19 symptoms? *bioRxiv.* 2021. https://doi.org/10.1101/2021.02.05.428650.

53. Tan Y, Schneider T, Leong M, et al. Novel Immunoglobulin Domain Proteins Provide Insights into Evolution and Pathogenesis of SARS-CoV-2-Related Viruses. *mBio.* 2020;11(3). https://doi.org/10.1128/mBio.00760-20.

54. Flower TG, Buffalo CZ, Hooy RM, et al. Structure of SARS-CoV-2 ORF8, a rapidly evolving immune evasion protein. *Proc Natl Acad Sci U S A.* 2021;118(2). https://doi.org/10.1073/pnas.2021785118.

55. Wang X, Lam JY, Wong WM, et al. Accurate Diagnosis of COVID-19 by a Novel Immunogenic Secreted SARS-CoV-2 orf8 Protein. *mBio.* 2020;11(5). https://doi.org/10.1128/mBio.02431-20.

56. Hachim A, Kavian N, Cohen CA, et al. ORF8 and ORF3b antibodies are accurate serological markers of early and late SARS-CoV-2 infection. *Nat Immunol.* 2020;21(10):1293–1301. https://doi.org/10.1038/s41590-020-0773-7.

57. Zhang Y, Chen Y, Li Y, et al. The ORF8 protein of SARS-CoV-2 mediates immune evasion through down-regulating MHC-I. *Proc Natl Acad Sci U S A.* 2021;118(23). https://doi.org/10.1073/pnas.2024202118.

58. Gordon, DE, Hiatt, J, Bouhaddou, M, et al. Comparative host-coronavirus protein interaction networks reveal pan-viral disease mechanisms. *Science.* 2020; 370(6521). https://doi.org/10.1126/science.abe9403

59. Lin X, Fu B, Yin S, et al. ORF8 contributes to cytokine storm during SARS-CoV-2 infection by activating IL-17 pathway. *iScience.* 2021;24(4):102293. https://doi.org/10.1016/j.isci.2021.102293.

60. Jiang HW, Zhang HN, Meng QF, et al. SARS-CoV-2 Orf9b suppresses type I interferon responses by targeting TOM70. *Cell Mol Immunol.* 2020;17(9):998–1000. https://doi.org/10.1038/s41423-020-0514-8.

61. Wu J, Shi Y, Pan X, et al. SARS-CoV-2 ORF9b inhibits RIG-I-MAVS antiviral signaling by interrupting K63-linked ubiquitination of NEMO. *Cell Rep.* 2021;34(7):108761. https://doi.org/10.1016/j.celrep.2021.108761.

62. Gordon DE, Jang GM, Bouhaddou M, et al. A SARS-CoV-2 protein interaction map reveals targets for drug repurposing. *Nature.* 2020;583(7816):459–468. https://doi.org/10.1038/s41586-020-2286-9.

63. Mena EL, Donahue CJ, Vaites LP, et al. ORF10-Cullin-2-ZYG11B complex is not required for SARS-CoV-2 infection. *Proc Natl Acad Sci U S A.* 2021;118(17). https://doi.org/10.1073/pnas.2023157118.

64. Finkel Y, Mizrahi O, Nachshon A, et al. The coding capacity of SARS-CoV-2. *Nature.* 2021;589(7840):125–130. https://doi.org/10.1038/s41586-020-2739-1.

65. Kim D, Lee JY, Yang JS, et al. The Architecture of SARS-CoV-2 Transcriptome. *Cell.* 2020;181(4):914–921.e910. https://doi.org/10.1016/j.cell.2020.04.011.

66. Davidson AD, Williamson MK, Lewis S, et al. Characterisation of the transcriptome and proteome of SARS-CoV-2 reveals a cell passage induced in-frame deletion of the furin-like cleavage site from the spike glycoprotein. *Genome Med.* 2020;12(1):68. https://doi.org/10.1186/s13073-020-00763-0.

67. Pancer K, Milewska A, Owczarek K, et al. The SARS-CoV-2 ORF10 is not essential in vitro or in vivo in humans. *PLoS Pathog.* 2020;16(12):e1008959. https://doi.org/10.1371/journal.ppat.1008959.

68. Wu F, Zhao S, Yu B, et al. A new coronavirus associated with human respiratory disease in China. *Nature.* 2020;

579(7798):265–269. https://doi.org/10.1038/s41586-020-2008-3.

69. Li X, Giorgi EE, Marichannegowda MH, et al. Emergence of SARS-CoV-2 through recombination and strong purifying selection. *Sci Adv.* 2020;6(27). https://doi.org/10.1126/sciadv.abb9153.

70. Bhatt PR, Scaiola A, Loughran G, et al. Structural basis of ribosomal frameshifting during translation of the SARS-CoV-2 RNA genome. *Science.* 2021;372(6548):1306–1313. https://doi.org/10.1126/science.abf3546.

71. Maxmen A. One million coronavirus sequences: popular genome site hits mega milestone. *Nature.* 2021;593(7857):21. https://doi.org/10.1038/d41586-021-01069-w.

72. Zhang YZ, Holmes EC. A Genomic Perspective on the Origin and Emergence of SARS-CoV-2. *Cell.* 2020;181(2):223–227. https://doi.org/10.1016/j.cell.2020.03.035.

73. Ferron F, Subissi L, Silveira De Morais AT, et al. Structural and molecular basis of mismatch correction and ribavirin excision from coronavirus RNA. *Proc Natl Acad Sci U S A.* 2018;115(2):E162–E171. https://doi.org/10.1073/pnas.1718806115.

74. Callaway E. The coronavirus is mutating - does it matter? *Nature.* 2020;585(7824):174–177. https://doi.org/10.1038/d41586-020-02544-6.

75. Liu C, Shi W, Becker ST, et al. Structural basis of mismatch recognition by a SARS-CoV-2 proofreading enzyme. *Science (New York, N.Y.).* 2021:eabi9310. Advance online publication. https://doi.org/10.1126/science.abi9310.

76. Su YCF, Anderson DE, Young BE, et al. Discovery and Genomic Characterization of a 382-Nucleotide Deletion in ORF7b and ORF8 during the Early Evolution of SARS-CoV-2. *mBio.* 2020;11(4). https://doi.org/10.1128/mBio.01610-20.

77. Holland LA, Kaelin EA, Maqsood R, et al. An 81-Nucleotide Deletion in SARS-CoV-2 ORF7a Identified from Sentinel Surveillance in Arizona. *J Virol.* January to March 2020;94(14). https://doi.org/10.1128/jvi.00711-20.

78. Muth D, Corman VM, Roth H, et al. Attenuation of replication by a 29 nucleotide deletion in SARS-coronavirus acquired during the early stages of human-to-human transmission. *Sci Rep.* 2018;8(1):15177. https://doi.org/10.1038/s41598-018-33487-8.

79. Young BE, Fong SW, Chan YH, et al. Effects of a major deletion in the SARS-CoV-2 genome on the severity of infection and the inflammatory response: an observational cohort study. *Lancet.* 2020;396(10251):603–611. https://doi.org/10.1016/s0140-6736(20)31757-8.

80. Harvey WT, Carabelli AM, Jackson B, et al. SARS-CoV-2 variants, spike mutations and immune escape. *Nat Rev Microbiol.* 2021;19(7):409–424. https://doi.org/10.1038/s41579-021-00573-0.

81. Piccoli L, Park YJ, Tortorici MA, et al. Mapping Neutralizing and Immunodominant Sites on the SARS-CoV-2 Spike Receptor-Binding Domain by Structure-Guided High-Resolution Serology. *Cell.* 2020;183(4):1024–1042.e1021. https://doi.org/10.1016/j.cell.2020.09.037.

82. Korber B, Fischer WM, Gnanakaran S, et al. Tracking Changes in SARS-CoV-2 Spike: Evidence that D614G Increases Infectivity of the COVID-19 Virus. *Cell.* 2020;182(4):812–827. e819. https://doi.org/10.1016/j.cell.2020.06.043.

83. Mercatelli D, Giorgi FM. Geographic and Genomic Distribution of SARS-CoV-2 Mutations. *Front Microbiol.* 2020;11:1800. https://doi.org/10.3389/fmicb.2020.01800.

84. Yang HC, Chen CH, Wang JH, et al. Analysis of genomic distributions of SARS-CoV-2 reveals a dominant strain type with strong allelic associations. *Proc Natl Acad Sci U S A.* 2020;117(48):30679–30686. https://doi.org/10.1073/pnas.2007840117.

85. Plante JA, Liu Y, Liu J, et al. Spike mutation D614G alters SARS-CoV-2 fitness. *Nature.* 2021;592(7852):116–121. https://doi.org/10.1038/s41586-020-2895-3.

86. Hou YJ, Chiba S, Halfmann P, et al. SARS-CoV-2 D614G variant exhibits efficient replication ex vivo and transmission in vivo. *Science.* 2020;370(6523):1464–1468. https://doi.org/10.1126/science.abe8499.

87. Yurkovetskiy L, Wang X, Pascal KE, et al. Structural and Functional Analysis of the D614G SARS-CoV-2 Spike Protein Variant. *Cell.* 2020;183(3):739–751.e738. https://doi.org/10.1016/j.cell.2020.09.032.

88. Li Q, Wu J, Nie J, et al. The Impact of Mutations in SARS-CoV-2 Spike on Viral Infectivity and Antigenicity. *Cell.* 2020;182(5):1284–1294.e1289. https://doi.org/10.1016/j.cell.2020.07.012.

89. Volz E, Hill V, McCrone JT, et al. Evaluating the Effects of SARS-CoV-2 Spike Mutation D614G on Transmissibility and Pathogenicity. *Cell.* 2021;184(1):64–75.e11. https://doi.org/10.1016/j.cell.2020.11.020.

90. Ozono S, Zhang Y, Ode H, et al. SARS-CoV-2 D614G spike mutation increases entry efficiency with enhanced ACE2-binding affinity. *Nat Commun.* 2021;12(1):848. https://doi.org/10.1038/s41467-021-21118-2.

91. Weissman D, Alameh MG, de Silva T, et al. D614G Spike Mutation increases SARS CoV-2 Susceptibility to Neutralization. *Cell Host Microbe.* 2021;29(1):23–31.e24. https://doi.org/10.1016/j.chom.2020.11.012.

92. Daniloski Z, Jordan TX, Ilmain JK, et al. The Spike D614G mutation increases SARS-CoV-2 infection of multiple human cell types. *Elife.* 2021:10. https://doi.org/10.7554/eLife.65365.

93. Shen X, Tang H, McDanal C, et al. SARS-CoV-2 variant B.1.1.7 is susceptible to neutralizing antibodies elicited by ancestral spike vaccines. *Cell Host Microbe.* 2021;29(4):529–539.e523. https://doi.org/10.1016/j.chom.2021.03.002.

94. Davies NG, Abbott S, Barnard RC, et al. Estimated transmissibility and impact of SARS-CoV-2 lineage B.1.1.7 in England. *Science.* 2021;372(6538). https://doi.org/10.1126/science.abg3055.

95. Leung K, Shum MH, Leung GM, et al. Early transmissibility assessment of the N501Y mutant strains of SARS-CoV-2 in the United Kingdom. *Euro Surveill.* October to November 2021;26(1). https://doi.org/10.2807/1560-7917.Es.2020.26.1.2002106.

96. Challen R, Brooks-Pollock E, Read JM, et al. Risk of mortality in patients infected with SARS-CoV-2 variant of concern 202012/1: matched cohort study. *Bmj.* 2021;372:n579. https://doi.org/10.1136/bmj.n579.

97. Davies NG, Jarvis CI, Edmunds WJ, et al. Increased mortality in community-tested cases of SARS-CoV-2 lineage B.1.1.7. *Nature.* 2021. https://doi.org/10.1038/s41586-021-03426-1.

98. Volz E, Mishra S, Chand M, et al. Assessing transmissibility of SARS-CoV-2 lineage B.1.1.7 in England. *Nature*. 2021;593(7858):266–269. https://doi.org/10.1038/s41586-021-03470-x.

99. Frampton D, Rampling T, Cross A, et al. Genomic characteristics and clinical effect of the emergent SARS-CoV-2 B.1.1.7 lineage in London, UK: a whole-genome sequencing and hospital-based cohort study. *Lancet Infect Dis*. 2021. S1473-3099(21)00170-5. Advance online publication. https://doi.org/10.1016/S1473-3099(21)00170-5.

100. Graham MS, Sudre CH, May A, et al. Changes in symptomatology, reinfection, and transmissibility associated with the SARS-CoV-2 variant B.1.1.7: an ecological study. *Lancet Public Health*. 2021;6(5):e335–e345. https://doi.org/10.1016/S2468-2667(21)00055-4.

101. Chan KK, Tan TJC, Narayanan KK, et al. An engineered decoy receptor for SARS-CoV-2 broadly binds protein S sequence variants. *Sci Adv*. 2021;7(8). https://doi.org/10.1126/sciadv.abf1738.

102. Starr TN, Greaney AJ, Hilton SK, et al. Deep Mutational Scanning of SARS-CoV-2 Receptor Binding Domain Reveals Constraints on Folding and ACE2 Binding. *Cell*. 2020;182(5):1295–1310. e1220. https://doi.org/10.1016/j.cell.2020.08.012.

103. Gu H, Chen Q, Yang G, et al. Adaptation of SARS-CoV-2 in BALB/c mice for testing vaccine efficacy. *Science*. 2020;369(6511):1603–1607. https://doi.org/10.1126/science.abc4730.

104. Niu Z, Zhang Z, Gao X, et al. N501Y mutation imparts cross-species transmission of SARS-CoV-2 to mice by enhancing receptor binding. *Signal Transduct Target Ther*. 2021;6(1):284. https://doi.org/10.1038/s41392-021-00704-2.

105. Li Q, Nie J, Wu J, et al. SARS-CoV-2 501Y.V2 variants lack higher infectivity but do have immune escape. *Cell*. 2021;184(9):2362–2371.e2369. https://doi.org/10.1016/j.cell.2021.02.042.

106. McCarthy KR, Rennick LJ, Nambulli S, et al. Recurrent deletions in the SARS-CoV-2 spike glycoprotein drive antibody escape. *Science*. 2021;371(6534):1139–1142. https://doi.org/10.1126/science.abf6950.

107. Kemp SA, Collier DA, Datir RP, et al. SARS-CoV-2 evolution during treatment of chronic infection. *Nature*. 2021;592(7853):277–282. https://doi.org/10.1038/s41586-021-03291-y.

108. McCallum M, De Marco A, Lempp FA, et al. N-terminal domain antigenic mapping reveals a site of vulnerability for SARS-CoV-2. *Cell*. 2021;184(9):2332–2347.e2316. https://doi.org/10.1016/j.cell.2021.03.028.

109. Rees-Spear C, Muir L, Griffith SA, et al. The effect of spike mutations on SARS-CoV-2 neutralization. *Cell Rep*. 2021;34(12):108890. https://doi.org/10.1016/j.celrep.2021.108890.

110. Xie X, Liu Y, Liu J, et al. Neutralization of SARS-CoV-2 spike 69/70 deletion, E484K and N501Y variants by BNT162b2 vaccine-elicited sera. *Nat Med*. 2021;27(4):620–621. https://doi.org/10.1038/s41591-021-01270-4.

111. Supasa P, Zhou D, Dejnirattisai W, et al. Reduced neutralization of SARS-CoV-2 B.1.1.7 variant by convalescent and vaccine sera. *Cell*. 2021;184(8):2201–2211.e7. https://doi.org/10.1016/j.cell.2021.02.033.

112. Tegally H, Wilkinson E, Giovanetti M, et al. Detection of a SARS-CoV-2 variant of concern in South Africa. *Nature*. 2021;592(7854):438–443. https://doi.org/10.1038/s41586-021-03402-9.

113. Wu K, Werner AP, Koch M, et al. Serum Neutralizing Activity Elicited by mRNA-1273 Vaccine. *N Engl J Med*. 2021;384(15):1468–1470. https://doi.org/10.1056/NEJMc2102179.

114. Shen X, Tang H, Pajon R, et al. Neutralization of SARS-CoV-2 Variants B.1.429 and B.1.351. *N Engl J Med*. 2021. https://doi.org/10.1056/NEJMc2103740.

115. Planas D, Bruel T, Grzelak L, et al. Sensitivity of infectious SARS-CoV-2 B.1.1.7 and B.1.351 variants to neutralizing antibodies. *Nat Med*. 2021. https://doi.org/10.1038/s41591-021-01318-5.

116. Zhou D, Dejnirattisai W, Supasa P, et al. Evidence of escape of SARS-CoV-2 variant B.1.351 from natural and vaccine-induced sera. *Cell*. 2021;184(9):2348–2361. e2346.

117. Chen RE, Zhang X, Case JB, et al. Resistance of SARS-CoV-2 variants to neutralization by monoclonal and serum-derived polyclonal antibodies. *Nat Med*. 2021;27(4):717–726. https://doi.org/10.1038/s41591-021-01294-w.

118. Baum A, Fulton BO, Wloga E, et al. Antibody cocktail to SARS-CoV-2 spike protein prevents rapid mutational escape seen with individual antibodies. *Science*. 2020;369(6506):1014–1018. https://doi.org/10.1126/science.abd0831.

119. Greaney AJ, Loes AN, Crawford KHD, et al. Comprehensive mapping of mutations in the SARS-CoV-2 receptor-binding domain that affect recognition by polyclonal human plasma antibodies. *Cell Host Microbe*. 2021;29(3):463–476.e466. https://doi.org/10.1016/j.chom.2021.02.003.

120. Starr TN, Greaney AJ, Dingens AS, et al. Complete map of SARS-CoV-2 RBD mutations that escape the monoclonal antibody LY-CoV555 and its cocktail with LY-CoV016. *Cell Rep Med*. 2021;2(4):100255. https://doi.org/10.1016/j.xcrm.2021.100255.

121. Collier DA, De Marco A, Ferreira I, et al. Sensitivity of SARS-CoV-2 B.1.1.7 to mRNA vaccine-elicited antibodies. *Nature*. 2021;593(7857):136–141. https://doi.org/10.1038/s41586-021-03412-7.

122. Starr TN, Greaney AJ, Addetia A, et al. Prospective mapping of viral mutations that escape antibodies used to treat COVID-19. *Science*. 2021;371(6531):850–854. https://doi.org/10.1126/science.abf9302.

123. Voloch CM, da Silva Francisco R Jr, de Almeida LGP, et al. Genomic characterization of a novel SARS-CoV-2 lineage from Rio de Janeiro, Brazil. *J Virol*. 2021. https://doi.org/10.1128/jvi.00119-21.

124. Sabino EC, Buss LF, Carvalho MPS, et al. Resurgence of COVID-19 in Manaus, Brazil, despite high seroprevalence. *Lancet*. 2021;397(10273):452–455. https://doi.org/10.1016/s0140-6736(21)00183-5.

125. Faria NR, Mellan TA, Whittaker C, et al. Genomics and epidemiology of the P.1 SARS-CoV-2 lineage in Manaus, Brazil. *Science*. 2021. https://doi.org/10.1126/science.abh2644.

126. Dejnirattisai W, Zhou D, Supasa P, et al. Antibody evasion by the P.1 strain of SARS-CoV-2. *Cell*. 2021;184(11):2939–2954.e9. https://doi.org/10.1016/j.cell.2021.03.055.

127. Singh J, Rahman SA, Ehtesham NZ, et al. SARS-CoV-2 variants of concern are emerging in India. *Nat Med*.

2021;27(7):1131–1133. https://doi.org/10.1038/s41591-021-01397-4.

128. Tchesnokova V, Kulasekara H, Larson L, et al. Acquisition of the L452R mutation in the ACE2-binding interface of Spike protein triggers recent massive expansion of SARS-CoV-2 variants. *J Clin Microbiol.* 2021. JCM0092121. Advance online publication. https://doi.org/10.1128/JCM.00921-21.

129. Deng X, Garcia-Knight MA, Khalid MM, et al. Transmission, infectivity, and neutralization of a spike L452R SARS-CoV-2 variant. *Cell.* 2021. https://doi.org/10.1016/j.cell.2021.04.025.

130. Motozono C, Toyoda M, Zahradnik J, et al. SARS-CoV-2 spike L452R variant evades cellular immunity and increases infectivity. *Cell Host Microbe.* 2021;29(7):1124–1136.e11. https://doi.org/10.1016/j.chom.2021.06.006.

131. Xu C, Wang Y, Liu C, et al. Conformational dynamics of SARS-CoV-2 trimeric spike glycoprotein in complex with receptor ACE2 revealed by cryo-EM. *Sci Adv.* 2021;7(1):eabe5575. https://doi.org/10.1126/sciadv.abe5575.

132. Liu Z, VanBlargan LA, Bloyet LM, et al. Identification of SARS-CoV-2 spike mutations that attenuate monoclonal and serum antibody neutralization. *Cell host & microbe.* 2021;29(3):477–488.e4. https://doi.org/10.1016/j.chom.2021.01.014.

133. Zahradník J., Marciano S., Shemesh M., et al. SARS-CoV-2 variant prediction and antiviral drug design are enabled by RBD in vitro evolution. Nat Microbiol. 2021;6:1188–1198. https://doi.org/10.1038/s41564-021-00954-4.

134. Li B, Deng A, Li K, et al. (2021). Viral infection and transmission in a large, well-traced outbreak caused by the SARS-CoV-2 Delta variant. *medRxiv* 2021. 2021.07.07.21260122. https://doi.org/10.1101/2021.07.07.21260122

135. Campbell F, Archer B, Laurenson-Schafer H, et al. Increased transmissibility and global spread of SARS-CoV-2 variants of concern as at June 2021. *Euro Surveill.* 2021;26(24):2100509. https://doi.org/10.2807/1560-7917.ES.2021.26.24.2100509.

136. Lopez Bernal J, Andrews N, Gower C, et al. Effectiveness of Covid-19 Vaccines against the B.1.617.2 (Delta) Variant. *New Engl J Med.* 2021. NEJMoa2108891. Advance online publication. https://doi.org/10.1056/NEJMoa2108891.

137. Planas D, Veyer D, Baidaliuk A, et al. Reduced sensitivity of SARS-CoV-2 variant Delta to antibody neutralization. *Nature.* 2021. 10.1038/s41586-021-03777-9. Advance online publication. https://doi.org/10.1038/s41586-021-03777-9.

138. Hoffmann M, Kleine-Weber H, Schroeder S, et al. SARS-CoV-2 Cell Entry Depends on ACE2 and TMPRSS2 and Is Blocked by a Clinically Proven Protease Inhibitor. *Cell.* 2020;181(2):271–280.e278. https://doi.org/10.1016/j.cell.2020.02.052.

139. Gheblawi M, Wang K, Viveiros A, et al. Angiotensin-Converting Enzyme 2: SARS-CoV-2 Receptor and Regulator of the Renin-Angiotensin System: Celebrating the 20th Anniversary of the Discovery of ACE2. *Circ Res.* 2020;126(10):1456–1474. https://doi.org/10.1161/CIRCRESAHA.120.317015.

140. Hoffmann M, Kleine-Weber H, Pöhlmann S. A Multibasic Cleavage Site in the Spike Protein of SARS-CoV-2 Is Essential for Infection of Human Lung Cells. *Mol Cell.* 2020;78(4):779–784. e775.https://doi.org/10.1016/j.molcel.2020.04.022.

141. Bestle D, Heindl MR, Limburg H, et al. TMPRSS2 and furin are both essential for proteolytic activation of SARS-CoV-2 in human airway cells. *Life Sci Alliance.* 2020;3(9). https://doi.org/10.26508/lsa.202000786.

142. Shang J, Wan Y, Luo C, et al. Cell entry mechanisms of SARS-CoV-2. *Proc Natl Acad Sci U S A.* 2020;117(21):11727–11734. https://doi.org/10.1073/pnas.2003138117.

143. Winstone H, Lista MJ, Reid AC, et al. The Polybasic Cleavage Site in SARS-CoV-2 Spike Modulates Viral Sensitivity to Type I Interferon and IFITM2. *J Virol.* 2021;95(9). https://doi.org/10.1128/jvi.02422-20.

144. Johnson BA, Xie X, Bailey AL, et al. Loss of furin cleavage site attenuates SARS-CoV-2 pathogenesis. *Nature.* 2021;591(7849):293–299. https://doi.org/10.1038/s41586-021-03237-4.

145. Papa G, Mallery DL, Albecka A, et al. Furin cleavage of SARS-CoV-2 Spike promotes but is not essential for infection and cell-cell fusion. *PLoS Pathog.* 2021;17(1):e1009246. https://doi.org/10.1371/journal.ppat.1009246.

146. Sungnak W, Huang N, Bécavin C, et al. SARS-CoV-2 entry factors are highly expressed in nasal epithelial cells together with innate immune genes. *Nat Med.* 2020;26(5):681–687. https://doi.org/10.1038/s41591-020-0868-6.

147. Hou YJ, Okuda K, Edwards CE, et al. SARS-CoV-2 Reverse Genetics Reveals a Variable Infection Gradient in the Respiratory Tract. *Cell.* 2020;182(2):429–446.e414. https://doi.org/10.1016/j.cell.2020.05.042.

148. Muus C, Luecken MD, Eraslan G, et al. Single-cell meta-analysis of SARS-CoV-2 entry genes across tissues and demographics. *Nat Med.* 2021;27(3):546–559. https://doi.org/10.1038/s41591-020-01227-z.

149. Sawicki SG, Sawicki DL, Siddell SG. A contemporary view of coronavirus transcription. *J Virol.* 2007;81(1):20–29. https://doi.org/10.1128/jvi.01358-06.

150. Snijder EJ, Limpens R, de Wilde AH, et al. A unifying structural and functional model of the coronavirus replication organelle: Tracking down RNA synthesis. *PLoS Biol.* 2020;18(6):e3000715. https://doi.org/10.1371/journal.pbio.3000715.

151. Oostra M, te Lintelo EG, Deijs M, et al. Localization and membrane topology of coronavirus nonstructural protein 4: involvement of the early secretory pathway in replication. *J Virol.* 2007;81(22):12323–12336. https://doi.org/10.1128/jvi.01506-07.

152. Subissi L, Posthuma CC, Collet A, et al. One severe acute respiratory syndrome coronavirus protein complex integrates processive RNA polymerase and exonuclease activities. *Proc Natl Acad Sci U S A.* 2014;111(37):E3900–E3909. https://doi.org/10.1073/pnas.1323705111.

153. Hillen HS, Kokic G, Farnung L, et al. Structure of replicating SARS-CoV-2 polymerase. *Nature.* 2020;584(7819):154–156. https://doi.org/10.1038/s41586-020-2368-8.

154. Gao Y, Yan L, Huang Y, et al. Structure of the RNA-dependent RNA polymerase from COVID-19 virus. *Science.* 2020;368(6492):779–782. https://doi.org/10.1126/science.abb7498.

155. Yin W, Mao C, Luan X, et al. Structural basis for inhibition of the RNA-dependent RNA polymerase from SARS-CoV-2 by remdesivir. *Science.* 2020;*368*(6498):1499–1504. https://doi.org/10.1126/science.abc1560.

156. Peng Q, Peng R, Yuan B, et al. Structural and Biochemical Characterization of the nsp12-nsp7-nsp8 Core Polymerase

Complex from SARS-CoV-2. *Cell Rep.* 2020;31(11):107774. https://doi.org/10.1016/j.celrep.2020.107774.

157. Wolff G, Limpens R, Zevenhoven-Dobbe JC, et al. A molecular pore spans the double membrane of the coronavirus replication organelle. *Science.* 2020;369(6509):1395–1398. https://doi.org/10.1126/science.abd3629.

158. Fehr AR, Perlman S. Coronaviruses: an overview of their replication and pathogenesis. *Methods Mol Biol.* 2015;1282:1–23. https://doi.org/10.1007/978-1-4939-2438-7_1.

159. Zhang K, Miorin L, Makio T, et al. Nsp1 protein of SARS-CoV-2 disrupts the mRNA export machinery to inhibit host gene expression. *Sci Adv.* 2021;7(6). https://doi.org/10.1126/sciadv.abe7386.

160. Schubert K, Karousis ED, Jomaa A, et al. SARS-CoV-2 Nsp1 binds the ribosomal mRNA channel to inhibit translation. *Nat Struct Mol Biol.* 2020;27(10):959–966. https://doi.org/10.1038/s41594-020-0511-8.

161. Thoms M, Buschauer R, Ameismeier M, et al. Structural basis for translational shutdown and immune evasion by the Nsp1 protein of SARS-CoV-2. *Science.* 2020;369(6508):1249–1255. https://doi.org/10.1126/science.abc8665.

162. Lapointe CP, Grosely R, Johnson AG, et al. Dynamic competition between SARS-CoV-2 NSP1 and mRNA on the human ribosome inhibits translation initiation. *Proc Natl Acad Sci U S A.* 2021;118(6). https://doi.org/10.1073/pnas.2017715118.

163. Banerjee AK, Blanco MR, Bruce EA, et al. SARS-CoV-2 Disrupts Splicing, Translation, and Protein Trafficking to Suppress Host Defenses. *Cell.* 2020;183(5):1325–1339.e1321. https://doi.org/10.1016/j.cell.2020.10.004.

164. Yin X, Riva L, Pu Y, et al. MDA5 Governs the Innate Immune Response to SARS-CoV-2 in Lung Epithelial Cells. *Cell Rep.* 2021;34(2):108628. https://doi.org/10.1016/j.celrep.2020.108628.

165. Rauch I, Müller M, Decker T. The regulation of inflammation by interferons and their STATs. *Jakstat.* 2013;2(1):e23820. https://doi.org/10.4161/jkst.23820.

166. Shin D, Mukherjee R, Grewe D, et al. Papain-like protease regulates SARS-CoV-2 viral spread and innate immunity. *Nature.* 2020;587(7835):657–662. https://doi.org/10.1038/s41586-020-2601-5.

167. Liu G, Lee JH, Parker ZM, et al. ISG15-dependent activation of the sensor MDA5 is antagonized by the SARS-CoV-2 papain-like protease to evade host innate immunity. *Nat Microbiol.* 2021;6(4):467–478. https://doi.org/10.1038/s41564-021-00884-1.

168. Lin MH, Chang SC, Chiu YC, et al. Structural, Biophysical, and Biochemical Elucidation of the SARS-CoV-2 Nonstructural Protein 3 Macro Domain. *ACS Infect Dis.* 2020;6(11):2970–2978. https://doi.org/10.1021/acsinfecdis.0c00441.

169. Alhammad YMO, Kashipathy MM, Roy A, et al. The SARS-CoV-2 Conserved Macrodomain Is a Mono-ADP-Ribosylhydrolase. *J Virol.* 2021;95(3). https://doi.org/10.1128/jvi.01969-20.

170. Claverie JM. A Putative Role of de-Mono-ADP-Ribosylation of STAT1 by the SARS-CoV-2 Nsp3 Protein in the Cytokine Storm Syndrome of COVID-19. *Viruses.* 2020;12(6). https://doi.org/10.3390/v12060646.

171. Fehr AR, Channappanavar R, Jankevicius G, et al. The Conserved Coronavirus Macrodomain Promotes Virulence and Suppresses the Innate Immune Response during

Severe Acute Respiratory Syndrome Coronavirus Infection. *mBio.* 2016;7(6). https://doi.org/10.1128/mBio.01721-16.

172. Yuen CK, Lam JY, Wong WM, et al. SARS-CoV-2 nsp13, nsp14, nsp15 and orf6 function as potent interferon antagonists. *Emerg Microbes Infect.* 2020;9(1):1418–1428. https://doi.org/10.1080/22221751.2020.1780953.

173. Chen K, Xiao F, Hu D, et al. SARS-CoV-2 Nucleocapsid Protein Interacts with RIG-I and Represses RIG-Mediated IFN-β Production. *Viruses.* 2020;13(1). https://doi.org/10.3390/v13010047.

174. Mu J, Fang Y, Yang Q, et al. SARS-CoV-2 N protein antagonizes type I interferon signaling by suppressing phosphorylation and nuclear translocation of STAT1 and STAT2. *Cell Discov.* 2020;6:65. https://doi.org/10.1038/s41421-020-00208-3.

175. Fu YZ, Wang SY, Zheng ZQ, et al. SARS-CoV-2 membrane glycoprotein M antagonizes the MAVS-mediated innate antiviral response. *Cell Mol Immunol.* 2021;18(3):613–620. https://doi.org/10.1038/s41423-020-00571-x.

176. Zheng Y, Zhuang MW, Han L, et al. Severe acute respiratory syndrome coronavirus 2 (SARS-CoV-2) membrane (M) protein inhibits type I and III interferon production by targeting RIG-I/MDA-5 signaling. *Signal Transduct Target Ther.* 2020;5(1):299. https://doi.org/10.1038/s41392-020-00438-7.

177. Fajgenbaum DC, June CH. Cytokine Storm. *N Engl J Med.* 2020;383(23):2255–2273. https://doi.org/10.1056/NEJMra2026131.

178. Mehta P, McAuley DF, Brown M, et al. COVID-19: consider cytokine storm syndromes and immunosuppression. *Lancet.* 2020;395(10229):1033–1034. https://doi.org/10.1016/s0140-6736(20)30628-0.

179. Ragab D, Salah Eldin H, Taeimah M, et al. The COVID-19 Cytokine Storm. What We Know So Far. *Front Immunol.* 2020;11:1446. https://doi.org/10.3389/fimmu.2020.01446.

180. Hadjadj J, Yatim N, Barnabei L, et al. Impaired type I interferon activity and inflammatory responses in severe COVID-19 patients. *Science.* 2020;369(6504):718–724. https://doi.org/10.1126/science.abc6027.

181. Blanco-Melo D, Nilsson-Payant BE, Liu WC, et al. Imbalanced Host Response to SARS-CoV-2 Drives Development of COVID-19. *Cell.* 2020;181(5):1036–1045.e1039. https://doi.org/10.1016/j.cell.2020.04.026.

182. Galani IE, Rovina N, Lampropoulou V, et al. Untuned antiviral immunity in COVID-19 revealed by temporal type I/III interferon patterns and flu comparison. *Nat Immunol.* 2021;22(1):32–40. https://doi.org/10.1038/s41590-020-00840-x.

183. Arunachalam PS, Wimmers F, Mok CKP, et al. Systems biological assessment of immunity to mild versus severe COVID-19 infection in humans. *Science.* 2020;369(6508):1210–1220. https://doi.org/10.1126/science.abc6261.

184. Lee JS, Park S, Jeong HW, et al. Immunophenotyping of COVID-19 and influenza highlights the role of type I interferons in development of severe COVID-19. *Sci Immunol.* 2020;5(49). https://doi.org/10.1126/sciimmunol.abd1554.

185. Israelow B, Song E, Mao T, et al. Mouse model of SARS-CoV-2 reveals inflammatory role of type I interferon signaling. *J Exp Med.* 2020;217(12). https://doi.org/10.1084/jem.20201241.

186. Liao M, Liu Y, Yuan J, et al. Single-cell landscape of bronchoalveolar immune cells in patients with COVID-19. *Nat Med*. 2020;26(6):842–844. https://doi.org/10.1038/s41591-020-0901-9.

187. Boudewijns R, Thibaut HJ, Kaptein SJF, et al. STAT2 signaling restricts viral dissemination but drives severe pneumonia in SARS-CoV-2 infected hamsters. *Nat Commun*. 2020;11(1):5838. https://doi.org/10.1038/s41467-020-19684-y.

188. Rodrigues TS, de Sá KSG, Ishimoto AY, et al. Inflammasomes are activated in response to SARS-CoV-2 infection and are associated with COVID-19 severity in patients. *J Exp Med*. 2021;218(3). https://doi.org/10.1084/jem.20201707.

189. Carsana L, Sonzogni A, Nasr A, et al. Pulmonary post-mortem findings in a series of COVID-19 cases from northern Italy: a two-centre descriptive study. *Lancet Infect Dis*. 2020;20(10):1135–1140. https://doi.org/10.1016/s1473-3099(20)30434-5.

190. Nieto-Torres JL, DeDiego ML, Verdiá-Báguena C, et al. Severe acute respiratory syndrome coronavirus envelope protein ion channel activity promotes virus fitness and pathogenesis. *PLoS Pathog*. 2014;10(5):e1004077. https://doi.org/10.1371/journal.ppat.1004077.

191. Ferreira AC, Soares VC, de Azevedo-Quintanilha IG, et al. SARS-CoV-2 engages inflammasome and pyroptosis in human primary monocytes. *Cell Death Discov*. 2021;7(1):43. https://doi.org/10.1038/s41420-021-00428-w.

192. Lee S, Channappanavar R, Kanneganti TD. Coronaviruses: Innate Immunity, Inflammasome Activation, Inflammatory Cell Death, and Cytokines. *Trends Immunol*. 2020;41(12):1083–1099. https://doi.org/10.1016/j.it.2020.10.005.

193. Li S, Zhang Y, Guan Z, et al. SARS-CoV-2 triggers inflammatory responses and cell death through caspase-8 activation. *Signal Transduct Target Ther*. 2020;5(1):235. https://doi.org/10.1038/s41392-020-00334-0.

194. Place DE, Lee S, Kanneganti TD. PANoptosis in microbial infection. *Curr Opin Microbiol*. 2021;59:42–49. https://doi.org/10.1016/j.mib.2020.07.012.

195. Karki R, Sharma BR, Tuladhar S, et al. Synergism of TNF-α and IFN-γ Triggers Inflammatory Cell Death, Tissue Damage, and Mortality in SARS-CoV-2 Infection and Cytokine Shock Syndromes. *Cell,*. 2021;184(1):149–168.e117. https://doi.org/10.1016/j.cell.2020.11.025.

196. Mudd PA, Crawford JC, Turner JS, et al. Distinct inflammatory profiles distinguish COVID-19 from influenza with limited contributions from cytokine storm. *Sci Adv*. 2020;6(50):eabe3024. https://doi.org/10.1126/sciadv.abe3024.

197. Sinha P, Matthay MA, Calfee CS. Is a "Cytokine Storm" Relevant to COVID-19? *JAMA Intern Med*. 2020;180(9):1152–1154. https://doi.org/10.1001/jamainternmed.2020.3313.

198. Patra T, Meyer K, Geerling L, et al. SARS-CoV-2 spike protein promotes IL-6 trans-signaling by activation of angiotensin II receptor signaling in epithelial cells. *PLoS Pathog*. 2020;16(12):e1009128. https://doi.org/10.1371/journal.ppat.1009128.

199. Abassi Z, Higazi A, Kinaneh S, et al. ACE2, COVID-19 Infection, Inflammation, and Coagulopathy: Missing Pieces in the Puzzle. *Front Physiol*. 2020;11:574753. https://doi.org/10.3389/fphys.2020.574753.

200. Iwasaki M, Saito J, Zhao H, et al. Inflammation Triggered by SARS-CoV-2 and ACE2 Augment Drives Multiple Organ Failure of Severe COVID-19: Molecular Mechanisms and Implications. *Inflammation*. 2021;44(1):13–34. https://doi.org/10.1007/s10753-020-01337-3.

201. Centers for Disease Control and Prevention. (2021a). Interim Guidelines for Collecting and Handling of Clinical Specimens for COVID-19 Testing. https://www.cdc.gov/coronavirus/2019-ncov/lab/guidelines-clinical-specimens.html

202. Sethuraman N, Jeremiah SS, Ryo A. Interpreting Diagnostic Tests for SARS-CoV-2. *Jama*. 2020;323(22):2249–2251. https://doi.org/10.1001/jama.2020.8259.

203. To KK, Tsang OT, Leung WS, et al. Temporal profiles of viral load in posterior oropharyngeal saliva samples and serum antibody responses during infection by SARS-CoV-2: an observational cohort study. *Lancet Infect Dis*. 2020;20(5):565–574. https://doi.org/10.1016/s1473-3099(20)30196-1.

204. Kevadiya BD, Machhi J, Herskovitz J, et al. Diagnostics for SARS-CoV-2 infections. *Nat Mater*. 2021;20(5):593–605. https://doi.org/10.1038/s41563-020-00906-z.

205. Butler-Laporte G, Lawandi A, Schiller I, et al. Comparison of Saliva and Nasopharyngeal Swab Nucleic Acid Amplification Testing for Detection of SARS-CoV-2: A Systematic Review and Meta-analysis. *JAMA Intern Med*. 2021;181(3):353–360. https://doi.org/10.1001/jamainternmed.2020.8876.

206. Teo AKJ, Choudhury Y, Tan IB, et al. Saliva is more sensitive than nasopharyngeal or nasal swabs for diagnosis of asymptomatic and mild COVID-19 infection. *Sci Rep*. 2021;11(1):3134. https://doi.org/10.1038/s41598-021-82787-z.

207. Diao B, Wen K, Zhang J, et al. Accuracy of a nucleocapsid protein antigen rapid test in the diagnosis of SARS-CoV-2 infection. *Clinical microbiology and infection: the official publication of the European Society of Clinical Microbiology and Infectious Diseases*. 2021;27(2):289.e281-289.e284. https://doi.org/10.1016/j.cmi.2020.09.057.

208. Barlev-Gross M, Weiss S, Ben-Shmuel A, et al. Spike vs nucleocapsid SARS-CoV-2 antigen detection: application in nasopharyngeal swab specimens. *Anal Bioanal Chem*. 2021;413(13):3501–3510. https://doi.org/10.1007/s00216-021-03298-4.

209. Lee JH, Choi M, Jung Y, et al. A novel rapid detection for SARS-CoV-2 spike 1 antigens using human angiotensin converting enzyme 2 (ACE2). *Biosens Bioelectron*. 2021;171:112715. https://doi.org/10.1016/j.bios.2020.112715.

210. Li D, Li J. Immunologic Testing for SARS-CoV-2 Infection from the Antigen Perspective. *J Clin Microbiol*. 2021;59(5). https://doi.org/10.1128/jcm.02160-20.

211. US Foods and Drug Administration. (2020, 11/03/2020). Potential for False Positive Results with Antigen Tests for Rapid Detection of SARS-CoV-2 - Letter to Clinical Laboratory Staff and Health Care Providers. https://www.fda.gov/medical-devices/letters-health-care-providers/potential-false-positive-results-antigen-tests-rapid-detection-sars-cov-2-letter-clinical-laboratory

212. Dao Thi VL, Herbst K, Boerner K, et al. A colorimetric RT-LAMP assay and LAMP-sequencing for detecting SARS-CoV-2 RNA in clinical samples. *Sci Transl Med*. 2020;12(556). https://doi.org/10.1126/scitranslmed.abc7075.

213. Fozouni P, Son S, Díaz de León Derby M, et al. Amplification-free detection of SARS-CoV-2 with CRISPR-Cas13a and mobile phone microscopy. *Cell*. 2021;184(2):323–333.e329. https://doi.org/10.1016/j.cell.2020.12.001.

214. Kellner MJ, Koob JG, Gootenberg JS, et al. SHERLOCK: nucleic acid detection with CRISPR nucleases. *Nat Protoc.* 2019;14(10):2986–3012. https://doi.org/10.1038/s41596-019-0210-2.

215. Broughton JP, Deng X, Yu G, et al. CRISPR-Cas12-based detection of SARS-CoV-2. *Nat Biotechnol.* 2020;38(7):870–874. https://doi.org/10.1038/s41587-020-0513-4.

216. Ning B, Yu T, Zhang S, et al. A smartphone-read ultrasensitive and quantitative saliva test for COVID-19. *Sci Adv.* 2021;7(2). https://doi.org/10.1126/sciadv.abe3703.

217. Centers for Disease Control and Prevention. (2021b). Interim Guidelines for COVID-19 Antibody Testing. https://www.cdc.gov/coronavirus/2019-ncov/lab/resources/antibody-tests-guidelines.html

218. Robbiani DF, Gaebler C, Muecksch F, et al. Convergent antibody responses to SARS-CoV-2 in convalescent individuals. *Nature.* 2020;584(7821):437–442. https://doi.org/10.1038/s41586-020-2456-9.

219. Suthar MS, Zimmerman MG, Kauffman RC, et al. Rapid Generation of Neutralizing Antibody Responses in COVID-19 Patients. *Cell Rep Med.* 2020;1(3):100040. https://doi.org/10.1016/j.xcrm.2020.100040.

220. Qu J, Wu C, Li X, et al. Profile of Immunoglobulin G and IgM Antibodies Against Severe Acute Respiratory Syndrome Coronavirus 2 (SARS-CoV-2). *Clin Infect Dis.* 2020;71(16):2255–2258. https://doi.org/10.1093/cid/ciaa489.

221. Iyer AS, Jones FK, Nodoushani A, et al. Persistence and decay of human antibody responses to the receptor binding domain of SARS-CoV-2 spike protein in COVID-19 patients. *Sci Immunol.* 2020;5(52). https://doi.org/10.1126/sciimmunol.abe0367.

222. Hou H, Wang T, Zhang B, et al. Detection of IgM and IgG antibodies in patients with coronavirus disease 2019. *Clin Transl Immunology.* 2020;9(5):e01136. https://doi.org/10.1002/cti2.1136.

223. Xiang F, Wang X, He X, et al. Antibody Detection and Dynamic Characteristics in Patients With Coronavirus Disease 2019. *Clin Infect Dis.* 2020;71(8):1930–1934. https://doi.org/10.1093/cid/ciaa461.

224. Dan JM, Mateus J, Kato Y, et al. Immunological memory to SARS-CoV-2 assessed for up to 8 months after infection. *Science.* 2021;371(6529). https://doi.org/10.1126/science.abf4063.

225. Pisanic N, Randad PR, Kruczynski K, et al. COVID-19 Serology at Population Scale: SARS-CoV-2-Specific Antibody Responses in Saliva. *J Clin Microbiol.* 2020;59(1). https://doi.org/10.1128/jcm.02204-20.

226. MacMullan MA, Ibrayeva A, Trettner K, et al. ELISA detection of SARS-CoV-2 antibodies in saliva. *Sci Rep.* 2020;10(1):20818. https://doi.org/10.1038/s41598-020-77555-4.

227. Garvin MR, E TP, Pavicic M, et al. Potentially adaptive SARS-CoV-2 mutations discovered with novel spatiotemporal and explainable AI models. *Genome Biol.* 2020;21(1):304. https://doi.org/10.1186/s13059-020-02191-0.

228. Cornillez-Ty CT, Liao L, Yates JR 3rd, et al. Severe acute respiratory syndrome coronavirus nonstructural protein 2 interacts with a host protein complex involved in mitochondrial biogenesis and intracellular signaling. *J Virol.* 2009;83(19):10314–10318. https://doi.org/10.1128/jvi.00842-09.

229. Rut W, Lv Z, Zmudzinski M, et al. Activity profiling and crystal structures of inhibitor-bound SARS-CoV-2 papain-like protease: A framework for anti-COVID-19 drug design. *Sci Adv.* 2020;6(42). https://doi.org/10.1126/sciadv.abd4596.

230. Angelini MM, Akhlaghpour M, Neuman BW, et al. Severe acute respiratory syndrome coronavirus nonstructural proteins 3, 4, and 6 induce double-membrane vesicles. *mBio.* 2013;4(4). https://doi.org/10.1128/mBio.00524-13.

231. Kneller DW, Galanie S, Phillips G, et al. Malleability of the SARS-CoV-2 3CL M(pro) Active-Site Cavity Facilitates Binding of Clinical Antivirals. *Structure.* 2020;28(12):1313–1320.e1313. https://doi.org/10.1016/j.str.2020.10.007.

232. Cottam EM, Maier HJ, Manifava M, et al. Coronavirus nsp6 proteins generate autophagosomes from the endoplasmic reticulum via an omegasome intermediate. *Autophagy.* 2011;7(11):1335–1347. https://doi.org/10.4161/auto.7.11.16642.

233. Cottam EM, Whelband MC, Wileman T. Coronavirus NSP6 restricts autophagosome expansion. *Autophagy.* 2014;10(8):1426–1441. https://doi.org/10.4161/auto.29309.

234. te Velthuis AJ, van den Worm SH, Snijder EJ. The SARS-coronavirus nsp7 + nsp8 complex is a unique multimeric RNA polymerase capable of both de novo initiation and primer extension. *Nucleic Acids Res.* 2012;40(4):1737–1747. https://doi.org/10.1093/nar/gkr893.

235. Imbert I, Guillemot JC, Bourhis JM, et al. A second, non-canonical RNA-dependent RNA polymerase in SARS coronavirus. *Embo j.* 2006;25(20):4933–4942. https://doi.org/10.1038/sj.emboj.7601368.

236. Littler DR, Gully BS, Colson RN, et al. Crystal Structure of the SARS-CoV-2 Non-structural Protein 9, Nsp9. *iScience.* 2020: 2589-0042 (Electronic).

237. Zhang C, Chen Y, Li L, et al. Structural basis for the multimerization of nonstructural protein nsp9 from SARS-CoV-2. *Molecular Biomedicine.* 2020;1(1):5. https://doi.org/10.1186/s43556-020-00005-0.

238. Krafcikova P, Silhan J, Nencka R, et al. Structural analysis of the SARS-CoV-2 methyltransferase complex involved in RNA cap creation bound to sinefungin. *Nat Commun.* 2020; 11(1):3717. https://doi.org/10.1038/s41467-020-17495-9.

239. Subissi L, Imbert I, Ferron F, et al. SARS-CoV ORF1b-encoded nonstructural proteins 12-16: replicative enzymes as antiviral targets. *Antiviral Res.* 2014;101:122–130. https://doi.org/10.1016/j.antiviral.2013.11.006.

240. Snijder EJ, Decroly E, Ziebuhr J. The Nonstructural Proteins Directing Coronavirus RNA Synthesis and Processing. *Adv Virus Res.* 2016;96:59–126. https://doi.org/10.1016/bs.aivir.2016.08.008.

241. Malone B, Chen J, Wang Q, et al. Structural basis for backtracking by the SARS-CoV-2 replication-transcription complex. *Proceedings of the National Academy of Sciences of the United States of America.* 2021;118(19):e2102516118. https://doi.org/10.1073/pnas.2102516118.

242. Pillon MC, Frazier MN, Dillard LB, et al. Cryo-EM structures of the SARS-CoV-2 endoribonuclease Nsp15 reveal insight into nuclease specificity and dynamics. *Nat Commun.* 2021;12(1):636. https://doi.org/10.1038/s41467-020-20608-z.

243. Escalera Alba, Gonzalez-Reiche Ana S, Aslam Sadaf, et al. Mutations in SARS-CoV-2 variants of concern link to

increased spike cleavage and virus transmission. *Cell Host Microbe.* 2022;30(3):373–387. doi:10.1016/j.chom.2022.01.006. 35150638 e7. 1934-6069.

244. Peacock Thomas P, Brown Jonathan C, Zhou Jie, et al. The SARS-CoV-2 variant, Omicron, shows rapid replication in human primary nasal epithelial cultures and efficiently uses the endosomal route of entry. *bioRxiv.* 2021. doi:10.1101/2021.12.31.474653.

245. Meng Bo, Kemp Steven A, Papa Guido, et al. COVID-19 Genomics UK (COG-UK) Consortium. Recurrent emergence of SARS-CoV-2 spike deletion H69/V70 and its role in the Alpha variant B.1.1.7. *Cell Rep.* 2021;35(13):109292. doi:10.1016/j.celrep.2021.109292. 34166617 2211-1247.

246. Saito Akatsuki, Irie Takashi, Suzuki Rigel, et al. Genotype to Phenotype Japan (G2P-Japan) Consortium. Enhanced fusogenicity and pathogenicity of SARS-CoV-2 Delta P681R mutation. *Nature.* 2022;602(7896):300–306. doi:10.1038/s41586-021-04266-9. 34823256 1476-4687.

247. Mlcochova Petra, Kemp Steven A, Dhar Mahesh Shanker, et al. Indian SARS-CoV-2 Genomics Consortium (INSACOG); Genotype to Phenotype Japan (G2P-Japan) Consortium; CITIID-NIHR BioResource COVID-19 Collaboration. SARS-CoV-2 B.1.617.2 Delta variant replication and immune evasion. *Nature.* 2021;599(7883):114–119. doi:10.1038/s41586-021-03944-y. 34488225 1476-4687.

248. Suryadevara Naveenchandra, Shrihari Swathi, Gilchuk Pavlo, et al. Neutralizing and protective human ™monoclonal antibodies recognizing the N-terminal domain of the SARS-CoV-2 spike protein. *Cell.* 2021;184(9):2316–2331. doi:10.1016/j.cell.2021.03.029. 33773105 e151097-4172.

249. McCallum Matthew, Czudnochowski Nadine, Rosen Laura E, et al. Structural basis of SARS-CoV-2 Omicron immune evasion and receptor engagement. *Science.* 2022;375(6583):864–868. doi:10.1126/science.abn8652. 35076256 1095-9203.

250. Ku Zhiqiang, Xie Xuping, Davidson Edgar, et al. Molecular determinants and mechanism for antibody cocktail preventing SARS-CoV-2 escape. *Nat Commun.* 2021;12(1):469. doi:10.1038/s41467-020-20789-7. 33473140 2041-1723.

251. Zhang Xiantao, Wu Shijian, Wu Bolin, et al. SARS-CoV-2 Omicron strain exhibits potent capabilities for immune evasion and viral entrance. *Signal Transduct Target Ther.* 2021;6(1):430. doi:10.1038/s41392-021-00852-5. 34921135 2059-3635.

252. Tseng Hung Fu, Ackerson Bradley K, Luo Yi, et al. Effectiveness of mRNA-1273 against SARS-CoV-2 Omicron and Delta variants. *Nat Med.* 2022:1546. doi:10.1038/s41591-022-01753-y. 35189624 -170X.

253. Cele Sandile, Jackson Laurelle, Khoury David S, et al. Omicron extensively but incompletely escapes Pfizer BNT162b2 neutralization. *Nature.* 2022;602(7898):654–656. doi:10.1038/s41586-021-04387-1. 35016196 1476-4687.

254. Mannar Dhiraj, Saville James W, Zhu Xing, et al. SARS-CoV-2 Omicron variant: Antibody evasion and cryo-EM structure of spike protein-ACE2 complex. *Science.* 2022;375(6582):760–764. doi:10.1126/science.abn7760. 35050643 1095-9203.

255. Gruell Henning, Vanshylla Kanika, Tober-Lau Pinkus, et al. mRNA booster immunization elicits potent neutralizing serum activity against the SARS-CoV-2 Omicron variant. *Nat Med.* 2022:1546. doi:10.1038/s41591-021-01676-0. 35046572 -170X.

256. Zou Jing, Xia Hongjie, Xie Xuping, et al. Neutralization against Omicron SARS-CoV-2 from previous non-Omicron infection. *Nat Commun.* 2022;13(1):852. doi:10.1038/s41467-022-28544-w. 35140233 2041-1723.

257. Buchrieser Julian, Dufloo Jérémy, Hubert Mathieu, et al. Syncytia formation by SARS-CoV-2-infected cells. *EMBO J.* 2020;39(23):e106267. doi:10.15252/embj.2020106267. 33051876 1460-2075.

258. Liu Lihong, Iketani Sho, Guo Yicheng, et al. Striking antibody evasion manifested by the Omicron variant of SARS-CoV-2. *Nature.* 2022;602(7898):676–681. doi:10.1038/s41586-021-04388-0. 35016198 1476-4687.

259. Han Pengcheng, Li Linjie, Liu Sheng, et al. Receptor binding and complex structures of human ACE2 to spike RBD from omicron and delta SARS-CoV-2. *Cell.* 2022;185(4):630–640. doi:10.1016/j.cell.2022.01.001. 35093192 e101097-4172.

260. Hui Kenrie P Y, Ho John C W, Cheung Man-Chun, et al. SARS-CoV-2 Omicron variant replication in human bronchus and lung ex vivo. *Nature.* 2022. doi:10.1038/s41586-022-04479-6. 35104836 1476-4687.

261. Shuai Huiping, Chan Jasper Fuk-Woo, Hu Bingjie, et al. Attenuated replication and pathogenicity of SARS-CoV-2 B.1.1.529 Omicron. *Nature.* 2022. doi:10.1038/s41586-022-04442-5. 35062016 1476-4687.

Part I

CHAPTER

3 Immunology of COVID-19

Robert S. Wallis, MD, FIDSA, FRCPE, Amit K. Srivastava, PhD, Andreas Wack, PhD, and Charles A. Knirsch, MD, MPH

The extraordinary global spread of SARS-CoV-2 through naïve populations provides compelling evidence of both the strengths and limitations of the human immune response: on the one hand, recognizing and eliminating a novel viral pathogen, while on the other, causing potentially lethal immunopathological conditions (Fig. 3.1). The pandemic also provided a striking opportunity to understand SARS-CoV-2 pathogenesis through a lens offered by multiple clinical trials. COVID-19 disease seems best considered in two phases: a brief early phase with high-level viral replication and limited immune responses, and a later phase in which these are reversed. A minority of infected persons progress to life-threatening illness in the later phase of infection, with striking consistency across diverse populations. Except for age, the risk for progression in most individuals cannot yet be attributed to a single critical social, economic, environmental, or genetic factor. For immunologists, the key emerging research questions regard how early responses to SARS-CoV-2 affect subsequent risks for severe disease and the underlying protective and pathogenic mechanisms. To this end, this chapter will discuss innate and adaptive immune responses to SARS-CoV-2 infection, the role of immune dysregulation and its contribution to severe pathological processes, and the potential role of endotypes to guide future studies of immunotherapy.

Innate Immune Responses

Early responses to many infections are driven by activation of cellular pattern recognition receptors (PRRs). Genetic sequences for these receptors are fixed: unlike immunoglobulin or T-cell receptor genes, they do not undergo rearrangement in somatic cells. PRRs located on cell membranes, such as Toll-like receptors (TLRs), are generally triggered by microbial ligands, whereas those in the cytoplasm may be triggered by indicators of molecular damage (damage-associated molecular patterns [DAMPs]) or by RNA or DNA with specific characteristics. As a single-stranded RNA virus, SARS-CoV-2 may be recognized by TLRs 7 or 8 (recognizing single-stranded RNA), retinoic acid–inducible gene I (RIG-Ia) (recognizing uncapped viral RNA), or melanoma differentiation–associated protein 5 (MDA5), an RIG-I–like PRR recognizing long double-stranded cytosolic RNA. PRR triggering results in a signaling cascade that includes production of interferons (IFNs), so named in the 1950s for their ability to interfere with virus propagation (Fig. 3.2).[1] Many IFN-stimulated genes (ISGs) encode proteins with direct antiviral effects[2] (Fig. 3.3). The breadth of ISG responses hampers the emergence of viral avoidance mechanisms,[3] although viruses nonetheless devote substantial genomic space in an attempt to do so.[4] This competition between viruses and host cells is one of the strongest drivers of protein adaptation in mammalian evolution.[5] Emerging evidence indicates that the enhanced transmissibility of new SARS-CoV-2 variants is due in part to enhanced evasion of innate responses.[6]

The IFN-driven innate response to viral infections has three important functions: creating an intracellular milieu that limits viral replication, recruiting immune cells to the site of infection, and priming an adaptive immune response through the expression of costimulatory molecules. However, the very breadth of the innate response can also pose significant costs to the host. This is best illustrated by clinical experience with various forms of recombinant IFN-α, which, for more than a decade, was combined with ribavirin for treatment of chronic hepatitis C virus infection. Together, these drugs could cure about half of patients; factors increasing the likelihood of cure included low pretreatment levels of IFN-induced protein 10 (IP-10).[7,8] However, IFN treatments were poorly tolerated, with black box warnings of fatal or life-threatening neuropsychiatric, hematological,

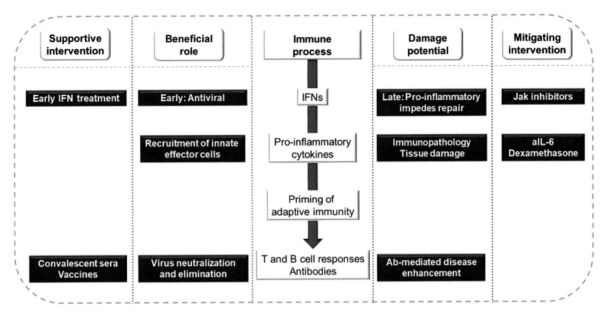

Fig. 3.1 The immune processes involved with beneficial and damaging responses to SARS-CoV-2 infection in humans is outlined with high level supportive and mitigating interventions.

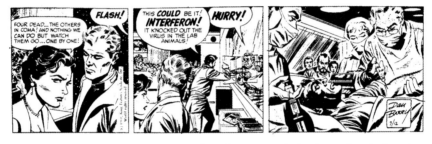

Fig. 3.2 A Flash Gordon comic strip from 1960 depicting the use of interferon to combat a virus outbreak aboard a space craft. (Flash Gordon © 1960 King Features Syndicate, Inc.)

autoimmune, ischemic, and infectious disorders. In routine clinical use, less than 25% of patients were able to complete a full course of treatment.[9] The IFN regimens have largely fallen out of use now that alternatives (direct-acting antiviral drugs) are available.[7]

IFN appears essential for protection against SARS-CoV-2, based on reports of life-threatening disease in persons with inborn errors or autoantibodies affecting pathways for type I IFNs (α and β).[10,11] Early IFN responses appear insufficient for optimal control of viral replication even in the absence of recognized immune defects. The clearest evidence for this comes from a small trial in which 60 newly diagnosed COVID-19 outpatients were administered a single dose of pegylated IFN-λ (PEG–IFN-λ) or placebo.[12] IFN recipients were more likely to have undetectable virus by day 7 (odds ratio [OR], 4.12; $P = .029$). The benefit was greatest in those with high viral loads at baseline. Receptors for IFN-λ (a type III IFN) are expressed on epithelial cells but not on lymphocytes, potentially preserving efficacy while increasing safety and tolerability.[13–15] Further

trials comparing subtypes of the IFN-α, β, or λ families are underway to test this hypothesis.

A trial conducted in Hong Kong examined the addition of IFN-β plus ribavirin to lopinavir/ritonavir in 127 patients.[16] Although subjects in this trial were inpatients, its patient population was similar to that of the IFN-λ trial, in that only 13% required supplemental oxygen at baseline. IFN treatment yielded a shorter median time to negative polymerase chain reaction (PCR) (7 vs. 12 days; $P = .0010$), and a shorter time to resolution of symptoms (4 vs. 8 days; $P < .0001$). In contrast, the World Health Organization Solidarity Trial examined IFN-β treatment in 243 hospitalized patients, most of whom already required oxygen therapy.[17] In this population with more advanced disease, IFN treatment tended to increase mortality risk compared with controls (relative risk [RR], 1.16; $P = .11$). Similarly, a retrospective study published early in the pandemic suggested that the likelihood of survival was increased by early IFN-α treatment (within 5 days of hospitalization), whereas survival was

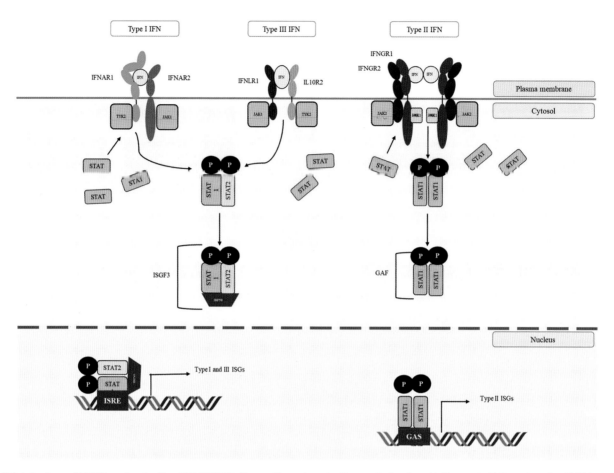

Fig. 3.3 Interferon (IFN) Signaling by the JAK-STAT Pathway. Reproduced with permission from Hoffman et al.[2] Once type I or III IFNs engage their cognate receptors at the cell surface, individual receptor chains are brought into close proximity. As a result, intracellular receptor-associated tyrosine kinases of the Janus kinase (JAK) family of proteins are juxtaposed and become activated. Activated JAK proteins subsequently phosphorylate (P) members of the signal transducer and activator of transcription (STAT) family of proteins, ultimately leading to the transcriptional activation of IFN-stimulated genes (ISGs). Inasmuch as is currently known, after receptor engagement, type I and III IFNs signal through the same pathway: activation of the two JAK proteins, JAK1 and TYK2, results in the phosphorylation of conserved tyrosine residues on STAT1 and STAT2, followed by formation of a heterotrimeric complex with IFN-regulatory factor 9 (IRF9). This complex, referred to as IFN-stimulated gene factor 3 (ISGF3), translocates to the nucleus and binds to a DNA sequence known as the IFN-stimulated response element (ISRE) in the promoters of ISGs. As a result, hundreds of ISGs are transcriptionally regulated. In addition to stimulating transcription of numerous genes, IFN signaling also leads to the transcriptional repression of a variety of genes; however, the underlying mechanisms and outcomes are comparatively underexplored. GAF, g-Interferon activation factor; GAS, g-interferon activation site. (Reproduced with permission from Hoffmann HH, Schneider WM, Rice CM. Interferons and viruses: an evolutionary arms race of molecular interactions. Trends Immunol. 2015;36[3]:124–138.)

reduced if IFN was started later.[18] Several studies have confirmed that IFN levels correlate generally with COVID-19 disease severity; that is, IFN levels are highest in persons with severe disease.[19–22] One study suggests that mutations outside of the spike coding region contributed to the evolutionary success of SARS-CoV-2 variants (most notably alpha) through the enhanced suppression of innate responses.[188] However, it seems that for later variants, evasion of antibody responses (induced by vaccination or prior infection with early lineage strains) may better account for evolutionary success (discussed below).

Together, these studies support a hypothesis that innate responses during early SARS-CoV-2 infection are insufficient for viral control, and that the subsequent amplification of these responses contributes to immunopathological processes.

Adaptive Immune Responses

The humoral and cellular arms of the adaptive immune system are integrally linked with innate immune mechanisms in the overall response to viral infection. Distinct mechanisms of each system are engaged differently depending on virus type, the timing of a response, and the cell types involved (Table 3.1). Unlike innate responses, which recognize patterns shared by many pathogens, adaptive immune responses recognize specific antigenic sequences of specific pathogens. The required receptor diversity is accomplished by gene rearrangements for antigen receptors or immunoglobulin regions early in the development of T and B cells, respectively. Antigen recognition triggers both cellular activation and clonal expansion. Depending on the frequency of precursor cells and the nature of the stimulus,

Table 3.1 Immune Cell Type Overview

	Dendritic Cells	Macrophage	B Cell	CD4+ T cell	CD8+ T cell
Location	Skin, mucosal epithelium (Langerhans cells), bone marrow, blood, spleen, thymus, tonsil, liver, lung, intestine, lymph nodes[165]	Throughout the body[166]	Blood, peripheral lymphoid organs[167]	Throughout body[168]	Throughout body[168]
Function	Antigen-presenting cell of innate immune system. Both extracellular and intracellular antigens[169]	Antigen-presenting cell of innate immune system. Extracellular antigens[170,171]	Adaptive immunity: Antibody production. Antigen-presenting cell. Effector cell killing of infected cells[172,173]	Effector cell terminating infection. B-cell help. CD8+ cell help. Cellular memory. Type 1 intracellular and type 2 extracellular (e.g., helminths) response to infections[174,175]	Effector cytotoxic killing of infected cells. Type 1 response to intracellular infections[174,176]
Specific antigen receptors	No[177]	No[170]	Surface immunoglobulins[178]	TCR[179]	TCR[174]
Differentiation	cDC1 and cDC2[180]	M1 and M2[181]	Memory B cells. Plasma cells[172]	Tfh-promoting B cell response in lymphoid tissue. Treg: Maintenance of immunological tolerance to self and foreign antigen. Th1: Eliminates intracellular pathogens and associated with organ-specific autoimmunity. Th2: Produces an immune response against extracellular parasites, and play major role in induction and persistence of asthma and other allergic diseases. Th17: Produces immune response against extracellular bacteria and fungi. Also involved in the generation of autoimmune diseases[175]	Tc1: Immune response against intracellular pathogens and tumors. Tc2: Th2-mediated allergic reaction, contributes to arthritis. Tc9: Inhibits CD4+ T-cell mediated colitis, propagates Th2-mediated allergic reaction, antitumor response. Tc17: Propagates autoimmunity, confers immunity to viral infections, antitumor response. CD8+ Treg: Regulates T-cell–mediated responses[182]
Costimulation/cytokines	ICOS,[183] CD28[177]	M1 is induced as a response to infectious stimuli (e.g., LPS and/or IFN-γ) and M2 is induced by resolving stimuli (e.g., IL-4)[184]	IL-21, IL-4, CD40L[178]	CD28[179]	CD28[185]
Interferon production	Type I and type III interferons[169]	Type I interferons[170]	IFN-γ[186]	IFN-γ[175]	Type I interferon protects antiviral CD8+ T cells from NK cell cytotoxicity[187]

cDC, Classic dendritic cells; ICOS, inducible T-cell costimulator; IFN-γ, interferon-gamma; LPS, lipopolysaccharides; MHC, major histocompatibility complex; TCR, T-cell receptor; Tfh, T follicular helper cells; Treg, regulatory T cells.

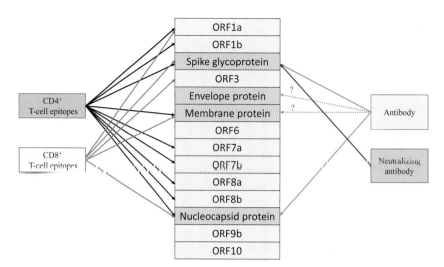

Fig. 3.4 SARS-CoV-2 Proteins Targeted by Adaptive Immune Responses. The four structural proteins are shown in the *red boxes*. Non-structural proteins and accessory factors are shown in the *blue boxes*. *Arrows* link antibodies to the viral proteins they target and identify viral proteins shown to contain epitopes targeted by CD4+ T cells or CD8+ T cells. *SARS-CoV-2,* severe acute respiratory syndrome coronavirus 2. (Reproduced with permission from Poland GA, Ovsyannikova IG, Kennedy RB. SARS-CoV-2 immunity: review and applications to phase 3 vaccine candidates. *Lancet.* 2020;396[10262]:1595-1606.)

a period of days to weeks must elapse for the evolution of a primary adaptive immune response.[23–25]

The neutralizing antibodies produced by B lymphocytes and plasma cells play a critical role in preventing SARS-CoV-2 infection in uninfected individuals and restricting viral replication in those already infected. Initial immunoglobulin M (IgM) antibody responses are often of limited binding avidity and functional capacity. The evolution of these responses to include other antibody isotypes with greater avidity and broader functionality (including IgA and IgG subtypes) requires the engagement of T helper (Th) cell lymphocytes. Antigens are presented in the form of short peptides by dendritic cells, macrophages, and B-lymphocytes. Presentation occurs in the context of major histocompatibility complex (MHC) (human leukocyte antigen [HLA]) determinants displayed on the cell surface together with appropriate costimulatory molecules. This process initiates the selection of antigen-specific naïve B and T lymphocytes for further clonal expansion (Fig. 3.4).

Variations in the character and timing of these responses give us clues to the relationship and relative roles of the innate and adaptive immune systems in defenses against COVID-19. Recovery is delayed in the absence of IgG responses (in persons with agammaglobulinemia), with cases reported in which disease progression continued until convalescent serum replacement therapy was administered.[26] Poor outcomes have been reported for individuals requiring treatment with anti–B-cell monoclonal antibodies, with the clinical severity of illness dependent on the extent of the humoral immune deficit.[27] Early decreases in the numbers of lymphocytes or dendritic cells (hindering the clonal expansion of pathogen-specific T and B cells) are similarly associated with sustained viral replication and

poor clinical outcomes.[28,29] These findings establish a critical role for neutralizing antibodies in defenses against SARS-CoV-2 infection.

Antibody Responses

Two key studies confirm the importance of the SARS-CoV-2 spike protein receptor binding domain (RBD) as a critical antigen for host immune responses. The first study found that RBD antibody accounted for 90% of neutralizing activity in convalescent patient sera.[30] The second found that most convalescent sera with high neutralizing titers specifically targeted the spike protein and its RBD.[31] These findings are consistent with current understanding of the role of the viral spike glycoprotein mediating cell entry by binding to the human angiotensin-converting enzyme-2 (ACE2) receptor.[32,33] Additional cross-sectional studies of hospitalized patients acutely infected with COVID-19 detected RBD-specific IgG neutralizing titers within a week of PCR diagnosis,[34] with their magnitude associated with disease severity.[35] In contrast, antibodies against the SARS-CoV-2 nucleocapsid protein are generally nonneutralizing and not associated with severity.[36] These studies confirm the importance of the spike protein as a critical antigen for a beneficial host immune response.

Although SARS-CoV-2 is a new pathogen, it belongs to a yet-evolving extended family of coronaviruses. Researchers have hypothesized that prior immunity to related pathogens might explain the wide diversity of SARS-CoV-2 clinical outcomes. Several studies have examined cross-reactivity of convalescent SARS-CoV-2 patient sera to previously characterized viruses. One study of the spike antigen found no cross-reactivity with the highly homologous pre-pandemic bat coronavirus

WIV1-CoV.[37] Another found little correlation between responses to the RBDs of SARS-CoV-2 and the endemic HKU1 and NL63 human coronaviruses or to antigens of influenza or respiratory syncytial virus.[38] A related hypothesis posits that even in the absence of detectable cross-reactivity, individuals with immune memory to related viruses might acquire adaptive responses to SARS-CoV-2 more rapidly.[39,40] However, a large study characterizing spike RBD antibody kinetics and isotype profiles in SARS-CoV-2 cases and pre-pandemic controls demonstrated no cross-reactivity with RBDs of Middle East respiratory syndrome coronavirus (MERS-CoV) or endemic human coronaviruses, although cross-reactivity was indeed found for SARS-CoV-1.[41] Together, these findings suggest that common prior viral infections, including endemic human coronaviruses, do not influence the functional evolution of immunity to SARS-CoV-2.

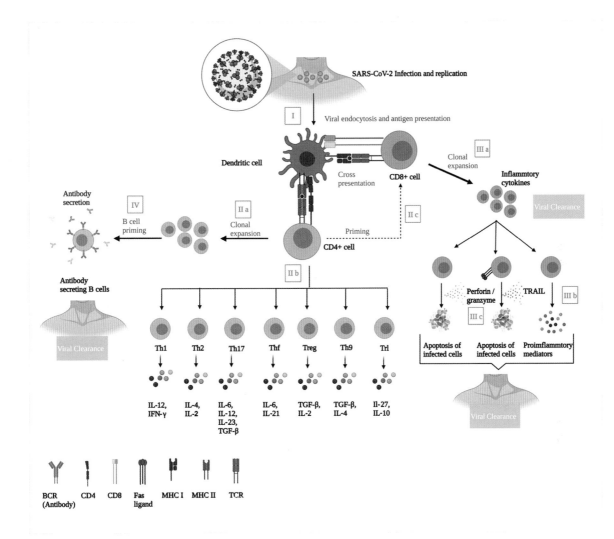

Fig. 3.5 SARS-CoV-2 and the Innate and Adaptive Immune System Responses. Stepwise explanation for the figure:
1. SARS-COV-2 infection leads to uptake by macrophages and dendritic cells for presentation to CD4+ and CD8+ cells.
2. **a.** CD4+ cells undergo clonal expansion.
   b. CD4+ cells undergo further differentiation to cells with distinct functional characteristics.
   c. CD4+ cells prime CD8+ cells.
3. **a.** CD8+ cells undergo clonal expansion.
   b. CD8+ cells further produce inflammatory cytokines.
   c. The inflammatory cytokines lead to apoptosis of cells.
4. CD4+ cells prime B cells to facilitate antibody secretion.
The dendritic cell presents peptide fragments to CD4+ cells complexed with MHC-II molecules. CD4+ cells undergo clonal expansion and further differentiation to prime B cells and CD8+ T cells; CD4+ cells differentiate further into functional cell types that produce inflammatory cytokines and regulatory molecules. CD8+ cells undergo clonal expansion when presented with peptide fragments complexed to MHC-I molecules and elaborate substances such as the cytokine TRAIL, perforin, granzyme, and other proinflammatory mediators. *BCR,* B-cell receptor; *IFN-γ,* interferon gamma; *IL,* interleukin; *MHC,* major histocompatibility complex; *SARS-CoV-2,* severe acute respiratory syndrome coronavirus 2; *TCR,* T-cell receptor; *TGF-β,* transforming growth factor-beta; *Th,* T helper cell; *Thf,* follicular T helper cell; *TNF,* tumor necrosis factor; *TRAIL,* TNF-related apoptosis-inducing ligand; *Treg,* regulatory T cell; *Trl,* type 1 regulatory T cell. (Figure created with BioRender.com.)

T-Cell Responses and Repertoire

T cells can be characterized according to expressed cell surface proteins detected by flow cytometry. The largest T-cell population, CD4+ helper lymphocytes, recognize peptide fragments from virus proteins complexed with MHC class II molecules (Fig. 3.5). CD4+ T cells can be differentiated further into T follicular helper (Tfh), Th1 or Th2 cells,[42] and others. Tfh cells are essential for antibody affinity maturation and isotype switching. They provide help to B cells in lymph nodes and influence naïve B cells to differentiate to become antibody-producing plasma cells.[43] Tfh cells also are able to provide help to accelerate responses in cases of reinfection or in vaccinated individuals. Th1 cells show antiviral properties such as IFN-γ production. T cells that are already optimized as a result of previous viral antigen exposure and often reside in respiratory epithelium are termed resident memory T cells (Trms). Their cellular properties and anatomic location facilitate rapid responses to infection. The Th2 signature pathway for CD4+ cells has not been a significant feature of SARS-CoV-2 infection. This is fortunate, given its relationship to antibody-dependent disease enhancement and cytokine profiles associated with poor clinical outcomes in other viral diseases, including the experience and lessons learned from respiratory syncytial virus (RSV) infection after formalin-inactivated RSV vaccine administration.[44,45] CD4+ T cells additionally recruit innate immune cells to sites of infection and support the clonal expansion of CD8+ T cells.[46] CD8+ T cells in turn can eliminate infected cells through the cytolytic activities of granzyme, perforin, IFN, and TNF-a.

Several elegant studies have examined adaptive immune responses and SARS-CoV-2 epitopes at different points of time in COVID-19 disease, from acute infection to convalescence or terminal illness.[24] Two studies paved the way for vaccine development by demonstrating that SARS-CoV-2 infection induces natural immunity and protects against reinfection in nonhuman primates and that neutralizing antibodies against the SARS-CoV-2 spike protein played a key role in protection.[47,48] T-cell responses to the spike protein can be detected within 7 days of infection; these are followed by B-cell responses associated with symptom onset (IgM and IgA by days 5–7, IgG by days 7–10). Antibody and T-cell levels decline after the acute phase of infection; serological memory is maintained by a small number of long-lived bone marrow plasma cells that constitutively secrete antibody and subsequently provide accelerated booster responses after reexposure.[23]

Studies of T cells in patients from the SARS-CoV-1 outbreak in 2003 showed evidence of long-lived recognition of the nucleocapsid (N) structural protein of the virus; when similar assays were performed in convalescent COVID-19 patients, there was evidence of CD4+ and CD8+ T-cell recognition of multiple epitopes on the SARS-CoV-2 N protein as well.[49] In studies with all proteins of SARS-CoV-2 represented, the transmembrane (M) and spike (S) proteins were codominant, with N proteins indicating a different pattern of response to epitopes than with the SARS-CoV-1 outbreak in 2003.[50] A small study of 12 patients characterized cellular immunity, antibody levels, and respiratory SARS-CoV-2 viral load by PCR cycle time and demonstrated that moderate and severe disease status had higher SARS-CoV-2 antibody responses compared with mild clinical syndromes in which early IFN-g production indicated a T-cell response correlated with mild disease and a shorter illness.[51] More recently in a study of nearly 100 convalescent COVID-19 patients evaluating T-cell immunodominance, the S and M SARS-CoV-2 proteins determined CD4+ helper cells' functional roles for both B-cell help producing RBD antibodies and to CD8+ T-cell responses.[52] CD8+ T cells also have been found to have an important role in decreasing severity of illness; in studies using peptide pools, CD8+ cells are notable for a broad response to viral protein epitopes albeit with different patterns of immunodominance compared with CD4+ cells.[52] CD4+ cell responses to SARS-CoV-2 antigens are most robust in persons recovering from mild COVID-19 disease, whereas antibody production and killing of infected cells by CD8+ T cells predominate in persons with severe disease.[46] Studies with candidate vaccines have demonstrated that SARS-CoV-2 spike induces multiple arms of the immune system, including specific CD4+ and CD8+ T cells and nonneutralizing antibodies that mediate antibody-dependent cytotoxicity.[51,53]

Coverage of Emerging Variants

As SARS-CoV-2 propagates among the global human and nonhuman population, the virus continues to accumulate mutations as a result of natural evolution and immune pressure. Although coronaviruses have been reported to be 10-fold less error-prone than other RNA viruses because of the presence of a proofreading replicase enzyme,[54] natural viral evolution during the pandemic has spawned SARS-CoV-2 variants with distinct mutations in the spike protein. For these emerging variants, we have different levels of scientific understanding of their transmissibility, pathogenicity, and ability for immune escape, though undoubtedly the variants have significantly changed our understanding and concerns regarding the COVID-19 pandemic.[55–57] Variants were noted, beginning with the notable D614G spike protein mutant that has shown a modest ability for faster spread,[58] and the mink variant with multiple mutations (e.g., "cluster 5") that demonstrate spillover transmission across species and highlights the risk for incrementally evolved SARS-CoV-2 viruses with broad host range and/or greater pathogenicity.[59–61] More recently the global public health community has increased the monitoring of emerging SARS-CoV-2 variants more purposefully with stepped up genomic surveillance and a classification scheme of (1) variant being monitored-primarily where data indicates association with increase in transmissibilty or disease severity but surveillance shows very low levels of circulation; (2) variant of interest—primarily with a predicted increase in transmissibility or disease severity; (2) variant of concern—primarily with evidence of an increase in transmissibility, pathogenicity (i.e., causing more severe disease), significant reduction in antibody neutralization, and vaccine effectiveness of treatments or vaccines; and (3) variant of high consequence—with clear evidence that prevention measures or medical countermeasures have significantly reduced effectiveness.[62,63] Among the prominent identified variants: alpha (B.1.1.7, first detected in the United Kingdom), beta (B.1.351; first detected in South Africa), and gamma (P.1; first detected in Brazil), were variants of concern but are now being monitored, and current variants of concern include delta (B.1.617.2 and AY lineages; first detected in India), but no identified variants of high consequence.[62–64,192,208] The latest nomenclature uses Greek letters for variants of concern[65] and is a departure from the influenza virus naming convention using place of origin and critical mutations.

One study of convalescent patient sera found cross-neutralization of both wild-type and D614G mutant SARS-CoV-2 spike antigens.[37] However, immune evasion was thought partly responsible for a resurgence of COVID-19 cases in Manaus, Brazil in November 2020, which occurred despite previously high levels of infection.[66] The resurgence was temporally associated with the emergence of new SARS-CoV-2 lineage (P.1) with three mutations in the spike protein, potentially increasing ACE2 binding and reducing neutralization by wild-type convalescent sera. Partial antibody resistance also has been described for variants alpha and beta causing second waves of infection in the United Kingdom and South Africa.[67,68]

Interpretation of these findings is handicapped by an incomplete understanding of the relationship of neutralizing antibody titers to protection from infection and/or disease. Neutralization assays may use either authentic SARS-CoV-2 viruses, or pseudoviruses in which specific SARS-CoV-2 proteins are expressed in other viral vectors such as human immunodeficiency virus-1 (HIV-1) or vesicular stomatitis virus, using well-characterized assay systems. A prototypical study early in the pandemic that collected convalescent sera from 149 patients of varying severity found a wide range of half-maximal neutralizing titers (NT_{50}s).[69] Only 1% of samples showed very high titers (>5000); the majority were less than 1000, and one-third were less than 50. Interestingly, nonhuman primate challenge studies have reported circulating neutralizing antibody titers of 1:20 or greater in animals protected from

SARS-CoV-2 infection.[25] Generally, however, the levels in most convalescent sera are broadly comparable to those after full vaccination in individuals receiving mRNA, adenoviral vector, or whole-virus inactivated vaccines.[215–217]

To date, all variants tested have been neutralized in vitro by immune sera from individuals vaccinated with mRNA, viral vector, or inactivated vaccines, although reduction in neutralization titers have been observed with particular variants.[70,188] Studies have shown that certain mutations and variants (E484K mutation in particular) are able to escape neutralization by convalescent plasma and monoclonal antibodies that target single epitopes.[67,71,72] Vaccine-elicited sera were able to neutralize engineered SARS-CoV-2 viruses containing key variant spike mutations in vitro, such as E484K, L452R, and N501Y mutations.[60,73–81] Studies of cellular immune responses to SARS-CoV-2 variants in recovered COVID-19 patients demonstrated that CD4+ and CD8+ T cells have broad responses to multiple epitopes compared with neutralizing antibodies to the S protein involved with humoral immunity;[48] this could bode well for the durability of vaccine-induced T-cell responses, given ongoing mutations of SARS-CoV-2 virus that have demonstrable effects in vitro on the amount of antibody needed to neutralize SARS-COV-2.

Reduced efficacy against clinical disease was observed in late-stage vaccine clinical trials in regions with high circulation of emerging variants. Interim analysis in January 2021 for an adenoviral vector vaccine (Ad26.COV2.S) in a single-dose regimen reported 66% efficacy overall against moderate to severe COVID-19, with 72% efficacy in the United States and 66% efficacy in Latin America cohorts, but efficacy dropped to 57% in the South African cohort, wherein 95% of the accrued cases were caused by the beta variant.[82,83] Similarly, phase III results for the adjuvanted protein subunit vaccine NVX-CoV2372 showed 89.3% efficacy in the UK cohort, in which more than 50% of accrued cases were caused by the alpha variant; efficacy in the South African cohort was 51%, with 93% of the accrued cases caused by the beta variant.[84] On the other hand, reassuring real-world vaccine effectiveness data have been accumulating from national immunization programs for COVID-19 vaccines. Two doses of BNT162b2 mRNA vaccine demonstrated high real-world vaccine effectiveness against circulating variants of concern: in Israel, BNT162b2 demonstrated 90% to 96% effectiveness against SARS-CoV-2 infection, asymptomatic infection, symptomatic COVID-19, severe and critical hospitalizations, and deaths during the period of high circulation (94%) of the alpha variant.[85] Similarly, from Qatar's national immunization program, a two-dose regimen of BNT162b2 demonstrated 89% effectiveness against alpha variant infection; 75% against beta variant infection; and 100% against severe, critical, or fatal COVID-19 caused by alpha or beta variants.[86] A two-dose regimen of mRNA-1273 demonstrated 100% effectiveness against alpha infection; 96% against beta infection; and 96% against severe, critical, or fatal COVID-19 caused by these two variants.[87] In the UK national immunization program, two-dose BNT162b2 mRNA effectiveness was 93.4%, with alpha cases and 87.9% with delta cases, and two-dose ChAdOx1 effectiveness was 66% with alpha cases and 59.8% with delta cases.[88] Vaccine effectiveness against the delta variant has been reported from national immunization programs in the United Kingdom and Canada. A two-dose regimen of BNT162b2 or ChAdOx1 vaccine demonstrated between 83% and 88% and 61% and 67% effectiveness, respectively, against symptomatic COVID-19. Scotland reported 79% and 60% effectiveness against SARs-CoV-2 infection; Canada reported that a two-dose regimen of BNT162b2 was 95% effective against hospitalization or death.[89–91] Data for two doses of an inactivated SARS-CoV-2 vaccine (Coronavac) from Chile indicated 66% to 90% effectiveness against COVID-19, hospitalization, intensive care unit (ICU) admission, and COVID-19–related death.[92] Brazil reported that in adults older than 70 years, effectiveness was 42% against symptomatic COVID-19, 59% against hospitalization, and 71% against death.[93] Systematic reviews of vaccine effectiveness data across multiple vaccine platforms, dosing intervals, varied geographies and assorted SARS-CoV-2 variants in circulation are now available.[189,190] In addition, the first real world data are now available for effectiveness of maternal vaccination using mRNA vaccines: 2-dose COVID-19 mRNA maternal vaccination during pregnancy showed 61% VE against COVID-19 hospitalization in infants <6 months, during a period of delta and omicron variant predominance in the USA.[214] Although no substantial clinical evidence of variant escape from vaccine-mediated protection has emerged,[192] vaccine manufacturers and regulatory bodies are building clinical evidence and frameworks for redesigning vaccines and/or booster vaccines using either the ancestral strain of SARS-CoV-2 or the emerging variants, if the need arises.[94] The most recently emerged SARS-CoV-2 variant – oicron (B.1.1.529 and BA lineages) has at least 30 mutations in the spike protein, half of which are in receptor binding domain[61–63,207] (RBD) that interacts with the host ACE2, receptor Furthermore, omicron does not appear to be the result of a linear progression from its immediate predecessor – delta, prevalent in 2021 – in an easily predictable fashion, but rather it appears to have evolved from the alpha variant prevalent in 2020.[193] In part due to it's significantly divergent sequence that enables immune evasion, omicron is highly transmissible and has spread rapidly to become the dominant circulating strain in most parts of the world.[194,195] Initial observations indicate a comparatively mild clinical *phenotype*,[196–201] and multiple studies have shown that neutralizing antibody responses are substantially diminished post-2-dose vaccination while T-cell responses appear to be preserved,[202] and a 3rd vaccine dose confers protection against omicron-related hospitalization and severe disease.[189,190,203–206]

Durability of Immunity

Early evidence indicated that protective immunity against seasonal CoVs is short term, that is, lasting 6 to 12 months, based on data derived from a 35-years-long epidemiological study examining frequency of reinfection with seasonal CoVs—NL63, 229E, OC43, and HKU1 in a cohort of individuals—as a measure of natural immunity.[95] In a 2020 large US serosurvey of more than 30,000 individuals who tested positive for SARS-CoV-2, more than 90% had detectable neutralizing antibody responses and antibody titers were stable over 3 months with modest declines at 5 months.[96] Another study measured risk of reinfection in a cohort of 12,000 health care workers based on the presence of antibodies to SARS-CoV-2 antibodies and found that postinfection immunity is associated with protection from reinfection for most individuals, for at least 6 months.[97] In population-level serosurveillance in Iceland of PCR-positive persons (n = 30,576), more than 90% remained seropositive 120 days after diagnosis, with no decline detected in antibody levels.[98] Two recent studies with convalescent patients showed that antibodies to SARS-CoV-2 persist for nearly 1 year after infection. One study with 77 convalescent individuals monitored regularly over 1 year showed that SARS-CoV-2 spike-specific antibodies were detectable 11 months after infection, showing a rapid decline for 4 months and a slower decline in the subsequent 7 months; furthermore, spike-specific bone marrow plasma cells persisted for 7 to 8 months in a subset of this convalescent cohort, indicating the stable presence of memory B cells.[99] A similar second study in convalescent patients (n = 63), approximately 40% of whom were vaccinated with at least one dose of mRNA vaccine, also demonstrated the stable presence of SARS-CoV-2 spike-specific antibodies and memory B cells 6 to 12 months after infection.[100] Very few reinfections with the wild-type or ancestral SARS-CoV-2 strain have been reported, and generally the subsequent disease episode has been less severe than the first, suggesting benefit from the protective immune responses triggered during the first infection.[100–102]

For SARS-CoV-2 mRNA vaccines authorized for emergency use, data on longer-term persistence of vaccine-elicited immune responses will become available as the participants from the phase III vaccine clinical studies are followed for 2 years after primary vaccination.[103] An interim readout of immune persistence has been reported for mRNA-1273[104] and BNT162b2[218] mRNA vaccines, suggesting that antibody binding and neutralization titers were maintained for 3-6 months after primary vaccination among study participants. An Ad vector vaccine against a related coronavirus, ChAdOx1-MERS, showed that vaccine-elicited neutralizing antibodies waned from peak postprimary immunization levels and remained stable above baseline for 1 year or longer.[105] Since COVID-19 mass vaccination programs began in late 2020, real world evidence for the duration of protection has been accumulating. The current state of understanding can be represented by the data available for vaccine effectiveness (VE) of the mRNA vaccine BNT162b2 against the latest circulating variant – omicron: against omicron infection – 2-doses of BNT162b2 conferred limited protection (~50% VE) for only one month and 3-doses increased VE up to 70-80%, with waning observed after the first few months; against omicron-mediated symptomatic COVID-19 – 2-doses of BNT162b2 demonstrated ~40-70% VE and 3-doses increased VE up to ~55-85%, both waning after the first few months; and finally against omicron-mediated hospitalization – 2-doses of BNT162b2 showed ~55-80% VE before 6 months and ~35-80% VE after 6 months after vaccination; 3-doses increased VE to ~75-90% with waning after the first few months.[203,204,206,208–213]

Correlates of Protection

Correlates of protection have been established for many different viral infections, such as influenza, measles, and hepatitis A and B viruses, and bacterial infections, such as pneumococcal and meningococcal disease, and are typically based on the level of antibody that is acquired from vaccination or natural infection that is able to significantly reduce the risk for infection or reinfection.[106,107] However, correlates of protection have yet to be defined for COVID-19,[108,109] in part because antibody and cellular immune responses may differentially affect risk for infection versus progression to severe disease. For a novel disease such as COVID-19, systems serological studies might potentially yield novel immune correlates based on composite antibody and cellular immune measurements. However, more familiar immune correlates, such as spike-specific neutralizing antibody titers, are being deduced from the immunogenicity data reported from the handful of COVID-19 vaccines authorized for emergency use during the pandemic. Modeling the relationship between vaccine-elicited neutralizing antibody titers and observed protection against SARS-CoV-2 infection, normalized against convalescent serum standards,[110,111] at least one study has deduced that a 50% protective titer was 20% of the convalescent level; 50% protective titer against severe disease was even lower, at 3% of the convalescent titer. mRNA vaccines ranked highest in terms of protective efficacy, followed by a protein vaccine; adenoviral vector vaccines ranked at or below convalescent protective titers, and inactivated vaccines ranked the lowest. Finally, modeling the duration of protection predicted that although protection against severe disease will persist, loss of protection against SARS-CoV-2 infection is likely over the first 250 days modeled; in addition, the model predicts erosion in protection against SARS-CoV-2 variants that elicit reduced neutralization titers.[111] Taken together, this would suggest the need for booster vaccine doses potentially on an annual basis to build up population protection against SARS-CoV-2. Development of an immune correlate of protection will catalyze rapid vaccine development for additional populations such as children younger than 12 years, pregnant and lactating women, and those with immunosuppressive conditions, in whom traditional field efficacy trials would be unfeasible. Potentially, it would also streamline the development of vaccines with updated compositions, which might be necessary to combat novel SARS-CoV-2 variants.

Systems Serology and Systems Immunology

Systems serology aims to define the breadth and depth of humoral responses to vaccine antigen(s) by measuring both polyclonal antibody features (antigen-binding portion, Fab and functional properties, and Fc portion) to clarify immune mechanisms and define multifactorial correlates of protection that can help assess vaccine candidates.[112] Molecular techniques have enabled higher resolution understanding of response determinants on both sides of the antigen–antibody reaction. Mining the antigenic proteome with antigen arrays enables screening for unique target epitopes—both linear sequences and conformationally defined epitopes, and the influence of posttranslational modifications such as glycosylation—that may have differential roles across the disease course and reveal the complex nature of elicited antibody response. On the other side, parallelized investigations of antibody downstream signaling, for example, activation of natural killer (NK) cells, monocytes, macrophages, neutrophils, dendritic cells, and effector responses, such as degranulation, cytokines secretion, cytotoxicity, and phagocytosis, help elucidate the complex information relay that triggers the comprehensive immune response to an antigen or pathogen and the dysfunction that often characterizes the deleterious inflammatory response.[112] For a brand-new pathogen such as SARS-CoV-2, this could help identify biomarkers for predicting the COVID-19 trajectory in infected persons. A comprehensive genome map of SARS-CoV-2 created by consensus of experts may facilitate such studies.[113]

Four distinctive immune response profiles that predicted divergent courses of COVID-19 within 10 days of SARS-CoV-2 infection were deduced from longitudinal immune profiling of peripheral blood mononuclear cells and plasma samples from 113 patients with moderate (n = 80) or severe (n = 33) COVID-19. An aberrant immune response with early, elevated proinflammatory cytokines was seen in patients with severe COVID-19 and poor clinical outcomes. In all COVID-19 patients, an overall increase in innate cell lineages such as monocytes, low-density neutrophils, and eosinophils was seen, with a parallel decrease in CD4+ and CD8+ T-cell levels.[19] Similarly, the ratio of neutrophils to lymphocytes emerged as a prognostic biomarker of COVID-19 severity and organ failure from comprehensive immunophenotyping of peripheral blood in 42 convalescent patients with divergent clinical trajectories of SARS-CoV-2 infection and COVID-19 (moderate n = 7, severe n = 28, recovered n = 7) that showed perturbations in multiple leukocyte populations, which distinguished cases of severe COVID-19 from healthy donors, cases of moderate COVID-19, and patients who have recovered from COVID-19.[114]

A study by Mathew et al.[115] found three distinct immunotypes in hospitalized COVID-19 patients that represent patterns of different suboptimal responses to infection: (1) robust activation of CD4+ T cells and highly activated or exhausted CD8+ T cells, (2) less robust CD4+ T cells and highly functional effector-like CD8+ T-cell responses, and (3) a lack of lymphocyte response.

In a cohort of 22 SARS-CoV-2–positive patients (recovered, n = 12; deceased, n = 10), Ateyo et al.[116] identified distinct humoral profiles comprising five antibody features that could differentiate between patients who went on to recover from or succumb to COVID-19. Although the two patient classes showed equivalent magnitude of the responses, convalescent patients showed a more spike-focused humoral response, including phagocytic and complement activity versus deceased patients who showed stronger nucleocapsid (N)-specific responses, poorly coordinated RBD-specific antibody-dependent complement deposition and NK cell functions. A prototypical biomarker—spike-to-N ratio—of humoral response was confirmed in a larger validation cohort of acutely infected individuals (recovered, n = 20; died, n = 20).[116] Similarly, neutralization potency indices predicted disease severity and survival in a cohort of 113 patients infected with SARS-CoV-2 stratified by disease severity and outcomes (i.e., nonhospitalized, hospitalized, intubated, immunosuppressed, and deceased), anti-RBD antibody levels and neutralization titers, indicating that potent SARS-CoV-2–specific neutralizing antibodies appear to increase survival and may protect against reinfection with variants of SARS-CoV-2.[36]

Finally, Dan et al.[24] combined five immune components to devise a composite measurement of SARS-CoV-2 immune memory: RBD-specific IgG, IgA, memory B cells, and SARS-CoV-2–specific CD4+ and CD8+ T cells. They measured circulating SARS-CoV-2 antigen-specific antibodies, memory B cells, and CD8+ and CD4+ T cells for more than 6 months after infection in a cohort of

patients with COVID-19 (n = 188) across a range of disease, including asymptomatic, mild (nonhospitalized), moderate (hospitalized), and severe (hospitalized). They determined that at 1 to 2 months after infection, 59% of individuals were positive for 5 of 5 components, and at 5 months or longer after infection, 40% were positive for 5 of 5 components; however, 96% of individuals were positive for 3 of 5 components.

Immune Dysregulation and Immunopathology

A significant minority of adult COVID-19 patients develop hypoxemic respiratory failure, with diffuse alveolar damage, inflammatory infiltrates, and intravascular thrombosis (involving both large and small blood vessels), often associated with lymphopenia and markedly increased levels of inflammatory markers, including C-reactive protein, D-dimers, interleukin-1 (IL-1), and IL-6.[28,114,117–119] Similar clinical and immunological features have been reported in other severe viral pneumonias, including pandemic influenza, severe acute respiratory syndrome (SARS), and Middle East respiratory syndrome (MERS).[120–123]

In a study of adaptive immune responses with serial paired sampling of systemic and lung compartments in severely ill COVID-19 patients compared with uninfected controls, investigators noted a chemokine signature CCL2-CCR2 associated with myeloid cell recruitment; cells of the innate immune system that in this study were associated with older patients and higher mortality whereas patients with Trm signature T-cell profiles were associated with younger age and lower mortality.[124] Replication of the study with larger numbers will be needed to differentiate among the effects of age, cell profiles, and mortality.

A study of coendemic diseases affecting T-cell function and SARS-CoV-2 described clinical features of 95 hospitalized COVID-19 patients of whom 38 patients were infected with HIV, tuberculosis (TB), or both and compared the CD4+ T-cell responses to 38 hospitalized patients without SARS-COV-2 infection.[125] Severe COVID-19 disease was associated with altered cellular immunity with deficits of CD4+ cell function potential and a reduced capacity to proliferate.

Antibodies may also participate in disease exacerbation, particularly through interactions with cells expressing Fc receptors. These risks, described as antibody-dependent enhancement (ADE) of disease, have been observed with SARS-CoV-1.[126] It is important to understand the balance between Fc signaling that promotes protective immunity and that which promotes inflammatory pathological processes and whether systems serology can identify those at risk. To date, there has been no evidence detected of ADE resulting from SARS-CoV-2 vaccines in preclinical studies or nonhuman primate studies.[127-130] Similarly, no evidence of ADE emerged in a phase III clinical study of an mRNA vaccine against SARS-CoV-2 after a median 2 months of follow-up.[103] Instead, it appears that immunopathological processes in severe COVID-19 mainly occur as a result of aberrant or excessive innate responses.

Clinical trials of antiinflammatory therapies in patients with severe COVID-19 can provide insights into the underlying pathological mechanisms.

Corticosteroids

As part of the RECOVERY trial, 2104 hospitalized COVID-19 patients assigned to receive dexamethasone 6 mg daily were compared with 4321 receiving usual care.[131] Findings differed substantially according to the degree of illness severity. The greatest benefit was observed in patients receiving invasive mechanical ventilation at the time of randomization, in whom adjunctive dexamethasone reduced the risk for death from 41% to 29% (RR, 0.64; 95% CI, 0.51–0.81). A smaller but still significant benefit was found in patients receiving oxygen without invasive mechanical ventilation (26% mortality in controls vs. 23% in dexamethasone recipients; RR, 0.82; 95% CI, 0.72–0.94). No benefit was found for patients not receiving respiratory support at randomization; indeed, in this subgroup, the trend was toward increased mortality risk attributable to dexamethasone (RR, 1.19; 95% CI, 0.92–1.55). Thus corticosteroids and IFN are each of greatest benefit to patients at the opposite polar extremes of disease stage and severity.

Corticosteroids exert dose-dependent antiinflammatory and immunosuppressive effects on nearly all immune cells, reducing production of proinflammatory cytokines, inhibiting cellular microbicidal responses, and increasing the risk for many bacterial, fungal, and viral infections after prolonged use.[132] Nonetheless, corticosteroids have become essential adjunctive treatments for several serious or life-threatening infections. In *Pneumocystis jiroveci* pneumonia, early adjunctive steroid treatment improves survival and decreases the need for mechanical ventilation, particularly in patients with the most profound immune dysregulation, for example, acquired immunodeficiency syndrome (AIDS) patients not yet on antiretroviral therapy (ART).[133-136] In patients beginning treatments for both AIDS and TB, corticosteroids reduce the risk for immune reconstitution inflammatory syndrome (IRIS), or alternatively can be used to treat IRIS once it has occurred.[137,138] IRIS is characterized by clinical worsening despite microbiological improvement; it is often accompanied by extrathoracic suppurative lymphadenopathy and is attributed to ART-associated recovery of immune function. Finally, a systematic review in 1997 and a formal meta-analysis in 2013 concluded that corticosteroids conferred a survival advantage in non-HIV central nervous system and pericardial TB and that in pulmonary TB, steroids hastened the resolution of constitutional, radiographic, and pulmonary function abnormalities.[139,140] The findings are striking in that, like in severe COVID-19, adjunctive corticosteroids provide a clinical benefit in selected patients despite their detrimental overall effects on host defenses against these infections.

Interleukin-6 Receptor Blockade

Interest in the role of IL-6 in COVID-19 pathogenesis in large part reflects the successes of IL-6 receptor blockade in the hyperinflammatory complications such as cytokine-release syndrome and macrophage activation syndrome associated with chimeric antigen receptor (CAR)-T cell therapy.[141] Although serum levels of IL-6 are indeed elevated in severe COVID-19, they are not strikingly so. A systematic review published in late 2020 compared serum IL-6 concentrations in 1245 patients with severe or critical COVID-19 to 8159 others with life-threatening conditions.[142] The mean IL-6 level in COVID-19 patients was 36.7 pg/mL (95% CI, 21.6–62.3 pg/mL). Mean concentrations were nearly 100 times higher in patients with CAR-T cytokine release syndrome, 27 times higher in patients with sepsis, and 12 times higher in patients with acute respiratory distress syndrome unrelated to COVID-19. One early study of IL-6 receptor blockade in hospitalized COVID-19 patients (COVACTA) found no benefit.[144] However, two subsequent studies—RECOVERY and REMAP-CAP—found that IL-6 receptor blockade improved clinical outcomes, including risk for progression to invasive mechanical ventilation and death.[144,145] The contrary findings of these studies may be due to the use of corticosteroids, which were given to a greater proportion of patients in the later studies. It appears the two treatments target complementary pathways and that the modest doses of dexamethasone given in COVID-19 are insufficient to fully inhibit the effects of IL-6.[146]

Signaling Pathway Inhibition

Successful viral pathogens face a challenge to take command of multiple cellular biosynthetic and metabolic processes using only limited genomic space. A strategy common to several viruses, including SARS, SARS-CoV-2, MERS, and pandemic influenza, is to seize control of two interrelated pathways—(Janus kinase–signal transducer and activator of transcription (JAK-STAT) and mammalian target of rapamycin (mTOR)—to promote cell activation, division, growth, and survival. Pharmacological inhibitors of these pathways therefore have two potential therapeutic properties, inhibiting viral replication and reducing immunopathological processes. In one study in 1033 hospitalized COVID-19 patients, baricitinib, a Jak1/2 inhibitor, shortened recovery time and tended to improve survival.[147] Benefit was greatest in the most seriously ill subset of patients. A second study in 83 seriously ill patients found baricitinib improved survival and inhibited viral replication.[148] A similar study in 289 hospitalized patients found that treatment with the Jak inhibitor tofacitinib led to a lower risk for death or respiratory failure through day 28 than placebo.[149] Antiinflammatory and antiviral effects of mTOR inhibitors have been reported in influenza,[150–152] but studies in COVID-19 have not yet been reported.

Pathogenesis of Multisystem Inflammatory Syndrome in Children

Children infected with SARS-CoV-2 are at reduced risk for pneumonia compared with adults but are at increased risk for subsequent multisystem inflammatory syndrome (MIS-C). This syndrome, which resembles Kawasaki disease, is a late phenomenon driven by inflammatory processes peaking at a time thought initially to be well after SARS-CoV-2 levels have declined. Its manifestations are mainly extrapulmonary, with vascular damage associated with autoantibodies directed against a specific set of autoantigens.[153,154] The antiinflammatory immunotherapy that is effective in Kawasaki disease appears similarly effective in MIS-C. The approach combines high-dose intravenous immunoglobulin that activates inhibitory Fc-receptors with administration of high-dose corticosteroids. In some cases, an anti–IL-6 receptor antibody or recombinant IL-1–receptor antagonist is also used. The report of a single patient treated with larazotide, a zonulin inhibitor, followed studies of a cohort of children with prolonged residence of SARS-CoV-2 in the gastrointestinal tract, with gut permeability changes and SARS-CoV-2 antigen presence in plasma, that provide further insight into the long-term manifestations in children.[10]

The Global Pandemic and Questions for Future Research

Advanced age is a consistent risk factor for severe disease and death and may indicate that the cellular immune system and immunosenescence are in play and important considerations for early prediction of poor outcomes and for constructing highly effective and durable vaccines.[155,156] Our ability to predict the risk for progression to severe or life-threatening COVID-19 in individual patients presently is limited. Although the hypothesis that severe disease is due to delayed IFN responses, heightened early viral replication, and exaggerated subsequent late innate responses is plausible, it remains to be confirmed and its underlying mechanisms determined. Further refinements will undoubtedly occur, such as a report documenting that some of

the risk for severe disease in men and in the elderly can be explained by the increased occurrence of anti-IFN autoantibodies.[10]

The burden of coendemic diseases, such as *Mycobacterium tuberculosis* (Mtb) infection, that have latent phases that may progress to clinical disease and are prevalent in low-income countries may also change. For example, a study of coendemic diseases affecting T-cell function and SARS-CoV-2, described clinical features of 95 hospitalized COVID-19 patients in which 38 patients were infected with HIV, TB, or both and compared the CD4+ T-cell responses to 38 hospitalized patients without SARS-COV-2 infection.[123] Severe COVID-19 disease was associated with deficits of CD4+ cell functional potential and a reduced capacity to proliferate. Larger studies of CD4+ cell function will be needed as the SARS-CoV-2 pandemic increasingly spreads to overlap endemic geographies with HIV and TB coinfections particularly since the investigators described a reduced frequency of Mtb-specific CD4+ cells that may indicate T-cell exhaustion with the potential implications for reactivation of latent TB in a large number of people. However, it was somewhat reassuring that the small number of patients with good control of HIV compared with HIV-negative patients did not have alterations in the functional profile of SARS-CoV-2 CD4+ T cells. Further studies in coendemic geographies are urgently needed to explore and expand on these observations.

The precise timing of interventions is crucial and must take into consideration comorbidities and coendemic diseases. Reliable biomarkers indicating the stage of disease would be extremely helpful. Because the early phase of infection is often asymptomatic, many of the direct antiviral interventions may come too late. Endotypes, defined as distinct molecular profiles based on metabolism, epigenetics, transcription, or immune function, have been proposed to guide the application of personalized immunotherapies.[157] One study, for example, found low serum levels of sphingosine-1-phosphate (S1P) to be a strong predictor of ICU admission and mortality in COVID-19.[158] S1P regulates endothelial integrity through its binding to high-affinity G protein–coupled receptors. In models of influenza and SARS-CoV-1 infection, agonists and antagonists of the S1P1 receptor had strong effects on cytokine storm and lethality.[159,160] Our understanding of specific endotypes in COVID-19 is incomplete. Interventions with greater specificity may be possible, for example, preserving the beneficial effects of cytokine families with pleiotropic functions such as IFNs and IL-6 while minimizing their proinflammatory signals.[161] This may be achieved by employing for therapy specifically those cytokine family members with the lowest inflammatory potential (e.g., IFN-III rather than type I)[162] or by targeting cytokine signaling modalities that specifically promote inflammation.[163] Similarly, pharmacological blockade of some but not all signaling pathways downstream of key cytokines may represent interventions with more specific effects.

Monitoring of vaccine efficacy and routine sequencing of SARS-CoV-2 will be essential to guide changes in vaccine constructs over time as expected changes in B-cell epitopes occur or if vaccinated patients develop severe diseases. This will be particularly urgent because it relates to the campaign for global vaccination in increasingly heterogenous populations with differences in comorbidities and coendemic diseases.

Conclusion

The SARS-CoV-2 genome was sequenced and placed in the GISAID repository before the awareness that a global pandemic causing disease (COVID-19), on the scale of the H1N1 influenza pandemic of 1918, was about to occur. In the early days, investigators naturally tried to understand the evolving pathogenesis and clinical profile of the disease by making comparisons to previous coronavirus infections. Human coronaviruses infect toddlers universally in the first years of life, and reinfection is the norm. More lethal coronavirus infections such as MERS and SARS-CoV-1 manifested as lethal full-blown infections with high mortality rates. As of this writing, vaccines created from mRNA, engineered adenovirus constructs expressing the spike protein, and more traditional subunit and inactivated vaccines have demonstrated a range of protective immunity against severe disease, death, and a decrease in spread from person to person. The interplay of innate, humoral, and cellular immunity is now better understood as investigators create models of infection and disease to find better means of protecting people and treating patients exposed to SARS-CoV-2. This chapter gave an overview of the current understanding of the immunology and pathogenesis of SARS-CoV-2 and focused on unique aspects that may provide rich areas of scientific exploration to advance our understanding of this pandemic. The rapid expansion of information on SARS-CoV-2 and COVID-19 clinical disease presents challenges to the student beginning study of this pandemic. We have aimed to provide a framework for understanding the immune system as it relates to a new virus spreading throughout humanity and the current understanding of how the virus interacts with different human hosts.

Acknowledgments

Thank you to Ms. Vaidehi Wadhwa M. Pharm. , Pfizer India Inc.for graphics and editorial assistance . Thank you to peer reviewers: Hernan Valdez, MD, Samuel H. Zwillich, MD, from Pfizer Global Development and Daniel Griffin, MD, PhD, Dickson D. Despommier PhD from Parasites without Borders.

REFERENCES

1. Isaacs A, Lindenmann J. Virus interference. I. The interferon. *Proc R Soc Lond B Biol Sci.* 1957;147(927):258–267.
2. Hoffmann HH, Schneider WM, Rice CM. Interferons and viruses: an evolutionary arms race of molecular interactions. *Trends Immunol.* 2015;36(3):124–138.
3. Davidson S. Treating influenza infection, from now and into the future. *Front Immunol.* 2018;9:1946.
4. Garcia-Sastre A. Ten strategies of interferon evasion by viruses. *Cell Host Microbe.* 2017;22(2):176–184.
5. Enard D, Cai L, Gwennap C, Petrov DA. Viruses are a dominant driver of protein adaptation in mammals. *Elife.* 2016:5.
6. Guo K, Barrett BS, Mickins KL, et al. Interferon resistance of emerging SARS-CoV-2 variants. *bioRxiv.* 2021: 2021.03.20. 436257.
7. Heim MH. 25 years of interferon-based treatment of chronic hepatitis C: an epoch coming to an end. *Nat Rev Immunol.* 2013;13(7):535–542.
8. Neesgaard B, Ruhwald M, Weis N. Inducible protein-10 as a predictive marker of antiviral hepatitis C treatment: A systematic review. *World J Hepatol.* 2017;9(14):677–688.
9. Butt AA, McGinnis KA, Skanderson M, Justice AC. Hepatitis C treatment completion rates in routine clinical care. *Liver Int.* 2010;30(2):240–250.
10. Bastard P, Rosen LB, Zhang Q, et al. Autoantibodies against type I IFNs in patients with life-threatening COVID-19. *Science.* 2020;370(6515).
11. Zhang Q, Bastard P, Liu Z, et al. Inborn errors of type I IFN immunity in patients with life-threatening COVID-19. *Science.* 2020;370(6515).
12. Feld JJ, Kandel C, Biondi MJ, et al. Peginterferon lambda for the treatment of outpatients with COVID-19: a phase 2, placebo-controlled randomised trial. *Lancet Respir Med.* 2021;9(5):498–510.
13. Prokunina-Olsson L, Alphonse N, Dickenson RE, et al. COVID-19 and emerging viral infections: The case for interferon lambda. *J Exp Med.* 2020;217(5):e20200653.
14. Davidson S, Crotta S, McCabe TM, Wack A. Pathogenic potential of interferon alphabeta in acute influenza infection. *Nat Commun.* 2014;5:3864.
15. Garcia-Del-Barco D, Risco-Acevedo D. Revisiting pleiotropic effects of type I interferons: rationale for its prophylactic and therapeutic use against SARS-CoV-2. *Front Immunol.* 2021;12:655528.
16. Hung IF, Lung K-C, Tso E Y-K, et al. Triple combination of interferon beta-1b, lopinavir-ritonavir, and ribavirin in the treatment of patients admitted to hospital with COVID-19: an open-label, randomised, phase 2 trial. *Lancet.* 2020;395(10238):1695–1704.
17. World Health Organization Solidarity Trial Consortium. Repurposed antiviral drugs for Covid-19: interim WHO solidarity trial results. *N Engl J Med.* 2021;384(6):497–511.
18. Wang N, Zhan Y, Zhu L, et al. Retrospective multicenter cohort study shows early interferon therapy is associated with favorable clinical responses in COVID-19 patients. *Cell Host Microbe.* 2020;28(3):455–464, e2.
19. Laing AG, Lorenc A, Del Molino Del Barrio I, et al. A dynamic COVID-19 immune signature includes associations with poor prognosis. *Nat Med.* 2020;26(10):1623–1635.
20. Lucas C, Wong P, Klein J, et al. Longitudinal analyses reveal immunological misfiring in severe COVID-19. *Nature.* 2020;584(7821):463–469.

21. Galani IE, Rovina N, Lampropoulou V, et al. Untuned anti-viral immunity in COVID-19 revealed by temporal type I/III interferon patterns and flu comparison. *Nat Immunol.* 2021;22(1):32–40.

22. Zhou Z, Ren L, Zhang L, et al. Heightened innate immune responses in the respiratory tract of COVID-19 patients. *Cell Host Microbe.* 2020;27(6):883–890, e2.

23. Stephens DS, McElrath MJ. COVID-19 and the path to immunity. *JAMA.* 2020;324(13):1279–1281.

24. Sette A, Crotty S. Adaptive immunity to SARS-CoV-2 and COVID-19. *Cell.* 2021,184(4):861–880.

25. Dan JM, Mateus J, Kato Y, et al. Immunological memory to SARS-CoV-2 assessed for up to 8 months after infection. *Science.* 2021;371(6529):eabf4063.

26. Hovey JG, Tolbert D, Howell D. Burton's Agammaglobulinemia and COVID-19. *Cureus.* 2020;12(11):e11701.

27. Jones JM, Faruqi AJ, Sullivan JK, et al. COVID-19 Outcomes in Patients Undergoing B Cell Depletion Therapy and Those with Humoral Immunodeficiency States: A Scoping Review. *Pathog Immun.* 2021;6(1):76–103.

28. Zhou R, To K K-W, Wong C-Y, et al. Acute SARS-CoV-2 Infection Impairs Dendritic Cell and T Cell Responses. *Immunity.* 2020;53(4):864–877, e5.

29. Fajnzylber J, Regan J, Coxen K, et al. SARS-CoV-2 viral load is associated with increased disease severity and mortality. *Nat Commun.* 2020;11(1):5493.

30. Piccoli L, Park Y-J, Tortorici MA, et al. Mapping Neutralizing and Immunodominant Sites on the SARS-CoV-2 Spike Receptor-Binding Domain by Structure-Guided High-Resolution Serology. *Cell.* 2020;183(4):1024–1042, e21.

31. Rogers TF, Zhao F, Huang D, et al. Isolation of potent SARS-CoV-2 neutralizing antibodies and protection from disease in a small animal model. *Science.* 2020;369(6506):956–963.

32. Tortorici MA, Veesler D. Structural insights into coronavirus entry. *Adv Virus Res.* 2019;105:93–116.

33. Wrapp D, Wang N, Corbett KS, et al. Cryo-EM structure of the 2019-nCoV spike in the prefusion conformation. *Science.* 2020;367(6483):1260–1263.

34. Suthar MS, Zimmerman MG, Kauffman RC, et al. Rapid Generation of Neutralizing Antibody Responses in COVID-19 Patients. *Cell Rep Med.* 2020;1(3):100040.

35. Lynch KL, Whitman JD, Lacanienta NP, et al. Magnitude and Kinetics of Anti-Severe Acute Respiratory Syndrome Coronavirus 2 Antibody Responses and Their Relationship to Disease Severity. *Clin Infect Dis.* 2021;72(2):301–308.

36. Anderson EM, Goodwin EC, Verman A, et al. Seasonal human coronavirus antibodies are boosted upon SARS-CoV-2 infection but not associated with protection. *Cell.* 2020; 11.06.20227215.

37. Garcia-Beltran WF, Lam EC, Astudillo MG, et al. COVID-19-neutralizing antibodies predict disease severity and survival. *Cell.* 2021;184(2):476–488, e11.

38. Loos C, Atyeo C, Fischinger S, et al. Evolution of Early SARS-CoV-2 and Cross-Coronavirus Immunity. *mSphere.* 2020;5(5): e00622-20.

39. Mateus J, Grifoni A, Tarke A, et al. Selective and cross-reactive SARS-CoV-2 T cell epitopes in unexposed humans. *Science.* 2020;370(6512):89–94.

40. Liu WJ, Zhao M, Liu K, et al. T-cell immunity of SARS-CoV: Implications for vaccine development against MERS-CoV. *Antiviral Res.* 2017;137:82–92.

41. Iyer AS, Jones FK, Nodoushani A, et al. Persistence and decay of human antibody responses to the receptor binding domain of SARS-CoV-2 spike protein in COVID-19 patients. *Sci Immunol.* 2020;5(52):eabe0367.

42. Crotty S, Follicular T. Helper Cell Biology: A Decade of Discovery and Diseases. *Immunity.* 2019;50(5):1132–1148.

43. Creech CB, Walker SC, Samuels RJ. SARS-CoV-2 Vaccines. *JAMA.* 2021;325(13):1318–1320.

44. Ruckwardt TJ, Morabito KM, Graham BS. Immunological Lessons from Respiratory Syncytial Virus Vaccine Development. *Immunity.* 2019;51(3):429–442.

45. DiPiazza AT, Graham BS, Ruckwardt TJ. T cell immunity to SARS-CoV-2 following natural infection and vaccination. *Biochem Biophys Res Commun.* 2021;538:211–217.

46. Rydyznski Moderbacher C, SI Ramirez, Dan JM, et al. Antigen-Specific Adaptive Immunity to SARS-CoV-2 in Acute COVID-19 and Associations with Age and Disease Severity. *Cell.* 2020;183(4):996–1012. e19.

47. Chandrashekar A, Liu J, Martinot AJ, et al. SARS-CoV-2 infection protects against rechallenge in rhesus macaques. *Science.* 2020;369(6505):812–817.

48. Deng W, Bao L, Liu J, et al. Primary exposure to SARS-CoV-2 protects against reinfection in rhesus macaques. *Science.* 2020;369(6505):818–823.

49. Le Bert N, Tan AT, Kunasegaran K, et al. SARS-CoV-2-specific T cell immunity in cases of COVID-19 and SARS, and uninfected controls. *Nature.* 2020;584(7821):457–462.

50. Grifoni A, Weiskopf D, Ramirez SI, et al. Targets of T Cell Responses to SARS-CoV-2 Coronavirus in Humans with COVID-19 Disease and Unexposed Individuals. *Cell.* 2020;181(7):1489–1501. e15.

51. Sahin U, Muik A, Vogler I, et al. BNT162b2 vaccine induces neutralizing antibodies and poly-specific T cells in humans. *Nature.* 2021;595(7868):572–577.

52. Tarke A, Sidney J, Kidd CK, et al. Comprehensive analysis of T cell immunodominance and immunoprevalence of SARS-CoV-2 epitopes in COVID-19 cases. *Cell Rep Med.* 2021;2(2):100204.

53. Tauzin A, Nayrac M, Benlarbi M, et al. A single BNT162b2 mRNA dose elicits antibodies with Fc-mediated effector functions and boost pre-existing humoral and T cell responses. *bioRxiv.* 2021: 2021.03.18.435972.

54. Rausch JW, Capoferri AA, Katusiime MG, et al. Low genetic diversity may be an Achilles heel of SARS-CoV-2. *Proc Natl Acad Sci U S A.* 2020;117(40):24614–24616.

55. Moore JP. Approaches for Optimal Use of Different COVID-19 Vaccines: Issues of Viral Variants and Vaccine Efficacy. *JAMA.* 2021;325(13):1251–1252.

56. Moore JP, Offit PA. SARS-CoV-2 Vaccines and the Growing Threat of Viral Variants. *JAMA.* 2021;325(9):821–822.

57. Neuzil KM. Interplay between Emerging SARS-CoV-2 Variants and Pandemic Control. *N Engl J Med.* 2021;384(20):1952–1954.

58. Korber B, Fischer WM, Gnanakaran S, et al. Tracking Changes in SARS-CoV-2 Spike: Evidence that D614G Increases Infectivity of the COVID-19 Virus. *Cell.* 2020;182(4):812–827, e19.

59. Oude Munnink BB, Sikkema RS, Nieuwenhuijse DF, et al. Transmission of SARS-CoV-2 on mink farms between humans and mink and back to humans. *Science.* 2021;371(6525):172–177.

60. Zhou D, Dejnirattisai W, Supasa P, et al. Evidence of escape of SARS-CoV-2 variant B.1.351 from natural and vaccine induced sera. *Cell.* 2021;184(9):2348–2361.

61. Lassaunière R, Fonager J, Rasmussen M, et al. SARS-CoV-2 spike mutations arising in Danish mink and their spread to humans (Working Paper 10 Nov 2020). *Statens Serum Institut,* 2020; p. https://files.ssi.dk/Mink-cluster-5-short-report_AFO2.

62. Centers for Disease Control and Prevention. SARS-CoV-2 Variant Classifications and Definitions. 2021 25 May 2021; Available from: https://www.cdc.gov/coronavirus/2019-ncov/variants/variant-info.html.

63. European Centre for Disease Control and Prevention. SARS-CoV-2 variants of concern. 2021; Available from: https://www.ecdc.europa.eu/en/covid-19/variants-concern.

64. World Health Organization, Tracking SARS-CoV-2 variants. 2021.

65. World Health Organization, WHO Naming SARS-CoV-2 variants – SARS-CoV-2 Variants of Concern and Variants of Interest, updated 31 May 2021. 2021: https://www.who.int/en/activities/tracking-SARS-CoV-2-variants/.

66. Faria NR, Mellan TA, Whittaker C, et al. Genomics and epidemiology of the P.1 SARS-CoV-2 lineage in Manaus, Brazil. *Science.* 2021;372(6544):815–821.

67. Wibmer CK, Ayres F, Hermanus T, et al. SARS-CoV-2 501Y. V2 escapes neutralization by South African COVID-19 donor plasma. *Nat Med.* 2021;27(4):622–625.

68. Wang P, Nair MS, Liu L, et al. Antibody resistance of SARS-CoV-2 variants B.1.351 and B.1.1.7. *Nature.* 2021; 593(7857):130–135.

69. Robbiani DF, Gaebler C, Muecksch F, et al. Convergent antibody responses to SARS-CoV-2 in convalescent individuals. *Nature.* 2020;584(7821):437–442.

70. Andreano E, Rappuoli R. SARS-CoV-2 escaped natural immunity, raising questions about vaccines and therapies. *Nat Med.* 2021;27(5):759–761.

71. Andreano E, Piccini G, Casalino L, et al. SARS-CoV-2 escape in vitro from a highly neutralizing COVID-19 convalescent plasma. *bioRxiv.* 2020: p. https://doi.org/10.1101/2020.12.28.424451.

72. Greaney AJ, Loes AN, Crawford KHD, et al. Comprehensive mapping of mutations in the SARS-CoV-2 receptor-binding domain that affect recognition by polyclonal human plasma antibodies. *Cell Host Microbe.* 2021;29(3):463–476, e6.

73. Liu Y, Liu J, Xia H, et al. Neutralizing Activity of BNT162b2-Elicited Serum. *N Engl J Med.* 2021;384(15):1466–1468.

74. Liu Y, Liu J, Xia H, et al. BNT162b2-Elicited Neutralization against New SARS-CoV-2 Spike Variants. *N Engl J Med.* 2021;385(5):472–474.

75. Wu K, Werner AP, Koch M, et al. Serum Neutralizing Activity Elicited by mRNA-1273 Vaccine. *N Engl J Med.* 2021;384(15):1468–1470.

76. Emary KRW, Golubchik T, Aley PA, et al. Efficacy of ChAdOx1 nCoV-19 (AZD1222) vaccine against SARS-CoV-2 variant of concern 202012/01 (B.1.1.7): an exploratory analysis of a randomised controlled trial. *Lancet.* 2021;397(10282):1351–1362.

77. Zhou P, Shi ZL. SARS-CoV-2 spillover events. *Science.* 2021;371(6525):120–122.

78. Sapkal G, Yadav P, Ella R, et al. Neutralization of B.1.1.28 P2 variant with sera of natural SARS-CoV-2 infection and recipients of BBV152 vaccine. *bioRxiv.* 2021: 2021.04.30.441559.

79. Sapkal GN, Yadav PD, Ella R, et al. Neutralization of UK-variant VUI-202012/01 with COVAXIN vaccinated human serum. *bioRxiv.* 2021: 2021.01.26.426986.

80. Yadav PD, Sapkal GN, Abraham P, et al. Neutralization of variant under investigation B.1.617 with sera of BBV152 vaccinees. *Clin Infect Dis.* 2021;74(2):366–368.

81. Huang B, Dai L, Wang H, et al. Neutralization of SARS-CoV-2 VOC 501Y.V2 by human antisera elicited by both inactivated BBIBP-CorV and recombinant dimeric RBD ZF2001 vaccines. *bioRxiv.* 2021: 2021.02.01.429069.

82. Sadoff J, Le Gars M, Shukarev G, et al. Interim Results of a Phase 1-2a Trial of Ad26.COV2.S Covid-19 Vaccine. *N Engl J Med.* 2021;384(19):1824–1835.

83. Janssen, EUA Application for Ad26.COV2.S Janssen Pharma Presentation (26 Feb 2021), in VRBPAC - FDA. 2021: https://www.fda.gov/advisory-committees/advisory-committee-calendar/vaccines-and-related-biological-products-advisory-committee-february-26-2021-meeting-announcement. p. 26 Feb 2021.

84. Shinde V, Bhikha S, Hoosain Z, et al. Efficacy of NVX-CoV2373 Covid-19 Vaccine against the B.1.351 Variant. *N Engl J Med.* 2021;384(20):1899–1909.

85. Haas EJ, Angulo F, McLaughlin JM, et al. Impact and effectiveness of mRNA BNT162b2 vaccine against SARS-CoV-2 infections and COVID-19 cases, hospitalisations, and deaths following a nationwide vaccination campaign in Israel: an observational study using national surveillance data. *Lancet.* 2021;397(10287):1819–1829.

86. Abu-Raddad LJ, Chemaitelly H, Butt AA, et al. Effectiveness of the BNT162b2 Covid-19 Vaccine against the B.1.1.7 and B.1.351 Variants. *N Engl J Med.* 2021;385(2):187–189.

87. Chemaitelly H, Yassine HM, Benslimane FM, et al. mRNA-1273 COVID-19 vaccine effectiveness against the B.1.1.7 and B.1.351 variants and severe COVID-19 disease in Qatar. *Nat Med.* 2021;27(9):1614–1621.

88. Lopez Bernal J, Andrews N, Gower C, et al. Effectiveness of COVID-19 vaccines against the B.1.617.2 variant. *medRxiv.* 2021: 2021.05.22.21257658.

89. Lopez Bernal J, Andrews N, Gower C, et al. Effectiveness of Covid-19 Vaccines against the B.1.617.2 (Delta) Variant. *N Engl J Med.* 2021;385(7):585–594.

90. Nasreen S, Chung H, He S, et al. Effectiveness of COVID-19 vaccines against variants of concern, Canada. *medRxiv.* 2021: 2021.06.28.21259420.

91. Sheikh A, Menamin J, Taylor B, et al. SARS-CoV-2 Delta VOC in Scotland: demographics, risk of hospital admission, and vaccine effectiveness. *Lancet.* 2021;397(10293):2461–2462.

92. Jara A, Undurraga EA, González C, et al. Effectiveness of an Inactivated SARS-CoV-2 Vaccine in Chile. *N Engl J Med.* 2021;385(10):875–884.

93. Ranzani OT, Hitchings MDT, Dorion M, et al. Effectiveness of the CoronaVac vaccine in the elderly population during a P.1 variant-associated epidemic of COVID-19 in Brazil: A test-negative case-control study. *medRxiv.* 2021: 2021.05.19.21257472.

94. US Food and Drug Administration. Updated guidance for Emergency Use Authorization for Vaccines to Prevent COVID-19 (22 Feb 2021). 2021: p. https://www.fda.gov/regulatory-information/search-fda-guidance-documents/emergency-use-authorization-vaccines-prevent-covid-19.

95. Edridge AWD, Kaczorowska J, Hoste ACR, et al. Seasonal coronavirus protective immunity is short-lasting. *Nat Med.* 2020;26(11):1691–1693.

96. Wajnberg A, Amanat F, Firpo A, et al. Robust neutralizing antibodies to SARS-CoV-2 infection persist for months. *Science.* 2020;370(6521):1227–1230.

97. Lumley SF, O'Donnell D, Stoesser NE, et al. Antibody Status and Incidence of SARS-CoV-2 Infection in Health Care Workers. *N Engl J Med.* 2021;384(6):533–540.

98. Gudbjartsson DF, Norddahl G, Melsted P, et al. Humoral Immune Response to SARS-CoV-2 in Iceland. *N Engl J Med.* 2020;383(18):1724–1734.

99. Turner JS, Kim W, al. Kaladinaet. SARS-CoV-2 infection induces long-lived bone marrow plasma cells in humans. *Nature.* 2021;595(7867):421–425.

100. Wang Z, Meucksch F, Schaefer-Babajew D, et al. Vaccination boosts naturally enhanced neutralizing breadth to SARS-CoV-2 one year after infection. *bioRxiv.* 2021: 2021.05.07.443175.

101. Kim AY, Gandhi RT. Reinfection with SARS-CoV-2: What Goes Around May Come Back Around. *Clin Infect Dis.* 2021;73(9):e23009–e3012.

102. Abu-Raddad LJ, Chemaitelly H, Malek JA, et al. Assessment of the risk of SARS-CoV-2 reinfection in an intense re-exposure setting. *Clin Infect Dis.* 2020;73(7):e1830–e1840.

103. Polack FP, Thomas SJ, Kitchin N, et al. Safety and Efficacy of the BNT162b2 mRNA Covid-19 Vaccine. *N Engl J Med.* 2020;383(27):2603–2615.

104. Widge AT, Rouphael NG, Jackson LA, et al. Durability of Responses after SARS-CoV-2 mRNA-1273 Vaccination. *N Engl J Med.* 2021;384(1):80–82.

105. Folegatti PM, Bittaye M, Flaxman A, et al. Safety and immunogenicity of a candidate Middle East respiratory syndrome coronavirus viral-vectored vaccine: a dose-escalation, open-label, non-randomised, uncontrolled, phase 1 trial. *Lancet Infect Dis.* 2020;20(7):816–826.

106. Plotkin SA, Gilbert P. Correlates of Protection. In: Orenstein W, Offit, Edwards K, Plotkin S, eds. *Plotkin's Vaccines.* Philadelphia: Elsevier; 2017:35–40. e4.

107. Plotkin SA. Updates on immunologic correlates of vaccine-induced protection. *Vaccine.* 2020;38(9):2250–2257.

108. Karim SSA. Vaccines and SARS-CoV-2 variants: the urgent need for a correlate of protection. *Lancet.* 2021; 397(10281):1263–1264.

109. Krammer F. Correlates of protection from SARS-CoV-2 infection. *Lancet.* 2021;397(10283):1421–1423.

110. Earle KA, Ambrosino DM, Fiore-Gartland A, et al. Evidence for antibody as a protective correlate for COVID-19 vaccines. *Vaccine.* 2021;39(32):4423–4428.

111. Khoury DS, Cromer D, Reynaldi A, et al. Neutralizing antibody levels are highly predictive of immune protection from symptomatic SARS-CoV-2 infection. *Nat Med.* 2021;27(7):1205–1211.

112. Loos C, Lauffenburger DA, Alter G. Dissecting the antibody-OME: past, present, and future. *Curr Opin Immunol.* 2020;65:89–96.

113. Jungreis, I., R. Sealfon, and M. Kellis, SARS-CoV-2 gene content and COVID-19 mutation impact by comparing 44 Sarbecovirus genomes. 3 2021;12(1):2642.

114. Kuri-Cervantes L, Pampena MB, Meng W, et al. Comprehensive mapping of immune perturbations associated with severe COVID-19. *Sci Immunol.* 2020;5(49):eabd7114.

115. Mathew D, Giles JR, Baxter AE, et al. Deep immune profiling of COVID-19 patients reveals distinct immunotypes with therapeutic implications. *Science.* 2020;369(6508). doi:10.1126/science.abc8511.

116. Atyeo C, Fischinger S, Zohar T, et al. Distinct Early Serological Signatures Track with SARS-CoV-2 Survival. *Immunity.* 2020;53(3):524–532, e4.

117. Carsana L, Sonzogni A, Nasr A, et al. Pulmonary post-mortem findings in a series of COVID-19 cases from northern Italy: a two-centre descriptive study. *Lancet Infect Dis.* 2020;20(10):1135–1140.

118. Moore JB, June CH. Cytokine release syndrome in severe COVID-19. *Science.* 2020;368(6490):473–474.

119. Ruan Q, Yang K, Wang W, et al. Clinical predictors of mortality due to COVID-19 based on an analysis of data of 150 patients from Wuhan, China. *Intensive Care Med.* 2020;46(5):846–848.

120. Wong CK, Lam CWK, Wu AKL, et al. Plasma inflammatory cytokines and chemokines in severe acute respiratory syndrome. *Clin Exp Immunol.* 2004;136(1):95–103.

121. Lam CW, Chan MH, Wong CK. Severe acute respiratory syndrome: clinical and laboratory manifestations. *Clin Biochem Rev.* 2004;25(2):121–132.

122. Liu J, Zheng X, Tong Q, et al. Overlapping and discrete aspects of the pathology and pathogenesis of the emerging human pathogenic coronaviruses SARS-CoV, MERS-CoV, and 2019-nCoV. *J Med Virol.* 2020;92(5):491–494.

123. Alsaad KO, Hajeer AH, Al Balwi M, et al. Histopathology of Middle East respiratory syndrome coronavirus (MERS-CoV) infection - clinicopathological and ultrastructural study. *Histopathology.* 2018;72(3):516–524.

124. Szabo PA, Dogra P, Gray JI, et al. Longitudinal profiling of respiratory and systemic immune responses reveals myeloid cell-driven lung inflammation in severe COVID-19. *Immunity.* 2021;54(4):797–814. e6.

125. Riou C, du Bruyn E, Stek C, et al. Profile of SARS-CoV-2-specific CD4 T cell response: Relationship with disease severity and impact of HIV-1 and active Mycobacterium tuberculosis co-infection. *medRxiv.* 2021:2021.02.16.21251838.

126. Poland GA, Ovsyannikova IG, Kennedy RB. SARS-CoV-2 immunity: review and applications to phase 3 vaccine candidates. *Lancet.* 2020;396(10262):1595–1606.

127. Vogel AB, et al. BNT162b vaccines protect rhesus macaques from SARS-CoV-2. *Nature.* 2021;592(7853):283–289.

128. Krammer F. SARS-CoV-2 vaccines in development. *Nature.* 2020;586(7830):516–527.

129. Corbett KS, Flynn B, Foulds KE, et al. Evaluation of the mRNA-1273 Vaccine against SARS-CoV 2 in Nonhuman Primates. *N Engl J Med.* 2020;383(16):1544–1555.

130. van Doremalen N, Lambe T, Spencer A, et al. ChAdOx1 nCoV-19 vaccine prevents SARS-CoV-2 pneumonia in rhesus macaques. *Nature.* 2020;586(7830):578–582.

131. Recovery Collaborative Group. Dexamethasone in Hospitalized Patients with Covid-19. *N Engl J Med.* 2021; 384(8):693–704.

132. Youssef J, Novosad SA, Winthrop KL. Infection Risk and Safety of Corticosteroid Use. *Rheum Dis Clin North Am.* 2016;42(1):157–176, ix-x.

133. MacFadden DK, Edelson JD, Rebuck AS. Pneumocystis carinii pneumonia in the acquired immune deficiency syndrome: response to inadvertent steroid therapy. *Can Med Assoc J.* 1985;132(10):1161–1163.

134. National Institutes of Health-University of California Expert Panel for Corticosteroids as Adjunctive Therapy for Pneumocystis, P. Consensus statement on the use of corticosteroids as adjunctive therapy for pneumocystis pneumonia in the acquired immunodeficiency syndrome. *N Engl J Med.* 1990;323(21):1500–1504.

135. Fujikura Y, Manabe T, Kawana A, Kohno S. Adjunctive Corticosteroids for *Pneumocystis jirovecii* Pneumonia in Non-HIV-infected Patients: A Systematic Review and Meta-analysis of Observational Studies. *Arch Bronconeumol.* 2017;53(2):55–61.

136. Ewald H, Raatz H, Boscacci R, et al. Adjunctive corticosteroids for Pneumocystis jiroveci pneumonia in patients with HIV infection. *Cochrane Database Syst Rev.* 2015;(4): CD006150.

137. Meintjes G, Wilkinson RJ, Morroni C, et al. Randomized placebo-controlled trial of prednisone for paradoxical tuberculosis-associated immune reconstitution inflammatory syndrome. *AIDS.* 2010;24(15):2381–2390.

138. Meintjes G, Stek C, Blumenthal L, et al. Prednisone for the Prevention of Paradoxical Tuberculosis-Associated IRIS. *N Engl J Med.* 2018;379(20):1915–1925.

139. Dooley DP, Carpenter JL, Rademacher S. Adjunctive corticosteroid therapy for tuberculosis: a critical reappraisal of the literature. *Clin Infect Dis.* 1997;25(4):872–887.

140. Critchley JA, Young F, Orton L, Garner P. Corticosteroids for prevention of mortality in people with tuberculosis: a systematic review and meta-analysis. *Lancet Infect Dis.* 2013;13(3):223–237.

141. Le RQ, Li L, Yuan W, et al. FDA Approval Summary: Tocilizumab for Treatment of Chimeric Antigen Receptor T Cell-Induced Severe or Life-Threatening Cytokine Release Syndrome. *Oncologist.* 2018;23(8):943–947.

142. Leisman DE, Ronner L, Pinotti R, et al. Cytokine elevation in severe and critical COVID-19: a rapid systematic review, meta-analysis, and comparison with other inflammatory syndromes. *Lancet Respir Med.* 2020;8(12):1233–1244.

143. Rosas IO, Bräu N, Waters M, et al. Tocilizumab in Hospitalized Patients with Severe Covid-19 Pneumonia. *N Engl J Med.* 2021;384(16):1503–1516.

144. Horby PW, et al. RECOVERY Collaborative Group. Tocilizumab in patients admitted to hospital with COVID-19 (RECOVERY): preliminary results of a randomised, controlled, open-label, platform trial. *medRxiv.* 2021: 2021.02.11.21249258.

145. Remap-Cap Investigators, et al. Interleukin-6 Receptor Antagonists in Critically Ill Patients with Covid-19. *N Engl J Med.* 2021;384(16):1491–1502.

146. Rubin EJ, Longo DL, Baden LR. Interleukin-6 Receptor Inhibition in Covid-19 - Cooling the Inflammatory Soup. *N Engl J Med.* 2021;384(16):1564–1565.

147. Kalil AC, Patterson TF, Mehta AK, et al. Baricitinib plus Remdesivir for Hospitalized Adults with Covid-19. *N Engl J Med.* 2021;384(9):795–807.

148. Stebbing J, Sánchez Nievas G, et al. JAK inhibition reduces SARS-CoV-2 liver infectivity and modulates inflammatory responses to reduce morbidity and mortality. *Sci Adv.* 2021;7(1):eabe4724.

149. Guimarães PO, Quirk D, Furtado RH, et al. Tofacitinib in Patients Hospitalized with Covid-19 Pneumonia. *N Engl J Med.* 2021;385(5):406–415.

150. Kuss-Duerkop SK, Wang J, Mena I, et al. Influenza virus differentially activates mTORC1 and mTORC2 signaling to maximize late stage replication. *PLoS Pathog.* 2017; 13(9):e1006635.

151. Buchkovich NJ, Yu Y, Zampieri CA, Alwine JC. The TORrid affairs of viruses: effects of mammalian DNA viruses on the PI3K-Akt-mTOR signalling pathway. *Nat Rev Microbiol.* 2008;6(4):266–275.

152. Mannick JB, Morris M, Hockey H-U P, et al. TORC1 inhibition enhances immune function and reduces infections in the elderly. *Sci Transl Med.* 2018;10(449):eaaq1564.

153. Consiglio CR, Cotugno N, Sardh F, et al. The Immunology of Multisystem Inflammatory Syndrome in Children with COVID-19. *Cell.* 2020;183(4):968–981, e7.

154. Gruber CN, Patel RS, Tractman R, et al. Mapping Systemic Inflammation and Antibody Responses in Multisystem Inflammatory Syndrome in Children (MIS-C). *Cell.* 2020;183(4):982–995, e14.

155. Zhou F, Yu T, Du R, et al. Clinical course and risk factors for mortality of adult inpatients with COVID-19 in Wuhan, China: a retrospective cohort study. *Lancet.* 2020; 395(10229):1054–1062.

156. Guan WJ, Ni Z-Y, Hu Y, et al. Clinical Characteristics of Coronavirus Disease 2019 in China. *N Engl J Med.* 2020;382(18):1708–1720.

157. DiNardo AR, Nishiguchi T, Grimm SL, et al. Tuberculosis endotypes to guide stratified host-directed therapy. *Med (N Y).* 2021;2:217–232.

158. Marfia G, Navone S, Guarnaccia L, et al. Decreased serum level of sphingosine-1-phosphate: a novel predictor of clinical severity in COVID-19. *EMBO Mol Med.* 2021; 13(1):e13424.

159. Teijaro JR, Walsh KB, Rice S, et al. Mapping the innate signaling cascade essential for cytokine storm during influenza virus infection. *Proc Natl Acad Sci U S A.* 2014;111(10):3799–3804.

160. Teijaro JR, Studer S, Leaf N, et al. S1PR1-mediated IFNAR1 degradation modulates plasmacytoid dendritic cell interferon-alpha autoamplification. *Proc Natl Acad Sci U S A.* 2016;113(5):1351–1356.

161. Garbers C, Heink S, Korn T, Rose-John S. Interleukin-6: designing specific therapeutics for a complex cytokine. *Nat Rev Drug Discov.* 2018;17(6):395–412.

162. Davidson S, McCabe TM, Crotta S, et al. IFNlambda is a potent anti-influenza therapeutic without the inflammatory side effects of IFNalpha treatment. *EMBO Mol Med.* 2016;8(9):1099–1112.

163. Rose-John S. Interleukin-6 Family Cytokines. *Cold Spring Harb Perspect Biol.* 2018;10(2):a028415.

164. Balan S, Saxena M, Bhardwaj N. Dendritic cell subsets and locations. *Int Rev Cell Mol Biol.* 2019;348:1–68.

165. Price JV, Vance RE. The macrophage paradox. *Immunity.* 2014;41(5):685–693.

166. Janeway CA, Travers Jr P, Walport M, Shlomchik MJ. The components of the immune system, in Immunobiology: The immune system in health and disease. New York: Garland Science; 2001.

167. Kumar BV, Connors TJ, Farber DL. Human T Cell Development, Localization, and Function throughout Life. *Immunity.* 2018;48(2):202–213.

168. Collin M, Bigley V. Human dendritic cell subsets: an update. *Immunology.* 2018;154(1):3–20.

169. Hirayama D, Iida T, Nakase H. The Phagocytic Function of Macrophage-Enforcing Innate Immunity and Tissue Homeostasis. *Int J Mol Sci.* 2018;19(1):92.

170. Mantegazza AR, Magalhaes JG, Amigorena S, Marks MS. Presentation of phagocytosed antigens by MHC class I and II. *Traffic*. 2013;14(2):135–152.

171. Seifert M, Kuppers R. Human memory B cells. *Leukemia*. 2016;30(12):2283–2292.

172. Antigen presenting cells. Nature Portfolio; Available from: https://www-nature-com.eu1.proxy.openathens.net/subjects/antigen-presenting-cells.

173. Spellberg B, Edwards Jr JE. Type 1/Type 2 immunity in infectious diseases. *Clin Infect Dis*. 2001;32(1):76–102.

174. Luckheeram RV, Zhou R, Verma AD, Xia B. CD4(+)T cells: differentiation and functions. *Clin Dev Immunol*. 2012;2012:925135.

175. Adamo S, Michler J, Zurbuchen Y, et al. Signature of long-lived memory CD8 + T cells in acute SARS-CoV-2 infection. *Nature* 2022;602:148–155. https://doi.org/10.1038/s41586-021-04280-x

176. Tanne A, Bhardwaj N. Dendritic cells: General overview and role in autoimmunity. In: *Kelley and Firestein's Textbook of Rheumatology*. Firestein GS, ed. Philadelphia: Elsevier; 2017:126–144.

177. Eibel H, Kraus H, Sic H, et al. B cell biology: an overview. *Curr Allergy Asthma Rep*. 2014;14(5):434.

178. Couture A, Garnier A, Docagne F, et al. HLA-Class II Artificial Antigen Presenting Cells in CD4(+) T Cell-Based Immunotherapy. *Front Immunol*. 2019;10:1081.

179. Patente TA, Pinho MP, Oliveira AA, et al. Human Dendritic Cells: Their Heterogeneity and Clinical Application Potential in Cancer Immunotherapy. *Front Immunol*. 2018;9:3176.

180. Zhang C, Yang M, Ericsson AC. Function of Macrophages in Disease: Current Understanding on Molecular Mechanisms. 2021;12:620510.

181. Mittrucker HW, Visekruna A, Huber M. Heterogeneity in the differentiation and function of CD8(+) T cells. *Arch Immunol Ther Exp (Warsz)*. 2014;62(6):449–458.

182. Gao X, Zhao L, Wang S, et al. Enhanced inducible costimulator ligand (ICOS-L) expression on dendritic cells in interleukin-10 deficiency and its impact on T-cell subsets in respiratory tract infection. *Mol Med*. 2013;19:346–356.

183. Munoz-Rojas AR, Kelsey I, Pappalardo J, et al. Co-stimulation with opposing macrophage polarization cues leads to orthogonal secretion programs in individual cells. *Nat Commun*. 2021;12(1):301.

184. Barber A. Costimulation of effector CD8 + T cells: Which receptor is optimal for immunotherapy? *MOJ Immunol*. 2014;1(2):00011.

185. Bao Y, Liu X, Han C, et al. Identification of IFN-gamma-producing innate B cells. *Cell Res*. 2014;24(2):161–176.

186. Xu HC, Grusdat M, Pandyra AA, et al. Type I interferon protects antiviral CD8 + T cells from NK cell cytotoxicity. *Immunity*. 2014;40(6):949–960.

187. Thorne L, Bouhaddou M, Mehdi R, Ann-Kathrin C, Zuliani-Alverez L, et al. Evolution of enhanced innate immune evasion by SARS-CoV-2. *Nature*. 2022;602:1915–1925. doi:10.1038/s41586-021-04352-y.

188. Muik A, Lui BG, Wallisch A-K, et al. Neutralization of SARS-CoV-2 Omicron by BNT162b2 mRNA vaccine-elicited human sera. *Science*. 2022;375(6581):678–680. 1095-9203. doi:10.1126/science.abn7591. 35040667.

189. Hatcher S, et al. COVID-19 Vaccine Effectiveness: A Review of the First 6 Months of COVID-19 Vaccine Availability (1 January–30 June 2021). *Vaccines*. 2022;10(3):393. doi: https://doi.org/10.3390/vaccines10030393.

190. Higdon M, et al. A systematic review of COVID-19 vaccine efficacy and effectiveness against SARS-CoV-2 infection and disease. *MedRxiv*. 2021. doi:10.1101/2021.09.17.21263549.

191. Tao K, Tzou PL, Nouhin J, et al. The biological and clinical significance of emerging SARS-CoV-2 variants. *Nat Rev Genet*. 2021;22(12):757–773. 1471-0064. doi:10.1038/s41576-021-00408-x. 34535792.

192. Harvey WT, Carabelli AM, Jackson B, et al. COVID-19 Genomics UK (COG-UK) Consortium. SARS-CoV-2 variants, spike mutations and immune escape. *Nat Rev Microbiol*. 2021;19(7):409–424. 1740-1534. doi:10.1038/s41579-021-00573-0. 34075212.

193. Kupferschmidt K. Where did "weird" Omicron come from? Science. 2021;374(6572):1179. 1095-9203. doi:10.1126/science.acx9738. 34855502.

194. Ingraham NE, Ingbar DH. The omicron variant of SARS-CoV-2: Understanding the known and living with unknowns. *Clin Transl Med*. 2021;11(12):e685. 1326–2001. doi:10.1002/ctm2.685. 34911167.

195. UK-HSA (2022). Technical briefing 35 SARS-CoV-2 variants of concern and variants under investigation in England (28 Jan 2022). https://assets.publishing.service.gov.uk/government/uploads/system/uploads/attachment_data/file/1050999/Technical-Briefing-35-28January2022.pdf. UK Health Security Agency.

196. Davies M-A, Kassanjee R, Rousseau P, et al. Outcomes of laboratory-confirmed SARS-CoV-2 infection in the Omicron-driven fourth wave compared with previous waves in the Western Cape Province, South Africa. *MedRxiv*. 2022. doi:10.1101/2022.01.12.22269148.35043121.

197. Maslo C, Friedland R, Toubkin M, Laubscher A, Akaloo T, Kama B. Characteristics and Outcomes of Hospitalized Patients in South Africa During the COVID-19 Omicron Wave Compared With Previous Waves. *JAMA*. 2022; 327(6):583–584. 1538-3598. doi:10.1001/jama.2021.24868. 34967859.

198. Wolter N, Jassat W, Walaza S, et al. Early assessment of the clinical severity of the SARS-CoV-2 omicron variant in South Africa: a data linkage study. *Lancet*. 2022;399(10323):437–446. 1474-547X. doi:10.1016/S0140-6736(22)00017-4. 35065011.

199. European Centre for Disease Prevention and Control. Assessment of the further spread and potential impact of the SARS-CoV-2 Omicron variant of concern in the EU/EEA, 19th update 2022. Available from: https://www.ecdc.europa.eu/sites/default/files/documents/RRA-19-update-27-jan-2022.pdf.

200. Bager P, Wohlfahrt J, Bhatt S, Edslev SM, Sieber RN, Ingham AC, et al. Reduced Risk of Hospitalisation Associated With Infection With SARS-CoV-2 Omicron Relative to Delta: A Danish Cohort Study 2022. Available from: https://papers.ssrn.com/sol3/papers.cfm?abstract_id=4008930.

201. UK Health Security Agency (UKHSA). SARS-CoV-2 variants of concern and variants under investigation in England. Technical briefing: Update on hospitalisation and vaccine effectiveness for Omicron VOC-21NOV01 (B.1.1.529) UKHSA; 2021. Available from: https://assets.publishing.service.gov.uk/government/uploads/system/uploads/

attachment_data/file/1045619/Technical-Briefing-31-Dec-2021-Omicron_severity_update.pdf.

202. Minka SO, Minka FHA. A tabulated summary of the evidence on humoral and cellular responses to the SARS-CoV-2 Omicron VOC, as well as vaccine efficacy against this variant. *Immunol Lett.* 2022;243:38–43.1879-0542. doi:10.1016/j.imlet.2022.02.002. 35131373.

203. Thompson MG, Natarajan K, Irving SA, et al. Effectiveness of a Third Dose of mRNA Vaccines Against COVID-19-Associated Emergency Department and Urgent Care Encounters and Hospitalizations Among Adults During Periods of Delta and Omicron Variant Predominance - VISION Network, 10 States, August 2021-January 2022. *MMWR Morb Mortal Wkly Rep.* 2022;71(4):139–145. 1545-861X. doi:10.15585/mmwr.mm7104e3. 35085224.

204. Accorsi EK, Britton A, Fleming-Dutra KE, et al. Association Between 3 Doses of mRNA COVID-19 Vaccine and Symptoma tic Infection Caused by the SARS-CoV-2 Omicron and Delta Variants. *MMWR JAMA.* 2022;327(7):639–651. 1538–3598. doi:10.1001/jama.2022.0470. 35060999.

205. Andrews, et al. Covid-19 Vaccine Effectiveness against the Omicron (B.1.1.529) Variant. *New England Journal of Medicine.* 2022. doi:10.1056/NEJMoa2119451.

206. Tartof Sara Y, Slezak Jeff M, Puzniak Laura, et al. Effectiveness of a third dose of BNT162b2 mRNA COVID-19 vaccine in a large US health system: A retrospective cohort study. *Lancet Reg Health Am.* 2022;100198. 2667-193X. doi:10.1016/j.lana.2022.100198. 35187521.

207. CDC (2022). "Science Brief: Omicron (B.1.1.529) Variant (02 Dec 2021)." From https://www.cdc.gov/coronavirus/2019-ncov/science/science-briefs/scientific-brief-omicron-variant.html.

208. Lauring AS, Tenforde MW, Chappell JD, et al. Influenza and Other Viruses in the Acutely Ill (IVY) Network. Clinical Severity and mRNA Vaccine Effectiveness for Omicron, Delta, and Alpha SARS-CoV-2 Variants in the United States: A Prospective Observational Study. *MedRxiv.* 2022. doi:10.1101/2022.02.06.22270558. 35169811.

209. Ferdinands JM, Rao S, Dixon BE, et al. Waning 2-Dose and 3-Dose Effectiveness of mRNA Vaccines Against COVID-19-Associated Emergency Department and Urgent Care Encounters and Hospitalizations Among Adults During Periods of Delta and Omicron Variant Predominance-VISION Network, 10 States, August 2021-January 2022. *MMWR Morb Mortal Wkly Rep.* 2022;71(7):255–263. 1545-861X. doi:10.15585/mmwr.mm7107e2. 35176007.

210. Collie S, Champion J, Moultrie H, Bekker L-G, Gray G. Effectiveness of BNT162b2 Vaccine against Omicron Variant in South Africa. *N Engl J Med.* 2022;386(5):494–496. 1533-4406. doi:10.1056/NEJMc2119270. 34965358.

211. Chemaitelly H, et al. "Duration of protection of BNT162b2 and mRNA-1273 COVID-19 vaccines against symptomatic SARS-CoV-2 Omicron infection in Qatar." *MedRxiv.* 2022 2002.2007.22270568.

212. UK-HSA. Week 6 COVID-19 vaccine surveillance report (10 Feb 2022). UK: Health Security Agency; 2022. https://assets.publishing.service.gov.uk/government/uploads/system/uploads/attachment_data/file/1054071/vaccine-surveillance-report-week-6.pdf.

213. Hansen CH, et al. (2021) "Vaccine effectiveness against SARS-CoV-2 infection with the Omicron or Delta variants following a two-dose or booster BNT162b2 or mRNA-1273 vaccination series: A Danish cohort study." *A Danish cohort study.* 2021 2012.2020.21267966.

214. Halasa NB, Olson SM, Staat MA, et al. Overcoming COVID-19 Investigators; Overcoming COVID-19 Network. Effectiveness of Maternal Vaccination with mRNA COVID-19 Vaccine During Pregnancy Against COVID-19-Associated Hospitalization in Infants Aged < 6 Months - 17 States, July 2021-January 2022. *MMWR Morb Mortal Wkly Rep.* 2022;71(7):264–270. 1545-861X. doi:10.15585/mmwr.mm7107e3. 35176002.

215. Walsh EE, Frenck Jr RW, Falsey AR, et al. Safety and Immunogenicity of Two RNA-Based Covid-19 Vaccine Candidates. *N Engl J Med.* 2020;383(25):2439–2450. 1533-4406. doi:10.1056/NEJMoa2027906. 33053279.

216. Ramasamy MN, Minassian AM, Ewer KJ, et al. Oxford COVID Vaccine Trial Group. Safety and immunogenicity of ChAdOx1 nCoV-19 vaccine administered in a prime-boost regimen in young and old adults (COV002): a single-blind, randomised, controlled, phase 2/3 trial. *Lancet.* 2021;396(10267):1979–1993. 1474-547X. doi:10.1016/S0140-6736(20)32466-1. 33220855.

217. Anderson EJ, Rouphael NG, Widge AT, et al. mRNA-1273 Study Group. Safety and Immunogenicity of SARS-CoV-2 mRNA-1273 Vaccine in Older Adults. *N Engl J Med.* 2020;383(25):2427–2438. 1533-4406. doi:10.1056/NEJMoa2028436. 32991794.

218. Thomas SJ, Moreira Jr ED, Kitchin N, et al. C4591001 Clinical Trial Group. Safety and Efficacy of the BNT162b2 mRNA Covid-19 Vaccine through 6 Months. *N Engl J Med.* 2021;385(19):1761–1773. 1533-4406. doi:10.1056/NEJMoa2110345.34525277.

CHAPTER

4 COVID-19: Natural History and Spectrum of Disease

Subramani Mani, MBBS, PhD, and Daniel Griffin, MD, PhD

OUTLINE

Coronavirus disease-2019 (COVID-19) caused by severe acute respiratory syndrome coronavirus 2 (SARS-CoV-2) was first described in the city of Wuhan, China in late 2019. After infecting tens of thousands of people in Wuhan and the province of Hubei, where Wuhan is located, the disease spread to various other cities of China and internationally. With multiple surges and peaks, it has infected individuals on every continent, even Antarctica (36 people testing positive at Chilean Bernardo O'Higgins research station in December 2020). It has spread rapidly to more than 200 countries and continues to challenge the health care resources of both the developed and developing world. With a global case count in hundreds of millions and with a death toll in multimillions over an 18-month period, the COVID-19 pandemic has become the most dangerous global infectious disease of the 21st century.[1]

Humans are susceptible to a range of microbes that include parasites, bacteria, and viruses. However, most of the newly identified emerging pathogens are viruses that are carried by vectors, or cause primary disease in animals and then "jump" to humans (zoonotic). These are opportunistic viruses that mutate at high rates, easily adapting to the new human host, thereby enabling human-to-human transmission. The most prominent of these emerging pathogens are the Zika virus and the newer zoonotic respiratory coronaviruses,[2,3] which also include the current pandemic-causing virus SARS-CoV-2.

Short Comparison of SARS-CoV-2 With SARS-CoV-1 and MERS-CoV

The first SARS-CoV outbreak occurred in late 2002 and soon became a pandemic in early 2003, resulting in the death of more than 700 people, with a large cluster of fatalities reported from Hong Kong. This SARS-CoV virus is thought to have originated in a single or multiple species of bats.[2] A more recent coronavirus (CoV) pathogen is the Middle Eastern respiratory syndrome (MERS) CoV, which first emerged in 2012 in Saudi Arabia, and spread to many countries in the region. By 2018, MERS-CoV had infected more than 2000 people, causing 803 deaths, the majority of them in Saudi Arabia. Camels and bats are considered to be reservoirs of this pathogen.[4]

Before the emergence of SARS, human coronaviruses typically caused only mild upper respiratory tract infections, resulting in the common cold. All of this changed with the emergence of SARS-CoV, MERS-CoV, and the newest member SARS-CoV-2, the causative agent of the COVID-19 pandemic.

The recently identified respiratory tract virus SARS-CoV-2 belongs to the viral family coronaviridae, also referred to as the coronavirus family.[5] Other prominent members of the respiratory tract group of viruses are the rhinovirus, the respiratory syncytial virus (RSV), and the influenza and parainfluenza viruses. The coronaviruses are positive-sense, single-stranded RNA viruses, containing an RNA inner core with an outer oily lipid envelope from which crown-like spikes of proteins project outward. These characteristic crown-like projections on their surface give the virions the appearance of a solar corona in electron micrographs and hence the nomenclature *corona*. For a detailed structure and other biological characteristics of SARS-CoV-2 the reader is referred to the specific chapter on the topic in this book. The coronaviruses are heat sensitive and are susceptible to lipid solvents such as acetone, ether, and vinegar (which contains acetic acid). The lipid envelope of the virus also breaks apart on contact with soap.

The viral sequence of SARS-CoV-2 identified by Zhu et al.[5] contains 29,892 nucleotides, and the viral genome reported by Wu et al.[6] contains 29,903 nucleotides. Phylogenetic analysis revealed the close relationship to SARS-like coronaviruses previously found in bats in China. The pangolin, a mammal also known as the scaly anteater, may be an intermediate host and a natural reservoir of SARS-CoV-2–like coronaviruses.[7] While initially there was the suggestion that the pangolin may be an intermediate host as it is a natural reservoir of SARS-CoV-2–like coronaviruses, it may be that in the case of SARS-CoV-2 that the raccoon dog was the critical host from which the virus spread into humans.[162–165] Also, a jump from a human to a tiger in New York City at the Bronx Zoo demonstrated that this pathogen also can be a reverse zoonosis. See Fig. 4.1 for an illustration of this zoonotic transmission model of SARS-CoV-2. There are also reports of domestic pets such as cats and dogs becoming susceptible to SARS-CoV-2 infection.[8]

Natural History

The manifestation and the course taken by the disease process without therapeutic intervention constitute the natural history of a disease. The evolution of a specific disease varies considerably based on host factors, and in the case of infectious diseases, agent characteristics can also play a major role. Agent factors are significantly more important for diseases caused by viruses that mutate rapidly with implications for pathogenicity and virulence.

The natural history of asymptomatic SARS-CoV-2 infection can be surmised from the outbreak characteristics of COVID-19 on the cruise ship *Diamond Princess*. Of the total number of 3711 passengers and crew members, 712 persons became infected based on the

A Transmission Model from Bat to Man with Pangolin as Reservoir

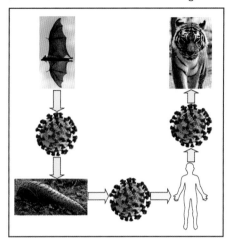

Fig. 4.1 A Zoonotic Transmission Model From Bat to Humans With the Pangolin as Reservoir. Phylogenetic analysis demonstrated the close similarity to other SARS-like coronaviruses found earlier in bats in China. The pangolin is suspected to be a natural reservoir of SARS-CoV-2–like coronaviruses and could be an intermediate host. (Image of SARS-CoV-2 from Centers for Disease Control and Prevention; Eckert and Higgins, in public domain images of bat, pangolin, and tiger from Wikimedia public domain images.)

reverse transcription polymerase chain reaction (RT-PCR) test. At the time of testing, 410 did not have any symptoms. A subset of 96 persons were observed subsequently for 7 days, and 11 became symptomatic.[9]

Incubation Period

The incubation period is the duration from the time of exposure to the pathogen to the manifestation of symptoms of the disease. The mean incubation period of SARS-CoV-2 infection is 5.5 days, with a range of 2 to 12 days. But there could be outliers, and Table 4.1[10] shows the number of positive cases that could be missed using a 14-day and 28-day protocol of isolation.

Transmission Characteristics SARS-CoV-2 is mainly transmitted by respiratory droplets; however, the virus also has been isolated from the patient stools,[11] and there have been many documented cases in which contact tracing supports infection secondary to inhalation of the virus in the air farther than 6 ft (or 2 m) from the source patient.[12–14] Both symptomatic patients and asymptomatic persons infected with SARS-CoV-2 can transmit the virus.[15] The virus

Table 4.1 Expected Number of Symptomatic SARS-CoV-2 Infections Missed During Active Monitoring Using 14-Day and 28-Day Protocols With Varying Risks for Infection After Exposure

	Missed Symptomatic Infections per 10,000 Monitored Persons			
Isolation Period	*Low Risk (1/10,000)*	*Medium Risk (1/1000)*	*High Risk (1/100)*	*Infected Sample (1/1)*
14 days	0	0.1	1	101
28 days	0	0	0	1.4

Modified from Lauer SA, Grantz KH, Bi Q, et al. The incubation period of coronavirus disease 2019 (COVID-19) from publicly reported confirmed cases: estimation and application. *Ann Intern Med.* 2020;172(9)577–582.

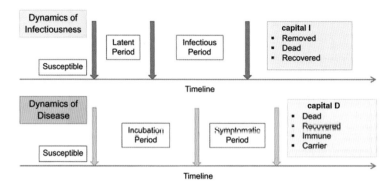

Fig. 4.2 Dynamics of Infection and Disease. Interactions of infectiousness and manifestations of disease and the connects and disconnects between the asymptomatic and symptomatic trajectories of the infectious process in susceptible individuals. Note that the incubation period subsumes the latent period and overlaps with part of the infectious period. The *top panel* shows how a person could get infected, remain asymptomatic, and be contagious. The *bottom panel* shows how a person can be contagious during a part of the incubation period when the symptoms have not manifested. (Modified from Weiss NS. Clinical epidemiology. In: Rothman KJ, Greenland SS [eds]. *Modern Epidemiology.* Philadelphia: Lippincott-Raven; 1998.)

can remain infectious suspended in aerosols for hours, and there is described transmission through the air in closed spaces and in a crowded and congested environment.[166] The virus can also remain viable for up to 72 hours on different surfaces as varied as plastic, steel, copper, and cardboard.[16] Despite detection on surfaces, the role of contact transmission (transmission involving fomites) appears to be minimal. Fig. 4.2 provides the dynamics of infectiousness, susceptibility to infection, and disease manifestation.

Table 4.2 provides the fatality rate and reproductive rate (R_0) of common and emerging virus infections.[17] The toll and the public health impact of major viral infections during the course of the 20th and early 21st centuries can be ascertained from the statistics.

Spectrum of COVID-19

The spectrum of disease can vary from asymptomatic without any clinical manifestations, through minimal symptoms causing just a mild limitation in activities of daily living, to more significant symptoms requiring hospitalization resulting in a mild, moderate, or severe disease trajectory. The spectral range also includes cases of persisting symptoms—weeks, months, or possibly even years after recovering from COVID-19, the long-hauler syndrome.

Pathogenicity and Virulence

Pathogenicity denotes the ability of a pathogen to induce disease. Smallpox, measles, and varicella have high pathogenicity.[18] Based on the Wuhan seroprevalence study of COVID-19 with only a third showing symptoms, the pathogenicity of SARS-CoV-2 can be considered moderate.[19]

Virulence is determined by the severity of the disease manifestation after the occurrence of infection. For example, smallpox and Ebola virus infections are highly virulent.[18] Based on available evidence, the virulence of SARS-CoV-2 infections, such as its pathogenicity, also can be considered moderate.

Table 4.2 Fatality Rate and Reproductive Rate (R_0) of Common and Emerging Virus Infections			
Virus	**Fatality rate (%)**	**Transmissibility Factor (R_0)**	**Deaths**
SARS-CoV-2 (2019)	3	2.2	4.7 million + (until September, 2021)
SARS-CoV (2002)	10	2–5	700
MERS-CoV (2012)	40	<1	800
H1N1 (2009)	0.03	1.2–1.6	18,600–300,000
H1N1 (1918)	3	1.4–3.8	17–50 million (1918–1920)
Measles virus	0.3	12–18	140,000 in 2018
Seasonal flu	<0.1	1.2–2.4	0.3–0.6 million/y currently
Ebola virus (2014–2016)	40	1.5–2.5	11,300 (2014–2016)
HIV	80 (without drug therapy)	2–4	30 million total deaths till 2020
Smallpox virus	17	5–7	300 million in 20th century

Modified from Chen J. Pathogenicity and transmissibility of 2019-nCoV: a quick overview and comparison with other emerging viruses. *Microbes Infect.* 2020;22(2):69-71.

Asymptomatic Trajectory

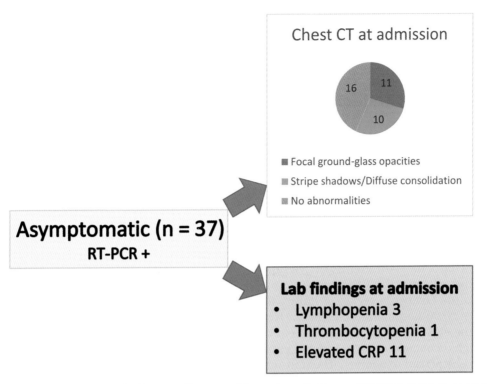

Fig. 4.3 Chest Computed Tomography and Laboratory Features of Asymptomatic Group of SARS-CoV-2–Infected Individuals (n = 37). Even though these 37 patients were SARS-CoV-2 positive *(RT-PCR+),* they did not have clinical symptoms. However, at admission many of the patients had significant laboratory findings and radiological features suggestive of COVID-19. *CRP,* C-Reactive protein; *CT,* computed tomography; *RT-PCR,* reverse transcriptase polymerase chain reaction. (Data from Long Q-X, Tang X-J, Shi Q-L, et al. Clinical and immunological assessment of asymptomatic SARS-CoV-2 infections. *Nat Med.* 2020;26[8]:1200-1204.)

Asymptomatic Disease and Carrier Status

COVID-19 was first reported in the city of Wuhan, China in December 2019.[9] Antibody tests performed on more than 11,000 healthy individuals from early March through early May 2020 showed a seroprevalence rate of 1.68% in Wuhan. Based on the seropositivity rate of 1.68% for the whole city of Wuhan, with a population of 10 million, the researchers estimated that 168,000 people were infected. However, the total number of hospitalized people in the first half of 2020 was only about 50,000—that is, a third of the total infected in Wuhan.[9] Wuhan had a clear policy of admitting all symptomatic people, which means that two-thirds of the infections were asymptomatic.[19] Transmission of COVID-19 by asymptomatic carriers has been demonstrated in different clusters.[20,21]

Asymptomatic Patient Trajectories

Long et al.[22] conducted a clinical and immunological study of SARS-CoV-2 RT-PCR–positive asymptomatic individuals who were isolated and hospitalized. This group of asymptomatic patients did not have any relevant clinical symptoms during the preceding 2 weeks and also during the period of hospitalization. The researchers also had two comparison groups—an age- and sex-matched control group and a symptomatic group. Fig. 4.3 summarizes the chest computed tomography (CT) and laboratory features of the asymptomatic group of 37 individuals. Of the 21 individuals with lung abnormalities based on chest CT imaging, two-thirds had unilateral radiological lung signs and in one-third the signs were bilateral. Of 16 who did not show any chest CT abnormalities, 5 developed focal ground-glass opacities or stripe shadows within 5 days of hospitalization.

Viral RNA detection was also prolonged in the asymptomatic group as measured by the median duration when compared with the symptomatic group. However, this increased viral RNA detection may not be correlated with higher infectivity of the virus.[22,23] The study by Long et al.[22] also showed that 18 proinflammatory and anti-inflammatory cytokines were elevated in the symptomatic group and the cytokine profiles were similar in the asymptomatic and control groups, pointing to a reduced inflammatory response in the asymptomatic group.

During the active phase of infection, the immunoglobulin (IgG) profiles in both the asymptomatic and symptomatic groups were similar. When the groups were seen 8 weeks after discharge from hospital (early convalescent phase), the IgG levels in the symptomatic group were significantly higher than those of the asymptomatic group.[22] This finding has implications for the duration of immunity resulting from asymptomatic versus symptomatic infection from SARS-CoV-2.

Symptomatic Patient Trajectories

The following description is based predominantly on these studies—the first based on 425 confirmed cases in Wuhan, China[24]; the second reporting data on 1099 patients admitted to various hospitals in mainland China[25]; the third on 138 hospitalized patients in Wuhan[26]; the fourth a review article based on 19 studies (18 from China and 1 from Australia), which also included the three primary studies[27]; the fifth a retrospective cohort study of 191 hospitalized patients in Wuhan with follow-up[28]; the sixth a retrospective study of 1591 consecutive patients admitted to an intensive care unit (ICU) in the Lombardy region of Italy[29]; the seventh a study of 5700 hospitalized patients in New York City[30]; and the eighth a review by Machhi et al.[31] COVID-19 is a highly contagious disease that is easily transmitted from one person to another. The transmissibility factor, also called the basic R_0, is defined as the number of new cases an existing case is likely to generate on average. The R_0 of COVID-19 is estimated to be 2.2.

Demographics

The median age of patients in different studies varied between 47 and 63 years. Males were disproportionately affected, ranging from 50% to 82%. Among the first 425 confirmed cases in Wuhan there were no children younger than 15 years.[24] In the study of 1099 patients, the number of children younger than 15 years was 9.[25] Of the 5700 hospitalized patients in New York City, only 26 were children below the age of 10 years.[30] About 15% of the hospitalized patients were categorized as severe and were on average older by 7 years and were more likely to have coexisting medical conditions compared with the less severe hospitalized group of patients.

Pathogenesis

The SARS-CoV2 virus enters the human body by droplets through the nose, mouth, or eyes. The virus enters the cells in the airway by binding the viral surface spike protein to the human angiotensin-converting enzyme-2 (ACE2) receptor. This follows activation of the spike protein by transmembrane protease serine 2 (TMPRSS2). ACE2 is expressed in the alveolar cells of the lung, heart, vascular endothelium, and kidneys, but the main portal of viral entry seems to be the lung alveolar cells.[32,33] Fig. 4.4 illustrates the tissue expression profile of ACE2 in the human host.

Clinical Characteristics

Fever was present in 40% of the patients on admission and in 80% of patients during the hospitalization period. Cough was the second most prevalent symptom and was reported by 70% of the patients. Half of the patients reported feeling fatigued. Breathlessness was observed in 30% of the patients. Nausea, vomiting, sore throat, and headache were uncommon (<10%). A third of the patients had one or more coexisting conditions such as high blood pressure, chronic obstructive pulmonary disease, diabetes, or coronary artery disease, and this was more pronounced among patients with severe disease. A large study of more than 8500 RT-PCR–positive COVID-19 patients treated in a large Chicago area academic medical center examined the risk factors leading to inpatient hospitalizations and critical illness (defined as requiring ICU admission).[34] The study found that increasing age, male sex, Hispanic/Latino ethnicity and comorbidities such as hypertension, diabetes mellitus, prior cerebrovascular accident, coronary artery disease, congestive heart failure (CHF), chronic kidney disease, and end-stage renal disease were risk factors associated with hospitalization.[34] Factors associated with elevated risk of critical illness included male sex, CHF, blood-borne cancer, leukocytosis, elevated neutrophil-to-lymphocyte ratio (absolute neutrophil count to absolute lymphocyte count), elevated aspartate transaminase (AST), elevated D-dimer, and elevated troponin.[34]

Another large study of 1150 RT-PCR–positive COVID-19 patients hospitalized at two New York hospitals affiliated with Columbia University Medical Center looked at the risk factors of in-hospital death.[35] The study found that older age per 10-year increase, chronic heart disease, chronic pulmonary disease, higher concentrations of interleukin-6 (IL-6) per decile rise, and higher concentrations of D-dimer per decile rise were independently associated with in-hospital death.[35] We now proceed to discuss the clinical manifestations of COVID-19 in the various systems of the human body.

Respiratory and Pulmonary Manifestations

The cardinal manifestation of COVID-19 is the triad of fever, cough, and breathlessness, because the primary transmission of the virus is by the respiratory tract.[25,27,36] With the enhancement of severity of the disease resulting in hypoxia, the trajectory of SARS marked by unilateral or bilateral pneumonia develops. A large meta-analysis showed that the incidence of acute respiratory distress syndrome (ARDS) was 20% in hospitalized patients.[36] COVID-19–associated ARDS results in high mortality. Based on a multicenter study of 301 hospitalized patients with COVID-19–associated ARDS in Italy, Grasselli et al.[37] reported that the pathophysiological injury was similar

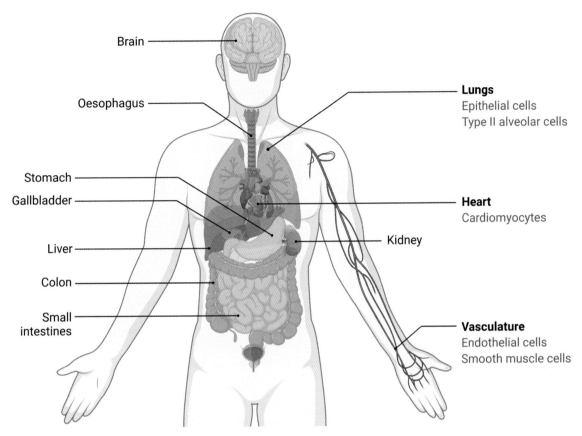

Fig. 4.4 Tissue Expression Profile of Angiotensin-Converting Enzyme-2 *(ACE2)* **in the Human Host.** ACE2 is the main host receptor that facilitates entry of SARS-CoV-2 into the host cells. The clinical manifestations of SARS-CoV-2 infection in various systems can be partly explained by the diversity in the expression profile of ACE2 expression in the human host. The main portal of viral entry seems to be the lung alveolar cells. (Figure adapted from Biorender.)

to that of ARDS from multiple causes unrelated to COVID-19. The study found that among patients with COVID-19–associated ARDS the subgroup who had reduced lung compliance and increased D-dimer concentrations had much higher mortality rates because SARS-CoV-2 affects the alveoli, the lung vasculature, and the coagulation pathway.[37] See Figs. 4.5 and 4.6 for illustrations of the effect of SARS-CoV-2 infection on the lung parenchyma and the pathophysiological processes of ARDS. Fig. 4.7 provides a summary of the mild, moderate, and severe respiratory system disease manifestations. The reader is referred to Chapter 5 for additional details.

Cardiovascular Manifestations

There have been some reports of patients with COVID-19 presenting with chest pain and showing ST-segment elevation on the electrocardiogram without any evidence of coronary artery disease. In these patients, echocardiography revealed left ventricular dysfunction with reduced

ejection fraction and elevated cardiac biomarkers such as troponin. Patients with SARS-CoV-2 infection also can present with myocarditis, stress cardiomyopathy, or cardiac failure, or they may present with palpitations and chest pain without fever and cough. Patients also can present with shortness of breath, supraventricular tachycardia, and cardiogenic shock.[38] The exact mechanism of cardiac pathogenesis is not clear,[33] but it could be a consequence of systemic hyperinflammation, lymphocytopenia, and elevated cardiac stress resulting from respiratory failure and hypoxemia.[39] The reader is referred to the specific chapter on cardiovascular manifestations (Chapter 6) in this volume for additional details.

Neurological Manifestations

Patients have presented with dizziness, headache, ataxia, altered sensorium, and other clinical features suggestive of brain inflammation.[40] A small subset of patients developed stroke and seizures. There are also

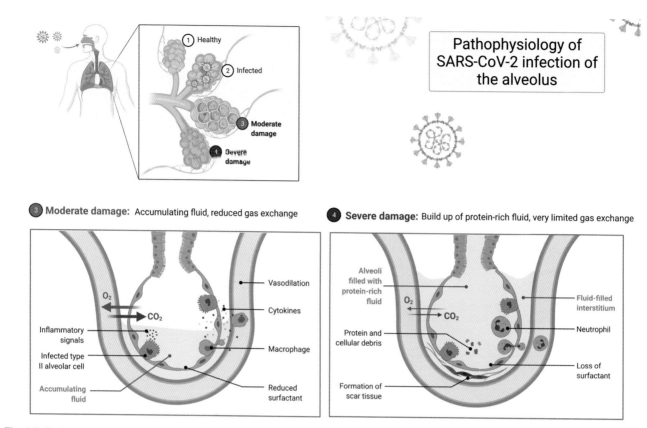

Fig. 4.5 Pathophysiology of SARS-CoV-2 Infection of the Alveolus and Its Effect on Respiration. The *top left panel* shows alveoli at four stages: (1) healthy through (4) severe damage after inhalation of SARS-CoV-2 viral particles. The *bottom two panels* show details of the pathophysiology of (3) moderate and (4) severe alveolar damage. In moderate damage, gas exchange (oxygenation of blood) is partially compromised, whereas in severe damage in which the alveolus and the interstitial space are filled with fluid, gas exchange and oxygenation are severely affected. (Figure adapted from Biorender.)

reports of acute necrotizing encephalopathy in COVID-19 patients. Some patients develop tingling and numbness in the upper and lower limbs, referred to as acroparesthesia. Patients have also presented with loss of smell and taste suggesting involvement of the olfactory, facial, and glossopharyngeal nerves.[41] In a study of COVID-19 patients in Wuhan, based on a sample of 113 patients who died and 161 patients who recovered, the researchers found that 20% of deceased patients developed hypoxic encephalopathy and among the recovered group of patients it was observed in only 1%.[42]

Pezzini et al.[43] proposed three underlying mechanisms for the neurological manifestations depicted in Fig. 4.8. These mechanistic postulates are shown in Fig. 4.9. However, there is no clear evidence of neurons being infected by SARS-CoV-2[44] and hence direct invasion of the central nervous system is probably the least likely pathway.[45]

Gastrointestinal Manifestations

Some patients with COVID-19 diagnosis exhibited digestive symptoms, with nausea, vomiting, diarrhea, and loss of appetite being the most common manifestation while and abdominal pain and bloating were less frequent.[46,47] Liver injury as evidenced by elevated AST,

alanine transaminase (ALT), or serum total bilirubin was present in 20% of COVID-19 patients undergoing liver function tests.[46,47] Of the 10 patients in the study sample, 1 presented with gastrointestinal (GI) features without concomitant respiratory manifestations, resulting in a delay in diagnosis of COVID-19. It was also noticed that patients who had GI manifestations showed an increased propensity for severe disease and subsequent development of ARDS.[46]

Clinical testing of samples from 205 patients with COVID-19 yielded a positivity rate of 29% (44/153 stool samples) and viable SARS-CoV-2 was observed in the stool samples from 2 patients who did not have diarrhea.[48] Some patients might have GI symptoms only during the course of their disease, with respiratory samples testing negative for the disease while shedding the virus in their stools.[5] See Fig. 4.10 for additional details of GI and hepatic manifestations of COVID-19 and Fig. 4.11 for the pathophysiological postulates underlying the hepatic manifestations of COVID-19.

Renal Manifestations

Kidney involvement in hospitalized patients with COVID-19 has been widely reported.[49–57] A large study

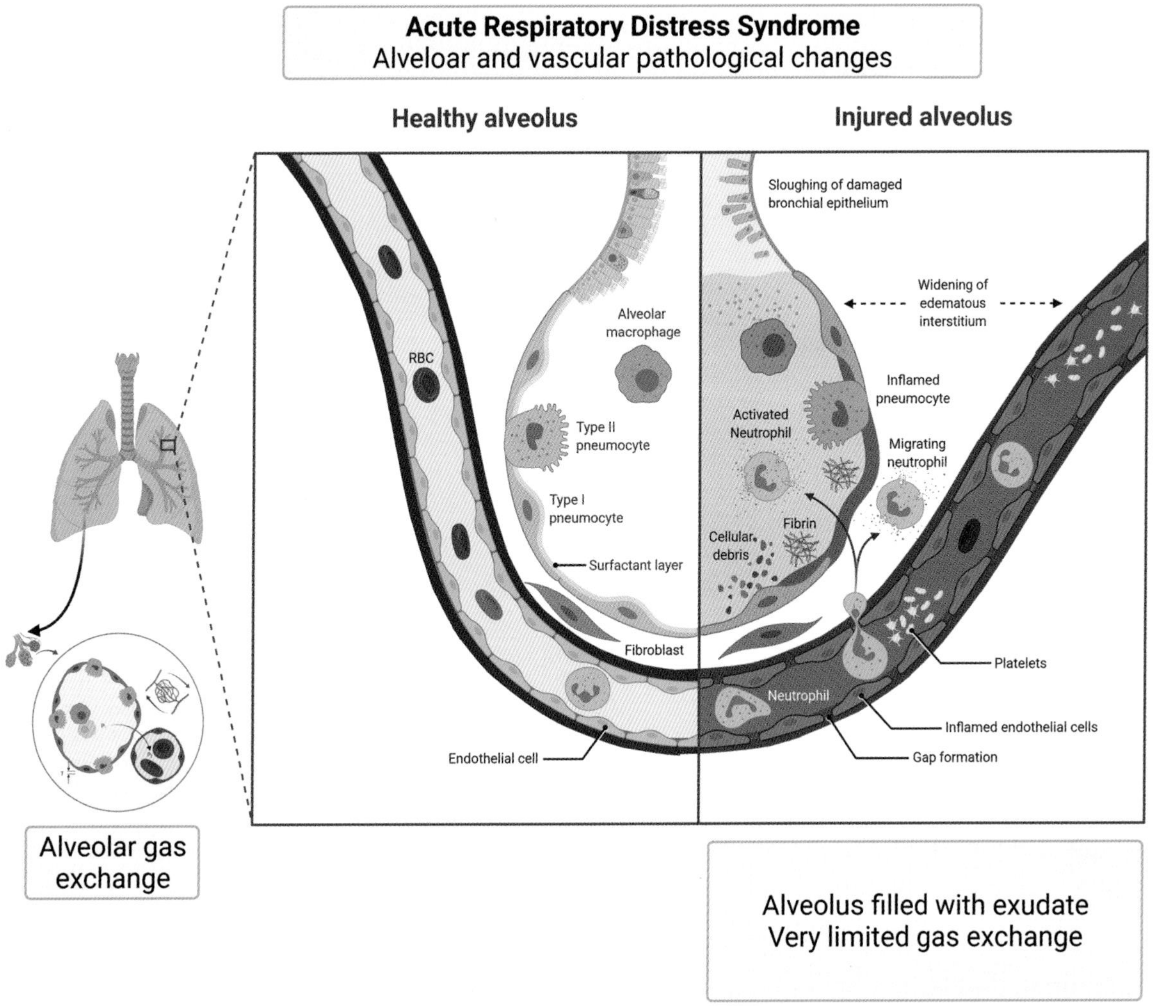

Acute Respiratory Distress Syndrome
Alveloar and vascular pathological changes

Healthy alveolus | Injured alveolus

Sloughing of damaged bronchial epithelium

Widening of edematous interstitium

Alveolar macrophage

Inflamed pneumocyte

RBC

Activated Neutrophil

Migrating neutrophil

Type II pneumocyte

Type I pneumocyte

Fibrin

Cellular debris

Surfactant layer

Fibroblast

Platelets

Neutrophil

Inflamed endothelial cells

Endothelial cell

Gap formation

Alveolar gas exchange

**Alveolus filled with exudate
Very limited gas exchange**

Fig. 4.6 Pathophysiology of Acute Respiratory Distress Syndrome (ARDS). The *right half of the main panel* shows the detailed pathological process in an alveolus when a patient develops ARDS after infection with SARS-CoV-2. Inflammatory changes in the alveolus and the capillary vessel show the extent of damage compromising alveolar gas exchange. Capillary endotheliitis causes migration of neutrophils and leakage of fluid into the alveolar sac, resulting in fluid accumulation and leading to pulmonary edema. (Figure adapted from Biorender.)

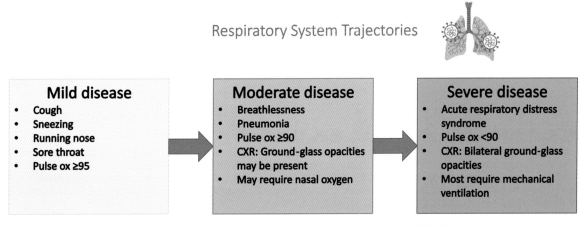

Respiratory System Trajectories

Mild disease
- **Cough**
- **Sneezing**
- **Running nose**
- **Sore throat**
- **Pulse ox ≥95**

Moderate disease
- **Breathlessness**
- **Pneumonia**
- **Pulse ox ≥90**
- **CXR: Ground-glass opacities may be present**
- **May require nasal oxygen**

Severe disease
- **Acute respiratory distress syndrome**
- **Pulse ox <90**
- **CXR: Bilateral ground-glass opacities**
- **Most require mechanical ventilation**

Fig. 4.7 Summary of the Mild, Moderate, and Severe Respiratory System Manifestations. *CXR,* Chest x-ray; *Pulse ox,* pulse oximeter. (Data from Machhi J, Herskovitz J, Senan AM, et al. The natural history, pathobiology, and clinical manifestations of SARS-CoV-2 infections. *J Neuroimmune Pharmacol.* 2020;15[3]:359-386; Gottlieb M, Sansom S, Frankenberger C, et al. Clinical course and factors associated with hospitalization and critical illness among COVID-19 patients in Chicago, Illinois. *Acad Emerg Med.* 2020;27[10]:963-973; and Cummings MJ, Baldwin MR, Abrams D, et al. Epidemiology, clinical course, and outcomes of critically ill adults with COVID-19 in New York City: a prospective cohort study. *Lancet.* 2020;395[10239]:1763-1770. Lung image from Biorender.)

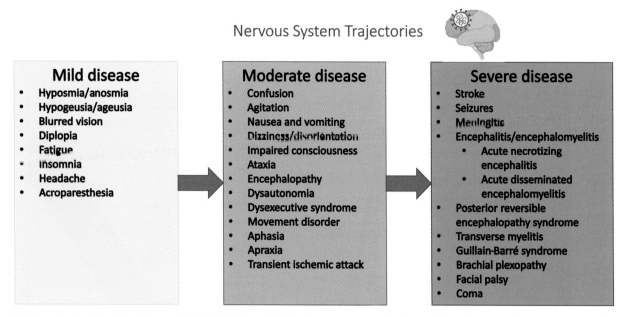

Fig. 4.8 **Neurological Manifestations of COVID-19.** The clinical features are categorized into mild, moderate, and severe versions of neurological disease resulting from SARS-CoV-2 infection. (Data from Machhi J, Herskovitz J, Senan AM, et al. The natural history, pathobiology, and clinical manifestations of SARS-CoV-2 infections. *J Neuroimmune Pharmacol.* 2020:15[3]:359-386; Pezzini A, Padovani A. Lifting the mask on neurological manifestations of COVID-19. *Nat Rev Neurol.* 2020;16[11]:636-644; Helms J, Kremer S, Merdji H, et al. Neurologic features in severe SARS-CoV-2 infection. *N Engl J Med* 2020;382;[23]:2268-2270; Mao L, Wang M, Chen S, et al. Neurological manifestations of hospitalized patients with COVID-19 in Wuhan, China: a retrospective case series study. *JAMA Neurol.* 2020;77[6]:683-690; Paterson RW, Brown RL, Benjamin L, et al. The emerging spectrum of COVID-19 neurology: clinical, radiological and laboratory findings. *Brain.* 2020;143[10]:3104-3120; and Ellul MA, Benjamin L, Singh B, et al. Neurological associations of COVID-19. *Lancet Neurol.* 2020;19[9]:767-783. Brain image from Biorender.)

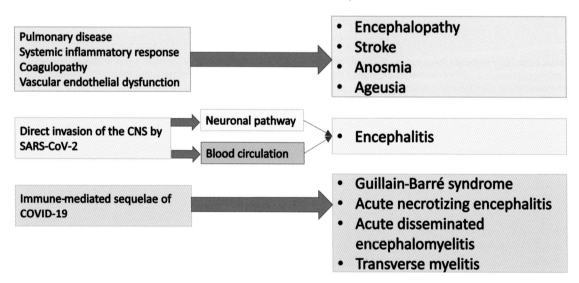

Fig. 4.9 **Key Postulated Mechanisms of Nervous System Manifestations.** The three potential pathways—direct invasion, immune-mediated sequelae, and impact from other diseased organs and systems—are illustrated. *CNS,* Central nervous system. (Data from Pezzini A, Padovani A. Lifting the mask on neurological manifestations of COVID-19. *Nat Rev Neurol.* 2020;16[11]:636-644; Solomon T. Neurological infection with SARS-CoV-2: the story so far. *Nat Rev Neurol.* 2021;17[2]:65-66; Ellul MA, Benjamin L, Singh B, et al. Neurological associations of COVID-19. *Lancet Neurol.* 2020;19[9]:767-783; and Bodro M, Compta Y, Sánchez-Valle R. Presentations and mechanisms of CNS disorders related to COVID-19. *Neurol Neuroimmunol.* 2021;8[1]:e923.)

of close to 4000 patients hospitalized for COVID-19 in the Mount Sinai hospital system in New York City showed that almost 1 in 2 developed acute kidney injury (AKI), with 20% of patients with AKI needing dialysis.[55]

Moreover, among patients who developed AKI, in-hospital mortality was 50% whereas the mortality rate was only 8% in patients who did not develop AKI.[55] Although there is a large variance in the reported occurrence of

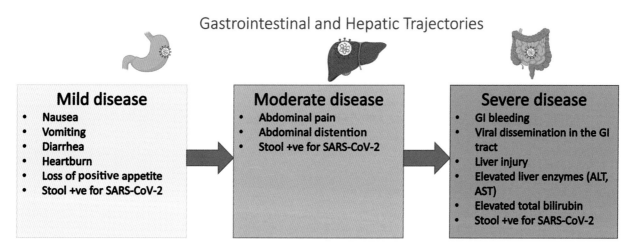

Fig. 4.10 Gastrointestinal *(GI)* and Hepatic Manifestations of COVID-19. The clinical features are categorized into expressions of mild, moderate, and severe disease. *+ve,* Positive; *ALT,* alanine transaminase; *AST,* aspartate transaminase. (Data from Machhi J, Herskovitz J, Senan AM, et al. The natural history, pathobiology, and clinical manifestations of SARS-CoV-2 infections. *J Neuroimmune Pharmacol.* 2020:15[3]:359-386; and Sultan S, Altayar O, Siddique SM, et al. AGA Institute rapid review of the GI and liver manifestations of COVID-19, meta-analysis of international data, and recommendations for the consultative management of patients with COVID-19. *Gastroenterology.* 2020;159[1]:320-334. Stomach, liver, and intestine images from Biorender.)

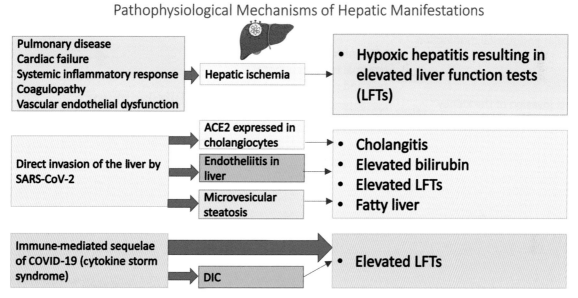

Fig. 4.11 Pathophysiological Mechanisms Underlying Hepatic Manifestations of COVID-19. The three potential pathways of liver injury—direct invasion, immune-mediated sequelae, and impact from other diseased organs and systems—are illustrated in the figure. *ACE2,* Angiotensin-converting enzyme-2; *DIC,* disseminated intravascular coagulation. (Data from Bertolini A, van de Peppel IP, Bodewes F, et al. Abnormal liver function tests in patients with COVID-19: relevance and potential pathogenesis. *Hepatology.* 2020;72[5]:1864-1872; and Nardo AD, Schneeweiss-Gleixner M, Bakail M, et al. Pathophysiological mechanisms of liver injury in COVID-19. *Liver Int.* 2021;41[1]:20-32. Liver image from Biorender.)

AKI in different studies, a consensus is emerging that AKI is a serious problem in patients hospitalized with COVID-19, affecting more than 20% of all hospitalized patients and possibly in excess of 50% of patients admitted to the ICU.[53] Proteinuria and hematuria are common predominant findings.

Risk factors for COVID-19 AKI include male sex, older age, Black race, higher body mass index (BMI), and preexisting conditions such as diabetes mellitus, high blood pressure, chronic kidney disease, and

cardiovascular disease (CVD).[53,58,59] Mortality rates for COVID-19 AKI varied from 35% to 80%, with a higher rate of 75% to 90% in patients requiring renal replacement therapy.[55,56,58,59]

A range of pathophysiological mechanisms have been postulated to account for the renal involvement. There is some evidence of viral tropism with direct infiltration of the kidney by SARS-CoV-2.[60,61] Other causal mechanisms implicated include endothelial dysfunction, coagulopathy, complement activation, systemic

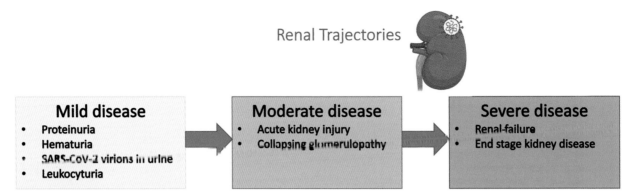

Fig. 4.12 **Renal Manifestations of COVID-19.** The three renal trajectories of mild, moderate, and severe presentations are summarized in the figure. (Data from Machhi J, Herskovitz J, Senan AM, et al. The natural history, pathobiology, and clinical manifestations of SARS-CoV-2 infections. *J Neuroimmune Pharmacol.* 2020:15[3]:359-386; and Chan L, Chaudhary K, Saha A, et al: AKI in hospitalized patients with COVID-19. *J Am Soc Nephrol.* 2021;32[1]:151-160. Kidney image from Biorender.)

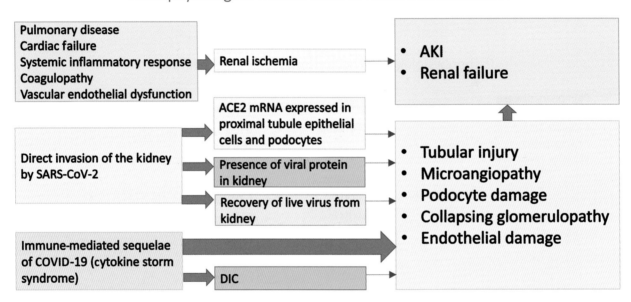

Fig. 4.13 **Pathophysiological Mechanisms Underlying Renal Manifestations of COVID-19.** The three potential pathways of kidney injury—direct invasion, immune-mediated sequelae, and impact from other diseased organs and systems—are illustrated. *ACE2,* Angiotensin-converting enzyme-2; *AKI,* acute kidney injury; *DIC,* disseminated intravascular coagulation. (Adapted from Khan S, Chen L, Yang C-R, et al. Does SARS-CoV-2 infect the kidney? *J Am Soc Nephrol.* 2020;31[12]:2746-2748; Batlle D, Soler MJ, Sparks MA, et al. Acute kidney injury in COVID-19: emerging evidence of a distinct pathophysiology. *J Am Soc Nephrol.* 2020;31[7]:1380-1383.)

inflammation, and immune dysfunction.[50,53] The immune-mediated sequelae of COVID-19 and organ crosstalk facilitated by the circulating chemokines, cytokines, and growth factors between vital organs can lead to AKI after severe lung injury with the release of damage-associated molecular patterns (DAMPs), cytokines, and chemokines.[53,62] When compared with COVID-19 patients who have normal kidney function, patients with COVID-19 AKI show higher levels of systemic inflammatory markers such as ferritin, C-reactive protein (CRP), procalcitonin, and lactate dehydrogenase.[59] See Fig. 4.12 for additional details of renal manifestations of COVID-19 and Fig. 4.13 for the pathophysiological postulates underlying the renal

manifestations of COVID-19. Fig. 4.14 illustrates pathological manifestations of COVID-19 leading to AKI.[52,63,64]

Currently, there is no evidence to suggest that COVID-19 AKI should be managed differently. However, it is recommended that the underlying disease pathological processes and mechanisms are considered carefully in the management of AKI in the setting of COVID-19.[53]

Cutaneous Manifestations

In a study of 88 patients in the Lombardy region of Italy, skin lesions were found in 20%.[65] The cutaneous manifestations reported were erythematous rash, urticaria,

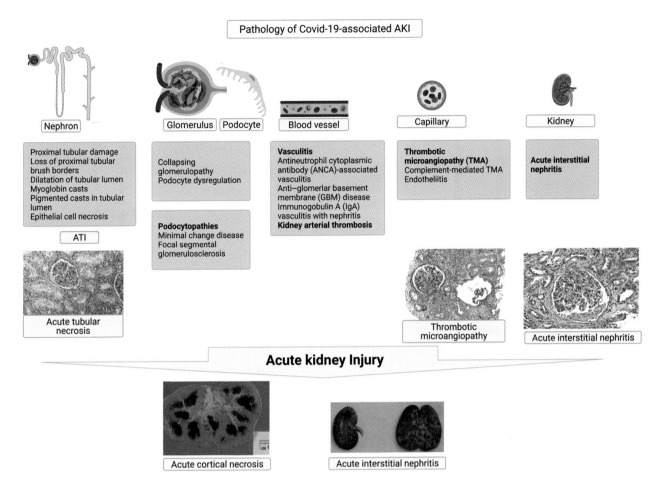

Fig. 4.14 Pathological Manifestations of COVID-19 Leading to Acute Kidney Injury *(AKI)*. The most common pathological condition is acute tubular injury *(ATI)*, followed by collapsing glomerulopathy, other podocytopathies, thrombotic microangiopathy, and vasculitis. A combination of these pathological processes results in AKI. (Adapted from Sharma P, Ng JH, Bijol V, et al. Pathology of COVID-19-associated acute kidney injury. *Clin Kidney J.* 2021;14[suppl. 1]:i30-i39; Izzedine H, Jhaveri KD. Acute kidney injury in patients with COVID-19: an update on the pathophysiology. *Nephrol Dial Transplant.* 2021;36[2]:224-226; and Shetty AA, Tawhari I, Safar-Boueri L, et al. COVID-19–associated glomerular disease. *J Am Soc Nephrol.* 2021;32[1]:33-40. Histopathology slides and gross pathology images from Wikimedia [creative common license]. Figure created using Biorender.)

and chickenpox-like vesicles distributed mainly on the trunk. There were also reports of erythematous chilblain-like lesions on feet and hands in asymptomatic coronavirus-positive patients.[66] Do et al.,[67] in their review of cutaneous manifestations in hospitalized patients, reported two broad types of lesions: vasculopathy-related cutaneous lesions and viral exanthematous eruptions.[67] The vasculopathy-related skin lesions were associated with severe disease manifestations and higher fatalities.[67] However, Marzano et al.,[68] in their study of 200 patients with COVID-19–associated cutaneous manifestations from 21 Italian dermatology units, did not find any significant association between type of skin manifestation and COVID-19 disease severity after adjusting for age. The study also reported an exception—chilblain-like acral lesions were more prevalent in younger patients who were asymptomatic or presented with mild symptoms of COVID-19.[68] Fig. 4.15 summarizes and illustrates the postulated pathophysiological mechanisms of skin manifestations.

Ocular Manifestations

There is a growing literature on ocular manifestations of COVID-19.[25,69–75] Specific retinal findings in COVID-19 patients also have been reported.[71,74,76–78] A set of potential mechanisms for ocular surface and retinal manifestations have been proposed.[25,79–83] Pooled data from 16 studies as part of a systematic review and meta-analysis consisting of more than 2300 patients revealed that 12% of the patients had ocular surface manifestations, with ocular pain in 30%, discharge in 20%, redness of the eyes in 11% and follicular conjunctivitis in 8%.[70] Another meta-analytic study that reported on 7300 COVID-19 patients found a similar prevalence of eye manifestations (11%) and the most prevalent ocular disease among those with eye symptoms was conjunctivitis (89%).[73] Some rare ophthalmic manifestations included keratitis (2%), keratoconjunctivitis (2%), and one case of posterior ischemic optic neuropathy.[73]

A study of 25 hospitalized patients in two referral hospitals of Rio de Janeiro, Brazil observed retinal

Postulated Pathophysiological Mechanisms of Skin Manifestations

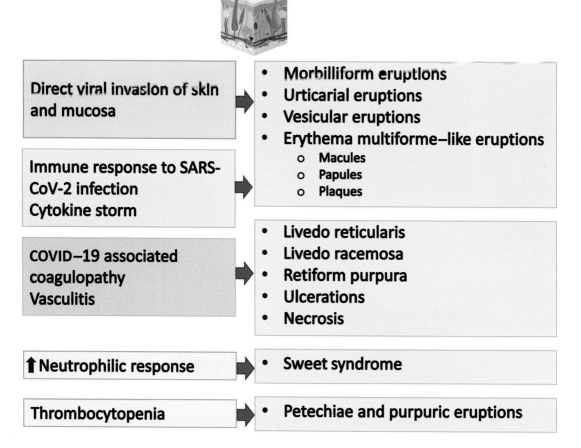

Fig. 4.15 Postulated Pathophysiological Mechanisms of Skin Manifestations. Five mechanisms are illustrated. (Data from Do MH, Stewart CR, Harp J. Cutaneous manifestations of COVID-19 in the inpatient setting. *Dermatol Clin.* 2021;39[4]:521-532; and Larenas-Linnemann D, Luna-Pech J, Navarrete-Rodríguez EM, et al. Cutaneous manifestations related to COVID-19 immune dysregulation in the pediatric age group. *Curr Allergy Asthma Rep.* 2021;21[2]:1-19. Skin cube image from Biorender.)

changes in 3 patients: the first patient with critical illness had bilateral nerve fiber layer infarcts and micro-hemorrhages, the second patient had isolated unilateral flame-shaped hemorrhages, and the third patient demonstrated bilateral discrete retinal dot and blot microhemorrhages.[77] It is likely that these retinal manifestations could be due to the systemic manifestations of COVID-19 and/or consequential to comorbidities and not necessarily to the direct involvement of the retina by the virus.[77]

Another study of 50 COVID-19–positive patients in a university hospital in Milan, Italy showed more retinal hemorrhages and an increase in mean arterial dimension and mean venous dimension based on fundus examination when compared with COVID-19–negative test control subjects.[76] But the investigators could not establish the cause of the retinal manifestations—a direct effect of the virus infiltration or the immune response triggered by the virus in the host.[76] A study of 18 patients hospitalized with COVID-19 in São Paulo,

Brazil revealed retinal abnormalities in 10 patients in the nature of flame-shaped hemorrhages and/or cotton wool spots.[78] See Fig. 4.16 for additional details of ocular surface and retinal manifestations of COVID-19.

However, a different study of 43 SARS-CoV-2–positive patients with pneumonia hospitalized in Rome, Italy that investigated retinal involvement did not find evidence of a causal link of the virus to the observed retinal changes, which the authors attributed to preexisting comorbidities.[74]

See Fig. 4.17 for the pathophysiological postulates underlying the ocular manifestations of COVID-19.

Musculoskeletal and Rheumatological Manifestations

Backache, muscle pain, and arthralgia have been reported in various studies of patients infected with SARS-CoV-2.[84–89] A few studies looked at the plight of

Eye Manifestations: Trajectories

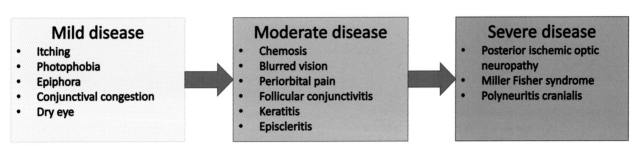

Fig. 4.16 Ocular Manifestations of COVID-19. The mild, moderate, and severe ophthalmic features. *ACE2,* Angiotensin-converting enzyme-2; *BSC,* basigin; *DIC,* disseminating intravascular coagulation; *MAD,* mean arterial dimension; *MVD,* mean venous dimension; *TMPRSS2,* transmembrane protease serine 2. (Data from Chen L, Deng C, Chen X, et al. Ocular manifestations and clinical characteristics of 535 cases of COVID-19 in Wuhan, China: a cross-sectional study. *Acta Ophthalmol.* 2020;98[8]:e951-e959; Abrishami M, Tohidinezhad F, Daneshvar R, et al. Ocular manifestations of hospitalized patients with COVID-19 in northeast of Iran. *Ocul Immunol Inflamm.* 2020;28[5]:739-744; Aggarwal K, Agarwal A, Jaiswal N, et al. Ocular surface manifestations of coronavirus disease 2019 (COVID-19): a systematic review and meta-analysis. *PloS One.* 2020;15[11]:e0241661; Nasiri N, Sharifi H, Bazrafshan A, et al. Ocular manifestations of COVID-19: a systematic review and meta-analysis. *J Ophthalmic Vis Res.* 2021;16[1]:103; and Ho D, Low R, Tong L, et al. COVID-19 and the ocular surface: a review of transmission and manifestations. *Ocul Immunol Inflamm.* 2020;28[5]:726-734. Eye image from Biorender.)

Proposed Mechanisms of Ocular Manifestations of SARS-CoV2

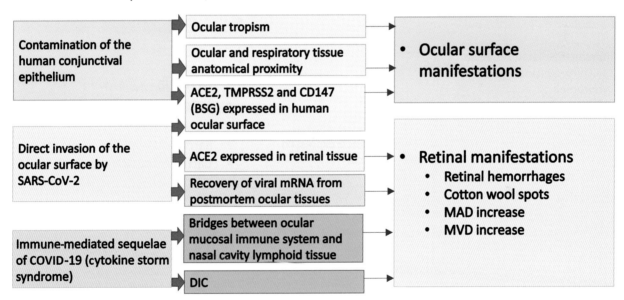

Fig. 4.17 Pathophysiological Mechanisms Underlying Ocular Manifestations of COVID-19. The three potential pathways of eye injury—direct invasion of the ocular surface by SARS-CoV-2, immune-mediated sequelae, and contamination of conjunctival epithelium—are illustrated. The pathways leading to ocular surface injury and retinal injury are delineated. *ACE2,* Angiotensin-converting enzyme-2; *BSG,* basigin; *CD147,* cluster of differentiation 147; *DIC,* disseminated intravascular coagulation; *MAD,* mean arteries diameter; *MVD,* mean veins diameter; *TMPRSS2,* transmembrane serine protease 2. (Data from Ho D, Low R, Tong L, et al. COVID-19 and the ocular surface: a review of transmission and manifestations. *Ocul Immunol Inflamm.* 2020;28[5]:726-734; Belser JA, Rota PA, Tumpey TM. Ocular tropism of respiratory viruses. *Microbiol Mol Biol Rev.* 2013;77[1]:144-156; Zhou L, Xu Z, Castiglione GM, et al. ACE2 and TMPRSS2 are expressed on the human ocular surface, suggesting susceptibility to SARS-CoV-2 infection. *Ocular Surf.* 2020;18[4]:537-544; Li Y-P, Ma Y, Wang N, Jin Z-B. Eyes on coronavirus. *Stem Cell Res.* 2021;51:102200; and Invernizzi A, Torre A, Parrulli S, et al. Retinal findings in patients with COVID-19: results from the SERPICO-19 study. *EClinicalMedicine* 2020;27:100550.)

people with rheumatological and musculoskeletal diseases during the pandemic and specifically when they get infected by SARS-CoV-2.[90,91] The study by Jorge et al.[92] specifically looked at temporal trends in outcomes of patients afflicted with severe COVID-19 who had

preexisting rheumatic disease. The study was conducted over a 6-month period in 2020 and reported that COVID-19 outcomes improved over time in patients with rheumatological and musculoskeletal diseases. Ahmed et al.[93] reported that COVID-19 can result in

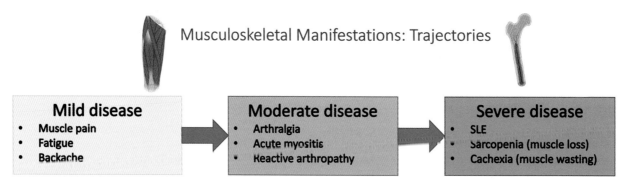

Fig. 4.18 Musculoskeletal Manifestations of COVID-19. *SLE,* Systemic lupus erythematosus. (Data from Ciaffi J, Meliconi R, Ruscitti P, et al. Rheumatic manifestations of COVID-19: a systematic review and meta-analysis. *BMC Rheumatol.* 2020;4[1]:65; Hoong CWS, Amin MNME, Tan TC, Lee JE. Viral arthralgia a new manifestation of COVID-19 infection? A cohort study of COVID-19-associated musculoskeletal symptoms. *Int J Infect Dis.* 2021;104:363-369; Abdullahi A, Candan SA, Abba MA, et al. Neurological and musculoskeletal features of COVID-19: a systematic review and meta-analysis. *Front Neurol.* 2020;11[687]; Zamani B, Moeini Taba S-M, Shayestehpour M. Systemic lupus erythematosus manifestation following COVID-19: a case report. *J Med Case Rep.* 2021;15[1]:29. Muscle and bone images from Biorender.)

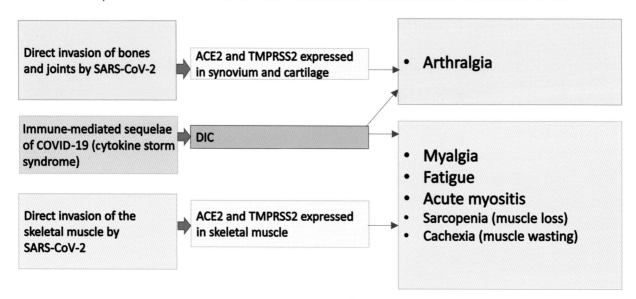

Fig. 4.19 Pathophysiological Mechanisms Underlying Musculoskeletal Manifestations of COVID-19. The three potential pathways of musculoskeletal injury—direct invasion of the skeletal muscle by SARS-CoV-2, immune-mediated sequelae, and direct invasion of bones and joints—are illustrated. *ACE2,* Angiotensin converting enzyme 2; *DIC,* disseminated intravascular coagulation; *TMPRSS2,* transmembrane serine protease 2. (Data from Disser NP, De Micheli AJ, Schonk MM, et al. Musculoskeletal consequences of COVID-19. *JBJS.* 2020;102[14]:1197-1204; and Shah S, Danda D, Kavadichanda C, et al. Autoimmune and rheumatic musculoskeletal diseases as a consequence of SARS-CoV-2 infection and its treatment. *Rheumatol Int.* 2020;40[10]:1539-1554.)

flare-ups of preexisting rheumatological diseases in many patients.

In their study of 80 hospitalized patients in Turkey, Batur et al.[94] found that 46% of them had myalgia and half of the patients reported fatigue. Myalgia was associated with elevated levels of creatine kinase and lymphocytosis.[94] D'Silva et al.,[95] in their study of hospitalized COVID-19 patients from Boston area hospitals reported that patients with preexisting rheumatological disease were three times more likely to require mechanical ventilation than hospitalized patients without preexisting rheumatological disease. However, another study from Wuhan reported a lesser need for mechanical

ventilation in patients hospitalized with COVID-19 who had preexisting rheumatological disease.[96]

A large study based on a registry of 3729 patients with rheumatological diseases and COVID-19 reported that known common factors such as older age, male sex, and comorbidities such as CVD and chronic lung disease were associated with mortality.[97] The study also found that moderate to high rheumatological disease activity and the drugs rituximab, sulfasalazine, and immunosuppressants were also associated with mortality.[97]

See Fig. 4.18 for additional details of musculoskeletal manifestations of COVID-19 and Fig. 4.19 for the pathophysiological postulates underlying the musculo-skeletal manifestations of COVID-19.

Impact of Comorbidities

Obesity and type 2 diabetes have been identified as important comorbidities resulting in adverse outcomes in patients hospitalized with COVID-19.[30,98–100] Obesity and type 2 diabetes do not increase susceptibility to SARS-CoV-2 infection but cause more severe disease.[101] Cai et al.,[102] based on a study of 383 hospitalized patients with COVID-19 in Shenzhen, China reported that obese patients were more than three times likely to develop severe COVID-19. Guo et al.,[103] in a study of 174 consecutive patients hospitalized with COVID-19 in Wuhan Union Hospital, in China, reported that 24 patients who had diabetes but no other comorbidities were at higher risk for severe pneumonia. Inflammatory biomarkers, including IL-6, CRP, serum ferritin, and D-dimer were also significantly elevated in these patients compared with patients without diabetes, indicating enhanced susceptibility to cytokine storm leading to adverse outcomes.[103] Based on their study of 605 hospitalized patients with COVID-19 in the city of Wuhan, China, Wang et al.[104] reported that elevated fasting blood glucose (FBG) at admission (≥ 7 mmol/L) was an independent risk factor for 28-day mortality in patients without a past diagnosis of diabetes. Based on a study of more than 19,000 patients hospitalized with COVID-19 in England, Dennis et al.[105] reported an increased risk for mortality with an adjusted hazard ratio (aHR) of 1.23 in patients with type 2 diabetes for 30-day in-hospital mortality. The aHR for younger patients with type 2 diabetes (18–49 years of age) was higher at 1.5.

Prolonged viral shedding has been reported in patients hospitalized with COVID-19 with obesity as a comorbidity[106] but not in patients with diabetes as a comorbidity.[107] Obesity also has been found to be associated with long-COVID syndrome.[108] The causal pathways responsible for the increased mortality and other adverse outcomes for patients hospitalized with COVID-19 who have obesity or type 2 diabetes as comorbidities have not been well understood,[101] but a few plausible mechanisms involving adipose tissue and ACE2 have been proposed.[98,109]

ACE2 performs three major roles, which Kuba et al.[110] refer to as the trilogy of ACE2. ACE2 acts as (1) the negative regulator of the renin-angiotensin system (RAS) in the cardiovascular system, playing a key role in the maintenance of cardiovascular homeostasis; (2) ACE2 acts as an essential amino acid transporter and is needed for the expression of these amino acid transporters in the intestines; and (3) ACE2 performs the role of a functional receptor for SARS-CoV-1 and SARS-CoV-2, facilitating viral entry into cells and tissues.[98,110] The postulated cascade of pathophysiological mechanisms resulting in severe heart and lung injury causing higher mortality in COVID-19 patients with obesity and/or diabetes is summarized from Kruglikov et al.[98] The increased expression of ACE2 in the adipose tissues of individuals with obesity and type 2 diabetes is protective against angiotensin-2. However, when SARS-CoV-2 infection sets in, viral load increases and ACE2 is engaged by the viral spike protein, which in turn causes increased levels of angiotensin-2 in circulating blood. This cascade of events creates a ripple effect in RAS-mediated cardiovascular homeostasis, causing inflammation of the heart and vasoconstriction in cardiac and lung tissue, aggravating heart and lung injury.[98]

Moreover, the dual impairment of vascular endothelial integrity and intestinal barrier breech cause extrusion of bacterial pathogens from the gut lumen, which then enter the circulation. The bacteremia in the lungs interacting with the viral particles also aggravate lung injury.[98] Fig. 4.20 illustrates the postulated pathophysiological pathways involved in the adverse outcomes of COVID-19 patients with underlying obesity and diabetes.

Based on autopsy studies of 26 hospitalized patients with COVID-19 who died during the course of their illness, Elezkurtaz et al.[111] reported on the causes of death and the contribution of preexisting health conditions to mortality. Even though many comorbidities, including high blood pressure, coronary artery disease, diabetes, and obesity, were present in the majority of the patients, the causes of death were directly linked to COVID-19 and its complications in 24 of 26 fatalities. The study also identified multiorgan failure, pneumonia, respiratory insufficiency, and right heart failure as a result of COVID-19 as the pathological mechanisms leading to death in these patients.

Radiology and Laboratory Features

Abnormal findings were reported in 80% of the CT scans of patients with nonsevere disease and 96% of the scans of patients in the severe disease category. The typical patterns on chest CT were ground-glass opacity and bilateral patchy shadowing. These abnormal patterns were also visible on chest radiographs. Lung opacities and patchy shadows were observed in multiple lobes, and the lung parenchymal involvement was peripherally distributed, which is a cardinal feature of SARS-CoV-2 infection.[112] As the lung infection progresses the diffuse lung opacities organize, evolving into coalescent or consolidation-type patterns over a period of 2 weeks.[112] Less frequent findings found toward the later stages of the disease include septal thickening, bronchiectasis, and thickening of the pleura. Other infrequent CT findings reported with disease progression were pleural effusion, pericardial effusion, lymphadenopathy, lung cavities, CT halo sign, and pneumothorax.[113] Pulmonary ultrasound also has been found useful in the workup of hospitalized critically ill COVID-19 patients for detection of pneumonia because it can be used at the bedside

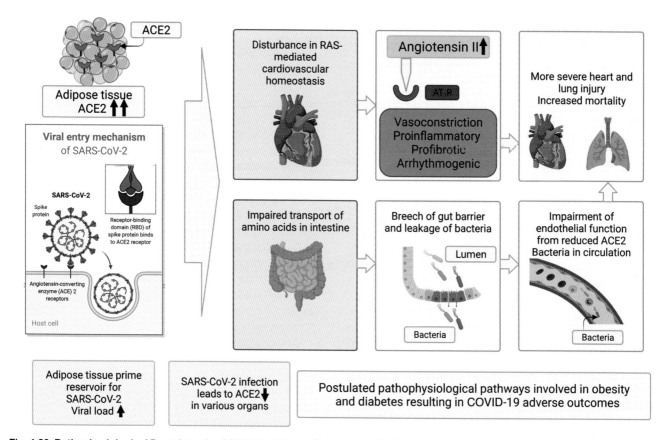

Fig. 4.20 Pathophysiological Postulates for COVID-19 Adverse Outcomes in Patients With Obesity and/or Diabetes. Adipose tissue acts as a reservoir for SARS-CoV-2, resulting in a viral overload that leads to a reduction in angiotensin-converting enzyme-2 *(ACE2)* in different organs. The resulting impairment in renin-angiotensin system *(RAS)*-mediated cardiovascular homeostasis causes heart and lung injury. The impaired amino acid transport in the intestine leads to bacteremia and vascular endothelial dysfunction. (Modified from Kruglikov IL, Shah M, Scherer PE. Obesity and diabetes as comorbidities for COVID-19: underlying mechanisms and the role of viral–bacterial interactions. *Elife.* 2020;9:e61330. Figure created using Biorender.)

and is less invasive.[112] When pulmonary embolism is suspected, a pulmonary CT angiography is undertaken to arrive at a definitive diagnosis. Thromboembolic manifestations can occur as a result of involvement of the arterial or venous vasculature and vascular imaging has a key role in assessment.[112]

Radiology also plays an important role in the evaluation of COVID-19 patients with underlying CVD and those who develop cardiovascular complications. Apart from routine imaging modalities such as chest x-ray, chest CT, and echocardiography, cardiac magnetic resonance imaging (MRI) is specifically recommended for assessment of myocardial injury.[112] Likewise, head CT and MRI of the brain are undertaken for evaluation of neurological complications of COVID-19. For GI manifestations of COVID-19, ultrasound and CT serve as key imaging modalities. The radiological features of COVID-19 are discussed further in the chapters dealing with specific systems.

More than 80% of patients had a low lymphocyte count.[25] Approximately one-third of patients had low white cell counts, and another third had low platelet counts.[25] Most patients also showed reduced albumin, high levels of CRP, and elevated erythrocyte sedimentation rate.[25–27,114] The laboratory findings were more pronounced in patients with a severe form of the disease. In a study of 2874 SARS-CoV-2–positive patients, RNAemia, that is, detection of viral RNA fragments in blood was positive in 97%.[27]

Based on pooled data from 10,491 confirmed COVID-19 patients from 32 studies, Malik et al.[115] identified 10 laboratory biomarkers—lymphopenia, thrombocytopenia, elevated CRP, creatine kinase, procalcitonin, D-dimer, lactate dehydrogenase, ALT, AST, creatinine—to be associated with adverse outcomes in hospitalized patients.[115] Table 4.3 provides the odds ratios and 95% confidence intervals for these biomarkers. Many of these biomarkers could be used to plan optimal treatment strategies to improve patient outcomes.

Treatment, Clinical Course, and Outcomes

Initially there was no specific evidence-based antiviral treatment available broadly for all patients at all stages of COVID-19. A majority of the patients (60%) were given intravenous antibiotics, and oxygen was administered to approximately 40% of the patients. Of the

Table 4.3 Laboratory Findings and COVID-19 Adverse Outcomes Based on 10,491 COVID-19 Patients

Laboratory Findings	Cutoff Values	Odds Ratio for Adverse Outcomes	95% Confidence Interval
Lymphopenia	<1500 cells/μL	3.3	2.51–4.41
Thrombocytopenia	<150000	2.36	1.64–3.40
Elevated D-dimer	≥0.5 mg/L	3.39	2.66–4.33
Elevated CRP	>10 mg/L	4.37	3.37–5.68
Elevated procalcitonin	>0.5 ng/L	6.33	4.24–9.45
Elevated creatine kinase	NA	2.42	1.35–4.32
Elevated AST	>40 IU/L	2.75	2.30–3.29
Elevated ALT	>40 IU/L	1.71	1.32–2.20
Elevated creatinine	>1.18	2.84	1.80–4.46
Elevated LDH	NA	5.48	3.89–7.71

ALT, Alanine transaminase; *AST*, aspartate transaminase; *CRP*, C-reactive protein; *LDH*, lactate dehydrogenase, *NA*, not available.
Data from Malik P, Patel U, Mehta D, et al. Biomarkers and outcomes of COVID-19 hospitalisations: systematic review and meta-analysis. *BMJ Evid Based Med.* 2021;26(3):107–108.

patients, 20% typically needed admission to the ICU and half had to be placed on a ventilator. More than 90% had pneumonia, 10% of patients developed ARDS, and 5% of patients went into shock. The median duration of hospitalization was 12 to 20 days in different studies, with the mortality rate varying from 2% to 20% in various studies. Details of treatment protocols are described under specific system chapters.

Drug Pipeline

Three drugs that underwent studies for effectiveness in the treatment of COVID-19 are remdesivir, hydroxychloroquine, and chloroquine. Despite preliminary evidence that these drugs had the potential to inhibit SARS-CoV-2,[116] only remdesivir ultimately demonstrated more benefit than harm. Remdesivir is an antiviral compound originally developed as a potential drug for Ebola, and hydroxychloroquine and chloroquine are in the category of repurposed drugs and have been used in the treatment of malaria. Hydroxychloroquine is also indicated in the treatment of discoid and systemic lupus erythematosus and rheumatoid arthritis. A placebo-controlled randomized trial of intravenous remdesivir in hospitalized COVID-19 patients reported a reduction in recovery time by 4 days (from 15 days to 11 days).[117] An observational study of more than 1300 hospitalized patients did not find any benefit resulting from hydroxychloroquine administration.[118] A multinational retrospective study of the efficacy of hydroxychloroquine and chloroquine for COVID-19 found higher mortality and increased occurrence of ventricular arrhythmias in both the hydroxychloroquine-treated group and chloroquine-treated group compared with the control group.[119] Another drug, tocilizumab, an IL-6 receptor antagonist used in the treatment of rheumatoid arthritis was also tested for the treatment of COVID-19.[33] In a randomized phase III trial in hospitalized patients with severe COVID-19 pneumonia, administration of tocilizumab did not result in significant clinical benefit or reduction in mortality at 28 days when compared with placebo.[120]

Under the auspices of the World Health Organization Solidarity Trial Consortium, randomized trials of four repurposed antiviral drugs—remdesivir, hydroxychloroquine, lopinavir, and interferon beta1a—were conducted in patients hospitalized with COVID-19 in multiple centers with reduction in mortality as the primary outcome measure.[121] Interim results showed that the drugs did not confer any benefit to hospitalized patients with COVID-19 based on outcome measures of overall mortality, need for ventilatory support, and duration of hospital stay.[121] Table 4.4 provides details of 28-day mortality in the drug and control arms of the trial.

A small study involving 10 seriously sick COVID-19 patients, who were administered a single dose of 200 mL of convalescent plasma (CP) from recently recovered donors, showed that CP therapy was well tolerated with resulting improvement in clinical symptoms.[122] CP may hold promise for improving clinical outcomes by neutralizing the virus circulating in blood if given very early in the course of disease, but studies in hospitalized patients to date has not supported its use.[123,124]

A randomized open-label trial in patients hospitalized with COVID-19 comparing oral or intravenous dexamethasone versus the regular standard care demonstrated a significant 28-day mortality reduction.[125] When patients were stratified based on respiratory support received, 28-day mortality reduction was observed in patients receiving mechanical ventilation or oxygen alone at randomization; there was no mortality reduction in the set of patients not receiving respiratory support at the time of randomization.[125]

Details of drugs administered in different clinical settings for the management of COVID-19 and its complications are discussed in the special chapter on therapeutics and the various system chapters.

Table 4.4 World Health Organization Solidarity Trial Results of Repurposed Antiviral Drugs Based on 11,330 Hospitalized COVID-19 Patients

Drug/Control	Number of Assigned Patients	28-Day Mortality (Drug Group) Died/Enrolled	28-Day Mortality (Control Group) Died/Enrolled	P Value
Remdesivir	2750	301/2743	303/2708	0.5
Hydroxychloroquine	954	104/947	84/906	0.23
Lopinavir	1411	148/1399	146/1372	0.97
Interferon	2063	243/2050	216/2050	0.11
Control (no trial drug)	4088			

Data abstracted from World Health Organization Solidarity Trial 2021.[121]

Vaccines

Various candidate vaccines based on RNA, DNA, or recombinant protein, viral vector–based, and the time-tested inactivated and live attenuated versions are undergoing preclinical evaluation, entered clinical trials or are being rolled out. Some of the leading vaccines have obtained authorization for emergency use, and a few have secured approval. There were no licensed human vaccines using RNA and DNA platforms till 2020.[126] However, the mRNA vaccine paradigm revolutionized the field of COVID-19 vaccines in 2020. Two vaccines based on mRNA developed by Moderna/ National Institute of Allergy and Infectious Diseases (NIAID) and Pfizer-BioNTech successfully completed phase III trials and secured emergency use authorization (EUA) from the US Food and Drug Administration. Two more vaccines, one from University of Oxford/Astra-Zeneca and another from CanSino Biological Inc/Beijing Institute of Biotechnology, based on a nonreplicating viral vector platform also successfully completed phase III trials and secured EUA from the regulatory agencies of the United Kingdome and China, respectively.

As of June 1, 2021, 51 COVID-19 candidate vaccines are in phase I, 34 in phase II, and 30 in phase III clinical trials.[127] EUA has been granted to 7 vaccines, and 8 vaccines have secured approval.[127] Additional details about the SARS-CoV-2 vaccines are discussed in Chapter 18.

Children and COVID-19

Compared with adults, children in general have been found to be less susceptible to serious manifestations of COVID-19. Worldwide, patients younger than 18 years initially have accounted for only 2% of the severely affected stratum even though they can be carriers and transmit the virus.[128] Based on an analysis of 2135 pediatric patients (728 laboratory-confirmed and 1407 suspected), Dong et al.[129] reported that more than 90% were asymptomatic, mild, or moderate cases. The distribution was similar in both sexes, and they found that younger children, particularly infants, were more

vulnerable. Researchers have hypothesized that this disparity in the susceptibility to COVID-19 between adults and children could be due to differences in the ACE2 receptors in the RAS (which are used by the SARS-CoV-2 virus to enter the respiratory epithelial cells), and altered inflammatory responses to the pathogen.[128,130]

A multisystem inflammatory syndrome in children (MIS-C) associated with SARS-CoV-2 infection in the United Kingdom, United States, and other countries have been reported and documented.[131–137] A small proportion of children came down with features of hyper-inflammatory shock 2 to 4 weeks after acute COVID-19.[138] The clinical manifestations were fever, rash, conjunctivitis, peripheral edema, GI symptoms, shock/hypotension, cardiac dysfunction, and elevated inflammatory markers.[132] A similar multisystem syndrome has been reported as a rare complication of COVID-19 in adults and designated MIS-A.[139,140]

Based on studies of four large cohorts of children and adolescents with MIS-C, two in the United States,[136,141] one each in the United Kingdom[142] and France,[134] Vogel et al.[143] reported that 100% of the patients had fever, 45% to 60% had rash, and more than 80% required ICU care.[143] The molecular mechanisms underlying the varied manifestations of MIS-C have not been delineated so far.[143]

Post Recovery Symptoms and the Long-Hauler Syndrome

Long-COVID, also referred to as the long-hauler syndrome or postacute sequelae of COVID (PASC), generally refers to individuals who have been sickened by COVID-19, but don't recover fully over a period of a few weeks[167] with some investigators defining this period as 60 days[144] or 12 weeks.[145,146] Carfi et al.[144] reported that of 143 patients followed for postacute care assessment for 60 days or more, only 13% were free of any symptom related to COVID-19, a third of the patients had one or two symptoms, and more than half of the patients had three or more persistent symptoms. The most common long-COVID manifestations have been cough, breathlessness,

Long-Covid Trajectories

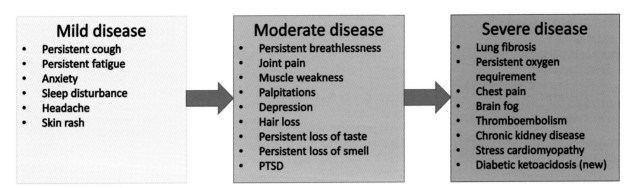

Mild disease
- Persistent cough
- Persistent fatigue
- Anxiety
- Sleep disturbance
- Headache
- Skin rash

Moderate disease
- Persistent breathlessness
- Joint pain
- Muscle weakness
- Palpitations
- Depression
- Hair loss
- Persistent loss of taste
- Persistent loss of smell
- PTSD

Severe disease
- Lung fibrosis
- Persistent oxygen requirement
- Chest pain
- Brain fog
- Thromboembolism
- Chronic kidney disease
- Stress cardiomyopathy
- Diabetic ketoacidosis (new)

Fig. 4.21 Long-COVID Manifestations. The clinical presentation and symptomatology of mild, moderate, and severe long-COVID trajectories. *PTSD,* Posttraumatic stress disorder. (Data from Mandal S, Barnett J, Brill SE, et al. "Long-COVID": a cross-sectional study of persisting symptoms, biomarker and imaging abnormalities following hospitalisation for COVID-19. *Thorax* 2021;76[4]:396-398; and Nalbandian A, Sehgal K, Gupta A, et al. Post-acute COVID-19 syndrome. *Nat Med.* 2021:1-15.)

fatigue, joint pain, and chest pain.[147] Other, more serious systemic long-COVID manifestations affecting the heart, brain, lung, liver, and the kidney are described in the respective chapters. In a follow-up study of more than 2000 hospitalized and nonhospitalized COVID-19 patients (RT-PCR confirmed, clinically assigned, clinically suspected) the persistence range of 29 symptoms was 10% to 90%.[146] The common symptoms that were persisting in more than 50% of the patients who originally reported them were fatigue, dyspnea, headache, muscle pain, pain between shoulder blades, heart palpitations, dizziness, hot flushes, and joint pains.[146] A study of 55 hospitalized COVID-19 patients evaluated after 12 weeks demonstrated persistence of GI symptoms in 31%, headache in 18%, fatigue and exertional dyspnea in 15%, and chest radiological abnormalities in 71% (39 patients).[148]

Based on an analysis of more than 4100 patients with COVID-19, Sudre et al.[108] reported that 13% of the patients had symptoms that lasted 4 or more weeks, 5% for 8 or more weeks, and 2% for 12 or more weeks. Older age, higher BMI, and female sex with a cluster of symptoms, including fatigue, headache, dyspnea, and anosmia, were characteristic of long-COVID.[108]

Nalbandian et al.[149] reviewed postacute COVID-19 by defining the condition as persistent symptoms or delayed complications beyond a 4-week cut-point from start of symptoms. The condition can be further categorized based on the timeline into symptoms during the 4- to 12-week period as subacute/ongoing symptomatic COVID-19 and symptoms persisting beyond 12 weeks as chronic or post–COVID-19.[145,149,150]

Fig. 4.21 summarizes common long-COVID trajectories based on data abstracted from Mandal et al.[147] and Nalbandian et al.[149] The postulated pathophysiological mechanisms of long-COVID manifestations abstracted from Nalbandian et al.[149] and Oronsky et al.[151] are included in Fig. 4.22.

Additional details about the long-COVID and long-hauler syndrome are presented in chapters elaborating the manifestations of COVID-19 in different systems.

Racial Disparities in Susceptibility to SARS-CoV-2

COVID-19 has had a disproportionate impact on individuals of different ages, different sexes, and different races. Differential susceptibility based on age was not surprising and has been explained by concepts such as immunosenescence and increasing incidence of comorbidities. Different infection rates and outcomes have consistently been observed between men and women, and several studies have looked at the effects of sex hormones on immune function.[152,153] Racial differences present communities and researchers with significant challenges because it is likely that multiple factors are involved ranging from socioeconomic to genetic factors.

It was observed in the United States that certain racial and ethnic minorities such as non-Hispanic Black and Hispanic individuals, were twice as likely to have a positive molecular test for SARS-CoV-2 compared with non-Hispanic White individuals.[154] This disparity was confirmed in multiple studies.[155] Not only were there differential rates of infection in certain racial and ethnic minorities such as non-Hispanic Black and Hispanic individuals, but this also resulted in increased hospitalization rates and mortality.

Several potential explanations for racial disparities in susceptibility to SARS-CoV-2 have been advanced. The possible explanations include different social determinants affecting exposures or baseline health status or genetic determinants that might result in different rates of infection given the same exposures. Several studies supported differential exposures affecting infection rates

Pathophysiological Mechanisms of Long COVID

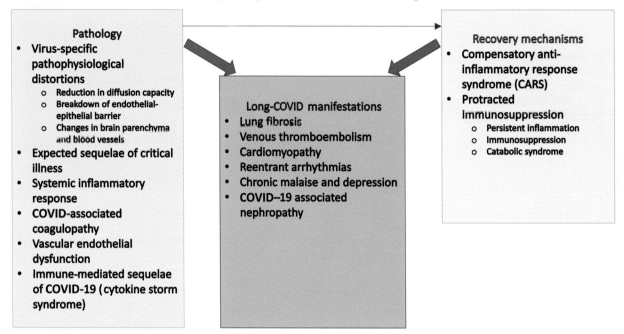

Fig. 4.22 Pathophysiological Mechanisms of Long-COVID. The systemic and virus-specific pathophysiological anomalies trigger recovery mechanisms and long-COVID manifestations. Both contribute to the sustained clinical picture of long-COVID. (Data from Nalbandian A, Sehgal K, Gupta A, et al. Post-acute COVID-19 syndrome. *Nat Med.* 2021:1-15; Oronsky B, Larson C, Hammond TC, et al. A review of persistent post-COVID syndrome (PPCS). *Clin Rev Allergy Immunol.* 2021:1-9.)

such as population density.[154] Other studies supported differential exposures and risk for infection as a result of occupational factors such as a higher rate of working in manual, essential, and public facing sectors.[156] Other compounding factors identified, including differences in baseline health status such as increased rates of high-risk comorbidities in these populations such as obesity, hypertension, and diabetes, may have contributed, but the evidence to date suggests a less significant impact.[157]

It has been suggested that intrinsic genetic differences might explain the disparities such as differential expression levels of ACE2, acetylcholinesterase, IL-6, or other genetic polymorphisms.[158] Other investigators have suggested that differences in aspects of the innate immune system such as baseline expression of IL-1-beta, IL-18 receptor, IL12R-beta1, TLR7, (Toll-like receptor 7) TLR9, (Toll-like receptor 9) and nuclear factor-kappa B might affect the events immediately after exposure to the virus and modulate whether infection occurs with a given exposure.[159] At this point the genetic basis of any difference in susceptibility is still being investigated, and it remains unclear how much such factors may have contributed to the racial disparities seen with SARS-CoV-2.[160,161]

Conclusion

COVID-19 showcases a wide spectrum of clinical presentations ranging from asymptomatic infection at one end to manifestations in multiple systems, including the rare syndromes of MIS-C and MIS-A. With the recent advances in vaccines and therapeutics, and the diligent application of nonpharmacological interventions, there is optimism that the SARS-CoV-2 pandemic can be gradually brought under control by coordinated national and global public health measures. Hopefully, the populace can soon return to their activities and pursue their interests without the threat of SARS-CoV-2 hanging over them.

REFERENCES

1. Worldometers.info: COVID-19 Coronavirus Pandemic: [https://ns.worldometers.info/coronavirus/]. Accessed July 1st, 2021.
2. Froude S, Hughes H. Newly discovered viruses. In: Firth J, Conlon C, Cox T, eds. *Oxford textbook of medicine.* 6th ed. Oxford, UK: Oxford University Press; 2020.
3. Peiris M. Respiratory tract viruses. In: Firth J, Conlon C, Cox T, eds. *Oxford textbook of Medicine.* 6th ed. Oxford, UK: Oxford University Press; 2020.
4. Al Mutair A, Ambani Z. Narrative review of Middle East respiratory syndrome coronavirus (MERS-CoV) infection: updates and implications for practice. *Journal of International Medical Research.* 2020;48(1):0300060519858030.
5. Zhu N, Zhang D, Wang W, Li X, Yang B, Song J, Zhao X, Huang B, Shi W, Lu R. A novel coronavirus from patients with pneumonia in China, 2019. *New England Journal of Medicine.* 2020;382(8):727–733.
6. Wu F, Zhao S, Yu B, Chen Y-M, Wang W, Song Z-G, Hu Y, Tao Z-W, Tian J-H, Pei Y-Y. A new coronavirus associated with human respiratory disease in China. *Nature.* 2020;579(7798):265–269.

7. Zhang T, Wu Q, Zhang Z. Probable pangolin origin of SARS-CoV-2 associated with the COVID-19 outbreak. *Current Biology.* 2020;30(7):1346–1351.

8. Shi J, Wen Z, Zhong G, Yang H, Wang C, Huang B, Liu R, He X, Shuai L, Sun Z. Susceptibility of ferrets, cats, dogs, and other domesticated animals to SARS–coronavirus 2. *Science.* 2020;368(6494):1016–1020.

9. Sakurai A, Sasaki T, Kato S, Hayashi M, Tsuzuki S-i, Ishihara T, Iwata M, Morise Z, Doi Y. Natural History of Asymptomatic SARS-CoV-2 Infection. *New England Journal of Medicine.* 2020;383(9):885–886.

10. Lauer SA, Grantz KH, Bi Q, Jones FK, Zheng Q, Meredith HR, Azman AS, Reich NG, Lessler J. The incubation period of coronavirus disease 2019 (COVID-19) from publicly reported confirmed cases: estimation and application. *Annals of internal medicine.* 2020;172(9):577–582.

11. Chen Y, Chen L, Deng Q, Zhang G, Wu K, Ni L, Yang Y, Liu B, Wang W, Wei C. The presence of SARS-CoV-2 RNA in the feces of COVID-19 patients. *Journal of medical virology.* 2020;92(7):833–840.

12. Scientific Brief: SARS-CoV-2 Transmission [https://www.cdc.gov/coronavirus/2019-ncov/science/science-briefs/sars-cov-2-transmission.html#anchor_1619805184733]

13. Hamner L. High SARS-CoV-2 attack rate following exposure at a choir practice—Skagit County, Washington, March 2020. *MMWR Morbidity and mortality weekly report.* 2020;69:606–610.

14. Jang S, Han SH, Rhee J-Y. Cluster of coronavirus disease associated with fitness dance classes, South Korea. *Emerging infectious diseases.* 2020;26(8):1917.

15. World Health Organization: Report of the WHO-China joint mission on coronavirus disease 2019 (Covid-19). In: Available on-line: https://wwwwhoint/docs/default-source/coronaviruse/who-china-joint-mission-on-covid-19-final-report.pdf, 2020.

16. van Doremalen N, Bushmaker T, Morris DH, Holbrook MG, Gamble A, Williamson BN, Tamin A, Harcourt JL, Thornburg NJ, Gerber SI. Aerosol and surface stability of SARS-CoV-2 as compared with SARS-CoV-1. *New England Journal of Medicine.* 2020;382(16):1564–1567.

17. Chen J. Pathogenicity and transmissibility of 2019-nCoV—a quick overview and comparison with other emerging viruses. *Microbes and infection.* 2020;22(2):69–71.

18. Nelson KE. Epidemiology of infectious disease: general principles. In: Nelson KE, Williams CM, eds. *Infectious disease epidemiology: theory and practice.* Burlington, MA: Jones and Bartlett; 2014:19–44.

19. Duan S, Zhou M, Zhang W, Shen J, Qi R, Qin X, Yu H, Zhou C, Hu Q, Yu X-J. Seroprevalence and asymptomatic carrier status of SARS-CoV-2 in Wuhan City and other places of China. *PLOS Neglected Tropical Diseases.* 2021;15(1):e0008975.

20. Hanley B, Naresh KN, Roufosse C, Nicholson AG, Weir J, Cooke GS, Thursz M, Manousou P, Corbett R, Goldin R, et al. Histopathological findings and viral tropism in UK patients with severe fatal COVID-19: a post-mortem study. *The Lancet Microbe.* 2020;1(6):e245–e253.

21. Sharfstein JM, Becker SJ, Mello MM. Diagnostic testing for the novel coronavirus. *JAMA.* 2020;323(15):1437–1438.

22. Long Q-X, Tang X-J, Shi Q-L, Li Q, Deng H-J, Yuan J, Hu J-L, Xu W, Zhang Y, Lv F-J. Clinical and immunological assessment of asymptomatic SARS-CoV-2 infections. *Nature Medicine.* 2020;26(8):1200–1204.

23. Atkinson B, Petersen E. SARS-CoV-2 shedding and infectivity. *The Lancet.* 2020;395(10233):1339–1340.

24. Li Q, Guan X, Wu P, Wang X, Zhou L, Tong Y, Ren R, Leung KS, Lau EH, Wong JY. Early transmission dynamics in Wuhan, China, of novel coronavirus–infected pneumonia. *New England Journal of Medicine.* 2020;382(13):1199–1207.

25. Guan W-j, Ni Z-y, Hu Y, Liang W-h, Ou C-q, He J-x, Liu L, Shan H, Lei C-l, Hui DS. Clinical characteristics of coronavirus disease 2019 in China. *New England Journal of Medicine.* 2020;382(18):1708–1720.

26. Wang D, Hu B, Hu C, Zhu F, Liu X, Zhang J, Wang B, Xiang H, Cheng Z, Xiong Y. Clinical characteristics of 138 hospitalized patients with 2019 novel coronavirus–infected pneumonia in Wuhan, China. *Jama.* 2020;323(11):1061–1069.

27. Rodriguez-Morales AJ, Cardona-Ospina JA, Gutiérrez-Ocampo E, Villamizar-Peña R, Holguin-Rivera Y, Escalera-Antezana JP, Alvarado-Arnez LE, Bonilla-Aldana DK, Franco-Paredes C, Henao-Martinez AF. Clinical, laboratory and imaging features of COVID-19: A systematic review and meta-analysis. *Travel Medicine and Infectious Disease.* 2020;34:101623.

28. Zhou F, Yu T, Du R, Fan G, Liu Y, Liu Z, Xiang J, Wang Y, Song B, Gu X. Clinical course and risk factors for mortality of adult inpatients with COVID-19 in Wuhan, China: a retrospective cohort study. *The Lancet.* 2020;395(10229):1054–1062.

29. Grasselli G, Zangrillo A, Zanella A, Antonelli M, Cabrini L, Castelli A, Cereda D, Coluccello A, Foti G, Fumagalli R. Baseline characteristics and outcomes of 1591 patients infected with SARS-CoV-2 admitted to ICUs of the Lombardy region, Italy. *Jama.* 2020;323(16):1574–1581.

30. Richardson S, Hirsch JS, Narasimhan M, Crawford JM, McGinn T, Davidson KW, Barnaby DP, Becker LB, Chelico JD, Cohen SL. Presenting characteristics, comorbidities, and outcomes among 5700 patients hospitalized with COVID-19 in the New York City area. *Jama.* 2020;323(20):2052–2059.

31. Machhi J, Herskovitz J, Senan AM, Dutta D, Nath B, Oleynikov MD, Blomberg WR, Meigs DD, Hasan M, Patel M. The natural history, pathobiology, and clinical manifestations of SARS-CoV-2 infections. *Journal of Neuroimmune Pharmacology.* 2020:1–28.

32. Hoffmann M, Kleine-Weber H, Schroeder S, Krüger N, Herrler T, Erichsen S, Schiergens TS, Herrler G, Wu N-H, Nitsche A. SARS-CoV-2 cell entry depends on ACE2 and TMPRSS2 and is blocked by a clinically proven protease inhibitor. *Cell.* 2020;181(2):271–280.

33. Clerkin KJ, Fried JA, Raikhelkar J, Sayer G, Griffin JM, Masoumi A, Jain SS, Burkhoff D, Kumaraiah D, Rabbani L. Coronavirus Disease 2019 (COVID-19) and Cardiovascular Disease. *Circulation.* 2020;141(20):1648–1655.

34. Gottlieb M, Sansom S, Frankenberger C, Ward E, Hota B. Clinical course and factors associated with hospitalization and critical illness among COVID-19 patients in Chicago, Illinois. *Academic Emergency Medicine.* 2020;27(10):963–973.

35. Cummings MJ, Baldwin MR, Abrams D, Jacobson SD, Meyer BJ, Balough EM, Aaron JG, Claassen J, Rabbani LE, Hastie J. Epidemiology, clinical course, and outcomes of critically ill adults with COVID-19 in New York City: a prospective cohort study. *The Lancet.* 2020;395(10239):1763–1770.

36. Zhu J, Ji P, Pang J, Zhong Z, Li H, He C, Zhang J, Zhao C. Clinical characteristics of 3,062 COVID-19 patients: a meta-analysis. *Journal of Medical Virology.* 2020;92(10):1902–1914.

37. Grasselli G, Tonetti T, Protti A, Langer T, Girardis M, Bellani G, Laffey J, Carrafiello G, Carsana L, Rizzuto C. Pathophysiology of COVID-19-associated acute respiratory distress syndrome: a multicentre prospective observational study. *The lancet Respiratory medicine.* 2020;8(12):1201–1208.

38. Fried JA, Ramasubbu K, Bhatt R, Topkara VK, Clerkin KJ, Horn E, Rabbani L, Brodie D, Jain SS, Kirtane A. The variety of cardiovascular presentations of COVID-19. *Circulation.* 2020;141(23):1930–1936.

39. Akhmerov A, Marbán E. COVID-19 and the Heart. *Circulation research.* 2020;126(10):1443–1455.

40. Mao L, Wang M, Chen S, He Q, Chang J, Hong C, Zhou Y, Wang D, Miao X, Hu Y. Neurological manifestations of hospitalized patients with COVID-19 in Wuhan, China: a retrospective case series study. *JAMA Neurol.* 2020;77(6):683–690.

41. Wu Y, Xu X, Chen Z, Duan J, Hashimoto K, Yang L, Liu C, Yang C. Nervous system involvement after infection with COVID-19 and other coronaviruses. *Brain, Behavior, and Immunity.* 2020;87:18–22.

42. Chen T, Wu D, Chen H, Yan W, Yang D, Chen G, Ma K, Xu D, Yu H, Wang H. Clinical characteristics of 113 deceased patients with coronavirus disease 2019: retrospective study. *BMJ.* 2020;368:m1091.

43. Pezzini A, Padovani A. Lifting the mask on neurological manifestations of COVID-19. *Nature Reviews Neurology.* 2020;16(11):636–644.

44. Solomon T. Neurological infection with SARS-CoV-2—the story so far. *Nature Reviews Neurology.* 2021:1–2.

45. Bodro M, Compta Y, Sánchez-Valle R. Presentations and mechanisms of CNS disorders related to COVID-19. *Neurology-Neuroimmunology Neuroinflammation.* 2021;8(1):e923.

46. Mao R, Qiu Y, He J-S, Tan J-Y, Li X-H, Liang J, Shen J, Zhu L-R, Chen Y, Iacucci M. Manifestations and prognosis of gastrointestinal and liver involvement in patients with COVID-19: a systematic review and meta-analysis. *The lancet Gastroenterology & hepatology.* 2020;5(7):667–678.

47. Sultan S, Altayar O, Siddique SM, Davitkov P, Feuerstein JD, Lim JK, Falck-Ytter Y, El-Serag HB. AGA Institute rapid review of the GI and liver manifestations of COVID-19, meta-analysis of international data, and recommendations for the consultative management of patients with COVID-19. *Gastroenterology.* 2020;159(1):320–334.

48. Wang W, Xu Y, Gao R, Lu R, Han K, Wu G, Tan W. Detection of SARS-CoV-2 in different types of clinical specimens. *Jama.* 2020;323(18):1843–1844.

49. Liu Y-F, Zhang Z, Pan X-L, Xing G-L, Zhang Y, Liu Z-S, Tu S-H. The chronic kidney disease and acute kidney injury involvement in COVID-19 pandemic: A systematic review and meta-analysis. *PLoS one.* 2021;16(1):e0244779.

50. Batlle D, Soler MJ, Sparks MA, Hiremath S, South AM, Welling PA, Swaminathan S. Acute kidney injury in COVID-19: emerging evidence of a distinct pathophysiology. *Journal of the American Society of Nephrology.* 2020;31(7):1380–1383.

51. Sharma P, Ng JH, Bijol V, Jhaveri KD, Wanchoo R. Pathology of COVID 19 associated acute kidney injury. *Clinical Kidney Journal.* 2021;14(Suppl 1):i30–i39.

52. Shetty AA, Tawhari I, Safar-Boueri L, Seif N, Alahmadi A, Gargiulo R, Aggarwal V, Usman I, Kisselev S, Gharavi AG, et al. COVID-19–associated glomerular disease. *Journal of the American Society of Nephrology.* 2021;32(1):33–40.

53. Nadim MK, Forni LG, Mehta RL, Connor MJ, Liu KD, Ostermann M, Rimmelé T, Zarbock A, Bell S, Bihorac A. COVID-19-associated acute kidney injury: consensus report of the 25th Acute Disease Quality Initiative (ADQI) Workgroup. *Nature reviews nephrology.* 2020:1–18.

54. Bruchfeld A. The COVID-19 pandemic: consequences for nephrology. *Nature Reviews Nephrology.* 2021;17(2):81–82.

55. Chan L, Chaudhary K, Saha A, Chauhan K, Vaid A, Zhao S, Paranjpe I, Somani S, Richter F, Miotto R, et al. AKI in Hospitalized Patients with COVID-19. *Journal of the American Society of Nephrology.* 2021;32(1):151–160.

56. Pei G, Zhang Z, Peng J, Liu L, Zhang C, Yu C, Ma Z, Huang Y, Liu W, Yao Y, et al. Renal involvement and early prognosis in patients with COVID-19 pneumonia. *Journal of the American Society of Nephrology.* 2020;31(6):1157–1165.

57. Ostermann M, Lumlertgul N, Forni LG, Hoste E. What every Intensivist should know about COVID-19 associated acute kidney injury. *Journal of critical care.* 2020;60:91–95.

58. Hirsch JS, Ng JH, Ross DW, Sharma P, Shah HH, Barnett RL, Hazzan AD, Fishbane S, Jhaveri KD, Abate M. Acute kidney injury in patients hospitalized with COVID-19. *Kidney international.* 2020;98(1):209–218.

59. Mohamed MM, Lukitsch I, Torres-Ortiz AE, Walker JB, Varghese V, Hernandez-Arroyo CF, Alqudsi M, LeDoux JR, Velez JCQ. Acute kidney injury associated with coronavirus disease 2019 in urban New Orleans. *Kidney360.* 2020 10.34067/KID.0002652020.

60. Puelles VG, Lütgehetmann M, Lindenmeyer MT, Sperhake JP, Wong MN, Allweiss L, Chilla S, Heinemann A, Wanner N, Liu S. Multiorgan and renal tropism of SARS-CoV-2. *New England Journal of Medicine.* 2020;383(6):590–592.

61. Khan S, Chen L, Yang C-R, Raghuram V, Khundmiri SJ, Knepper MA. Does SARS-CoV-2 Infect the Kidney?. *Journal of the American Society of Nephrology.* 2020;31(12):2746–2748.

62. Perico L, Benigni A, Casiraghi F, Ng LFP, Renia L, Remuzzi G. Immunity, endothelial injury and complement-induced coagulopathy in COVID-19. *Nature Reviews Nephrology.* 2021;17(1):46–64.

63. Izzedine H, Jhaveri KD. Acute kidney injury in patients with COVID-19: an update on the pathophysiology. *Nephrology Dialysis Transplantation.* 2021;36(2):224–226.

64. Sharma P, Ng JH, Bijol V, Jhaveri KD, Wanchoo R. Pathology of COVID-19-associated acute kidney injury. *Clinical kidney journal.* 2021;14(Suppl 1):i30–i39.

65. Recalcati S. Cutaneous manifestations in COVID-19: a first perspective. *Journal of the European Academy of Dermatology and Venereology.* 2020;34(50):e212–e213.

66. Landa N, Mendieta-Eckert M, Fonda-Pascual P, Aguirre T. Chilblain-like lesions on feet and hands during the COVID-19 Pandemic. *International Journal of Dermatology.* 2020;59(6):739–743.

67. Do MH, Stewart CR, Harp J. Cutaneous Manifestations of COVID-19 in the Inpatient Setting. *Dermatologic Clinics.* 2021;39(4):521–532.

68. Marzano AV, Genovese G, Moltrasio C, Gaspari V, Vezzoli P, Maione V, Misciali C, Sena P, Patrizi A, Offidani A. The clinical spectrum of COVID-19–associated cutaneous manifestations: An Italian multicenter study of 200 adult patients. *Journal of the American Academy of Dermatology.* 2021;84(5):1356–1363.

69. Abrishami M, Tohidinezhad F, Daneshvar R, Omidtabrizi A, Amini M, Sedaghat A, Amini S, Reihani H, Allahyari A, Seddigh-Shamsi M, et al. Ocular Manifestations of Hospitalized

Patients with COVID-19 in Northeast of Iran. *Ocular Immunology and Inflammation.* 2020;28(5):739–744.

70. Aggarwal K, Agarwal A, Jaiswal N, Dahiya N, Ahuja A, Mahajan S, Tong L, Duggal M, Singh M, Agrawal R, et al. Ocular surface manifestations of coronavirus disease 2019 (COVID-19): A systematic review and meta-analysis. *PLOS ONE.* 2020;15(11):e0241661.

71. Bertoli F, Veritti D, Danese C, Samassa F, Sarao V, Rassu N, Gambato T, Lanzetta P. Ocular Findings in COVID-19 Patients: A Review of Direct Manifestations and Indirect Effects on the Eye. *Journal of Ophthalmology.* 2020;2020:4827304.

72. Chen L, Deng C, Chen X, Zhang X, Chen B, Yu H, Qin Y, Xiao K, Zhang H, Sun X. Ocular manifestations and clinical characteristics of 535 cases of COVID-19 in Wuhan, China: a cross-sectional study. *Acta ophthalmologica.* 2020;98(8):e951–e959.

73. Nasiri N, Sharifi H, Bazrafshan A, Noori A, Karamouzian M, Sharifi A. Ocular Manifestations of COVID-19: A Systematic Review and Meta-analysis. *Journal of Ophthalmic & Vision Research.* 2021;16(1):103.

74. Pirraglia MP, Ceccarelli G, Cerini A, Visioli G, d'Ettorre G, Mastroianni CM, Pugliese F, Lambiase A, Gharbiya M. Retinal involvement and ocular findings in COVID-19 pneumonia patients. *Scientific Reports.* 2020;10(1):17419.

75. Wu P, Duan F, Luo C, Liu Q, Qu X, Liang L, Wu K. Characteristics of Ocular Findings of Patients With Coronavirus Disease 2019 (COVID-19) in Hubei Province, China. *JAMA Ophthalmology.* 2020;138(5):575–578.

76. Invernizzi A, Torre A, Parrulli S, Zicarelli F, Schiuma M, Colombo V, Giacomelli A, Cigada M, Milazzo L, Ridolfo A, et al. Retinal findings in patients with COVID-19: Results from the SERPICO-19 study. *EClinicalMedicine.* 2020;27:100550.

77. Lani-Louzada R, do Val Ferreira Ramos C, Cordeiro RM, Sadun AA. Retinal changes in COVID-19 hospitalized cases. *PLOS ONE.* 2020;15(12):e0243346.

78. Pereira LA, Soares LCM, Nascimento PA, Cirillo LRN, Sakuma HT, GLd Veiga, Fonseca FLA, Lima VL, Abucham-Neto JZ. Retinal findings in hospitalised patients with severe COVID-19. *British Journal of Ophthalmology.* 2020;106(1):102–105.

79. Al-Sharif E, Strianese D, AlMadhi NH, D'Aponte A, dell'Omo R, Di Benedetto R, Costagliola C. Ocular tropism of coronavirus (CoVs): a comparison of the interaction between the animal-to-human transmitted coronaviruses (SARS-CoV-1, SARS-CoV-2, MERS-CoV, CoV-229E, NL63, OC43, HKU1) and the eye. *International Ophthalmology.* 2021;41(1):349–362.

80. Belser JA, Rota PA, Tumpey TM. Ocular Tropism of Respiratory Viruses. *Microbiology and Molecular Biology Reviews.* 2013;77(1):144–156.

81. Collin J, Queen R, Zerti D, Dorgau B, Georgiou M, Djidrovski I, Hussain R, Coxhead JM, Joseph A, Rooney P, et al. Co-expression of SARS-CoV-2 entry genes in the superficial adult human conjunctival, limbal and corneal epithelium suggests an additional route of entry via the ocular surface. *The Ocular Surface.* 2021;19:190–200.

82. Li Y-P, Ma Y, Wang N, Jin Z-B. Eyes on coronavirus. *Stem Cell Research.* 2021;51:102200.

83. Zhou L, Xu Z, Castiglione GM, Soiberman US, Eberhart CG, Duh EJ. ACE2 and TMPRSS2 are expressed on the human ocular surface, suggesting susceptibility to SARS-CoV-2 infection. *The Ocular Surface.* 2020;18(4):537–544.

84. Abdullahi A, Candan SA, Abba MA, Bello AH, Alshehri MA, Afamefuna Victor E, Umar NA, Kundakci B. Neurological and

Musculoskeletal Features of COVID-19: A Systematic Review and Meta-Analysis. *Frontiers in Neurology.* 2020;11:687.

85. Ciaffi J, Meliconi R, Ruscitti P, Berardicurti O, Giacomelli R, Ursini F. Rheumatic manifestations of COVID-19: a systematic review and meta-analysis. *BMC Rheumatology.* 2020;4(1):65.

86. Cipollaro L, Giordano L, Padulo J, Oliva F, Maffulli N. Musculoskeletal symptoms in SARS-CoV-2 (COVID-19) patients. *J Orthop Surg Res.* 2020;15(1):178.

87. Disser NP, De Micheli AJ, Schonk MM, Konnaris MA, Piacentini AN, Edon DL, Toresdahl BG, Rodeo SA, Casey EK, Mendias CL. Musculoskeletal consequences of COVID-19. *JBJS.* 2020;102(14):1197–1204.

88. Hoong CWS, Amin MNME, Tan TC, Lee JE. Viral arthralgia a new manifestation of COVID-19 infection? A cohort study of COVID-19-associated musculoskeletal symptoms. *International Journal of Infectious Diseases.* 2021;104:363–369.

89. Schenker HM, Hagen M, Simon D, Schett G, Manger B. Reactive arthritis and cutaneous vasculitis after SARS-CoV-2 infection. *Rheumatology.* 2021;60(1):479–480.

90. Stradner MH, Dejaco C, Zwerina J. Fritsch-Stork RD: Rheumatic Musculoskeletal Diseases and COVID-19 A Review of the First 6 Months of the Pandemic. *Frontiers in medicine.* 2020;7:562142.

91. Nikiphorou E, Alpizar-Rodriguez D, Gastelum-Strozzi A, Buch M. Peláez-Ballestas I: Syndemics & syndemogenesis in COVID-19 and rheumatic and musculoskeletal diseases: old challenges, new era. *Rheumatology.* 2021;60(5):2040–2045.

92. Jorge A, D'Silva KM, Cohen A, Wallace ZS, McCormick N, Zhang Y, Choi HK. Temporal trends in severe COVID-19 outcomes in patients with rheumatic disease: a cohort study. *The Lancet Rheumatology.* 2021;3(2):e131–e137.

93. Ahmed S, Zimba O, Gasparyan AY. COVID-19 and the clinical course of rheumatic manifestations. *Clinical Rheumatology.* 2021:1–9.

94. Batur EB, Korez MK, Gezer IA, Levendoglu F, Ural O. Musculoskeletal symptoms and relationship with laboratory findings in patients with COVID-19. *International Journal of Clinical Practice.* 2021:e14135.

95. D'Silva KM, Serling-Boyd N, Wallwork R, Hsu T, Fu X, Gravallese EM, Choi HK, Sparks JA, Wallace ZS. Clinical characteristics and outcomes of patients with coronavirus disease 2019 (COVID-19) and rheumatic disease: a comparative cohort study from a US 'hot spot. *Annals of the rheumatic diseases.* 2020;79(9):1156–1162.

96. Zhao J, Pang R, Wu J, Guo Y, Yang Y, Zhang L, Xia X. Clinical characteristics and outcomes of patients with COVID-19 and rheumatic disease in China 'hot spot' versus in US 'hot spot': similarities and differences. *Annals of the Rheumatic Diseases.* 2021;80(5) e63-e63.

97. Strangfeld A, Schäfer M, Gianfrancesco MA, Lawson-Tovey S, Liew JW, Ljung L, Mateus EF, Richez C, Santos MJ, Schmajuk G. Factors associated with COVID-19-related death in people with rheumatic diseases: results from the COVID-19 Global Rheumatology Alliance physician-reported registry. *Annals of the rheumatic diseases.* 2021;80(7):930–942.

98. Kruglikov IL, Shah M, Scherer PE. Obesity and diabetes as comorbidities for COVID-19: Underlying mechanisms and the role of viral–bacterial interactions. *Elife.* 2020;9: e61330.

99. Petrilli CM, Jones SA, Yang J, Rajagopalan H, O'Donnell L, Chernyak Y, Tobin KA, Cerfolio RJ, Francois F, Horwitz LI. Factors associated with hospital admission and critical

illness among 5279 people with coronavirus disease 2019 in New York City: prospective cohort study. *BMJ.* 2020;369:m1966.

100. Williamson EJ, Walker AJ, Bhaskaran K, Bacon S, Bates C, Morton CE, Curtis HJ, Mehrkar A, Evans D, Inglesby P, et al. Factors associated with COVID-19-related death using Open-SAFELY. *Nature.* 2020;584(7821):430–436.

101. Drucker DJ: Diabetes, obesity, metabolism and SARS-CoV-2 infection: The end of the beginning. *Cell Metabolism.* 2021;33(3):479–498.

102. Cai Q, Chen F, Wang T, Luo F, Liu X, Wu Q, He Q, Wang Z, Liu Y, Liu L. Obesity and COVID-19 severity in a designated hospital in Shenzhen, China. *Diabetes care.* 2020;43(7):1392–1398.

103. Guo W, Li M, Dong Y, Zhou H, Zhang Z, Tian C, Qin R, Wang H, Shen Y, Du K. Diabetes is a risk factor for the progression and prognosis of COVID-19. *Diabetes/metabolism research and reviews.* 2020;36(7):e3319.

104. Wang S, Ma P, Zhang S, Song S, Wang Z, Ma Y, Xu J, Wu F, Duan L, Yin Z. Fasting blood glucose at admission is an independent predictor for 28-day mortality in patients with COVID-19 without previous diagnosis of diabetes: a multi-centre retrospective study. *Diabetologia.* 2020;63(10):2102–2111.

105. Dennis JM, Mateen BA, Sonabend R, Thomas NJ, Patel KA, Hattersley AT, Denaxas S, McGovern AP, Vollmer SJ. Type 2 diabetes and COVID-19–Related mortality in the critical care setting: a national cohort study in England, March–July 2020. *Diabetes care.* 2021;44(1):50–57.

106. Moriconi D, Masi S, Rebelos E, Virdis A, Manca ML, De Marco S, Taddei S, Nannipieri M. Obesity prolongs the hospital stay in patients affected by COVID-19, and may impact on SARS-COV-2 shedding. *Obesity research & clinical practice.* 2020;14(3):205–209.

107. Cano E, Campioli CC, O'Horo JC. Nasopharyngeal SARS-CoV-2 viral RNA shedding in patients with diabetes mellitus. *Endocrine.* 2021;71(1):26–27.

108. Sudre CH, Murray B, Varsavsky T, Graham MS, Penfold RS, Bowyer RC, Pujol JC, Klaser K, Antonelli M, Canas LS. Attributes and predictors of long COVID. *Nature Medicine.* 2021;27(4):626–631.

109. Touyz RM, Li H, Delles C. ACE2 the Janus-faced protein–from cardiovascular protection to severe acute respiratory syndrome-coronavirus and COVID-19. *Clinical Science.* 2020;134(7):747–750.

110. Kuba K, Imai Y, Ohto-Nakanishi T, Penninger JM. Trilogy of ACE2: A peptidase in the renin–angiotensin system, a SARS receptor, and a partner for amino acid transporters. *Pharmacology & therapeutics.* 2010;128(1):119–128.

111. Elezkurtaj S, Greuel S, Ihlow J, Michaelis EG, Bischoff P, Kunze CA, Sinn BV, Gerhold M, Hauptmann K, Ingold-Heppner B. Causes of death and comorbidities in hospitalized patients with COVID-19. *Scientific Reports.* 2021;11(1):1–9.

112. Revzin MV, Raza S, Warshawsky R, D'agostino C, Srivastava NC, Bader AS, Malhotra A, Patel RD, Chen K, Kyriakakos C. Multisystem imaging manifestations of covid-19, part 1: Viral pathogenesis and pulmonary and vascular system complications. *Radiographics.* 2020;40(6):1574–1599.

113. Salehi S, Abedi A, Balakrishnan S, Gholamrezanezhad A. Coronavirus disease 2019 (COVID-19): a systematic review of imaging findings in 919 patients. *American Journal of Roentgenology.* 2020:1–7.

114. Pormohammad A, Ghorbani S, Baradaran B, Khatami A, Turner RJ, Mansournia MA, Kyriacou DN, Idrovo J-P, Bahr NC. Clinical characteristics, laboratory findings, radiographic signs and outcomes of 61,742 patients with confirmed COVID-19 infection: A systematic review and meta-analysis. *Microbial pathogenesis.* 2020;147:104390.

115. Malik P, Patel U, Mehta D, Patel N, Kelkar R, Akrmah M, Gabrilove JL, Sacks H. Biomarkers and outcomes of COVID-19 hospitalisations: systematic review and meta analysis. *BMJ evidence based medicine.* 2021;26(3):107–108.

116. Wang M, Cao R, Zhang L, Yang X, Liu J, Xu M, Shi Z, Hu Z, Zhong W, Xiao G. Remdesivir and chloroquine effectively inhibit the recently emerged novel coronavirus (2019-nCoV) in vitro. *Cell research.* 2020;30(3):269–271.

117. Beigel JH, Tomashek KM, Dodd LE, Mehta AK, Zingman BS, Kalil AC, Hohmann E, Chu HY, Luetkemeyer A, Kline S. Remdesivir for the Treatment of Covid-19—Preliminary Report. *New England Journal of Medicine.* 2020;383(19):1813–1826.

118. Geleris J, Sun Y, Platt J, Zucker J, Baldwin M, Hripcsak G, Labella A, Manson D, Kubin C, Barr RG. Observational study of hydroxychloroquine in hospitalized patients with Covid-19. *New England Journal of Medicine.* 2020;382(25):2411–2418.

119. Mehra MR, Desai SS, Ruschitzka F, Patel AN. Hydroxychloroquine or chloroquine with or without a macrolide for treatment of COVID-19: a multinational registry analysis. *The Lancet.* 2020 S0140-6736(20)31180-6.

120. Rosas IO, Bräu N, Waters M, Go RC, Hunter BD, Bhagani S, Skiest D, Aziz MS, Cooper N, Douglas IS. Tocilizumab in hospitalized patients with severe Covid-19 pneumonia. *New England Journal of Medicine.* 2021;384(16):1503–1516.

121. Consortium WST. Repurposed antiviral drugs for COVID-19—interim WHO SOLIDARITY trial results. *New England journal of medicine.* 2021;384(6):497–511.

122. Duan K, Liu B, Li C, Zhang H, Yu T, Qu J, Zhou M, Chen L, Meng S, Hu Y. Effectiveness of convalescent plasma therapy in severe COVID-19 patients. *Proceedings of the National Academy of Sciences.* 2020;117(17):9490–9496.

123. Janiaud P, Axfors C, Schmitt AM, Gloy V, Ebrahimi F, Hepprich M, Smith ER, Haber NA, Khanna N, Moher D. Association of convalescent plasma treatment with clinical outcomes in patients with COVID-19: a systematic review and meta-analysis. *Jama.* 2021;325(12):1185–1195.

124. Sostin OV, Rajapakse P, Cruser B, Wakefield D, Cruser D, Petrini J. A matched cohort study of convalescent plasma therapy for COVID-19. *Journal of clinical apheresis.* 2021;36(4):523–532.

125. Group RC. Dexamethasone in hospitalized patients with Covid-19. *New England Journal of Medicine.* 2021;384(8):693–704.

126. Amanat F, Krammer F. SARS-CoV-2 vaccines: status report. *Immunity.* 2020;52(4):583–589.

127. Coronavirus vaccine tracker [https://www.nytimes.com/interactive/2020/science/coronavirus-vaccine-tracker.html]

128. Molloy EJ, Bearer CF. COVID-19 in children and altered inflammatory responses. *Pediatr Res.* 2020;88:340–341.

129. Dong Y, Mo X, Hu Y, Qi X, Jiang F, Jiang Z, Tong S. Epidemiology of COVID-19 among children in China. *Pediatrics.* 2020;145(6):e20200702.

130. Zhu L, Lu X, Chen L. Possible causes for decreased susceptibility of children to coronavirus. *Pediatr Res.* 2020;88(3):342.

131. Mahase E. Covid-19: concerns grow over inflammatory syndrome emerging in children In.:. *British Medical Journal Publishing Group*. 2020;369:m1710.

132. Riphagen S, Gomez X, Gonzalez-Martinez C, Wilkinson N, Theocharis P. Hyperinflammatory shock in children during COVID-19 pandemic. *The Lancet*. 2020;395(10237):1607–1608.

133. Bautista-Rodriguez C, Sanchez-de-Toledo J, Clark BC, Herberg J, Bajolle F, Randanne PC, Salas-Mera D, Foldvari S, Chowdhury D, Munoz R. Multisystem inflammatory syndrome in children: an international survey. *Pediatrics*. 2021;147(2):e2020024554.

134. Belhadjer Z, Méot M, Bajolle F, Khraiche D, Legendre A, Abakka S, Auriau J, Grimaud M, Oualha M, Beghetti M. Acute heart failure in multisystem inflammatory syndrome in children in the context of global SARS-CoV-2 pandemic. *Circulation*. 2020;142(5):429–436.

135. Diorio C, Henrickson SE, Vella LA, McNerney KO, Chase J, Burudpakdee C, Lee JH, Jasen C, Balamuth F, Barrett DM. Multisystem inflammatory syndrome in children and COVID-19 are distinct presentations of SARS–CoV-2. *The Journal of clinical investigation*. 2020;130(11):5967–5975.

136. Dufort EM, Koumans EH, Chow EJ, Rosenthal EM, Muse A, Rowlands J, Barranco MA, Maxted AM, Rosenberg ES, Easton D. Multisystem inflammatory syndrome in children in New York State. *New England Journal of Medicine*. 2020;383(4):347–358.

137. Esposito S, Principi N. Multisystem inflammatory syndrome in children related to SARS-CoV-2. *Pediatric Drugs*. 2021;23(2):119–129.

138. Godfred-Cato S, Bryant B, Leung J, Oster ME, Conklin L, Abrams J, Roguski K, Wallace B, Prezzato E, Koumans EH. COVID-19–associated multisystem inflammatory *syndrome in children—United States, March–July 2020. Morbidity and Mortality Weekly Report*. 2020;69(32):1074.

139. Morris SB, Schwartz NG, Patel P, Abbo L, Beauchamps L, Balan S, Lee EH, Paneth-Pollak R, Geevarughese A, Lash MK. Case series of multisystem inflammatory syndrome in adults associated with SARS-CoV-2 infection—United Kingdom and United States, March–August 2020. *Morbidity and Mortality Weekly Report*. 2020;69(40):1450.

140. Weatherhead JE, Clark E, Vogel TP, Atmar RL, Kulkarni PA. Inflammatory syndromes associated with SARS-CoV-2 infection: dysregulation of the immune response across the age spectrum. *The Journal of clinical investigation*. 2020;130(12):6194–6197.

141. Feldstein LR, Tenforde MW, Friedman KG, Newhams M, Rose EB, Dapul H, Soma VL, Maddux AB, Mourani PM, Bowens C. Characteristics and outcomes of US children and adolescents with multisystem inflammatory syndrome in children (MIS-C) compared with severe acute COVID-19. *Jama*. 2021;325(11):1074–1087.

142. Davies P, Evans C, Kanthimathinathan HK, Lillie J, Brierley J, Waters G, Johnson M, Griffiths B, du Pré P, Mohammad Z. Intensive care admissions of children with paediatric inflammatory multisystem syndrome temporally associated with SARS-CoV-2 (PIMS-TS) in the UK: a multicentre observational study. *The Lancet Child & Adolescent Health*. 2020;4(9):669–677.

143. Vogel TP, Top KA, Karatzios C, Hilmers DC, Tapia LI, Moceri P, Giovannini-Chami L, Wood N, Chandler RE, Klein NP. Multisystem inflammatory syndrome in children and adults (MIS-C/A): Case definition & guidelines for data collection, analysis, and presentation of immunization safety data. *Vaccine*. 2021;39(22):3037–3049.

144. Carfi A, Bernabei R, Landi F. Persistent symptoms in patients after acute COVID-19. *Jama*. 2020;324(6):603–605.

145. Greenhalgh T, Knight M, Buxton M, Husain L. Management of post-acute covid-19 in primary care. *BMJ*. 2020;370:m3026.

146. Goërtz YM, Van Herck M, Delbressine JM, Vaes AW, Meys R, Machado FV, Houben-Wilke S, Burtin C, Posthuma R, Franssen FM. Persistent symptoms 3 months after a SARS-CoV-2 infection: the post-COVID-19 syndrome?. *ERJ open research*. 2020;6(4):00542–02020.

147. Mandal S, Barnett J, Brill SE, Brown JS, Denneny EK, Hare SS, Heightman M, Hillman TE, Jacob J, Jarvis HC. Long-COVID': a cross-sectional study of persisting symptoms, biomarker and imaging abnormalities following hospitalisation for COVID-19. *Thorax*. 2021;76(4):396–398.

148. Zhao Y-m, Shang Y-m, Song W-b, Li Q-q, Xie H, Xu Q-f, Jia J-l, Li L-m, Mao H-l, Zhou X-m. Follow-up study of the pulmonary function and related physiological characteristics of COVID-19 survivors three months after recovery. *EClinicalMedicine*. 2020;25:100463.

149. Nalbandian A, Sehgal K, Gupta A, Madhavan MV, McGroder C, Stevens JS, Cook JR, Nordvig AS, Shalev D, Sehrawat TS. Post-acute COVID-19 syndrome. *Nature Medicine*. 2021:1–15.

150. Shah W, Hillman T, Playford ED, Hishmeh L. Managing the long term effects of covid-19: summary of NICE, SIGN, and RCGP rapid guideline. *BMJ*. 2021;372:n136.

151. Oronsky B, Larson C, Hammond TC, Oronsky A, Kesari S, Lybeck M, Reid TR. A review of persistent post-COVID syndrome (PPCS). *Clinical reviews in allergy & immunology*. 2021:1–9.

152. Channappanavar R, Fett C, Mack M, Ten Eyck PP, Meyerholz DK, Perlman S. Sex-based differences in susceptibility to severe acute respiratory syndrome coronavirus infection. *The Journal of Immunology*. 2017;198(10):4046–4053.

153. Wray S, Arrowsmith S. The physiological mechanisms of the sex-based difference in outcomes of COVID19 infection. *Frontiers in Physiology*. 2021;12:627260.

154. Vahidy FS, Nicolas JC, Meeks JR, Khan O, Pan A, Jones SL, Masud F, Sostman HD, Phillips R, Andrieni JD. Racial and ethnic disparities in SARS-CoV-2 pandemic: analysis of a COVID-19 observational registry for a diverse US metropolitan population. *BMJ open*. 2020;10(8):e039849.

155. Mackey K, Ayers CK, Kondo KK, Saha S, Advani SM, Young S, Spencer H, Rusek M, Anderson J, Veazie S. Racial and ethnic disparities in COVID-19–related infections, hospitalizations, and deaths: a systematic review. *Annals of internal medicine*. 2021;174(3):362–373.

156. Lewis NM, Friedrichs M, Wagstaff S, Sage K, LaCross N, Bui D, McCaffrey K, Barbeau B, George A, Rose C. Disparities in COVID-19 incidence, hospitalizations, and testing, by area-level deprivation—Utah, March 3–July 9, 2020. *Morbidity and Mortality Weekly Report*. 2020;69(38):1369.

157. Azar KM, Shen Z, Romanelli RJ, Lockhart SH, Smits K, Robinson S, Brown S, Pressman AR. Disparities In Outcomes Among COVID-19 Patients In A Large Health Care System In California: Study estimates the COVID-19 infection fatality rate at the US county level. *Health Affairs*. 2020;39(7):1253–1262.

158. Phillips N, Park I-W, Robinson JR, Jones HP. The perfect storm: COVID-19 health disparities in US Blacks. *Journal of racial and ethnic health disparities*. 2020:1–8.

159. Jacob CO. On the genetics and immunopathogenesis of COVID-19. *Clinical Immunology*. 2020:108591.

160. Sironi M, Hasnain SE, Rosenthal B, Phan T, Luciani F, Shaw M-A, Sallum MA, Mirhashemi ME, Morand S, González-Candelas F. SARS-CoV-2 and COVID-19: A genetic, epidemiological, and evolutionary perspective. *Infection, Genetics and Evolution*. 2020;84:104384.

161. Anastassopoulou C, Gkizarioti Z, Patrinos GP, Tsakris A. Human genetic factors associated with susceptibility to SARS-CoV-2 infection and COVID-19 disease severity. *Human genomics*. 2020;14(1):1–8.

162. Maxmen Amy Wuhan market was epicentre of pandemic's start, studies suggest. Nature. 2022;603(7899):15–16.

163. He Wan-Ting, Hou Xin, Zhao Jin, et al. Virome characterization of game animals in China reveals a spectrum of emerging pathogens. Cell. 2022.

164. v3. https://zenodo.org/record/6342616#.YjXWay-B23W, 2022. [Accessed 20 March 2022].

165. v2. https://zenodo.org/record/6299600,2022. [Accessed 20 March 2022].

166. Li Yuguo, Qian Hua, Hang Jian, et al. Probable airborne transmission of SARS-CoV-2 in a poorly ventilated restaurant. Building and Environment. 2021;196.

167. https://www.nih.gov/about-nih/who-we-are/nih-director/statements/nih-launches-new-initiative-study-long-covid#:~:text=While%20still%20being%20defined,%20these,-2%20infection%20(PASC), 2021. [Accessed 20 March 2022].

The Clinical: Manifestations in Systems and Domains of the Body

CHAPTER

5 Pulmonary Manifestations of COVID-19

Sivakumar Nagaraju, MD, Sathishkumar Ramalingam, MD, FACP, FHM, and Subramani Mani, MBBS, PhD

The severe acute respiratory syndrome coronavirus 2 (SARS-CoV-2), the causative pathogen for coronavirus disease 2019 (COVID-19), as its name signifies, predominantly infects the lung, resulting in mild to severe lung injury. Most of the mortality and morbidity attributed to COVID-19 is a direct consequence of the lung pathological processes and the resulting complications. The cardinal clinical manifestation of COVID-19, ARDS, and in the severest form of the disease, multiorgan failure, paint a grave picture of the damage that a SARS-CoV-2 infection can do to infected individuals.

COVID-19 Manifestations in the Respiratory System

Clinical Presentation

The classic symptom complex of COVID-19 such as fever, cough, sore throat, and difficulty in breathing with underlying hypoxemia, pneumonia, and the varied manifestations in different systems of the body have been covered extensively in other chapters of this book. The common symptoms, including comorbidities and other medical conditions that can predispose SARS-CoV-2–infected individuals to severe forms of COVID-19 are summarized in Table 5.1, which is adapted from published Centers for

Disease Control and Prevention (CDC) documents.[1,2] The incubation period of COVID-19 is generally within 14 days after exposure, with most cases occurring approximately 4 to 5 days after exposure.[3,4] The pulmonary spectrum of pathological conditions ranges from mild upper respiratory tract involvement to ARDS leading to respiratory failure, with the spread of the infection to the lower respiratory tract. The range of associated symptoms of COVID-19 was illustrated in a report of 370,000 confirmed COVID-19 cases nationwide provided by the CDC.[5] Cough was found in 50% of all reported cases with other associated symptoms, including fever (43%), myalgia (36%), headache (34%), dyspnea (29%), sore throat (20%), diarrhea (19%), nausea and vomiting (12%), and loss of smell or taste, abdominal pain, and rhinorrhea (10% each).[5] Of all patients presenting with SARS-CoV-2 infection, 33% were asymptomatic, many of whom still had objective clinical manifestations such as ground-glass opacities (GGOs) visible on computed tomography (CT) scan and other nonspecific imaging abnormalities.[6] The spectrum of the clinical disease varied from mild to critical, depending on age, other risk factors, and comorbidities. Almost all critically ill patients required hospitalization. In a study conducted in New York in May 2020, of 2741 critically hospitalized patients, 664 (24%) patients died or were transferred to hospice.[7]

Table 5.1 Common Symptoms Reported in COVID-19 and a List of Medical Conditions That Make Individuals More Susceptible to Severe COVID-19

Symptomatology and Comorbidities of COVID-19	
Category	**Listing**
Symptoms	Fever, cough, shortness of breath, fatigue, body pain, headache, new loss of taste or smell, sore throat, running nose, nausea and/or vomiting, diarrhea
Comorbidities and medical conditions predisposing individuals to severe COVID-19	Cancer
	Cerebrovascular disease
	Chronic kidney disease
	Chronic lung diseases • Interstitial lung disease • Pulmonary embolism • Pulmonary hypertension • Bronchopulmonary dysplasia • Bronchiectasis • Chronic obstructive pulmonary disease
	Chronic liver diseases • Cirrhosis • Nonalcoholic fatty liver disease • Alcoholic liver disease • Autoimmune hepatitis
	Diabetes mellitus (types 1 and type 2)
	Heart conditions 1. Heart failure 2. Coronary artery disease 3. Cardiomyopathies
	Mental health disorders 1. Mood disorders including depression 2. Schizophrenia spectrum disorders
	Obesity (BMI ≥30 kg/m²)
	Pregnancy and recent pregnancy
	Smoking (past and present)
	Tuberculosis

Data from Centers for Disease Control and Prevention (CDC). Symptoms of Covid-19 https://www.cdc.gov/coronavirus/2019-ncov/symptoms-testing/symptoms.html; and CDC. People with certain medical conditions at increased risk for severe Covid-19. https://www.cdc.gov/coronavirus/2019-ncov/need-extra-precautions/people-with-medical-conditions.html.

Table 5.2 Laboratory Abnormalities Associated With Severe Outcome in COVID-19[a]

Laboratory Abnormality	Possible Threshold	Reference Range
D-Dimer	1000 ng/ml	≤500 ng/mL
C-Reactive protein (CRP)	100 mg/L	0.0–0.9 mg/dL
Lactate dehydrogenase (LDH)	245 U/L	117–224 U/L
Troponin	2 × upper limits	0.00–0.05 ng/mL
Ferritin	500 µg/L	30–490 ng/mL
Creatine phosphokinase (CPK)	2 × upper limits	35–232 U/L
Absolute lymphocyte count	<800 µL	1000–800 µL

[a]Elevated laboratory biomarkers such as D-dimer, CRP, LDH, troponin, ferritin, and CPK are associated with severe COVID-19.[9]

laboratory abnormalities have been associated with severe outcomes, as shown in Table 5.2.[9] A genome-wide association study raised concern for the higher risk for specific host genetic factors associated with the ABO blood group system for severe disease.[10] Ray et al.[11] looked at the association between ABO/Rh blood groups and susceptibility to SARS-CoV-2 infection and severe COVID-19 and reported that individuals with O and Rh-negative blood groups have a lower risk for both.[11]

Complications

Drake et al.[12] performed a prospective, multicenter cohort study of more than 70,000 patients admitted with COVID-19 to 302 hospitals across the United Kingdom (UK) over 7 months in 2020 and characterized the organ-specific and systemic complications of COVID-19, which are shown in Table 5.3.[12] Systemic, respiratory, and renal problems were the top three most frequent complications of COVID-19 among all the hospitalized patients with COVID-19 and among the patients who survived the disease; respiratory, renal, and cardiovascular complications topped the list among hospitalized patients who did not survive (see Table 5.3). Respiratory system complications were observed in 18% of all hospitalized patients; it was 14% among the survival group and twice that rate (28%) among the nonsurvival cohort (see Table 5.3). Among the various respiratory system complications presented in Table 5.4, ARDS was the most prevalent; 13% of all hospitalized patients with COVID-19 satisfied the criteria for likely ARDS, which the investigators assigned clinically or based on fulfilling one or more of the following: (1) receiving extracorporeal membrane oxygenation (ECMO), (2) nursed in a prone position and receiving mechanical ventilation, and (3) receiving mechanical

Based on the Chinese Centers for Disease Control and Prevention data, 81% of patients had a mild infection, 14% had a severe infection, and 5% manifested critical illness.[8] The criteria for severe cases were described as patients presenting with dyspnea, hypoxia, or more than 50% lung involvement on imaging within 24 to 48 hours of hospitalization; critical cases were determined based on respiratory failure and multiorgan failure. The overall case fatality reported was 2.3%.[8]

Severe illness can occur at any age but was more prominent in advanced age and in patients with significant comorbidities. Certain demographic populations have been associated with severe illness and primarily constitute communities of color, such as African Americans, Hispanics, and South Asians. Additionally, some

Table 5.3 Systemic and Organ-Specific Complications in Hospitalized Adult Patients With COVID-19 Based on a Large Multicenter Prospective Cohort Study Characterizing Systemic and Organ-Specific Complications of the Disease With Survival as Outcome

Systemic/ Organ	Systemic and Organ-Specific Complications Based on Outcomes: Survived (n = 50,105)/ Died (n = 23,092)/Total (n = 73,197)		
	Survived Cohort Complications n (%)	Died Cohort Complications n (%)	Total Complications n (%)
Systemic	7423 (14.8)	4472 (19.4)	11,895 (16.3)
Respiratory system	7028 (14.0)	6458 (28.0)	13,486 (18.4)
Renal	10,059 (20.1)	7693 (33.3)	17,762 (24.3)
Gastrointestinal (including liver)	4837 (9.7)	3064 (13.3)	7901 (10.8)
Cardiovascular	4035 (8.1)	4938 (21.4)	8973 (12.3)
Neurological	1880 (3.8)	1235 (5.3)	3115 (4.3)

Data from Drake TM, Riad AM, Fairfield CJ, et al. Characterisation of in-hospital complications associated with COVID-19 using the ISARIC WHO Clinical Characterisation Protocol UK: a prospective, multicentre cohort study. *Lancet.* 2021;398(10296):223-237.

Table 5.4 Types of Respiratory Complications Observed in Hospitalized Adult Patients With COVID-19 Based on the Cohort in Table 5.3

Respiratory System Complications	Males (n = 41,025) n (%)	Females (n = 31,977) n (%)	Total (n = 73,002) n (%)
Cryptogenic organizing pneumonia	50 (0.1)	42 (0.1)	92 (0.1)
Likely acute respiratory distress syndrome	6417 (15.6)	3251 (10.2)	9668 (13.2)
Pneumothorax	466 (1.1)	227 (0.7)	693 (0.9)
Pleural effusion	2583 (6.3)	1940 (6.1)	4523 (6.2)
Likely bacterial pneumonia	260 (0.6)	99 (0.3)	359 (0.5)
Pulmonary embolism	622 (1.5)	382 (1.2)	1004 (1.4)

Data from Drake TM, Riad AM, Fairfield CJ, et al. Characterisation of in-hospital complications associated with COVID-19 using the ISARIC WHO Clinical Characterisation Protocol UK: a prospective, multicentre cohort study. *Lancet.* 2021;398(10296):223-237.

ventilation with a ratio of partial pressure of arterial oxygen to fraction of inspired air of 300 mm Hg or less ($PaO_2/FiO_2 \leq 300$ mm Hg).[12]

After presentation of the basic clinical picture of COVID-19, including symptomatology and potential complications, we provide a detailed description of ARDS, its epidemiology, pathogenesis, clinical presentation, and management as a foundation for understanding the pulmonary pathological processes and specific complications of COVID-19.

Acute Respiratory Distress Syndrome

The ARDS syndromic complex is characterized by pulmonary edema, ventilation-perfusion (V/Q) defects, breathlessness, hypoxemia, and significant alveolar damage. The original description of the syndrome goes back more than 50 years to 1967.[13] A consensus definition of ARDS in adults was proposed in 2012 and referred to as the Berlin definition[14]; it was modified in 2016 and called the Kigali modification.[15] The definitions are based on four parameters as depicted in Table 5.5. ARDS, briefly, is hypoxemia with a partial pressure of arterial oxygen (PaO_2) to fraction of inspired oxygen (FiO_2) ratio of 300 mm Hg or less and presence of bilateral lung infiltrates seen on chest imaging (x-ray, CT), in the absence of supporting evidence for left heart failure.

Epidemiology of Acute Respiratory Distress Syndrome

One of the largest pre-COVID ARDS studies, the LUNG-SAFE study, conducted in 2014 assessed an in-hospital

Table 5.5 Acute Respiratory Distress Syndrome (ARDS) Berlin Definition With Kigali Tweak for Resource-Constrained Settings

Berlin Definition	
Characteristics	**Description**
Timing of respiratory failure	Within 1 wk of a known clinical insult or new or worsening respiratory symptoms
Origin of pulmonary edema	Respiratory failure not fully explained by cardiac failure or fluid overload. Need objective assessment, such as echocardiography, to exclude hydrostatic edema if no risk factor is present
Chest imaging	Bilateral opacities on chest radiograph or chest computed tomography not fully explained by effusion, collapse, or nodules
Oxygenation	Acute onset of hypoxemia defined as $PaO_2/FiO_2 \leq 300$ mm Hg on at least PEEP 5 cm H_2O
Mild	PaO_2/FiO_2 201–300 mm Hg
Moderate	PaO_2/FiO_2 101–200 mm Hg
Severe	$PaO_2/FiO_2 \leq 100$ mm Hg
Kigali Modification	
Timing and origin	Same as the Berlin criteria given above
Chest imaging	Bilateral opacities on chest radiograph or chest *ultrasound* not fully explained by effusion, collapse, or nodules
Oxygenation	$SpO_2/FiO_2 \leq 315$ and no PEEP requirement

FiO_2, Fraction of inspired oxygen; PaO_2, partial pressure of arterial oxygen; *PEEP*, positive end-expiratory pressure; SpO_2, peripheral capillary oxygen saturation.
Modified from Force ADT, Ranieri V, Rubenfeld G, et al. Acute respiratory distress syndrome. *JAMA.* 2012;307(23):2526-2533; and Riviello ED, Kiviri W, Twagirumugabe T, et al. Hospital incidence and outcomes of the acute respiratory distress syndrome using the Kigali modification of the Berlin definition. *Am J Respir Crit Care Med.* 2016;193(1):52-59.

mortality of 40% with a range of 35% to 46% based on severity of ARDS at the time of diagnosis.[16,17] The study estimated the prevalence of ARDS among patients hospitalized in intensive care units (ICUs) based on data from 50 countries to be 10.4% and also concluding that ARDS appeared to be underrecognized, undertreated, and underreported.[16] In the United States the annual incidence of ARDS was estimated to be 190,000 cases, with a reported mortality of 38.5%.[18] Several comorbidities, including alcohol abuse, cigarette smoking, polluted air, and hypoalbuminemia, have been recognized as contributing to the severity of the syndrome.[18] There are also significant racial, ethnic, and sex disparities, as well as differences in susceptibility based on population density and socioeconomic status for ARDS morbidity and mortality, with higher rates among the Black and Hispanic populace, males, low-income groups, and people living in high-density population regions.[16,19,20]

Cause of Acute Respiratory Distress Syndrome

The causative risk factors for ARDS, which generally occurs in the setting of pneumonia can be broadly categorized as local and systemic. Respiratory bacterial, viral, fungal, and secondary infections that cause pneumonia, aspiration pneumonia, lung trauma resulting from blunt or penetrating injuries, and inhalation injuries are common local causes; systemic causes include nonpulmonary sepsis, acute pancreatitis, blood or blood product transfusion, drug overdose, major burns, cardiopulmonary bypass, graft-versus-host disease, and high-altitude pulmonary edema (HAPE).[21,22]

Pathophysiology of Acute Respiratory Distress Syndrome

Histopathology With Alveolar Focus

The characteristic pathological hallmark of ARDS is diffuse alveolar damage which compromises the basic lung physiology of ventilation and perfusion, leading to hypoxemia.[18,21,23-25] The temporal evolution of the alveolar damage occurs over weeks in three phases. The first or the exudative phase starts in the first week with alveolar epithelial injury affecting both type I and type II pneumocytes. This causes denudation of the alveolar membrane and increased permeability. Eosinophilic deposits result in hyaline membrane formation along the denuded alveolar basement membrane, a classic finding in diffuse alveolar damage along with white blood cell agglutination and formation of platelet-fibrin thrombi.[18] Alveolar fluid reabsorption by ion transport, a normal function of alveolar cells, is affected resulting in accumulation of exudative fluid in the alveolar cavity. Macrophages residing in the alveolus secrete proinflammatory factors such as interleukin-8 (IL-8) and monocyte chemoattractant protein-1, which attract neutrophils and other macrophages into the lung, aggravating the lung injury.[18] Concomitant endothelial damage to the capillaries lining the alveolus results in

the disruption of endothelial barrier leading to interstitial flooding, with the excess fluid finding its way to the alveolar space and causing intraalveolar flooding and exacerbation of edema. The nature of insult to the endothelial cells is not well understood but apoptosis and pyroptosis have been proposed as plausible mechanisms.[18,26] Endothelial cell activation results in release of angiopoietin-2, leading to formation of neutrophil-platelet aggregates that pass through the weakened endothelial barrier and infiltrate the alveolar space.[18] The neutrophil-platelet aggregates manifest thromboinflammatory mechanisms such as neutrophil extracellular traps (NETs), which are implicated in both capillary endothelial and alveolar epithelial barrier perturbations.[27,28] Other causative factors responsible for endothelial wall damage are pathogens and circulating toxins, alveolar macrophage factors, and proinflammatory cytokines and chemokines.[21,27] The cascade of events set in motion by epithelial and endothelial injury causing alveolar flooding with exudate results in surfactant dysfunction, which promotes atelectasis and biophysical injury to the lung.[29]

The second phase, called the proliferative phase, sets in motion the repair mechanisms to tackle the intraalveolar and interstitial exudative edema of phase 1. Beginning in the second week, the proliferative phase lasts for about 2 weeks. The key events of this phase include interstitial fibroblast proliferation with secretion of epithelial growth factors, alveolar type II cell hyperplasia with differentiation into alveolar type I cells, phagocytosis of apoptotic neutrophils, and reestablishment of junctions between epithelial cells with restoration of the integrity of the epithelial barrier.[21] Epithelial barrier repair enables reabsorption of edematous fluid into the interstitial space. Fibroblasts transform the exudate to cellular granulation tissue with matrix morphology, which eventually turns into fibrous tissue with the deposition of collagen.[24] Likewise, in the lung capillaries endothelial cell proliferation sets in with repair of endothelial disruption and restoration of the endothelial barrier function.[21] The pathogenetic mechanisms of the three phases of ARDS are enumerated in Figs. 5.1 and 5.2, which illustrate the pathological process of the injured alveolus in the exudative phase and the repair mechanisms of the proliferative phase with the healthy alveolus as reference.

The third or fibrotic phase necessitates mechanical ventilation and is typically seen in patients surviving beyond 3 to 4 weeks from the onset of ARDS. This phase is marked by significant interstitial and intraalveolar fibrosis with lung remodeling by thick collagenous connective tissue.[21,24] The process of fibrosis acts as a nonspecific response to the lung injury and resembles the lung tissue reorganization that occurs in typical organizing pneumonia.[24]

Additional pathological features of ARDS are summarized in Table 5.6 and salient histopathological changes observed in the temporal evolution of diffuse alveolar damage are shown in Table 5.7. After exploration of the

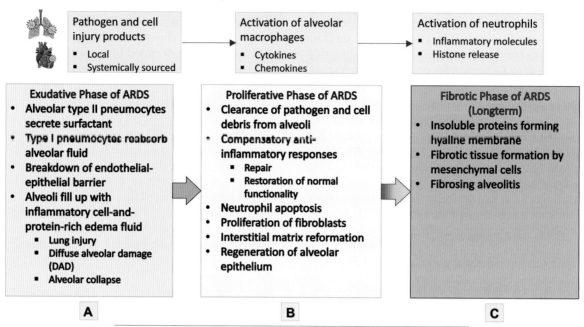

Fig. 5.1 Pathogenetic Mechanisms of Acute Respiratory Distress Syndrome *(ARDS).* The pathogenic and cell injury products activate the macrophages residing in the alveolus resulting in the release of cytokines and chemokines, which in turn trigger the neutrophils causing inflammatory molecules and histone to be released. *Panels A, B,* and *C* list the features of the three critical phases of ARDS, the near-term exudative and proliferative and the long-term fibrotic. The proliferative phase sets up the repair and regenerative mechanisms to counter the alveolar injury. (Contents modified from the descriptions in Swenson KE, Swenson ER. Pathophysiology of ARDS and COVID-19 lung injury. *Crit Care Clin.* 2021;37[4]:749-776; and Huppert LA, Matthay MA, Ware LB. Pathogenesis of acute respiratory distress syndrome. *Semin Respir Crit Care Med.* 2019;40[1]:31-39.)

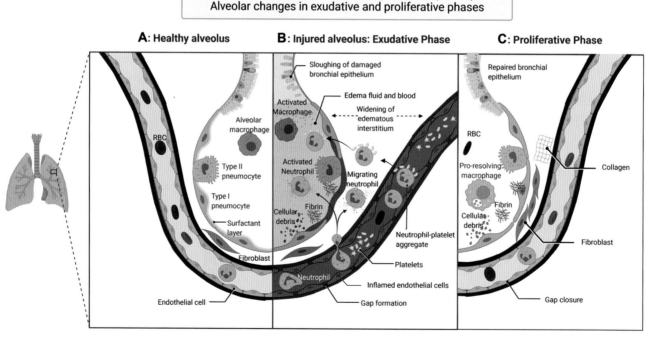

Fig. 5.2 Acute Respiratory Distress Syndrome (ARDS) Alveolar Changes. *Panel A* shows a healthy alveolus, and *panel B* shows an injured alveolus in the exudative phase. In this phase the enhanced alveolar epithelial and capillary endothelial permeability causes the alveolus to fill up with protein-rich edema fluid. Fluid also accumulates in the interstitial space, causing widening. These pathological changes induce labored breathing, hypoxia, and accumulation of carbon dioxide, which can lead to respiratory failure. *Panel C* shows the proliferative phase, which initiates the repair process. Type II pneumocytes proliferate initially and then differentiate into type I cells. Immune cells and their mediators play a role in initiating alveolar epithelial repair. Fibroblasts secrete epithelial growth factors and collagen deposition in this phase. (Figure created using Biorender.)

Table 5.6 Acute Respiratory Distress Syndrome (ARDS) Salient Pathophysiological Mechanisms

ARDS	
Pathophysiological Characteristics	**Description**
Diffuse alveolar damage (DAD)	The predominant pathological condition is epithelial injury that involves types I and II pneumocytes and dissociation of junctions between these alveolar cells resulting in increased permeability. Neutrophil migration resulting from endothelial injury leads to alveolar epithelial injury by the perturbation of intercellular junctions and causing enhanced epithelial permeability. See Table 5.7 for a list of additional histopathological details of DAD and its three phases.
Impaired alveolar fluid clearance	Alveolar fluid reabsorption is performed by types I and II alveolar pneumocytes by active ion transport into the interstitium from which clearance occurs by lymphatic channels. Because of alveolar cell damage, permeability is lost, affecting ion transport resulting in accumulation of exudative fluid in alveolar spaces.
Ventilation-perfusion abnormalities (gas exchange anomalies)	Type II alveolar cells secrete surfactant, which plays a key role in gas exchange in the lungs by keeping the alveoli open based on its capacity to lower surface tension. The loss of surfactant causes ventilation-perfusion mismatch and impairs carbon dioxide elimination.
Reduction in lung compliance	Increased permeability, loss of surfactant resulting from damage to type II pneumocytes and accumulation of fluid in the alveolus leads to reduction in lung volume available for gas exchange. This in turn causes increased dead space in the lungs and lowering of lung compliance.
Increased pulmonary vascular resistance	Impaired carbon dioxide elimination causes hypercapnia leading to pulmonary vasoconstriction. This, along with thromboembolism and interstitial edema, results in increased pulmonary vascular resistance and pulmonary hypertension.
Endothelial injury	Endothelial cell damage results in leakage of fluid across the capillary barrier into the interstitial space. This results in an edematous interstitium with fluid moving into the alveoli through the damaged epithelial barrier.
Thromboembolism	Postmortem studies of lungs from patients dying of ARDS have consistently demonstrated thromboembolic lesions. Macrothrombi and microthrombi have been extensively observed in arterioles and capillaries of the lung. Two types of microthrombi have been reported: (1) composed of hyaline platelet-fibrin seen in capillaries and arterioles and (2) laminated fibrin clots visualized in preacinar and intraacinar arteries.
Ventilatory support injury	See Table 5.8

Data from Matthay MA, Zemans RL, Zimmerman GA, et al. Acute respiratory distress syndrome. *Nat Rev Dis Primers*. 2019;5(1):1-22; Tomashefski JF Jr. Pulmonary pathology of acute respiratory distress syndrome. *Clin Chest Med*. 2000;21(3):435-466; Swenson KE, Swenson ER. Pathophysiology of ARDS and COVID-19 lung injury. *Crit Care Clin*. 2021;37(4):749-776; and Huppert LA, Matthay MA, Ware LB. Pathogenesis of acute respiratory distress syndrome. *Semin Respir Crit Care Med*. 2019;40(1):31-39.

Table 5.7 Chronology of Acute Respiratory Distress Syndrome (ARDS) Diffuse Alveolar Damage (DAD)

ARDS DAD		
Exudative Phase (wk 1)	**Proliferative Phase (wk 2 and 3)**	**Fibrotic Phase (>3 wk)**
1. Interstitial edema 2. Alveolar edema 3. Leukocyte infiltration and agglutination 4. Pneumocyte type I necrosis 5. Endothelial cell necrosis 6. Alveolar basement membrane denudation 7. Hyaline membrane formation 8. Platelet-fibrin thrombi	1. Interstitial fibroblast proliferation 2. Pneumocyte type II proliferation and differentiation into pneumocyte type I 3. Reestablishment of tight junctions and adherent junctions 4. Restoration of epithelial barrier function 5. Parenchymal necrosis 6. Phagocytosis of apoptotic neutrophils 7. Endothelial cell proliferation 8. Restoration of endothelial barrier function 9. Obliterative endarteritis 10. Macrothrombi	1. Prolonged proliferation of fibroblasts 2. Collagenous fibrosis 3. Microcystic honeycombing 4. Traction bronchiectasis 5. Obliteration of microcapillaries 6. Arterial tortuosity with mural fibrosis and medial hypertrophy

Modified from Tomashefski JF Jr. Pulmonary pathology of acute respiratory distress syndrome. *Clin Chest Med*. 2000;21(3):435-466. See also references 25, 31, and 32. wk: week.

pathophysiology of ARDS, the chapter discusses alterations in respiratory mechanics. To formulate a rational approach to the management of ARDS it is necessary to understand the changes in respiratory mechanics in ARDS.

Respiratory Physiology and ARDS

The honeycomb-like structure of the lung composed of a multitude of small air sacs or alveoli, capillaries, and interstitial tissue confers the lung parenchyma its elastance and compliance, enabling it to expand without ballooning during inspiration and contract without collapsing during expiration. As diffuse alveolar damage sets in, the increased permeability across the alveolar membrane and vascular endothelium results in alveolar flooding. Alveolar fluid accumulation combined with loss of surfactant results in alveoli becoming unrecruitable, leading to shrinkage of lung volume available for gas exchange and loss of compliance.[30] This alveolar derecruitment, that is, exclusion from gas exchange, causes a physiological division of the lung into nonaerated diseased regions and aerated healthy regions.[30] Because the number of recruitable lung units, that is, aerated healthy regions, are reduced in toto, the phenomenon has been labeled "baby lung."[33]

The two key blood gas anomalies of ARDS are hypoxemia and hypercapnia. The basic respiratory physiological measure that modulates these two blood gas values is the alveolar V/Q ratio, denoted by V_A/Q, where V_A refers to alveolar ventilation and Q is perfusion. For normal gas exchange to occur, an optimal V_A/Q is needed, which is disrupted in ARDS because of the V/Q mismatch, resulting in some regions of the lung with low V_A/Q ratios and other regions with high V_A/Q ratios.[34] In regions with low V_A/Q ratios, perfusion is much higher with respect to ventilation, leading to hypoxemia; in regions where the V_A/Q ratios are higher, ventilation is markedly more compared with perfusion, resulting in hypercapnia. Low V_A/Q ratios cause shunting, the gas partial pressures reflecting those of the mixed venous blood, whereas high V_A/Q ratios result in dead spaces with gas partial pressures similar to those of inspired air.[34] In short, hypoxemia of ARDS results from blood flow to alveoli that are not ventilated and hypercapnia sets in when alveoli have proper ventilation but lack perfusion.

Lung Injury From Mechanical Ventilation

Ventilator-induced lung injury (VILI) has garnered a lot of attention over the last decade[30,35-39] and continues to do so with the advent of the COVID-19 pandemic. In this section we will introduce the salient types of VILI and examine how mechanical ventilation exacerbates evolving lung injury of ARDS. At the end of inspiration when there is no air flowing into the lungs, lung inflation is maintained by what is referred to as the transpulmonary pressure, which is the difference between alveolar and pleural pressures and is closely linked with VILI.[35] Details of transpulmonary pressure and how it can be estimated in the clinical setting are illustrated in Fig. 5.3. Lung volume and transpulmonary pressure are interrelated, and the type of injury resulting from mechanical ventilation is based on whether ventilation occurs at high or low lung volumes.[35,36] Four types of

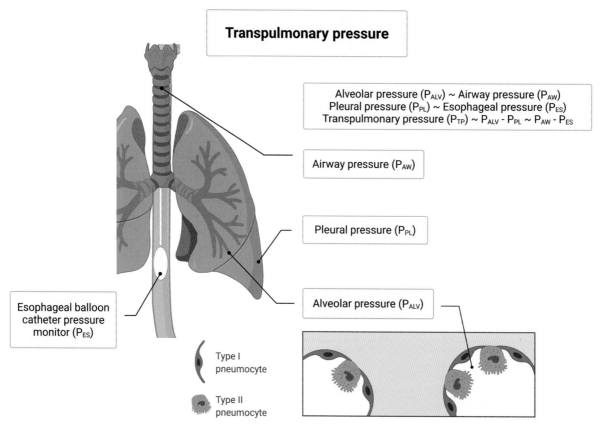

Transpulmonary pressure

Alveolar pressure (P_{ALV}) ~ Airway pressure (P_{AW})
Pleural pressure (P_{PL}) ~ Esophageal pressure (P_{ES})
Transpulmonary pressure (P_{TP}) ~ P_{ALV} - P_{PL} ~ P_{AW} - P_{ES}

Airway pressure (P_{AW})

Pleural pressure (P_{PL})

Alveolar pressure (P_{ALV})

Esophageal balloon catheter pressure monitor (P_{ES})

Type I pneumocyte

Type II pneumocyte

Fig. 5.3 Transpulmonary Pressure. Transpulmonary pressure *(P_TP)* is clinically estimated as the difference between airway pressure *(P_AW)* and esophageal pressure *(P_ES)* measured at two time points in the respiratory cycle: end of inspiration and end of expiration. P_{TP} measurement is critical for positive end-expiratory pressure (PEEP) calculation in mechanical ventilation, for example, to maintain P_{TP} less than 25 cm H_2O at the end of inspiration and P_{TP} greater than 0 cm H_2O at the end of expiration to minimize ventilator-induced lung injury while facilitating lung recruitment. (Modified from Fig. 5.1, Coleman MH, Aldrich JM. Acute respiratory distress syndrome: ventilator management and rescue therapies. *Crit Care Clin* 2021;37[4]:851-866. Created using Biorender.)

Table 5.8 Ventilator-Induced Lung Injury (VILI) Mechanisms, Types, and Manifestations[a]

Mechanism of Injury	Type of Injury	Manifestations
Mechanical ventilation at high lung volumes • Overdistension of the alveoli • Repetitive strain	Barotrauma (air leaks) Volutrauma	Pneumothorax Pneumomediastinum Air embolism Subcutaneous emphysema Pulmonary edema
MV at low lung volumes 1. Lung injury from opening and closing of alveoli 2. Parenchymal shear injury 3. Aggravated by heterogeneity	Atelectrauma	
Patient self-inflicted lung injury (P-SILI), that is, spontaneous breathing during MV causing lung injury • High tidal volumes from effort • High transpulmonary pressure from vigorous efforts (pendelluft effect) • Negative pleural pressure leading to increased transvascular pressure resulting in alveoli filling up with edematous fluid • Asynchrony between spontaneous effort and MV • Forced expiration causes diaphragmatic shift leading to lower end-expiratory lung volume and hypoxemia	Barotrauma	Pneumothorax
Downstream biological effects of all types of lung injury 1. High lung volume 2. Low lung volume 3. Molecular and cellular events of lung parenchymal stress 4. Increased alveolar-capillary permeability	Biotrauma	Pulmonary edema Pulmonary fibrosis (long-term) Multiple-organ failure from proinflammatory mediators entering systemic circulation

Data from Swenson KE, Swenson ER. Pathophysiology of ARDS and COVID-19 lung injury. *Crit Care Clin*. 2021;37(4):749-776; Slutsky AS, Ranieri VM. Ventilator-induced lung injury. *N Engl J Med*. 2013;369(22):2126-2136; Curley GF, Laffey JG, Zhang H, Slutsky AS. Biotrauma and ventilator-induced lung injury: clinical implications. *Chest*. 2016, 150(5):1109-1117; and Yoshida T, Fujino Y, Amato MB, Kavanagh BP. Fifty years of research in ARDS: spontaneous breathing during mechanical ventilation—risks, mechanisms, and management. *Am J Respir Crit Care Med*. 2017;195(8):985–992.

[a]The table also includes patient self-inflicted lung injury (P-SILI). Both VILI and P-SILI are "ventilation"-induced lung injury.[41]

VILI have been described—barotrauma, volutrauma, atelectrauma, and biotrauma. VILI is also related to lung injury that results from the efforts to breathe spontaneously on the part of the patient during mechanical ventilation and is described as patient self-inflicted lung injury (P-SILI).[40,41] Both VILI and P-SILI are "ventilation"-induced lung injury.[41] Table 5.8 and Fig. 5.4 summarize the types of VILI, the mechanisms underlying the injury, and their clinical manifestations.

Following up on the observation that VILI originates in isolated and scattered regions of the lung parenchyma based on heterogeneity, Gaver III et al.[37] proposed a permeability-originated obstruction response framework with four features: (1) enhanced endothelial permeability, (2) alveolar surfactant deactivation, (3) alveolar and interstitial edema, and (4) repetitive recruitment/derecruitment resulting in decreased compliance leading to atelectrauma, which has implications for mechanical ventilation management. Unless effective interventions are promptly undertaken, the proponents of the model warn that a repetitive cycle of these four steps will induce a vicious cycle resulting in increasing VILI.

Clinical Features and Diagnosis of Acute Respiratory Distress Syndrome

ARDS is characterized by the triad of rapid-onset hypoxemia, bilateral lung infiltrates, and pulmonary edema

not attributable to a pathological cardiac condition. As the syndromic nomenclature based on clinical and pathophysiological criteria signifies, there is considerable heterogeneity in terms of cause, comorbidities, pathophysiology, and biology of ARDS. There is no specific biomarker to diagnose ARDS; moreover, no set of findings by themselves—molecular, clinical, radiological, or pathological—can be considered a sufficient set of markers for the diagnosis of ARDS.[42] Thus there is a need for consensus diagnostic criteria for uniformity in approach to the diagnosis of ARDS.

ARDS diagnosis follows the Berlin definition criteria presented earlier in Table 5.1. To recapitulate, the clinical recognition is based on (1) the onset of acute respiratory failure within 1 week of clinical insult, (2) noncardiac origin of respiratory failure, (3) bilateral opacities on chest radiograph or chest CT, and (4) hypoxemia. Although the diffuse alveolar damage feature is implicitly incorporated into the definition, autopsy studies of the lung identified diffuse alveolar damage features in only half of the patients dying from the syndrome.[22,43] Likewise, lung biopsy samples of patients hospitalized with ARDS demonstrated histological evidence of diffuse alveolar damage in similar proportions.[22,44,45]

Clinically, ARDS can be broadly categorized into two clinical phenotypes based on local or systemic

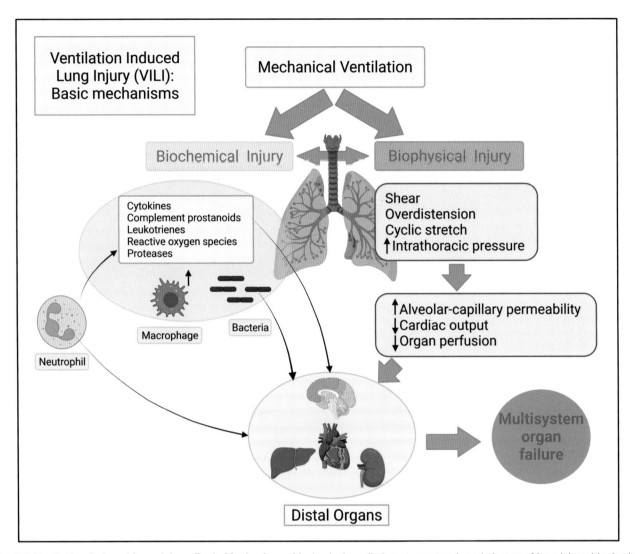

Fig. 5.4 Ventilation-Induced Lung Injury: Basic Mechanisms. Mechanical ventilation causes two broad classes of lung injury: biophysical injury and biochemical injury, also referred to as biotrauma. The biophysical injury types constitute the spectrum of barotrauma, volutrauma, and atelectrauma. Both the biochemical and biophysical pathways of injury can affect the distal organs leading to multisystem organ failure. (Modified from reference Slutsky AS, Tremblay LN. Multiple system organ failure: is mechanical ventilation a contributing factor? *Am J Respir Crit Care Med.* 1998;157[6]:1721-1725. Created using Biorender. See also reference 236.)

etiological factors. See Fig. 5.5 for an illustration of these clinical phenotypes and their risk/causative factors. It has been shown that the risk for developing ARDS increases when the insult is local when compared with systemic factors.[46]

Morphological phenotypes have been postulated based on radiological patterns observed in chest CT of patients with ARDS. Two distinct subgroups have been identified: (1) focal ARDS evidenced by consolidations in the lower lobes and dependent dorsal regions and (2) nonfocal ARDS with diffuse patchy opacities; the two groups had significant differences in lung physiological processes, with the lungs of the nonfocal ARDS group more recruitable than the focal ARDS group.[22,47,48] Researchers have developed a noninvasive method to estimate the extent of pulmonary edema based on chest x-rays. The radiographic assessment of lung edema (RALE) score, which evaluates the extent and density

of alveolar opacities on chest radiographs, was found to be highly correlated with the severity of ARDS and increased mortality from ARDS.[49] However, the relationship of the RALE score to the focal and nonfocal ARDS groups based on chest CT findings has not been established.[48]

Investigators have also explored protein biomarkers to stratify and discover ARDS phenotypes. In particular, Forel et al.[50] identified a specific protein biomarker, procollagen peptide (PCP-III), with the best cutoff value from bronchoalveolar lavage fluid in persistent ARDS to identify patients with lung fibroproliferation who could likely benefit from the administration of corticosteroids.[50] Hamon et al.[51] used the threshold level of PCP-III greater than 9 μG/L, indicating lung fibroproliferation, and compared chest scans of 228 patients with ARDS who had a bronchoalveolar lavage fluid PCP-III level and a chest CT scan; the study

Clinical Phenotypes of ARDS

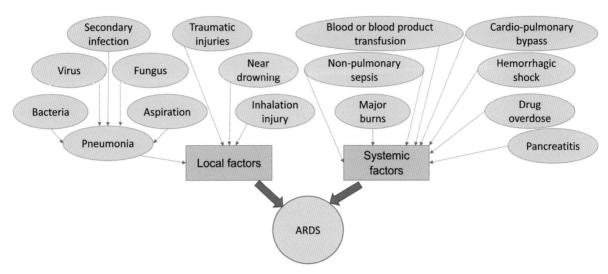

Fig. 5.5 Clinical Phenotypes of Acute Respiratory Distress Syndrome *(ARDS)*. Broadly, two clinical phenotypes of ARDS are recognized based on the locality of the factors causing the lung injury. A constellation of local and/or systemic factors contribute to the development of the syndrome of ARDS and these are depicted here. (Data from Thompson BT, Chambers RC, Liu KD. Acute respiratory distress syndrome. *N Engl J Med.* 2017;377[6]:562-572.)

demonstrated significant association between high levels of PCP-III and CT scan fibrosis scores.[51]

Using data from two randomized controlled trials (RCTs), the ARMA and ALVEOLI, and applying a latent class analytics approach, Calfee et al.[52] identified two subphenotypes: the hyperinflammatory, characterized by severe inflammation, shock, and metabolic acidosis, leading to worse outcomes and labeled subphenotype 2, and the less inflammatory type, denoted subphenotype 1; the distribution was 30% for subphenotype 2 and 70% for subphenotype 1.[52] The hyperinflammatory subphenotype 2 had higher plasma levels of inflammatory biomarkers, greater vasopressor use, lower sodium bicarbonate levels, and a higher prevalence of sepsis compared with subphenotype 1; subphenotype 2 also had a differential response to positive end-expiratory pressure (PEEP).[52]

Using a different ARDS cohort from another trial, the Fluid and Catheter Treatment Trial (FACTT), Famous et al.[53] identified the two subphenotypes, hyperinflammatory subphenotype 2 and the less inflammatory subphenotype 1, based on levels of IL-8, bicarbonate, and tumor necrosis factor receptor-1, and reported that fluid management protocols had significantly different effects on 90-day mortality outcomes in the two subphenotypes. A fluid conservative strategy resulted in lower 90-day mortality in subphenotype 1, whereas the same approach caused an increase in 90-day mortality in subphenotype 2.

There is currently no clinically valid biological marker for detecting ARDS with high sensitivity and specificity. However, markers of epithelial[54] and

endothelial[55] injuries have been shown to be elevated in ARDS and they could be useful in distinguishing ARDS from local and systemic insults.[22] Plasma biomarkers of epithelial injury such as surfactant protein-D and soluble receptor for advanced glycation end products are found to be elevated in ARDS from local causes.[54] Likewise, plasma biomarkers of endothelial injury, for example, angiopoietin-2 and von Willebrand factor antigen, are higher in ARDS from systemic causes such as nonpulmonary sepsis.[55]

Because bacterial and viral infections are common causes, a typical ARDS workup involves blood culture, sputum or tracheal aspirate Gram staining, and culture. However, identification of the causative pathogen may not be straightforward. Nucleic acid detection methods might help improve detection and can help with the identification of both bacterial and viral pathogens.[48,56]

Conditions that can mimic ARDS include congestive heart failure, interstitial lung diseases, connective tissue disorders such as polymyositis, vasculitis, lymphomas, and endobronchial tuberculosis; these are commonly referred to as ARDS mimics and would require additional investigations for a precise diagnosis.[21]

Treatment and Prevention

The treatment for ARDS is evolving, but it is still mostly preventive and supportive. Once the patient has transitioned from lung injury to the stage of ARDS, effective treatments are still in experimental stages. Hence the focus of investigators has broadened to include identification and treatment of patients who are at risk for developing ARDS and show early evidence of lung

Management of ARDS: Recent Trends

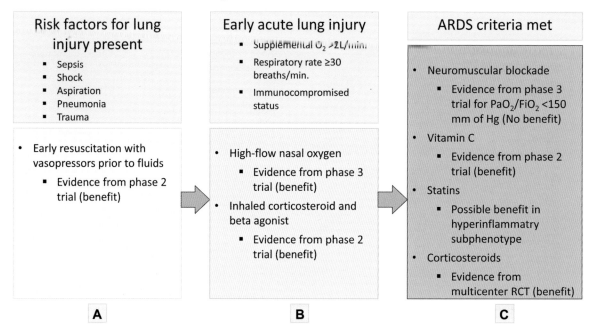

Fig. 5.6 Management of Acute Respiratory Distress Syndrome *(ARDS):* Recent Trends. The protocol categorizes intervention approaches based on the evolution of lung injury. *Panel A* points to the value of early resuscitation when risk factors for lung injury are noted. *Panel B* shows the value of high-flow nasal oxygen, corticosteroid, and beta agonist during the early phase of acute lung injury. *Panel C* provides the intervention strategies shown to be beneficial/not beneficial when ARDS criteria are met in a specific patient. *FiO₂*, Fraction of inspired oxygen; *PaO₂*, partial pressure of arterial oxygen; *RCT,* randomized controlled trial. (Modified from Matthay MA, Arabi YM, Siegel ER, et al. Phenotypes and personalized medicine in the acute respiratory distress syndrome. *Intensive Care Med.* 2020:1-17; see also reference 237.)

Table 5.9 Acute Respiratory Distress Syndrome

Clinical Practice Guideline Recommendations for Mechanical Ventilation Proposed by ATS, ESICM, and SCCM for Adults[58]

ARDS: Mechanical Ventilation Guideline Recommendations				
Intervention	**Severity of ARDS**	**Quality of Evidence**	**Strength of Recommendation**	**Recommendation Type (For/Against)**
Mechanical ventilation using lower tidal volumes • 4–8 mL/kg PBW • Plateau pressure <30 cm H₂0	Mild, moderate, and severe	Moderate	Strong	For
Prone positioning • >12 hr/day	Severe	Moderate	Strong	For
Routine use of high-frequency oscillatory ventilation	Moderate and severe	High	Strong	Against
Higher positive end-expiratory pressure (T)	Moderate and severe	Moderate	Conditional	For
Recruitment maneuvers	Moderate and severe	Low	Conditional	For
Extracorporeal membrane oxygenation (ECMO)	Severe	Not applicable	Not applicable	More evidence needed for recommendation

ᵃSee also reference 58. Quality of evidence was assigned based on GRADE guidelines 3.[59]

ATS, American Thoracic Society; *ARDS,* acute respiratory distress syndrome; *ESICM,* European Society of Intensive Care Medicine; *PBW,* predicted body weight; *SCCM,* Society of Critical Care Medicine.

injury.[48] Based on this approach, three categories have been developed: (1) patients with risk factors for lung injury such as sepsis, shock, or pneumonia; (2) patients in the early stage of acute lung injury; and (3) patients meeting ARDS criteria.[48] These categories and modified approaches for treating them are presented in Fig. 5.6.

Table 5.9 provides the protective ventilation and intervention strategies and their rationale.[57,58]

To summarize, the various strategies to reduce VILI include (1) low tidal volume ventilation to limit overdistention, (2) moderate to high PEEP to prevent derecruitment and injury from low lung volume, and

(3) recruitment maneuvers with application of greater than 35 cm H_2O airway pressure to open collapsed lung segments.[35]

There has been a recent trend toward finding subphenotypes of ARDS with the goal of personalization of treatment based on cause, various types of biomarkers, or gene expression data.[48,60,61] Sinha et al.[62] proposed a method of clinical stratification of ARDS for subphenotype identification based on a machine learning method called latent class analysis using clinically available data. Once the model is validated using clinical data from different centers, it is possible that the machine learning model could be useful at the bedside for phenotype identification. Wick et al.[63] discuss the promises and challenges of developing a personalized medicine approach for the management of ARDS. The review specifically identified the heterogeneity in the presentation and manifestation of ARDS and the differences in the cause of ARDS in developed and developing countries as two significant challenges for developing a patient-specific paradigm of treatment.

As Kotas and Thompson[64] have nicely put it, ARDS is a syndrome and not a disease. To maximize desirable outcomes, it is important to identify the cause of ARDS in a patient-specific manner while following the general principles and guidelines for the management of ARDS.

Long-Term Outcomes

Patients recovering from ARDS suffer from significant long-term health consequences. Muscular weakness, anxiety, depression, and posttraumatic stress disorder (PTSD) have been reported in survivors.[65]

With this basic layout of the different facets of ARDS, which hopefully will serve as a foundation for understanding the lung pathological processes and management of COVID-19 respiratory manifestations, the chapter will proceed to discussion of the pathophysiology, management, and complications of lung injury resulting from SARS-CoV-2 infection. The focus will be on the pathophysiology of COVID-19 lung injury, similarities and differences between COVID-19 ARDS and classic ARDS, pulmonary complications of COVID-19, management protocols, and long-term sequelae after SARS-CoV-2 infection.

COVID-19 Acute Respiratory Distress Syndrome

Epidemiology of COVID-19 Acute Respiratory Distress Syndrome

The epidemiology of SARS-CoV-2 and COVID-19 has been covered in detail in an earlier chapter. As mentioned earlier, the annual incidence of ARDS in the United States before the advent of the COVID-19 pandemic was 190,000. Based on the mortality figure of 650,000 in the United States from March 2020 to September 2021 and assuming that 80% had severe pneumonia/ARDS and attributing a mortality of 20% from COVID-19 ARDS, Wick et al.[63] estimate an incidence of 2.5 million cases of COVID-19–associated ARDS over 18 months or about 1.7 million over a period of 12 months.

Pathophysiology of COVID-19 Acute Respiratory Distress Syndrome

In the early months of the SARS-CoV-2 pandemic, a controversy emerged on whether the pathophysiological mechanisms of COVID-19 ARDS and classic ARDS were significantly different to warrant an alternative approach to the management of the condition.[66-69] However, a consensus later emerged signifying that there are more similarities than differences between COVID-19 ARDS and ARDS from other causes and that COVID-19–related lung injury should be managed based on the lung-protective strategies recommended for classic ARDS.[30,70-72]

Hypoxemia and COVID-19 Lung Injury

The key manifestation in COVID-19 lung injury is hypoxemia. COVID-19 patients presenting with "silent hypoxemia," that is, hypoxemia measured by SpO_2 or PaO_2 values disproportionate to dyspnea and/or radiological evidence of lung injury on chest radiograph or chest CT, has been widely reported[73-80] but has never been observed in classic non-COVID ARDS.[71] Various hypotheses have been put forward to explain the silent hypoxemia of COVID-19 lung injury: (1) vascular damage resulting from endotheliitis, with macrothrombi and microthrombi more pronounced in COVID-19 pneumonia compared with other viral or bacterial pneumonias resulting in lung injury[81,82]; (2) diffuse alveolar damage might not be the predominant pathological condition of COVID-19 lung injury leading to hypoxemia because lung compliance compromise is not significant[83]; (3) pulmonary vascular dilatation and evidence of perfusion in areas of the lung with GGOs on chest radiograph and chest CT as evidence of possible failure of the compensatory mechanism of physiological hypoxic pulmonary vasoconstriction[84]; and (4) impaired central and peripheral oxygen sensing and dyspnea perception based on the presence of angiotensin-converting enzyme-2 (ACE2) receptors in the carotid body and brain, with potential direct viral effects and accounting for the observation that dyspnea is less prevalent.[85-87] Other pandemic-causing coronaviruses such as SARS-CoV and MERS-CoV have been shown to infect brainstem respiratory centers leading to respiratory failure.[88,89]

Swenson et al.,[71] in their review of silent hypoxemia and its pathophysiology in COVID-19, discussed these four hypotheses and argued that the evidence is not compelling enough to conclude that the pathophysiology of COVID-19 is unique to advocate a different

Table 5.10 Pathophysiology of Hypoxemia in COVID-19 Lung Injury Versus Acute Respiratory Distress Syndrome (ARDS) From Other Causes

Pathophysiological Measures	COVID-19 Lung Injury	Non–COVID-19 ARDS	Comment
Vascular regulation	No direct evidence of HPV impairment	Intact vascular responsiveness	Vascular endotheliitis and microthrombi much more prevalent in COVID-19 lung injury
Lung compliance	Compliance reduced	Compliance greatly reduced	Clinically nonsignificant difference in reported values of C_{ST} ranges
Neural oxygen sensing and dyspnea perception	Impaired central and peripheral oxygen sensing and dyspnea perception postulated based on the presence of ACE2 receptors in carotid body and brain and potential direct viral effects Dyspnea less prevalent	Preserved oxygen sensing at both peripheral and central chemoreceptors with intact dyspnea perception Dyspnea more prevalent	No direct HVR testing has been performed in both groups

ARDS, Acute respiratory distress syndrome; C_{ST}, static total respiratory system compliance; *HPV*, hypoxic pulmonary vasoconstriction; *HVR*, hypoxic ventilatory response.
(Modified from Swenson KE, Ruoss SJ, Swenson ER. The pathophysiology and dangers of silent hypoxemia in COVID-19 lung injury. *Ann Am Thorac Soc.* 2021;18(7):1098–1105.)

therapeutic approach from the current protocols of care for classic ARDS.[71] The perceived differences and uncertainties in the pathophysiology of COVID-19 lung injury in comparison with the pathological manifestations of classic ARDS are summarized in Table 5.10, which is adapted from reference 72.

The principal causes of gas exchange abnormalities leading to hypoxemia in COVID-19 are the same as those of other infectious viral and bacterial pneumonias and ARDS: V/Q mismatch and intrapulmonary shunt.[73] As mentioned earlier, endothelial damage, macrothrombi, and microthrombi could be more preponderant in COVID-19–induced hypoxemia.[81,82]

Phenotypes of COVID-19–Associated ARDS

In the early months of the pandemic, Gattinoni et al.[69] described two distinct phenotypes of COVID-19 pneumonia, type L (standing for low elastance, i.e., high compliance), and type H standing for high elastance, that is, low compliance. Type L pneumonia is characterized by the following features: (1) low elastance (preserved compliance) and hence normal aeration/ventilation; (2) low V/Q ratio and hypoxia, possibly resulting from impairment of hypoxic pulmonary vasoconstriction; (3) low lung weight because GGOs are found predominantly in the subpleural regions; and (4) low lung recruitability because most alveoli are ventilated.[69] Type H pneumonia showcases classic ARDS features: (1) high elastance (greatly reduced compliance) and severely compromised ventilation, (2) high right-to-left shunt resulting from perfusion of nonventilated regions, (3) high lung weight resulting from alveolar edema; and (4) high recruitability resulting from nonventilated regions.[69] The phenotype categorization has implications for respiratory management; however, type L could be an earlier manifestation in the timeline of the evolution of COVID-19 lung injury.

COVID-19 Lung Injury Versus High-Altitude Pulmonary Edema

There have been some comparisons of lung involvement in COVID-19 with HAPE,[90-92] so it is appropriate to look into the similarities and differences between the two pathological conditions because it has implications for clinical management of COVID-19 lung injury. HAPE and COVID-19 pneumonia are both *not* of cardiogenic origin, which is because of left heart decompensation with elevation of left atrial pressure, for example, from mitral/aortic valve stenosis. Both HAPE and COVID-19 lung injury are characterized by evidence of fluid accumulation in the interstitial space and alveoli, visualized as bilateral opacities on chest radiographs and chest CT. However, the similarities end there because the basic pathophysiological mechanisms of pulmonary edema are different for the two conditions.[93] The differences in the pathophysiology of HAPE and COVID-19 lung injury are summarized in Table 5.11.[94] HAPE can be typically managed by supplemental oxygen or descending to lower elevations. This intervention quickly increases alveolar partial pressure of alveolar oxygen (PO_2) and PaO_2 (partial pressure of arterial oxygen) leading to a reversal of the basic pathophysiology of HAPE: (1) reduction in hypoxic pulmonary vasoconstriction, (2) lowering of pulmonary arterial pressure, and (3) a reduction in hydrostatic pressure responsible for interstitial and alveolar fluid accumulation.[91] However, an increase in FiO_2 alleviates the hypoxemia of COVID-19 but cannot reverse the pathological changes of diffuse alveolar damage, endotheliitis, and thromboembolic changes of COVID-19 lung injury.[91]

Pathogenesis of Lung Injury in COVID-19

Lung injury in COVID-19 is a consequence of two mechanisms: (1) direct viral damage to the lung and (2) damage resulting from immunological host defenses

Table 5.11 Comparison of the Pathophysiology of High-Altitude Pulmonary Edema (HAPE) and COVID-19 Lung Injury

Pathophysiological Measures	High-Altitude Pulmonary Edema	COVID-19 Lung Injury
HPV and pulmonary hypertension	1. High pulmonary pressure (40–60 mm Hg) 2. HPV occurs unevenly 3. Increase in capillary hydrostatic pressure leads to interstitial and alveolar edema (overperfusion edema)	1. HPV absent 2. Mild pulmonary hypertension (25–30 mm Hg)
Alveolar fluid clearance	1. Sodium transport decreased 2. Reduction in alveolar fluid reabsorption	Alveolar epithelial fluid reabsorption impaired
Inflammatory changes	1. No inflammation in early stages 2. No neutrophil infiltration or proinflammatory cytokines 3. Mild alveolar hemorrhage with escape of plasma proteins 4. More of a hemodynamic problem than inflammation	1. Cytokine mediated injury 2. Neutrophil and macrophage infiltration 3. Pneumocyte death
Surfactant	No impairment in production or function	Impaired surfactant production and function
Ventilation-perfusion (V/Q) mismatch	Moderate	Severe V/Q mismatch and right to left shunt
Thromboembolic changes	Not observed	Microthrombi and embolism

HPV, Hypoxic pulmonary vasoconstriction.
Adapted from COVID-19 rapid guideline: managing COVID-19, NICE guideline [NG191], 2021.

triggered locally and systemically by the involvement of immune cells such as macrophages, lymphocytes, and neutrophils and the inflammatory mediators, cytokines, and chemokines. In the respiratory system the expression of ACE2, the membrane receptor used by the virus for binding and cell entry, follows a variable pattern with higher levels of expression reported in the upper respiratory tract such as the epithelial cells of the nasopharynx when compared with the lower respiratory tract structures, including the bronchial tree and alveolar sacs.[95] However, the alveolar epithelial cells (types I and II pneumocytes) and the pulmonary vascular endothelial cells are targets for SARS-CoV-2 because both express ACE2.[96] When the viral load is high there is a greater probability of aspiration of fluid containing the virus from the oropharynx into the lung, infecting the alveolar epithelial cells and macrophages.[95,97] Alveolar epithelial and capillary endothelial cell damage caused by SARS-CoV-2 infection and inflammatory mediators result in breeches and breaks in the alveolar basal membrane and capillary wall. These in turn cause transmigration of plasma proteins, leading to interstitial edema with fluid then slowly entering the alveolus and filling it up with edematous fluid.

Pathological Findings of COVID-19 Lung Injury

Histopathological findings based on autopsy investigations from more than 200 patients who died of COVID-19 are summarized here from three published reports.[98-100] Diffuse alveolar damage was observed in 87% to 100% of the cohorts. Borczuk et al.[99] reported large vessel thrombi in more than 40% of cases, whereas platelet and fibrin microthrombi were found in more than 80%.[99] Of note, Bryce et al.[100] found macrothrombi

and microthrombi in less than 10% of their autopsy samples. However, Carsana et al.[98] reported finding platelet-fibrin microthrombi in 87% of their study samples. Based on ultrastructure investigation of a subsample of 10 cases they also reported finding viral particles in 9 that were predominantly found in types I and II pneumocytes and occasionally in alveolar macrophages, but not in polymorphs or capillary endothelial cells.[98] Borczuk et al.[99] reported detection of the virus in airway epithelium and type II pneumocytes based on immunohistochemistry or lung culture. Typical histological findings of the ARDS exudative phase, such as capillary congestion, interstitial edema, alveolar flooding, alveolar duct dilatation, hyaline membrane formation with collapse/loss of alveoli, and features of the proliferative phase characteristic of ARDS, such as type II pneumocyte hyperplasia, interstitial myofibroblast aggregation, and alveolar granulation tissue formation were observed in a majority of lung samples.[98,99] Likewise, organizing pneumonia and squamous metaplasia were seen in more than a third of the autopsied lung specimens.[99] Inflammation of the trachea and bronchi in 90% of the samples with the observation of diffuse alveolar damage in the majority of autopsies suggest a progressive pathological pattern starting in the large airways and extending to the alveoli.[99]

It is notable that the exudative and proliferative phases of COVID-19 ARDS may not occur throughout the lung sequentially. There could be disparities, with some regions in one phase, for example, the exudative, whereas certain other regions might exhibit lung tissue organizing itself to repair the pathology, thus entering the proliferative phase.[42]

COVID-19 Lung Injury, Coagulation, and Thrombosis

Vascular injury in the form of endotheliitis and thrombi are widely prevalent in the small and medium vessels of the pulmonary vasculature.[81,101-105] The microthrombosis resulting from endothelial injury is referred to as thromboinflammation because it is characterized by microvascular thrombosis–associated inflammation.[102] As noted earlier, the vascular and endothelial damage from SARS-CoV-2 infection coupled with the pathophysiological responses to the vascular insult result in acute lung injury. Iba et al.[106] describe the mechanics of coagulation activation and thromboinflammation resulting in COVID-19–associated coagulopathy (CAC) based on the activation of monocytes by SARS-CoV-2 and damage-associated molecular patterns (DAMPs) released from infected and injured host cells. This results in a cascade of events: (1) activated monocytes release proinflammatory cytokines and chemokines; (2) cytokines and chemokines stimulate other immune cells such as neutrophils and lymphocytes, as well as platelets and endothelial cells of the pulmonary vascular bed; and (3) the monocytes and these immune cells then express tissue factor and phosphatidylserine, causing the formation of fibrin-platelet aggregation, which eventually leads to CAC.[106] Vascular thrombi composed of both fibrin and platelets form part of the lung injury manifestation of diffuse alveolar damage but the CAC cascade seems to be markedly predominant in the setting of COVID-19.[99] CAC is marked by elevated levels of D-dimer and thrombocytopenia and can evolve into disseminated intravascular coagulation.[107]

Although three factors play a role in the pathogenesis of lung injury—the viral infection of vascular endothelial cells, CAC, and systemic immune response—in COVID-19 severe disease, the initial response seems to be a localized lung injury with inflammatory changes and microvascular thrombi without the systemic endothelial injury and vasoplegia of disseminated intravascular coagulation seen, for example, in sepsis.[102] Although recruitment of neutrophils is typically associated with secondary bacterial infections, they do seem to play a significant role in alveolar epithelial injury, pneumocyte apoptosis, and microthrombi formation. This pathogenetic mechanism is thought to be mediated by the release of what are referred to as NETs; these web-like structures of DNA and proteins are extruded from the neutrophil to snare pathogens and are implicated in the development of acute tracheobronchitis, ARDS, and thrombosis as collateral damage.[108] When inflammation enters a vicious cycle, for example, during a cytokine storm contributing to ARDS, severe lung injury and respiratory failure, a closed loop signaling between macrophages and neutrophils (macrophage → IL-1B → NETs → macrophage) has been postulated that initiates an uncontrollable, progressively worse inflammatory cycle.[108] Based on their

investigation of patients hospitalized with severe COVID-19 pneumonia, using CT pulmonary angiography, dual-energy CT (DECT), and thromboelastography, Patel et al.[109] demonstrated the presence of a hypercoagulable phenotype with significant impairment of lung perfusion, possibly a consequence of pulmonary angiopathy and thrombosis.

Magro et al.[110] succinctly described severe COVID-19 as a multifaceted viral vasculopathy proposing three distinct patterns of injury: (1) small vessel microangiopathy with a predilection for pulmonary capillaries and carrying a high viral load with endothelial cell destruction, which leads to the release of pseudovirions, that is, virions without viral RNA such as spike, envelope, and membrane proteins, into systemic circulation; (2) systemic vascular disease with large vessel thrombi and microthrombi in small vessels and endothelial damage occurring in various other organs; and (3) host response triggered by complement activation from infectious virus particles and pseudovirions.

COVID-19 ARDS or Organizing Pneumonia?

Although a consensus has recently emerged that the later stages of lung injury in COVID-19 resemble ARDS, albeit with much more pronounced pulmonary angiopathy, microangiopathy, and thromboembolism resulting from severe endotheliitis and CAC in COVID-19 ARDS,[30,42,111-113] there is some debate regarding the nature of COVID-19 lung injury and how it should be characterized. Marik et al.[97] have argued that COVID-19 pneumonia and related pulmonary manifestations are better termed COVID-19 organizing pneumonia and not ARDS. However, other investigators consider organizing pneumonia to be a later manifestation of COVID-19 lung injury, possibly as a result of a secondary bacterial infection.[114-116] On the other hand, Kory et al.[117] have argued that early COVID-19 lung injury is SARS-CoV-2–induced secondary organizing pneumonia based on clinical picture, radiological features, histopathological findings from autopsy reports, and steroid responsiveness.

Lung Microbiome and COVID-19

Traditionally, healthy lungs have been considered microbe free, but that view has been transformed by the discovery of various microbes in the lower respiratory tract based on microbial immigration through inhalation, aspiration, and mucosal dispersion.[118] Khatiwada and Subedi proposed that the spectrum of COVID-19 pulmonary manifestations could be influenced by the lung microbiome acting by innate and adaptive immune mechanisms.[119] The dysbiosis occurring in the lung microbiome, that is, loss of microbial diversity with a shift in balance toward harm-causing microbes from beneficial ones, could modify the risk for the development of severe lung injury after SARS-CoV-2 infection by provoking a dysregulated and uncontrolled immune response causing inflammation.[119,120]

Sulaiman et al.[121] in their study of 142 hospitalized COVID-19 patients requiring mechanical ventilation investigated the relationship of SARS-CoV-2 viral load, lower respiratory tract microbiome (using bronchoalveolar lavage and metagenomic and metatranscriptomic approaches), host immune response, and patient outcomes. The study authors reported that high viral load and low anti-SARS-CoV-2 antibody response (anti–spike immunoglobulin G [IgG]) were predictive of increased mortality, indicating that high levels of SARS-CoV-2 replication in the lower respiratory tract and poor SARS-CoV-2–specific immune responses are the cause of adverse outcomes in these patients. Significantly, the study did not find any association between secondary infection with other respiratory pathogens and mortality.

Tsitsiklis et al.[122] studied the lower respiratory tract microbiome and immune responses using tracheal aspirate in 28 hospitalized patients on mechanical ventilation focusing on the outcome of the development of ventilator-associated pneumonia (VAP). The study reported finding dysregulated immune signaling 2 weeks before the development of VAP and a transcriptional signature of bacterial infection 2 days before the occurrence of VAP, and a metatranscriptomic analysis revealed a dysbiosis of the lung microbiome up to 3 weeks before the development of VAP.

Both the Sulaiman study[121] and Tsitsiklis study[122] have implications for the management of patients with COVID-19–associated acute respiratory failure, with both the studies reporting downregulated immune responses associated with poor outcomes.

Specific COVID-19 Pulmonary Complications

Pneumonia

COVID-19 pneumonia is part of the syndrome complex of ARDS, with a more prominent vascular pathological condition necessitating therapeutic anticoagulation.[123] Note that there is considerable overlap between COVID-19 pneumonia and COVID-19–induced ARDS, and the literature does not clearly distinguish between the two. The aggravated silent hypoxemia observed in the early stage of COVID-19 pneumonia has been explained by a combination of embolization in pulmonary vasculature, V/Q mismatch in the healthy parts of the lung, and normal perfusion of the injured sections of the lung by modeling.[124] Based on an evaluation of 108 patients with COVID-19 pneumonia confirmed by reverse transcription polymerase chain reaction (RT-PCR) testing for SARS-CoV-2, Han et al.[125] reported that fever (87%), cough (60%), and fatigue (39%) were the predominant symptoms, with normal WBC count in 90%,

lymphopenia in 60%, and elevated C-reactive protein (CRP) in 97%. Chest CT findings were present in multiple lobes in the majority of patients, typically with a peripheral distribution and showing patchy consolidation, GGOs, vascular thickening, crazy-paving patterns, and air bronchogram signs.[125-128] Less common radiological findings reported were reverse halo sign, signs of lobar or segmental consolidation in the absence of GGOs, discrete small pulmonary nodular patterns, pleural effusion, cavities, pneumothorax and septal thickening.[128,129] Based on their study of 48 RT-PCR–confirmed patients with COVID-19 pneumonia who underwent CT pulmonary angiography, Lang et al.[130] reported various pulmonary vascular abnormalities such as pulmonary emboli, vessel enlargement, and regional mosaic perfusion patterns. Zheng et al.[131] performed a meta-analysis using 15 published studies of COVID-19 pneumonia involving more than 2000 patients and reported chest CT findings based on severity of the disease. The investigators reported that although vascular enlargement and GGOs were common chest CT findings, patients with severe disease were more likely to show CT features of traction bronchiectasis, interlobular septal thickening, consolidation, crazy-paving pattern, reticular pattern, pleural effusion, and lymphadenopathy.[131]

Pneumothorax and Pneumomediastinum

Pneumothorax is a well-recognized complication of COVID-19 lung injury.[132-139] Investigators have also reported pneumothorax along with pneumomediastinum in hospitalized patients with COVID-19.[133,140-144] Chong et al.[144] performed a systematic review of papers published between January 1, 2020 and January 30, 2021 and reported on COVID-19–induced pneumothorax. Based on their analysis of nine observational studies the investigators reported an incidence of 0.3% for pneumothorax in patients hospitalized with COVID-19 and a much higher incidence of 12.8% to 23.8% in those requiring mechanical ventilation, resulting in increased mortality. A single institutional study of 1595 patients hospitalized with COVID-19 in a teaching hospital in the United States reported an incidence of 7.4% for pneumothorax, with 80% of the patients developing the complication while on mechanical ventilation.[136] The study also reported that a large majority of patients who developed pneumothorax (92/118) required tube thoracostomy drainage of air; the mortality rate was 58% for patients who developed pneumothorax and 13% for hospitalized patients without pneumothorax.[136] Another single institutional study of hospitalized COVID-19 patients who were also intubated reported an incidence of 14% (18/132) for pneumothorax.[146] A large prospective observational study of 131,679 patients hospitalized with COVID-19 in the United Kingdom found an overall incidence of 0.97% for pneumothorax while it was much higher (6.1%) in patients receiving invasive mechanical ventilation; pneumothorax was also associated with a higher mortality in general.[137]

Cut et al.[140] in their evaluation of 1648 patients hospitalized with COVID-19 reported the occurrence of spontaneous pneumomediastinum (SPM) in 11 patients (0.66%); 8 patients had associated pneumothorax, 1 had pneumopericardium, and 7 had subcutaneous emphysema. These patients underwent prolonged hospitalization, with only 3 of 11 surviving. In their study of 976 patients hospitalized with COVID-19, Eperjesiova et al.[142] identified 20 patients with air leak; 3 were traumatic or postprocedure, 10 were intubated and mechanically ventilated, 5 developed SPM, and 2 had spontaneous pneumothorax. All of the 10 mechanically ventilated patients who developed air leak died, whereas death occurred in 1 of 7 who developed spontaneous air leak.

Although barotrauma after intubation and mechanical ventilation has been recognized as a cause of pneumothorax and pneumomediastinum, the mechanisms underlying the occurrence of spontaneous pneumothorax and pneumomediastinum are not well understood. The postulated mechanisms include pulmonary infarction and cyst formation resulting from diffuse alveolar damage of ARDS.[138,143]

Pulmonary Embolism

Pulmonary embolism (PE) resulting from COVID-19 lung injury has been reported in various case reports and clinical studies.[147-156] Suh et al.[157] in their systematic review of 27 studies involving 3342 patients hospitalized with COVID-19 reported an incidence of 16.5% for PE with a higher incidence in patients admitted to the ICU (25%) compared with non-ICU patients (10.5%). The study also reported that PE was confined to the peripheral pulmonary arteries in the majority of patients and D-dimer levels 500 μg/L or greater were predictive of PE. Planquette et al.,[158] in their study of 1042 patients hospitalized with COVID-19 in two French hospitals reported an incidence of 5.6% for PE. The investigators also reported that patients with PE required invasive ventilation more often when compared with demographically matched patients hospitalized with COVID-19; D-dimer levels were also five times higher in patients with PE. Garcia-Ortega et al.[152] in their institutional study based on a random cohort of 119 of 372 patients hospitalized with COVID-19 reported an incidence of 35.6% for PE and identified heart rate, room-air oxygen saturation (SpO$_2$), D-dimer, and CRP values at the time of admission as predictors of PE. Another single-institution study based on 107 patients admitted to the ICU for COVID-19 pneumonia reported an incidence 20.6% for PE.[148]

Miró et al.[155] in their study of PE in COVID-19 patients reporting to emergency departments (EDs) found an incidence of 0.5% (368/74,814) for PE, whereas the incidence of PE in the non–COVID-19 ED population was 0.12% (1707/1,388,879). The study reported D-dimer values greater than 1000 μg/L and chest pain as risk factors for PE in COVID-19 patients and thrombi typically affecting peripheral pulmonary arteries when compared with non–COVID-19 PE manifestations. The investigators did not find any significant differences in in-hospital mortality between patients with and without PE in the COVID-19 patient cohort; however, mortality was significantly higher in COVID-19 patients with PE compared with non–COVID-19 patients with PE.

Embolization from deep vein thrombosis (DVT) observed in COVID-19 patients resulting from CAC and pulmonary microthrombosis secondary to pulmonary vascular endotheliitis are likely causes of pulmonary thromboembolic manifestations.[159]

Secondary Lung Infections Complicating COVID-19

Secondary infections of the lung can follow COVID-19 pneumonia/pneumonitis/ARDS. In their narrative review of hospitalized patients with COVID-19 based on published literature, Chong et al.[160] reported an incidence of 16% (range 4.8–2.8%) for secondary bacterial infection of the lung and an incidence of 6.3% (range 0.9–33.3%) for secondary fungal infection of the lung. Some of the most common bacterial infections are due to VAP. Invasive aspergillosis has been noticed in some immunocompetent patients with COVID-19 ARDS.[161] The microbial profile of VAP of COVID-19 is similar to that in non–COVID-19 patients.

COVID-19 Long-Term Pulmonary Complications

An understanding of the long-term respiratory system complications of COVID-19 is gradually evolving. Long-term respiratory effects of COVID-19 survivors are an active area of concern and investigation.[162-168] Based on a systematic review of 65 articles, SeyedAlinaghi et al.[169] identified lung injuries as the most prevalent long-term complication of COVID-19. Blanco et al.[162] conducted a prospective study to assess pulmonary function in patients discharged from hospital after treatment for COVID-19. Based on their hospital course the study sample of 100 patients were categorized into two groups: those who had experienced severe disease and those who had nonsevere disease and evaluated using pulmonary function tests, chest CT, and a standardized 6-minute walk test (6MWT). The investigators reported that diffusing capacity for carbon monoxide (DLCO) less than 80% persisted in some patients and was associated with a severe historical course of COVID-19. The authors postulated that DLCO could be a potential biomarker to predict individuals at risk for pulmonary sequelae.[162] Wu et al.[168] followed patients hospitalized for COVID-19 after they were discharged at 3-, 6-, and

12-month intervals. Their study also found a significant reduction in DLCO at these follow-up intervals, and even after 12 months radiological changes persisted in 20 of 83 patients studied. The radiological changes were also correlated with high-resolution CT pneumonia scores of the patients, and they underwent hospitalization for COVID-19 earlier.[168] The reduction in DLCO reported in both these studies could be a result of interstitial pathological processes, pulmonary vascular endotheliitis, pulmonary angiopathy, and thrombosis.[84,109,130] The UK Interstitial Lung Disease Consortium (UKILD) has proposed to undertake longitudinal observational studies of patients suspected to have both fibrosing and nonfibrosing interstitial lung disease by enrolling 12,000 patients in the United Kingdom.[170]

We now proceed to describe salient respiratory system sequelae of COVID-19 with widely different postulated pathophysiological mechanisms.

Persistent Cough

Cough and fever are the most common manifesting symptoms of COVID-19 in the early stages of the disease. However, cough can persist in COVID-19 survivors and is an important manifestation of long COVID, with a varied range of reported prevalence between 2% and 42%.[167,171,172] Song et al.[167] postulated two potential mechanisms for the persistent post-COVID cough: (1) a neurogenic mechanism of direct infection of vagal sensory neurons by the SARS-CoV-2 virus and (2) a consequence of a neuroinflammatory response, triggering peripheral and central pathways of cough. The neuroinflammatory process can involve the vagus nerve and its branches innervating the respiratory tract inducing cough.

Pulmonary Fibrosis

Pulmonary fibrosis causes scarring of the lung parenchyma leading to loss of lung compliance and compromised pulmonary function. COVID-19 lung injury, including ARDS, during SARS-CoV-2 infection can cause pulmonary fibrosis in the post-COVID recovery phase. Concerns of pulmonary fibrosis, a serious long-term complication of COVID-19, have been raised by the scientific community,[173-179] and reports documenting the problem are increasingly becoming available.[180-182] Based on a follow-up evaluation of 81 COVID-19 survivors who had been previously hospitalized with severe COVID-19 pneumonia, Huang et al.[182] reported chest CT evidence of extensive pulmonary fibrosis such as parenchymal bands, reticular opacities, crazy-paving patterns, and traction bronchiectasis in 52% (42/81) of patients.[182] Yu et al.[183] studied 32 patients hospitalized with COVID-19 who had undergone thin-section CT scans during their hospital stay and reported that follow-up revealed 14 patients had CT evidence of fibrosis and 18 did not show evidence of fibrosis. The study also found that fibrosis was more likely in patients with

severe disease characterized by elevated inflammatory markers such as CRP and IL-6.

Li et al.[184] studied the progression of fibrosis in the lungs of 30 patients who died after COVID-19 pneumonia by performing minimally invasive autopsies and reported finding evidence of diffuse alveolar damage in 28 samples (93%), with 43% of them showing fibrosing patterns. It is possible that many of these patients would have gone on to develop pulmonary fibrosis if they had survived.

Etiological factors of post–COVID-19 pulmonary fibrosis (PCPF) include viral pneumonias, COVID-19 lung injury, COVID-19 sepsis, thromboembolism, and trauma from mechanical ventilation.[180] The pathological mechanism underlying PCPF is thought to be an aberrant repair process of COVID-19 lung injury.[180] Tanni et al.[181] categorized the risk factors for PCPF as (1) those before SARS-CoV-2 infection: male sex, old age, history of smoking, and comorbidities such as diabetes, lung disease, and heart disease; and (2) risk factors pertaining to severe disease: high-flow nasal oxygen, mechanical ventilation, ARDS, severe dyspnea, and systemic inflammation. The postulated pathophysiological pathways of PCPF are depicted in Fig. 5.7.

Chronic Hypoxic Respiratory Failure With Long-Term Oxygen Use

Many COVID-19 patients who remained hospitalized even after they became negative for SARS-CoV-2 still required prolonged oxygen administration. Some of these patients needed long-term usage of oxygen even after the acute phase of COVID-19 had resolved. Based on a prospective study of 93 patients admitted to a teaching hospital in India, Ray et al.[185] identified the following risk factors for prolonged oxygen administration even after testing negative for COVID-19 in the post–COVID-19 phase:

- Patients older than 60 years of age
- Males affected more than females
- Patients with more than three comorbidities: diabetes mellitus, coronary artery disease, and obesity (with a body mass index [BMI] >35 kg/m²)
- Patients admitted to ICU with ARDS secondary to COVID-19
- Previous pulmonary disease
- History of tobacco use disorder

COVID-19–Induced Secondary Organizing Pneumonia

A review of COVID-19 CT scan imaging and the postmortem lung biopsies and autopsies indicated that most of the patients with COVID-19 pulmonary involvement showed secondary organizing pneumonia.[117]

The clinical course of COVID-19 and secondary organizing pneumonia follows a subacute respiratory illness, although a rapid-onset progression to fulminant respiratory failure is possible in both conditions.

Pathophysiology of Post-Covid-19 Pulmonary Fibrosis

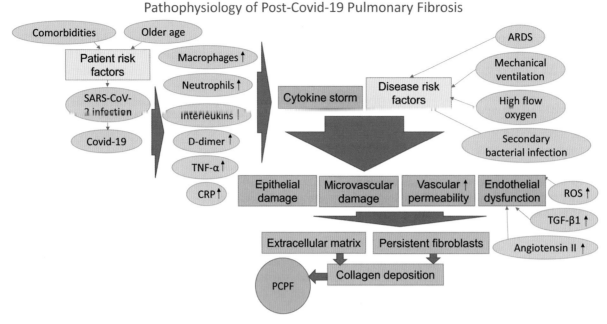

Fig. 5.7 Postulated Pathophysiological Pathways of Post–COVID-19 Pulmonary Fibrosis (PCPF). Patient risk factors increase the susceptibility to SARS-CoV-2 infection and severe COVID-19, which can lead to an exacerbated immunological response of cytokine storm. Severe pneumonia and acute respiratory distress syndrome (ARDS) increase the need for interventions such as mechanical ventilation, high-flow oxygen, and the development of secondary bacterial infections. Cytokine storm, disease risk factors, and the renin-angiotensin system (RAS)-mediated responses such as elevated angiotensin II, which is proinflammatory and accompanied by elevated levels of transforming growth factor-beta 1 (TGF-β1) and reactive oxygen species (ROS) result in endothelial dysfunction, increased vascular permeability, and microvascular pathological conditions. Alveolar epithelial damage is a consequence of both cytokine storm and ARDS. These in turn lead to proliferation of fibroblasts and extracellular matrix formation followed by collagen deposition in the alveoli causing pulmonary fibrosis. CRP, C-reactive protein; TNF-α: tumor necrosis factor-alpha. (Modified from Tanni SE, Fabro AT, de Albuquerque A, et al. Pulmonary fibrosis secondary to COVID-19: a narrative review. Exp Rev Resp Med. 2021:1-13; and Vianello A, Guarnieri G, Braccioni F, et al. The pathogenesis, epidemiology and biomarkers of susceptibility of pulmonary fibrosis in COVID-19 survivors. Clin Chem Lab Med. 2021;60[3]:307-316.)

Wang et al.[186] reported that 74.5% of organizing pneumonia cases were nonsevere, and 97.1% had a good prognosis with recovery. The dominant radiological finding in organizing pneumonia was GGO, followed by mixed GGO and consolidation, with peripheral and lower lobes distribution. Although cases of COVID-19 with organizing pneumonia had a favorable prognosis, early monitoring and detection of adverse outcomes and radiological sequelae could facilitate early intervention in those with the potential risk for fibrosis, respiratory failure, and death. Although steroids still play a significant role in the treatment of COVID-19, the optimal duration of steroid administration is unclear and its administration needs to be carefully monitored.

Treatment and Management of Salient Pulmonary Manifestations and Complications of COVID-19

This section addresses the treatment and management principles for various pulmonary manifestations and provides specific guidelines for the important clinical problems encountered in COVID-19 patients.

Treatment of Hypoxemia

A cardinal reason for admission to hospital for COVID-19 patients is hypoxemia, and even younger patients without any significant comorbidities can present with severe hypoxemia. Hypoxemia has been the leading predictor of admission to the ICU, need for mechanical ventilation, and death in COVID-19 patients. The degree of worsening of hypoxemia mostly determines the different stages of worsening of COVID-19 pulmonary manifestations. However, half the number of patients with COVID-19 discharged from the ED who subsequently recorded an oxygen saturation less than 92% on home pulse oximeter did not report worsening of symptoms. The home pulse oximeter serves as an adjunct to home monitoring in World Health Organization guidelines. All patients developing hypoxemia with less than 94% oxygen saturation can be supplemented through various modalities, including nasal cannula, oxygen mask, and high-flow oxygen therapy. On high-flow oxygen therapy, it is possible to give 100% of oxygen to the patients (normal room air contains 21%). When the patient's oxygen saturation does not improve even with high-flow oxygen, it is necessary to evaluate for respiratory failure, ARDS, and thromboembolic pulmonary disease complications.

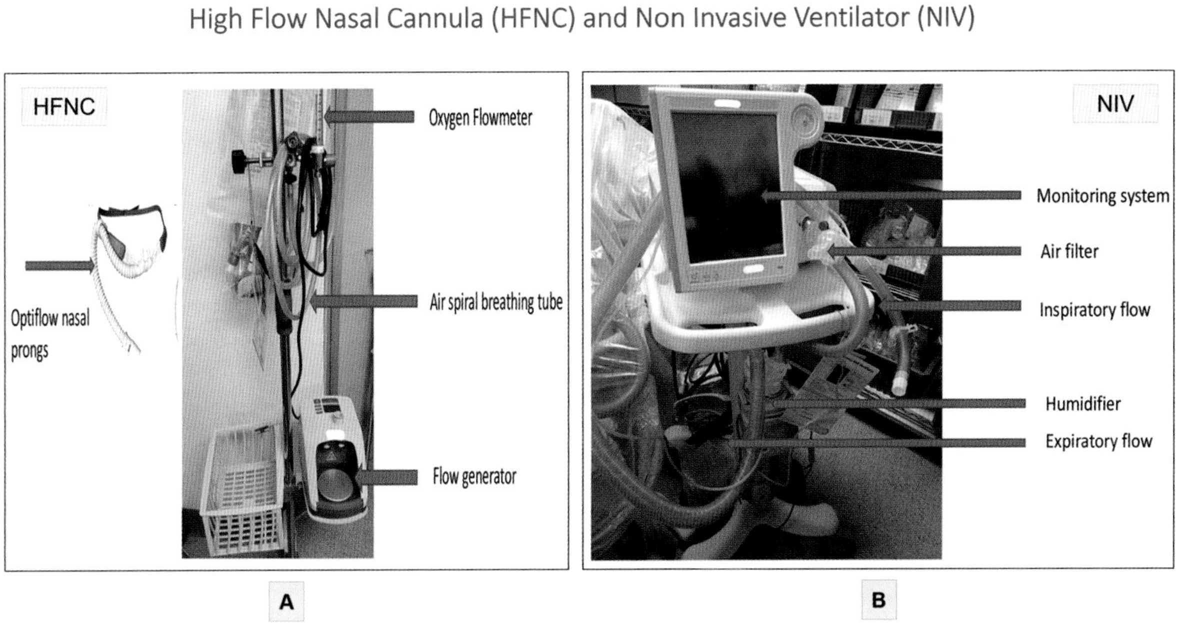

High Flow Nasal Cannula (HFNC) and Non Invasive Ventilator (NIV)

HFNC

Oxygen Flowmeter

Optiflow nasal prongs

Air spiral breathing tube

Flow generator

A

NIV

Monitoring system

Air filter

Inspiratory flow

Humidifier

Expiratory flow

B

Fig. 5.8 High-Flow Nasal Cannula *(Panel A)* and Noninvasive Ventilator *(Panel B)*. With HFNC, a flow generator is used to generate humidified oxygen, which is delivered through the air spiral breathing tube using Optiflow nasal prongs. The noninvasive ventilator works by delivering oxygen by the face mask (not shown) by creating positive airway pressure, which causes air to be forced into the lungs, reducing respiratory effort and work of breathing.

Management of Respiratory Failure

Respiratory failure is of three different types: (1) hypoxemic respiratory failure; (2) hypercapnic respiratory failure, that is, $PaCO_2$ greater than 55 mm Hg; and (3) mixed respiratory failure. COVID-19 commonly manifests as hypoxemic respiratory failure. Hypoxemic respiratory failure is defined as partial pressure of oxygen in arterial blood (PaO_2) or oxygen saturation in arterial blood (SpO_2) less than 90 or PaO_2/FiO_2 ratio, that is, P/F ratio less than 300 mm Hg. Hypoxemic respiratory failure might be a manifesting feature of (1) pneumonia/pneumonitis, (2) ARDS, (3) thromboembolic lung disease, (4) cytokine release syndrome, and (5) secondary infections of the lung.

Management Guidelines for the Treatment of Hypoxemic Respiratory Failure

The management guidelines and precautions while treating hypoxemic respiratory failure in COVID-19 discussed in the following text are based on these two studies.[187,188]

The goal SpO_2 of 90% to 96% should be reached while treating COVID-19 hypoxemic respiratory failure. Patients may use a nasal cannula that delivers up to 6 L or a nonrebreather mask for up to 10 L of oxygen. High-flow nasal cannula (HFNC) and noninvasive ventilation (NIV) increase the risk for aerosolization and spread of COVID-19 to the treating team. HFNC is generally preferred over NIV. However, NIV is more effective in the management of hypercapnic (high $PaCO_2$) respiratory failure. Reassessment of patients on HFNC and NIV is usually done regularly for ascertaining the response to therapy. If the described measures fail because of worsening of disease, patients might require endotracheal intubation and mechanical ventilation. Self-proning in nonintubated patients has been found to be helpful in COVID-19 patients to improve oxygenation.

Indications for tracheal intubation and mechanical ventilation in COVID-19 patients with hypoxemic respiratory failure are (1) signs of respiratory distress, (2) rapid progression of the disease, (3) oxygen saturation less than 90% despite maximum supplemental oxygen, (4) persistent arterial pH less than 7.3 with $PaCO_2$ greater than 50 mm Hg even on NIV, and (5) hemodynamic instability and multiple organ system failure.

High-Flow Nasal Cannula

HFNC delivers 100% heated and humidified oxygen and is being increasingly used in patients with respiratory failure. Fig. 5.8A presents for a representative HFNC device. HFNC has four main components: (1) air-oxygen blender, (2) active humidifier, (3) a heating circuit for warming the inspiratory air-oxygen mixture to normal body temperature, and (4) a nasal cannula.[189] An HFNC device can deliver oxygen up to 60 L/min and has many advantages compared with a low-flow nasal cannula. Cold and dry oxygen delivery by low-flow nasal cannula can cause airway inflammation, mucosal irritation, increased airway resistance, and mucociliary dysfunction. HFNC has been shown to reduce the frequency and work of breathing and prevent worsening of respiratory failure. HFNC improves oxygenation by decreasing respiratory rate, increasing tidal and end-expiratory volume, increasing positive end-expiratory pressure, and physiological wash out of dead space. HFNC has been used in hypoxemic respiratory failure, hypercapnic respiratory failure, preintubation, and postextubation oxygenation.[189-191] Patients with COVID-19 develop acute respiratory failure and require a high amount of oxygen to reverse the hypoxemia. HNFC has been shown to reduce intubation and subsequent ventilation.[192] The median duration of HFNC in COVID-19 patients was 6 days. Patients had successful outcomes with HFNC if they had higher oxygen saturation, lower heart and respiratory rate, and lower oxygen requirement within 6 hours of commencement of HFNC.[193] HFNC failure leading to intubation and mechanical ventilation occurs in patients with increased respiratory rate and reduced ROX index within the first 3 days of HFNC. ROX index is the ratio of oxygen saturation as measured by pulse oximetry/fraction of inspired oxygen (SpO_2/FiO_2) to respiratory rate (RR), that is, $(SpO_2/FiO_2)/RR$.[194,195] HFNC can be used outside the ICU and in smaller hospitals with no ICU, where patients are unstable to be transferred to a tertiary center.

Noninvasive Ventilation

NIV provides ventilatory support without an invasive endotracheal airway. Fig. 5.8B presents an illustration of the device and setup. Bilevel positive airway pressure (BPAP) NIV is commonly used to treat hypoxemic and hypercapnic respiratory failure such as acute exacerbation of chronic obstructive pulmonary disease (COPD) and acute respiratory failure secondary to pneumonia and asthma. The patient spontaneously breathes during BPAP, which provides inspiratory positive airway pressure (IPAP) and expiratory positive airway pressure (EPAP). Continuous positive airway pressure (CPAP) is used in patients with acute cardiogenic pulmonary edema. Oronasal masks are used for NIV to provide a tight seal and prevent air leaks. NIV has been used to treat acute respiratory failure and prevent intubation in COVID-19.

Moreover, NIV is associated with a shorter length of stay, fewer cases of hospital-acquired infection, and lower mortality than in patients on mechanical ventilation.[196,197] The noninvasive ventilator has been increasingly used outside the ICU. Early intubation and mechanical ventilation were used during the initial periods of the COVID-19 pandemic, but recent studies have demonstrated the utility of NIV in the early phase of the disease in preventing intubation.[198] The use of NIV with a good interface in patients with COVID-19 has been shown to mitigate the risk for airborne transmission to health care workers.[199]

Prone Positioning in COVID-19

Prone positioning has been shown to improve oxygenation in patients with ARDS who are on mechanical ventilation. In patients with severe ARDS, prolonged initial prone positioning decreases mortality. The mechanism by which prone positioning helps intubated patients with ARDS is poorly understood; it may reduce the overinflated lung areas while promoting alveolar recruitment.[188,200] Prone positioning has been used only in intubated patients in the ICU before the COVID-19 pandemic, and it requires a considerable team effort. However, the prone position has been increasingly used in COVID-19 patients who are awake, not intubated, and not in severe respiratory failure. Various studies have shown improved oxygenation and some mortality reduction with prone positioning in patients with COVID-19; more RCTs are needed to validate these findings.[201-203] Self-proning protocols have been implemented in many hospitals and need considerable staff training.

Management of COVID-19 Pneumonia and Pneumonitis

It is important to distinguish COVID-19 pneumonia and pneumonitis from other bacterial and viral pneumonias.

COVID-19 pneumonia/pneumonitis can be a rapidly progressive disease resulting in significant mortality. Lymphocytopenia (decreased lymphocytes) and thrombocytopenia (decreased platelets) are common hematological abnormalities. CRP is typically greater than 10 mg/mL in 80% of patients with severe disease and 56% of patients with nonsevere manifestations.[204] However, procalcitonin remains in the normal range in COVID-19 pneumonia, unlike in bacterial pneumonia. Lactate dehydrogenase, D-dimer, and creatinine kinase can be significantly elevated in severe COVID-19 pneumonia/pneumonitis.[204] Imaging studies show GGOs, local or patchy bilateral shadows, and interstitial abnormalities in the majority of the patients with COVID-19 pneumonia/pneumonitis. Consolidations, nodular opacities, and reticulations are also seen in COVID-19 pneumonitis. See Fig. 5.9 for an illustration of these pathological conditions.

Differentiating COVID-19 pneumonia/pneumonitis from community-acquired viral or bacterial pneumonia is important from a management perspective. In the United Kingdom, the National Institute for Health and Care Excellence (NICE) has provided rapid guidelines for differentiating COVID-19 pneumonia and bacterial pneumonia in the clinical setting.[205] Table 5.12 provides a list of the clinical features that help discriminate the causes. Differentiating COVID-19 from primary bacterial lung infection is of great importance, because early detection and intervention tailored to the patient's condition are essential for better clinical outcomes.

Based on their experience of treating patients hospitalized with severe COVID-19 pneumonia, Attaway et al.[206] proposed that a large number of patients with COVID-19 pneumonia could be treated efficiently using HFNC or NIV. The authors argued that such an approach

Chest CT and Chest X-ray of a Patient with Covid-19 Pneumonia

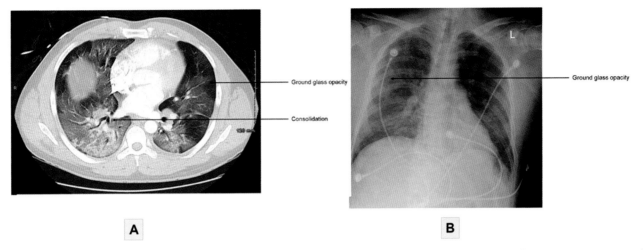

Fig. 5.9 COVID-19 Pneumonia. Chest computed tomography *(CT)* (A) and chest radiograph (B) showing ground-glass appearance as a result of COVID-19 pneumonia. Chest CT also shows features of consolidation.

Table 5.12 Differentiating COVID-19 Pneumonia and Bacterial Pneumonia in the Clinical Setting	
COVID-19 viral pneumonia may be more likely if the patient:	A bacterial cause of pneumonia may be more likely if the patient:
1. Presents with a history of typical COVID-19 symptoms for about a week 2. Has severe muscle pain (myalgia) 3. Has a loss of sense of smell (anosmia) 4. Is breathless but has no pleuritic pain 5. Has a history of exposure to known or suspected COVID-19, such as a household or workplace contact	1. Becomes rapidly unwell after only a few days of symptoms 2. Does not have a history of typical COVID-19 symptoms 3. Has pleuritic pain 4. Has purulent sputum

Data from Pulsetoday. Differentiating viral Covid-19 pneumonia from bacterial pneumonia. https://www.pulsetoday.co.uk/covid-19-primary-care-resources/guides/differentiating-viral-covid-19-pneumonia-from-bacterial-pneumonia/.

would also allow for optimal use of mechanical ventilators, which could quickly become scarce during surges of hospitalizations for COVID-19. They proposed a smart algorithm combining noninvasive and invasive ventilatory approaches for respiratory management of a patient with COVID-19 pneumonia, illustrated in Fig. 5.10.[206]

Management of COVID-19 Acute Respiratory Distress Syndrome

ARDS typically does not have any specific chest radiographic or chest CT scan findings but usually has evolving pulmonary infiltrates in both lungs. Fig. 5.11 shows bilateral lung infiltrates in the chest radiograph of a patient with COVID-19 ARDS discussed in detail in Case Report 2.

There is no specific therapy for ARDS other than treating the underlying cause, providing supportive care, administering noninvasive or invasive mechanical ventilation based on respiratory function parameters, and initiating conservative fluid management. These recommendations for the management of ARDS are based on the following studies. A fluid conservative strategy showed improved oxygenation index and an increase in ventilator-free days in patients with ARDS.[207]

HFNC systems that can deliver up to 50 to 60 L per minute of oxygen demonstrated a decreased incidence of intubation and mechanical ventilation and improved 90-day mortality in pure hypoxemic nonhypercapnic patients compared with the use of just nasal canula or NIV.[208] The goal of mechanical ventilation in ARDS is to maintain oxygenation while avoiding oxygen toxicity. The strategies for mechanical ventilation in ARDS resulting from COVID-19 do not differ from the mechanical ventilation standards for ARDS from other causes—a low-tidal volume 4 to 6 mL/kg predicted body weight (PBW) using the best PEEP to improve oxygenation and keep plateau pressure on the ventilator less than 30 mm Hg.[209] Prone positioning of the patient and mechanical ventilation have shown improvement in oxygenation in ARDS; the approach reduced the 28-day mortality in the prone position group of patients with ARDS. Venovenous ECMO has been tried in some patients with ARDS resulting from COVID-19. Indications for ECMO in patients with ARDS secondary to COVID-19 are similar to ECMO indications for ARDS resulting from other causes. The data regarding ECMO use in COVID-19 patients are very scant. Absolute contraindications for ECMO in COVID-19 patients include severe comorbidities such as multiorgan failure, advanced metastatic

Algorithm for the respiratory management of a patient with Covid-19 pneumonia

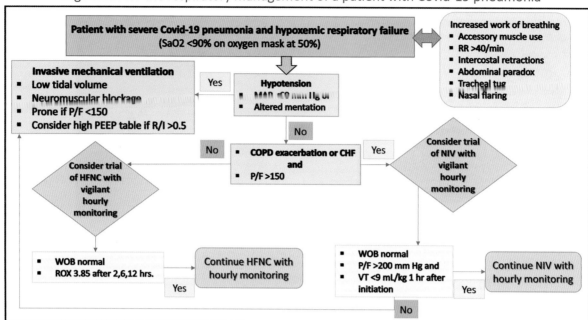

Fig. 5.10 Algorithm for the Respiratory Management of a Patient With COVID-19 Pneumonia. *CHF,* Congestive heart failure; *COPD,* chronic obstructive pulmonary disease; *HFNC,* high-flow nasal cannula; *MAP,* mean arterial pressure; *NIV,* noninvasive ventilation; *PEEP,* positive end-expiratory pressure; *P/F,* PaO_2/FiO_2 ratio; *R/I,* recruitment/inflation ratio; *RR,* respiratory rate; *WOB,* work of breathing. (Redrawn from Fig. 5.2, Attaway AH, Scheraga RG, Bhimraj A, et al. Severe covid-19 pneumonia: pathogenesis and clinical management. *BMJ.* 2021;372:n436.)

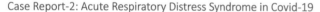

Case Report-2: Acute Respiratory Distress Syndrome in Covid-19

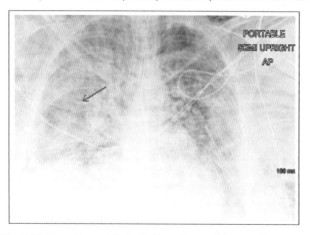

Fig. 5.11 Case Report 2: Acute Respiratory Distress Syndrome in COVID-19. Chest radiograph of patient discussed in Case Report 5.2 showing extensive bilateral lung infiltrates due to COVID-related ARDS.

cancers and brain hemorrhages; relative contraindications are age older than 70 years, severely immunocompromised status, and BMI greater than 40 kg/m². Investigators have studied the use of stem cell–based therapies, specifically mesenchymal cells in the treatment of COVID-19 lung injury and ARDS.[210-213] Zanirati et al.[211] performed a systematic review of 29 studies and reported alleviation of lung injury in COVID-19 and ARDS based on the impact of stem cell therapies on immunological and inflammatory processes causing injury. Lanzoni et al.[213] reported a survival benefit in COVID-19 ARDS for mesenchymal stem cell treatment based on a randomized controlled phase II study of 12 patients. However, additional validation based on larger studies is needed for the therapy to be included in standard protocols for the management of COVID-19 lung injury.

Management of Barotrauma

Barotrauma can be an isolated and important manifestation of COVID-19 lung injury. The clinical presentations can vary from pulmonary interstitial emphysema, pneumothorax, subcutaneous emphysema, pneumopericardium, and pneumomediastinum. Fig. 5.12 illustrates these pathological conditions.

Chest radiograph and CT scan findings lead to the diagnosis of barotrauma, and interpreting the mechanics of the mechanical ventilator settings can also help arrive at the diagnosis. Only rarely, surgical repair of the lung is required for the management of barotrauma. If the patient has a pneumothorax, the patient might need a tube thoracostomy as an urgent intervention. Prevention can be accomplished by optimizing ventilator settings and maintaining low tidal volume and low plateau pressure. Interestingly, in their study of patients with barotrauma, McGuinness et al.[214] reported no difference in survival rates in patients with COVID-19 with and without barotrauma; however, the survival rate was lower in patients with barotrauma and ARDS without COVID-19.

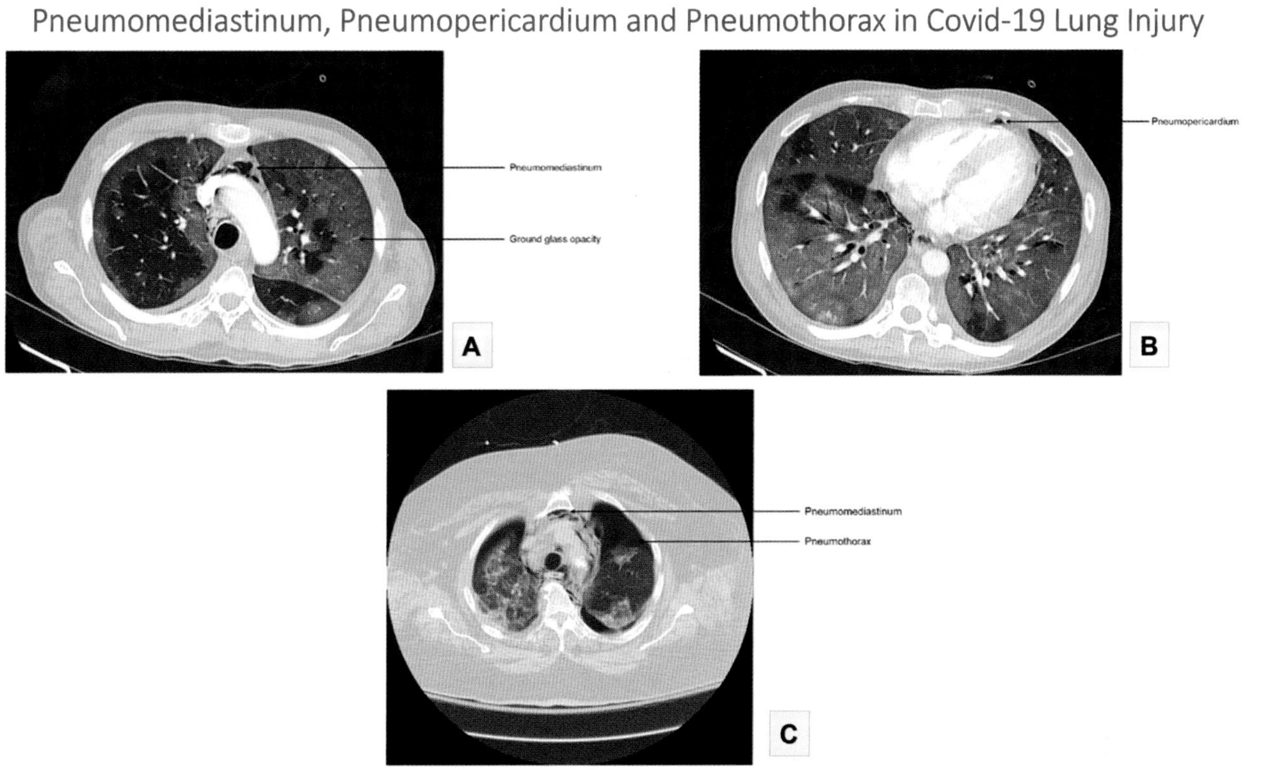

Pneumomediastinum, Pneumopericardium and Pneumothorax in Covid-19 Lung Injury

Fig. 5.12 COVID-19 Lung Injury: Pneumomediastinum, Pneumopericardium, and Pneumothorax. Chest computed tomography (CT) (A) shows air around the aorta (pneumomediastinum) and ground-glass infiltrates in the left lung. Chest CT (B) shows air around the heart (pneumopericardium). Chest CT (C) shows air under the sternum and in front of the aorta (pneumomediastinum) and air around the lungs causing compression of the lungs (pneumothorax).

Management of Spontaneous Pneumothorax

Spontaneous pneumothorax occurs without any obvious trauma or iatrogenic causes, and primary spontaneous pneumothorax (PSP) refers to pneumothorax occurring in individuals without any underlying pulmonary disease. Subpleural blebs and smoking have been shown to increase the risk for developing spontaneous pneumothorax. Secondary spontaneous pneumothorax (SSP) occurs in patients with underlying lung conditions such as COPD, cystic fibrosis, lung malignancy, and necrotizing lung infections such as *Pneumocystis jiroveci* infection, bacterial pneumonia, and tuberculosis. Spontaneous pneumothorax in lung infection may be due to direct invasion by microorganisms and necrosis of the lung tissue. Patients with pneumothorax typically present with increasing shortness of breath, chest pain, and worsening of respiratory status. Patients with COVID-19 experiencing an acute deterioration and worsening hypoxia will need a chest radiograph to rule out pneumothorax. Stable patients with small secondary spontaneous pneumothorax (<2 cm) and minimal symptoms can be treated with supplemental oxygen and observation. Patients with small SSP (<2 cm) with symptoms and patients with large SSP (>2 cm) will need tube or catheter thoracostomy.

Patients with PSP present with shortness of breath and chest and neck pain. PSP is usually self-limiting,

but patients may be treated with rest, supplemental oxygen, and analgesics.

Management of Spontaneous Pneumomediastinum

SPM is a rare condition characterized by free air in the mediastinum not associated with trauma or surgical procedures. SPM is caused by alveolar rupture as a result of increased alveolar pressure, and air dissects through the pulmonary interstitium into the mediastinum. SPM has been reported in patients with COVID-19, but their exact causative mechanism is not known. SPM also has been reported secondary to barotrauma caused during mechanical ventilation.[215] In addition, there are case reports of SPM in nonventilated patients coinfected with SARS-CoV-2 and influenza B.[216] Surgical intervention (thoracostomy) or conservative nonsurgical management can be undertaken based on clinician assessment of the patient's overall clinical status.[215]

Management of Thromboembolic Pulmonary Manifestations of COVID-19

Patients with COVID-19 have a high incidence of DVT and PE. In patients with COVID-19 the hypercoagulative state is characterized by elevated D-dimer and fibrinogen, mild prolonged prothrombin time and activated partial

Algorithm for the management of thromboembolism in patients with Covid-19

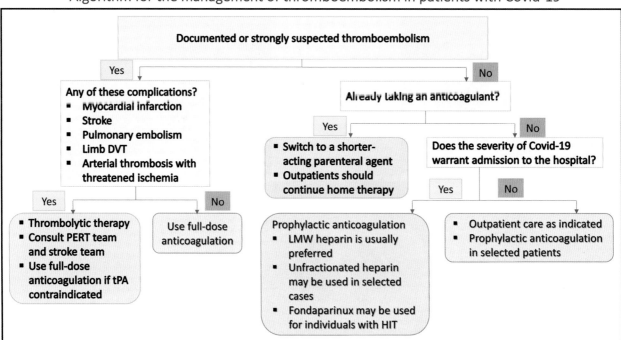

Fig. 5.13 Algorithm for the Management of Thromboembolism in Patients With COVID-19. *DVT,* Deep vein thrombosis; *HIT,* heparin-induced thrombocytopenia; *LMW,* low molecular weight; *tPA,* tissue plasminogen activator. (Data from Cuker A, Tseng EK, Nieuwlaat R, et al. American Society of Hematology 2021 guidelines on the use of anticoagulation for thromboprophylaxis in patients with COVID-19. *Blood Adv.* 2021;5[3]:872-888.)

thromboplastin time. The diagnosis of PE in COVID-19 patients is challenging, because patients present with dyspnea, which may be due to COVID-19. Patients with worsening respiratory status having elevated D-dimer, low oxygen saturation, hypotension, and right ventricular dysfunction must prompt the physician to consider PE. Computed tomography pulmonary angiogram (CTPA) is considered the gold standard in diagnosing PE. Currently, the recommendations in the setting of COVID-19 are to start with prophylaxis for DVT. Fig. 5.13 presents the management protocol of suspected or documented thromboembolism.

The American Society of Hematology recommends that all critically ill patients admitted to the ICU with COVID-19 receive prophylactic anticoagulation, preferably low molecular weight heparin or unfractionated heparin unless they have a high risk for bleeding.[217] Patients with thrombocytopenia as a result of heparin administration can be started on fondaparinux. A recent multiplatform trial by the National Institutes of Health (NIH) addresses more intensive anticoagulation in critically ill patients.[218] The study also found that full-dose anticoagulation is superior to prophylactic dose anticoagulation in moderately ill patients with COVID-19 in reducing multiorgan failure and mortality. An individual patient's risk for developing thrombosis and bleeding must be considered before deciding on anticoagulation intensity. Hospitalized patients with medical illness, in general, have an increased risk for developing venous thromboembolism (VTE) 90 days

after being discharged. Therefore postdischarge anticoagulation in patients with COVID-19 should be carefully weighed against the risk for bleeding and the feasibility of administering the drug. Therapeutic anticoagulation with low molecular weight heparin is preferred in patients with PE, but unfractionated heparin can be used in patients with severe renal impairment. Antivirals used to treat COVID-19 may interfere with direct oral anticoagulant levels, so low molecular weight heparin is preferred for therapeutic anticoagulation.

Management of Cytokine Storm and Systemic Inflammatory Response Secondary to COVID-19

COVID-19 causes cytokine storm syndrome (CSS) by two mechanisms: (1) macrophage activation syndrome and (2) secondary hemophagocytic lymphohistiocytosis, resulting in excessive proinflammatory and inadequate antiinflammatory stimuli. The most common inflammatory stimuli include foreign antigens, interleukins, tumor necrosis factor-alpha (TNF-α) interferon-gamma, and granulocyte colony-stimulating factor (GCSF).[219] The CSS inflammatory response is characterized by accelerated fever and multiorgan involvement with rapid progression of ARDS, acute cardiac injury, and acute kidney injury. CSS is associated with increased morbidity and mortality. This condition can be diagnosed based on laboratory findings of leukopenia; increased IL-6, IL-7,

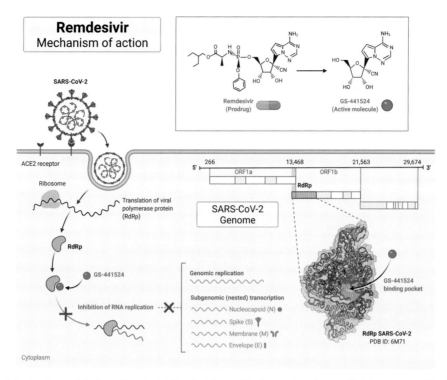

Fig. 5.14 Remdesivir: Mechanism of Action. Remdesivir is administered in its prodrug form, which is converted in vivo in the host cell into the active molecule monophosphate nucleoside analog (GS-441524). It acts as a viral RNA-dependent RNA polymerase (RdRp) inhibitor and blocks the replication of SARS-CoV-2 genomic RNA inside the host cell. (Created using Biorender.)

TNF-α, and ferritin; and elevated concentrations of D-dimer. Elevated IL-6 and ferritin levels greater than 1200 ng/mL were associated with significant mortality.[220]

Tocilizumab, a recombinant humanized monoclonal antibody against the IL-6 receptor, is used to manage cytokine storm syndrome. A multicenter cohort study showed that tocilizumab used within 2 days of ICU admission resulted in lower in-hospital mortality.[221] Two other studies also showed lesser likelihood of disease progression or death when tocilizumab was administered.[222,223]

Current Guidelines and Medications Available for Management of COVID-19

Anti-inflammatory and Antiviral Medications Used in COVID-19

Dexamethasone 6 mg daily for 10 days has been shown to lower 28-day mortality in patients with COVID-19 on mechanical ventilation and patients hospitalized with COVID-19 and receiving oxygen.[224] Various studies, including the RECOVERY trial, have confirmed the benefits of dexamethasone.[225] The use of dexamethasone did not provide any benefit in patients who did not require oxygen. Dexamethasone has strong antiinflammatory and immunosuppressive properties, and it helps control severe inflammation, ARDS, and diffuse alveolar damage caused by COVID-19. A significant side effect of steroids is hyperglycemia, and blood glucose needs to be monitored closely. Secondary infections, including bacterial and fungal infections, are also associated with the use of steroids. There have been increasing case reports of rhino-orbital mucormycosis in people with COVID-19, especially in India; diabetes and the use of steroids are major risk factors for mucormycosis.[226]

Remdesivir is an antiviral medication that inhibits RNA-dependent RNA polymerase of coronaviruses demonstrated with in-vitro inhibitory activity against SARS-CoV-2. Fig. 5.14 illustrates the mechanism of action of remdesivir. Remdesivir has been shown to shorten the recovery time in hospitalized patients with COVID-19.[227] However, administration of remdesivir was not effective in reducing mortality in patients with COVID-19. Remdesivir is administered intravenously with a loading dose of 200 mg followed by a maintenance dose of 100 mg daily for a total of 5 days. The physician should monitor hepatic and renal functions while administering remdesivir.

Tocilizumab is an anti–IL-6 receptor monoclonal antibody that has been approved in the treatment of moderate to severe COVID-19 with high serum levels of CRP.[228] Tocilizumab inhibits the IL-6 receptor, which plays a significant role in cytokine storm. Tocilizumab has been used in treating patients with rheumatoid arthritis, giant cell arteritis, and cytokine release syndrome. Tocilizumab is used as a single intravenous dose of 8 mg/kg of actual body weight up to 800 mg.

Table 5.13 Current Guidelines for the Management of COVID-19	
Disease Severity	**Recommendations**
Not hospitalized, Mild to moderate COVID-19	Not high risk for disease progression: supportive and symptomatic management High risk for disease progression: • Bamlanivimab plus etesevimab • Casirivimab plus imdevimab
Hospitalized but does not require supplemental oxygen	Patients with high risk for disease progression, use of remdesivir may be appropriate
Hospitalized and requires supplemental oxygen	Use one of the following options: • Remdesivir with minimal oxygen supplementation • Dexamethasone plus remdesivir with an increase in requirement of supplemental oxygen • Dexamethasone administration when remdesivir cannot be used
Hospitalized and requires oxygen delivery through a high-flow device or noninvasive ventilation	Use one of the following: • Dexamethasone • Dexamethasone plus remdesivir • When corticosteroids cannot be used, baricitinib plus remdesivir can be used
Recently hospitalized with increased oxygen requirement and systemic inflammation	Add tocilizumab to any one of the above options • When corticosteroids cannot be used, baricitinib plus remdesivir can be used
Hospitalized and requires invasive mechanical ventilation or ECMO	Dexamethasone • Within 24 hours of ICU admission, dexamethasone plus tocilizumab • When corticosteroids cannot be used, baricitinib plus remdesivir can be used

ECMO, Extracorporeal membrane oxygenation; *ICU*, intensive care unit.
(Modified from National Institutes of Health. Therapeutic management of nonhospitalized and hospitalized patients with confirmed coronavirus disease (COVID-19). https://www.covid19treatmentguidelines.nih.gov/management/clinical-management/nonhospitalized-adults-therapeutic-management/. https://www.covid19treatmentguidelines.nih.gov/management/clinical-management/hospitalized-adults-therapeutic-management/.)

Tocilizumab must be used in combination with dexamethasone.

Baricitinib, an inhibitor of Janus kinase (JAK) used with remdesivir in COVID-19 patients on high-flow oxygen, and NIV has reduced recovery time and improved clinical status.[229] Baricitinib is administered 4 mg orally daily for 14 days or till hospital discharge, whichever comes first. Baricitinib is used to treat patients with moderate to severe rheumatoid arthritis who have an inadequate response to one or more anti-cytokine biologicals such as anti–TNF-α and anti–IL-6 antibodies. Hyperglycemia, anemia, decreased lymphocyte count, and acute kidney injury were the most common side effects of baricitinib observed in COVID-19 patients.

The current guidelines for managing pulmonary manifestations of COVID-19 do not differ much from those for the overall treatment of COVID-19 (Table 5.13). Medications such as remdesivir, dexamethasone, and baricitinib are used in hospitalized patients. Bamlanivimab plus etesevimab or casirivimab plus imdevimab were used in nonhospitalized patients with COVID-19.[230]

Antibiotic Use in COVID-19

Broad-spectrum antibiotics have been increasingly used in patients with COVID-19 pneumonia. Antibiotics to treat community-acquired pneumonia were commonly used in patients with COVID-19. Early recognition of bacterial superinfection is vital in treating patients with COVID-19. The clinical presentation with fever and cough, chest radiograph findings of lung infiltrates, and elevated inflammatory markers in COVID-19 make it challenging to diagnose bacterial superinfection.[231] Inappropriate use of antibiotics can lead to bacterial resistance. The most commonly used antibiotic in patients with COVID-19 is the piperacillin-tazobactam combination.[232] Antibiotic stewardship based on well-thought-out antibiotic use guidelines plays a significant role in preventing unnecessary use of antibiotics in COVID-19.[233]

General Principles of Management of Long-Term Pulmonary Sequelae

While performing clinical evaluation and assessment after recovery from acute COVID-19, it is recommended that follow-up of patients be undertaken based on clinical history, chest radiograph, and pulmonary function studies to determine residual deficits in pulmonary function. Patients who had thromboembolic pulmonary complications should be carefully monitored for the duration of anticoagulant use. Evaluation for the need for outpatient or inpatient rehabilitation should be determined before the patient's discharge from the hospital. Most of the patients who were admitted to the ICU for acute COVID-19 might require long-term acute care, inpatient rehabilitation care, or skilled nursing care. A majority of the patients managed in the ICU who underwent tracheostomy might require postdischarge tracheostomy care. Health care providers should observe for COVID-19–related laryngotracheal stenosis.[165] Likewise, they would need support and rehabilitation for post-ICU syndrome, including physical impairment from critical illnesses such as polyneuropathy, myopathy, and neuropsychological problems. The ability of patients to return to work or exercise should be addressed on an individual basis.

Case Reports Highlighting the Varied Pulmonary Manifestations of COVID-19

This section introduces three case reports from our (SN and SR) hospital practice that illustrate the varied pulmonary manifestations and complications resulting from COVID-19.

■ Case Report 5.1 COVID-19–Associated Pneumonia and Pneumomediastinum

A 58-year-old man with a past medical history of polymyositis and type 2 diabetes mellitus who developed a fever and shortness of breath presented to his primary care physician. His oxygen saturation was 70% on room air, and he was admitted to an outside hospital. He was found to have a temperature of 101°F, respiratory rate of 29 breaths per minute, and saturating 56% on room air in the emergency department. His white blood count was 10.4 K/μL (normal range, 4.0–11 K/μL), D-dimer 7650 ng/mL (normal <500 ng/mL), C-reactive protein sodium was 23.8 mg/dL (normal range, 0.0–0.9 mg/dL), lactate dehydrogenase was 754 U/L (normal range, 117–224 U/L). SARS-CoV-2 reverse transcription polymerase chain reaction and influenza B tests were positive. He was started on high-flow oxygen because of low oxygen saturation and had a radiograph that showed diffuse interstitial and alveolar airspace disease suggestive of multifocal pneumonia and pneumomediastinum. CT angiogram of the chest was negative for PE but demonstrated ground-glass appearance and pneumomediastinum. Fig. 5.15 illustrates these radiological features. He was transferred to our hospital for pulmonary consultation.

The patient was admitted to the step-down unit and required a high flow of oxygen. He was treated with dexamethasone, oseltamivir, and remdesivir. He was started on enoxaparin for DVT prophylaxis and prone positioning. A repeat chest radiograph done on day 3 showed the resolution of the pneumomediastinum. On day 5, he completed treatment with remdesivir and oseltamivir and was placed on 15 L of oxygen by a nonrebreather mask. On day 10 of hospitalization, he completed the dexamethasone course, and his oxygen requirement was better, requiring 12 L of oxygen by nasal cannula. He was discharged home on 3 L of oxygen by nasal cannula on day 14 of hospitalization.

■ Case Report 5.2 COVID-19–Associated Acute Respiratory Distress Syndrome

A 35-year-old woman with a medical history of asthma and obesity was admitted to an outside hospital with shortness of

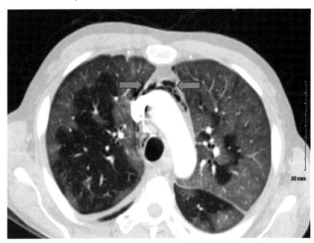

Fig. 5.15 Case Report 5.1 Showing Pneumomediastinum. Computed tomography (CT) scan of chest demonstrating bilateral lung infiltrates resulting acute respiratory distress syndrome related to COVID-19 infection complicated by air between the sternum and aortic arch (pneumomediastinum) shown with *orange arrows*. Chest CT in patient discussed in Case Report 5.1.

breath and a positive SARS-CoV-2 reverse transcription polymerase chain reaction test. Her oxygen saturation was 76% on room air, and she was started on 3 L of oxygen by nasal cannula. She was treated with dexamethasone and remdesivir. A chest radiograph showed extensive bilateral opacities. See Fig. 5.11 for the chest radiograph findings. On day 3 of hospitalization, her oxygen requirement worsened, she required noninvasive ventilation, and she was subsequently intubated and transferred to our hospital. She was admitted to the ICU, and a repeat chest radiograph showed severe subcutaneous emphysema and bilateral lung opacities; she was too unstable for a CT scan of the chest. Arterial blood gas showed a PaO_2 of 64 mm Hg (normal range 70–90 mm Hg) on 100% FiO_2 with a PaO_2/FiO_2 (PF) ratio of 64, consistent with acute respiratory distress syndrome (ARDS). She was treated with dexamethasone, remdesivir, and tocilizumab. She completed 5 days of treatment with remdesivir and 10 days with dexamethasone, but she remained in critical condition and on mechanical ventilation in the ICU.

■ Case Report 5.3 COVID-19–Associated Pulmonary Embolism

An 80-year-old man with a medical history of coronary artery disease, hypertension, and hyperlipidemia was admitted with increased shortness of breath, oxygen saturation of 70% on room air, and positive SARS-CoV-2 reverse transcription polymerase chain reaction test. A chest radiograph showed interstitial and ground-glass densities throughout the lungs. D-Dimer was 4974 ng/mL (normal <500 ng/mL), C-reactive protein was 11.4 mg/dL (normal range 0.0–0.9 mg/dL), and troponin was 0.03 ng/dL (normal range 0.0–0.05 ng/dL). He was started on dexamethasone and remdesivir. CT chest showed a nonocclusive pulmonary embolus in a subsegmental branch going to the left lower lobe. See Fig. 5.16 for an illustration of the CT findings.

Case Report-3: Pulmonary Embolism in Covid-19

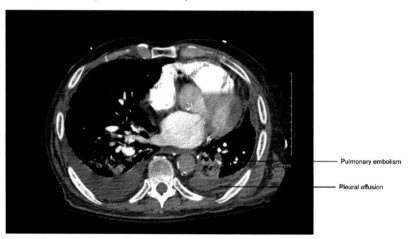

Fig. 5.16 Case Report 5.3: Pulmonary Embolism in COVID-19. Computed tomography (CT) scan of the chest showing pulmonary embolism resulting from COVID-19 infection complicated by fluid surrounding the lung (pleural effusion). CT chest of patient discussed in Case Report 5.3.

Venous duplex ultrasound of bilateral lower extremities was negative for deep vein thrombosis. He was treated with antico-agulation therapy with 1 mg/kg of enoxaparin (low molecular weight heparin) twice daily and was on 8 L of oxygen by nasal cannula. He completed treatment with remdesivir on the day 5 and dexamethasone on day 10. On day 12 of his hospitalization, his oxygen requirement increased and he required 15 L of oxygen by nonrebreather mask. A repeat chest radiograph done on the day 12 showed worsening bilateral airspace disease. On day 13, his clinical condition worsened, requiring high-flow oxygen, and he was transferred to the ICU. His clinical condition deteriorated further, and he died on the 18th day of hospitalization.

CONCLUSION

Patients infected with SARS-CoV-2 usually present with fever and shortness of breath, and many are admitted to the hospital with progressive respiratory failure. Refractory respiratory failure is the most common cause of death in patients with COVID-19. Clinicians should be aware of various pulmonary manifestations of COVID-19 and management strategies, including supplemental oxygen administration modalities and commonly employed drugs to mitigate the disease pathological processes. The management protocols and guidelines are likely to evolve as the pandemic changes course, but the basic principles of treatment we have laid out can be expected to remain valid.

After the SARS-CoV-2 outbreak, an increasing number of patients worldwide survived the spectrum of COVID-19 manifestations with a range of long-term consequences, which are being evaluated and documented. Health care providers face enormous challenges in caring for the patients who survived COVID-19 but continue to suffer. After recovery from the acute phase of COVID-19, a persisting problem is the management of a range of COVID-19 sequelae, which could vary from fatigue and body aches to severe lung damage leading to extensive pulmonary fibrosis and requiring lung transplantation.

REFERENCES

1. Centers for Disease Control and Prevention. Symptoms of Covid-19 [https://www.cdc.gov/coronavirus/2019-ncov/symptoms-testing/symptoms.html]
2. Centers for Disease Control and Prevention. People with certain medical conditions at increased risk for severe Covid-19 [https://www.cdc.gov/coronavirus/2019-ncov/need-extra-precautions/people-with-medical-conditions.html]
3. Chan JF-W, Yuan S, Kok K-H, To KK-W, Chu H, Yang J, Xing F, Liu J, Yip CC-Y, Poon RW-S. A familial cluster of pneumonia associated with the 2019 novel coronavirus indicating person-to-person transmission: a study of a family cluster. *The Lancet.* 2020;395(10223):514–523.
4. Fauci AS, Lane HC, Redfield RR. COVID-19: navigating the uncharted. *N Engl J Med. Soc.* 2020;382:1268–1269.
5. Stokes EK, Zambrano LD, Anderson KN, Marder EP, Raz KM, Felix SEB, Tie Y, Fullerton KE. Coronavirus disease 2019 case surveillance—United States. *Morbidity and Mortality Weekly Report.* 2020;69(24):759.
6. Oran DP, Topol EJ. The proportion of SARS-CoV-2 infections that are asymptomatic: a systematic review. *Annals of internal medicine.* 2021;174(5):655–662.
7. Petrilli CM, Jones SA, Yang J, Rajagopalan H, O'Donnell L, Chernyak Y, Tobin KA, Cerfolio RJ, Francois F, Horwitz LI. Factors associated with hospital admission and critical illness among 5279 people with coronavirus disease 2019 in New York City: prospective cohort study. *Bmj.* 2020;369:m1966.
8. Wu Z, McGoogan JM. Characteristics of and important lessons from the coronavirus disease 2019 (COVID-19) outbreak in China: summary of a report of 72 314 cases from the Chinese Center for Disease Control and Prevention. *Jama.* 2020;323(13):1239–1242.

9. Castro VM, McCoy TH, Perlis RH. Laboratory findings associated with severe illness and mortality among hospitalized individuals with coronavirus disease 2019 in eastern Massachusetts. *JAMA network open*. 2020;3(10):e2023934.

10. Ellinghaus D, Degenhardt F, Bujanda L, Group SC-G. Genomewide association study of severe Covid-19 with respiratory failure. *New England Journal of Medicine*. 2020;383(16):1522–1534.

11. Ray JG, Schull MJ, Vermeulen MJ, Park AL. Association between ABO and Rh blood groups and SARS-CoV-2 infection or severe COVID-19 illness: a population-based cohort study. *Annals of internal medicine*. 2021;174(3):308–315.

12. Drake TM, Riad AM, Fairfield CJ, Egan C, Knight SR, Pius R, Hardwick HE, Norman L, Shaw CA, McLean KA. Characterisation of in-hospital complications associated with COVID-19 using the ISARIC WHO Clinical Characterisation Protocol UK: a prospective, multicentre cohort study. *The Lancet*. 2021;398(10296):223–237.

13. Ashbaugh D, Bigelow DB, Petty T, Levine B. Acute respiratory distress in adults. *The Lancet*. 1967;290(7511):319–323.

14. Force ADT, Ranieri V, Rubenfeld G, Thompson B, Ferguson N, Caldwell E, Fan E, Camporota L, Slutsky A. Acute respiratory distress syndrome. *Jama*. 2012;307(23):2526–2533.

15. Riviello ED, Kiviri W, Twagirumugabe T, Mueller A, Banner-Goodspeed VM, Officer L, Novack V, Mutumwinka M, Talmor DS, Fowler RA. Hospital incidence and outcomes of the acute respiratory distress syndrome using the Kigali modification of the Berlin definition. *American journal of respiratory and critical care medicine*. 2016;193(1):52–59.

16. Bellani G, Laffey JG, Pham T, Fan E, Brochard L, Esteban A, Gattinoni L, Van Haren F, Larsson A, McAuley DF. Epidemiology, patterns of care, and mortality for patients with acute respiratory distress syndrome in intensive care units in 50 countries. *Jama*. 2016;315(8):788–800.

17. Pham T, Rubenfeld GD. Fifty years of research in ARDS. The epidemiology of acute respiratory distress syndrome. A 50th birthday review. *American journal of respiratory and critical care medicine*. 2017;195(7):860–870.

18. Matthay MA, Zemans RL, Zimmerman GA, Arabi YM, Beitler JR, Mercat A, Herridge M, Randolph AG, Calfee CS. Acute respiratory distress syndrome. *Nature reviews Disease primers*. 2019;5(1):1–22.

19. Cochi SE, Kempker JA, Annangi S, Kramer MR, Martin GS. Mortality trends of acute respiratory distress syndrome in the United States from 1999 to 2013. *Annals of the American Thoracic Society*. 2016;13(10):1742–1751.

20. Laffey JG, Madotto F, Bellani G, Pham T, Fan E, Brochard L, Amin P, Arabi Y, Bajwa EK, Bruhn A. Geo-economic variations in epidemiology, patterns of care, and outcomes in patients with acute respiratory distress syndrome: insights from the LUNG SAFE prospective cohort study. *The Lancet Respiratory Medicine*. 2017;5(8):627–638.

21. Thompson BT, Chambers RC, Liu KD. Acute respiratory distress syndrome. *New England Journal of Medicine*. 2017;377(6):562–572.

22. Sinha P, Bos LD. Pathophysiology of the acute respiratory distress syndrome: insights from clinical studies. *Critical Care Clinics*. 2021;37(4):795–815.

23. Katzenstein A, Bloor CM, Leibow AA. Diffuse alveolar damage–the role of oxygen, shock, and related factors. A review. *The American Journal of Pathology*. 1976;85(1):209.

24. Tomashefski JF Jr. Pulmonary pathology of acute respiratory distress syndrome. *Clinics in chest medicine*. 2000;21(3):435–466.

25. Thille AW, Esteban A, Fernández-Segoviano P, Rodriguez J-M, Aramburu J-A, Vargas-Errázuriz P, Martín-Pellicer A, Lorente JA. Frutos-Vivar F: Chronology of histological lesions in acute respiratory distress syndrome with diffuse alveolar damage: a prospective cohort study of clinical autopsies. *The Lancet Respiratory Medicine*. 2013;1(5):395–401.

26. Cheng KT, Xiong S, Ye Z, Hong Z, Di A, Tsang KM, Gao X, An S, Mittal M, Vogel SM. Caspase-11–mediated endothelial pyroptosis underlies endotoxemia-induced lung injury. *The Journal of Clinical Investigation*. 2017;127(11):4124–4135.

27. Matthay MA, Ware LB, Zimmerman GA. The acute respiratory distress syndrome. *The Journal of Clinical Investigation*. 2012;122(8):2731–2740.

28. Lefrançais E, Mallavia B, Zhuo H, Calfee CS, Looney MR. Maladaptive role of neutrophil extracellular traps in pathogen-induced lung injury. *JCI Insight*. 2018;3(3):e98178.

29. Albert RK. The role of ventilation-induced surfactant dysfunction and atelectasis in causing acute respiratory distress syndrome. *American Journal of Respiratory and Critical Care Medicine*. 2012;185(7):702–708.

30. Swenson KE, Swenson ER. Pathophysiology of ARDS and COVID-19 lung injury. *Crit Care Clin*. 2021;37(4):749–776.

31. Cardinal-Fernández P, Lorente JA, Ballén-Barragán A, Matute-Bello G. Acute respiratory distress syndrome and diffuse alveolar damage. New insights on a complex relationship. *Annals of the American Thoracic Society*. 2017;14(6):844–850.

32. Middleton EA, Zimmerman GA. COVID-19–associated acute respiratory distress syndrome: lessons from tissues and cells. *Critical Care Clinics*. 2021;37(4):777–793.

33. Gattinoni L, Marini JJ, Pesenti A, Quintel M, Mancebo J, Brochard L. The "baby lung" became an adult. *Intensive Care Medicine*. 2016;42(5):663–673.

34. Radermacher P, Maggiore SM, Mercat A. Fifty years of research in ARDS. Gas exchange in acute respiratory distress syndrome. *American Journal of Respiratory and Critical Care Medicine*. 2017;196(8):964–984.

35. Slutsky AS, Ranieri VM. Ventilator-induced lung injury. *New England Journal of Medicine*. 2013;369(22):2126–2136.

36. Curley GF, Laffey JG, Zhang H, Slutsky AS. Biotrauma and ventilator-induced lung injury: clinical implications. *Chest*. 2016;150(5):1109–1117.

37. Gaver III DP, Nieman GF, Gatto LA, Cereda M, Habashi NM, Bates JH. The POOR Get POORer: A hypothesis for the pathogenesis of ventilator-induced lung injury. *American Journal of Respiratory and Critical Care Medicine*. 2020;202(8):1081–1087.

38. Coleman MH, Aldrich JM. Acute respiratory distress syndrome: ventilator management and rescue therapies. *Critical Care Clinics*. 2021;37(4):851–866.

39. Gattinoni L, Tonetti T, Cressoni M, Cadringher P, Herrmann P, Moerer O, Protti A, Gotti M, Chiurazzi C, Carlesso E. Ventilator-related causes of lung injury: the mechanical power. *Intensive Care Medicine*. 2016;42(10):1567–1575.

40. Yoshida T, Fujino Y, Amato MB, Kavanagh BP. Fifty years of research in ARDS. Spontaneous breathing during mechanical ventilation. Risks, mechanisms, and management. *American Journal of Respiratory and Critical Care Medicine*. 2017;195(8):985–992.

41. Yoshida T, Grieco DL, Brochard L, Fujino Y. Patient self-inflicted lung injury and positive end-expiratory pressure for safe spontaneous breathing. *Current Opinion in Critical Care.* 2020;26(1):59–65.

42. Batah SS, Fabro AT. Pulmonary pathology of ARDS in COVID-19: A pathological review for clinicians. *Respiratory Medicine.* 2020:106239.

43. Thille AW, Esteban A, Fernández-Segoviano P, Rodríguez J-M, Aramburu J-A, Peñuelas O, Cortés-Puch I, Cardinal-Fernández P, Lorente JA. Frutos-Vivar F: Comparison of the Berlin definition for acute respiratory distress syndrome with autopsy. *American Journal of Respiratory and Critical Care Medicine.* 2013;187(7):761–767.

44. Guerin C, Bayle F, Leray V, Debord S, Stoian A, Yonis H, Roudaut J-B, Bourdin G, Devouassoux-Shisheboran M, Bucher E. Open lung biopsy in nonresolving ARDS frequently identifies diffuse alveolar damage regardless of the severity stage and may have implications for patient management. *Intensive Care Medicine.* 2015;41(2):222–230.

45. Park J, Lee YJ, Lee J, Park SS, Cho Y-J, Lee S-M, Kim YW, Han SK, Yoo C-G. Histopathologic heterogeneity of acute respiratory distress syndrome revealed by surgical lung biopsy and its clinical implications. *The Korean Journal of Internal Medicine.* 2018;33(3):532.

46. Sheu C-C, Gong MN, Zhai R, Bajwa EK, Chen F, Thompson BT, Christiani DC. The influence of infection sites on development and mortality of ARDS. *Intensive Care Medicine.* 2010;36(6):963–970.

47. Constantin J-M, Grasso S, Chanques G, Aufort S, Futier E, Sebbane M, Jung B, Gallix B, Bazin JE, Rouby J-J. Lung morphology predicts response to recruitment maneuver in patients with acute respiratory distress syndrome. *Critical Care Medicine.* 2010;38(4):1108–1117.

48. Matthay MA, Arabi YM, Siegel ER, Ware LB, Bos LD, Sinha P, Beitler JR, Wick KD, Curley MA, Constantin J-M. Phenotypes and personalized medicine in the acute respiratory distress syndrome. *Intensive Care Medicine.* 2020:1–17.

49. Warren MA, Zhao Z, Koyama T, Bastarache JA, Shaver CM, Semler MW, Rice TW, Matthay MA, Calfee CS, Ware LB. Severity scoring of lung oedema on the chest radiograph is associated with clinical outcomes in ARDS. *Thorax.* 2018;73(9):840–846.

50. Forel J-M, Guervilly C, Hraiech S, Voillet F, Thomas G, Somma C, Secq V, Farnarier C, Payan M-J, Donati S-Y. Type III procollagen is a reliable marker of ARDS-associated lung fibroproliferation. *Intensive Care Medicine.* 2015;41(1):1–11.

51. Hamon A, Scemama U, Bourenne J, Daviet F, Coiffard B, Persico N, Adda M, Guervilly C, Hraiech S, Chaumoitre K. Chest CT scan and alveolar procollagen III to predict lung fibroproliferation in acute respiratory distress syndrome. *Annals of Intensive Care.* 2019;9(1):1–8.

52. Calfee CS, Delucchi K, Parsons PE, Thompson BT, Ware LB, Matthay MA, Network NA. Subphenotypes in acute respiratory distress syndrome: latent class analysis of data from two randomised controlled trials. *The Lancet Respiratory Medicine.* 2014;2(8):611–620.

53. Famous KR, Delucchi K, Ware LB, Kangelaris KN, Liu KD, Thompson BT, Calfee CS. Acute respiratory distress syndrome subphenotypes respond differently to randomized fluid management strategy. *American Journal of Respiratory and Critical Care Medicine.* 2017;195(3):331–338.

54. Calfee CS, Janz DR, Bernard GR, May AK, Kangelaris KN, Matthay MA, Ware LB. Distinct molecular phenotypes of direct vs indirect ARDS in single-center and multicenter studies. *Chest.* 2015;147(6):1539–1548.

55. Hendrickson CM, Matthay MA. Endothelial biomarkers in human sepsis: pathogenesis and prognosis for ARDS. *Pulmonary Circulation.* 2018;8(2):2045894018769876.

56. Arabi YM, Fowler R, Hayden FG. Critical care management of adults with community-acquired severe respiratory viral infection. *Intensive Care Medicine.* 2020;46(2):315–328.

57. Fan E, Del Sorbo L, Goligher EC, Hodgson CL, Munshi L, Walkey AJ, Adhikari NK, Amato MB, Branson R, Brower RG. An official American Thoracic Society/European Society of Intensive Care Medicine/Society of Critical Care Medicine clinical practice guideline: mechanical ventilation in adult patients with acute respiratory distress syndrome. *American Journal of Respiratory and Critical Care Medicine.* 2017;195(9):1253–1263.

58. Fan E, Brodie D, Slutsky AS. Acute respiratory distress syndrome: advances in diagnosis and treatment. *JAMA.* 2018;319(7):698–710.

59. Balshem H, Helfand M, Schünemann HJ, Oxman AD, Kunz R, Brozek J, Vist GE, Falck-Ytter Y, Meerpohl J, Norris S. GRADE guidelines: 3. Rating the quality of evidence. *Journal of Clinical Epidemiology.* 2011;64(4):401–406.

60. Bos LD, Scicluna BP, Ong DS, Cremer O, van Der Poll T, Schultz MJ. Understanding heterogeneity in biologic phenotypes of acute respiratory distress syndrome by leukocyte expression profiles. *American Journal of Respiratory and Critical Care Medicine.* 2019;200(1):42–50.

61. Calfee CS, Delucchi KL, Sinha P, Matthay MA, Hackett J, Shankar-Hari M, McDowell C, Laffey JG, O'Kane CM, McAuley DF. Acute respiratory distress syndrome subphenotypes and differential response to simvastatin: secondary analysis of a randomised controlled trial. *The Lancet Respiratory Medicine.* 2018;6(9):691–698.

62. Sinha P, Churpek MM, Calfee CS Machine learning classifier models can identify acute respiratory distress syndrome phenotypes using readily available clinical data. *American Journal of Respiratory and Critical Care Medicine.* 2020;202(7):996–1004.

63. Wick KD, McAuley DF, Levitt JE, Beitler JR, Annane D, Riviello ED, Calfee CS, Matthay MA. Promises and challenges of personalized medicine to guide ARDS therapy. *Critical Care.* 2021;25(1):1–15.

64. Kotas ME, Thompson BT. Toward optimal acute respiratory distress syndrome outcomes: recognizing the syndrome and identifying its causes. *Critical Care Clinics.* 2021;37(4):733–748.

65. Bein T, Weber-Carstens S, Apfelbacher C. Long-term outcome after the acute respiratory distress syndrome: different from general critical illness?. *Current Opinion in Critical Care.* 2018;24(1):35–40.

66. Gattinoni L, Chiumello D, Rossi S. COVID-19 pneumonia: ARDS or not?. *BioMed Central.* 2020;24(1):154.

67. Goligher EC, Ranieri VM, Slutsky AS. *Is severe COVID-19 pneumonia a typical or atypical form of ARDS? And does it matter?.* New York: Springer; 2021.

68. Chiumello D, Busana M, Coppola S, Romitti F, Formenti P, Bonifazi M, Pozzi T, Palumbo MM, Cressoni M, Herrmann P. Physiological and quantitative CT-scan characterization of COVID-19 and typical ARDS: a matched cohort study. *Intensive Care Medicine.* 2020;46(12):2187–2196.

69. Gattinoni L, Chiumello D, Caironi P, Busana M, Romitti F, Brazzi L, Camporota L. *COVID-19 pneumonia: different respiratory treatments for different phenotypes?*. New York: Springer; 2020.

70. Welker C, Huang J, Gil IJN, Ramakrishna H. 2021 acute respiratory distress syndrome update, with coronavirus disease 2019 Focus. *Journal of Cardiothoracic and Vascular Anesthesia*. 2021;S1053(21):001188–001189.

71. Swenson KE, Ruoss SJ, Swenson ER. The pathophysiology and dangers of silent hypoxemia in COVID-19 lung injury. *Annals of the American Thoracic Society*. 2021;18(7):1098–1105.

72. Fan E, Beitler JR, Brochard L, Calfee CS, Ferguson ND, Slutsky AS, Brodie D. COVID-19-associated acute respiratory distress syndrome: is a different approach to management warranted?. *The Lancet Respiratory Medicine*. 2020;8(8):816–821.

73. Bickler PE, Feiner JR, Lipnick MS, McKleroy W. Silent" presentation of hypoxemia and cardiorespiratory compensation in COVID-19. *Anesthesiology*. 2021;134(2):262–269.

74. Brouqui P, Amrane S, Million M, Cortaredona S, Parola P, Lagier J-C, Raoult D. Asymptomatic hypoxia in COVID-19 is associated with poor outcome. *International Journal of Infectious Diseases*. 2021;102:233–238.

75. García-Grimshaw M, Flores-Silva FD, Chiquete E, Cantú-Brito C, Michel-Chávez A, Vigueras-Hernández AP, Domínguez-Moreno R, Chávez-Martínez OA, Sánchez-Torres S, Marché-Fernández OA. Characteristics and predictors for silent hypoxemia in a cohort of hospitalized COVID-19 patients. *Autonomic Neuroscience*. 2021;235:102855.

76. Okuhama A, Ishikane M, Hotta M, Sato L, Akiyama Y, Morioka S, Suzuki S, Tajima T, Yamamoto M, Teruya K. Clinical and radiological findings of silent hypoxia among COVID-19 patients. *Journal of Infection and Chemotherapy*. 2021;27(10):1536–1538.

77. Simonson TS, Baker TL, Banzett RB, Bishop T, Dempsey JA, Feldman JL, Guyenet PG, Hodson EJ, Mitchell GS, Moya EA. Silent hypoxaemia in COVID-19 patients. *The Journal of Physiology*. 2021;599(4):1057–1065.

78. Tobin MJ, Laghi F, Jubran A. Why COVID-19 silent hypoxemia is baffling to physicians. *American Journal of Respiratory and Critical Care Medicine*. 2020;202(3):356–360.

79. Wilkerson RG, Adler JD, Shah NG, Brown R: Silent hypoxia: a harbinger of clinical deterioration in patients with COVID-19. The American Journal of Emergency Medicine 2020, 38(10):2243. e2245-2243. e2246.

80. Xie J, Covassin N, Fan Z, Singh P, Gao W, Li G, Kara T, Somers VK. Association between hypoxemia and mortality in patients with COVID-19. *In: Mayo Clinic Proceedings:*. 2020;95(6):1138–1147.

81. Ackermann M, Verleden SE, Kuehnel M, Haverich A, Welte T, Laenger F, Vanstapel A, Werlein C, Stark H, Tzankov A, et al. Pulmonary vascular endothelialitis, thrombosis, and angiogenesis in COVID-19. *New England Journal of Medicine*. 2020;383(2):120–128.

82. Chan NC, Weitz JI. COVID-19 coagulopathy, thrombosis, and bleeding. *Blood*. 2020;136(4):381–383.

83. Gattinoni L, Coppola S, Cressoni M, Busana M, Rossi S, Chiumello D. COVID-19 does not lead to a "typical" acute respiratory distress syndrome. *American Journal of Respiratory and Critical Care Medicine*. 2020;201(10):1299–1300.

84. Lang M, Som A, Mendoza DP, Flores EJ, Reid N, Carey D, Li MD, Witkin A, Rodriguez-Lopez JM, Shepard J-AO: Hypoxaemia related to COVID-19: vascular and perfusion abnormalities on dual-energy CT. *The Lancet Infectious Diseases 2020*, 20(12):1365-1366.

85. Villadiego J, Ramírez-Lorca R, Cala F, Labandeira-García JL, Esteban M, Toledo-Aral JJ, López-Barneo J. *Is carotid body infection responsible for silent hypoxemia in COVID-19 patients?*. Oxford, UK: Oxford University Press; 2021.

86. Manganelli F, Vargas M, Iovino A, Iacovazzo C, Santoro L, Servillo G. Brainstem involvement and respiratory failure in COVID-19. *Neurological Sciences*. 2020;41:1663–1665.

87. Li YC, Bai WZ, Hashikawa T. The neuroinvasive potential of SARS-CoV2 may play a role in the respiratory failure of COVID-19 patients. *Journal of Medical Virology*. 2020;92(6):552–555.

88. Li K, Wohlford-Lenane C, Perlman S, Zhao J, Jewell AK, Reznikov LR, Gibson-Corley KN, Meyerholz DK, McCray Jr PB. Middle East respiratory syndrome coronavirus causes multiple organ damage and lethal disease in mice transgenic for human dipeptidyl peptidase 4. *The Journal of Infectious Diseases*. 2016;213(5):712–722.

89. Netland J, Meyerholz DK, Moore S, Cassell M, Perlman S. Severe acute respiratory syndrome coronavirus infection causes neuronal death in the absence of encephalitis in mice transgenic for human ACE2. *Journal of Virology*. 2008;82(15):7264–7275.

90. Strapazzon G, Hilty MP, Bouzat P, Pratali L, Brugger H, Rauch S. To compare the incomparable: COVID-19 pneumonia and high-altitude disease. *European Respiratory Journal*. 2020;55(6).

91. Luks AM, Swenson ER. COVID-19 lung injury and high-altitude pulmonary edema. A false equation with dangerous implications. *Annals of the American Thoracic Society*. 2020;17(8):918–921.

92. Solaimanzadeh I. Acetazolamide, nifedipine and phosphodiesterase inhibitors: rationale for their utilization as adjunctive countermeasures in the treatment of coronavirus disease 2019 (COVID-19). *Cureus*. 2020;12(3):e7343.

93. Allado E, Poussel M, Valentin S, Kimmoun A, Levy B, Nguyen DT, Rumeau C, Chenuel B. The fundamentals of respiratory physiology to manage the COVID-19 pandemic: an overview. *Frontiers in Physiology*. 2021;11:1862.

94. Archer SL, Sharp WW, Weir EK. Differentiating COVID-19 pneumonia from acute respiratory distress syndrome and high altitude pulmonary edema: therapeutic implications. *Circulation*. 2020;142(2):101–104.

95. Hou YJ, Okuda K, Edwards CE, Martinez DR, Asakura T, Dinnon III KH, T Kato, RE Lee, BL Yount, TM Mascenik. SARS-CoV-2 reverse genetics reveals a variable infection gradient in the respiratory tract. *Cell*. 2020;182(2):429–446 e414.

96. Clerkin KJ, Fried JA, Raikhelkar J, Sayer G, Griffin JM, Masoumi A, Jain SS, Burkhoff D, Kumaraiah D, Rabbani L. Coronavirus disease 2019 (COVID-19) and cardiovascular disease. *Circulation*. 2020;141(20):1648–1655.

97. Marik PE, Iglesias J, Varon J, Kory P. A scoping review of the pathophysiology of COVID-19. *International Journal of Immunopathology and Pharmacology*. 2021;35: 20587384211048026.

98. Carsana L, Sonzogni A, Nasr A, Rossi RS, Pellegrinelli A, Zerbi P, Rech R, Colombo R, Antinori S, Corbellino M. Pulmonary post-mortem findings in a series of COVID-19 cases from northern Italy: a two-centre descriptive study. *The Lancet Infectious Diseases*. 2020;20(10):1135–1140.

99. Borczuk AC, Salvatore SP, Seshan SV, Patel SS, Bussel JB, Mostyka M, Elsoukkary S, He B, Del Vecchio C, Fortarezza F. COVID-19 pulmonary pathology: a multi-institutional autopsy cohort from Italy and New York City. *Modern Pathology.* 2020;33(11):2156–2168.

100. Bryce C, Grimes Z, Pujadas E, Ahuja S, Beasley MB, Albrecht R, Hernandez T, Stock A, Zhao Z. AlRasheed MR: Pathophysiology of SARS-CoV-2: the Mount Sinai COVID-19 autopsy experience. *Modern Pathology.* 2021:1–12.

101. Beigee FS, Toutkaboni MP, Khalili N, Nadji SA, Dorudinia A, Rezaei M, Askari E, Farzanegan B, Marjani M, Rafiezadeh A. Diffuse alveolar damage and thrombotic microangiopathy are the main histopathological findings in lung tissue biopsy samples of COVID-19 patients. *Pathology-Research and Practice.* 2020;216(10):153228.

102. Levy JH, Iba T, Olson LB, Corey KM, Ghadimi K, Connors JM. COVID-19: Thrombosis, thromboinflammation, and anticoagulation considerations. *International Journal of Laboratory Hematology.* 2021;43:29–35.

103. Mitchell WB. Thromboinflammation in COVID-19 acute lung injury. *Paediatric Respiratory Reviews.* 2020;35:20–24.

104. Zuo Y, Zuo M, Yalavarthi S, Gockman K, Madison JA, Shi H, Woodard W, Lezak SP, Lugogo NL, Knight JS. Neutrophil extracellular traps and thrombosis in COVID-19. *Journal of Thrombosis and Thrombolysis.* 2021;51(2):446–453.

105. Nicolai L, Leunig A, Brambs S, Kaiser R, Weinberger T, Weigand M, Muenchhoff M, Hellmuth JC, Ledderose S, Schulz H. Immunothrombotic dysregulation in COVID-19 pneumonia is associated with respiratory failure and coagulopathy. *Circulation.* 2020;142(12):1176–1189.

106. Iba T, Levy JH, Levi M, Thachil J. Coagulopathy in COVID-19. *Journal of Thrombosis and Haemostasis.* 2020;18(9):2103–2109.

107. Terpos E, Ntanasis-Stathopoulos I, Elalamy I, Kastritis E, Sergentanis TN, Politou M, Psaltopoulou T, Gerotziafas G, Dimopoulos MA. Hematological findings and complications of COVID-19. *American Journal of Hematology.* 2020;95(7):834–847.

108. Barnes BJ, Adrover JM, Baxter-Stoltzfus A, Borczuk A, Cools-Lartigue J, Crawford JM, Daßler-Plenker J, Guerci P, Huynh C, Knight JS. Targeting potential drivers of COVID-19: Neutrophil extracellular traps. *Journal of Experimental Medicine.* 2020;217(6).

109. Patel BV, Arachchillage DJ, Ridge CA, Bianchi P, Doyle JF, Garfield B, Ledot S, Morgan C, Passariello M, Price S. Pulmonary angiopathy in severe COVID-19: physiologic, imaging, and hematologic observations. *American Journal of Respiratory and Critical Care Medicine.* 2020;202(5):690–699.

110. Magro CM, Mulvey J, Kubiak J, Mikhail S, Suster D, Crowson AN, Laurence J, Nuovo G. Severe COVID-19: a multifaceted viral vasculopathy syndrome. *Annals of Diagnostic Pathology.* 2021;50:151645.

111. Grasselli G, Tonetti T, Protti A, Langer T, Girardis M, Bellani G, Laffey J, Carrafiello G, Carsana L, Rizzuto C. Pathophysiology of COVID-19-associated acute respiratory distress syndrome: a multicentre prospective observational study. *The Lancet Respiratory Medicine.* 2020;8(12):1201–1208.

112. Bertelli M, Fusina F, Prezioso C, Cavallo E, Nencini N, Crisci S, Tansini F, Mari LM, Hoxha L, Lombardi F. COVID-19 ARDS is characterized by increased dead space ventilation compared with non-COVID ARDS. *Respiratory Care.* 2021;66(9):1406–1415.

113. Sinha P, Calfee CS, Cherian S, Brealey D, Cutler S, King C, Killick C, Richards O, Cheema Y, Bailey C. Prevalence of phenotypes of acute respiratory distress syndrome in critically ill patients with COVID-19: a prospective observational study. *The Lancet Respiratory Medicine.* 2020;8(12):1209–1218.

114. Arrossi AV, Farver C. The pulmonary pathology of COVID-19. *Cleveland Clinic Journal of Medicine.* 2020.

115. Vadász I, Husain-Syed F, Dorfmüller P, Roller FC, Tello K, Hecker M, Morty RE, Gattenlöhner S, Walmrath H-D, Grimminger F. Severe organising pneumonia following COVID-19. *Thorax.* 2021;76(2):201–204.

116. Colorado JMC, Ardila LFC, Vásquez NA, Calderón KCG, Álvarez SLL, Bayona JAC. Organizing pneumonia associated with SARS-CoV-2 infection. *Radiology Case Reports.* 2021;16(9):2634–2639.

117. Kory P, Kanne JP. SARS-CoV-2 organising pneumonia: Has there been a widespread failure to identify and treat this prevalent condition in COVID-19?. *BMJ Open Respiratory Research.* 2020;7(1):e000724.

118. Dickson RP, Erb-Downward JR, Martinez FJ, Huffnagle GB. The microbiome and the respiratory tract. *Annual Review of Physiology.* 2016;78:481–504.

119. Khatiwada S, Subedi A. Lung microbiome and coronavirus disease 2019 (COVID-19): possible link and implications. *Human Microbiome Journal.* 2020;17:100073.

120. Yang D, Xing Y, Song X, Qian Y. The impact of lung microbiota dysbiosis on inflammation. *Immunology.* 2020;159(2):156–166.

121. Sulaiman I, Chung M, Angel L, Koralov S, Wu B, Yeung S, Krolikowski K, Li Y, Duerr R, Schluger R. Microbial signatures in the lower airways of mechanically ventilated COVID19 patients associated with poor clinical outcome. *Res Sq..* 2021:rs.3.rs-266050.

122. Tsitsiklis A, Zha B, Byrne A, DeVoe C, Levan S, Rackaityte E, Sunshine S, Mick E, Ghale R, Jauregui A. Impaired immune signaling and changes in the lung microbiome precede secondary bacterial pneumonia in COVID-19. *Research Square.* 2021:rs.3.rs-380803.

123. Horie S, McNicholas B, Rezoagli E, Pham T, Curley G, McAuley D, O'Kane C, Nichol A, Dos Santos C, Rocco PR. Emerging pharmacological therapies for ARDS: COVID-19 and beyond. *Intensive care medicine.* 2020;46(12):2265–2283.

124. Herrmann J, Mori V, Bates JH, Suki B. Modeling lung perfusion abnormalities to explain early COVID-19 hypoxemia. *Nature communications.* 2020;11(1):1–9.

125. Han R, Huang L, Jiang H, Dong J, Peng H, Zhang D. Early clinical and CT manifestations of coronavirus disease 2019 (COVID-19) pneumonia. *American Journal of Roentgenology.* 2020;215(2):338–343.

126. Hani C, Trieu NH, Saab I, Dangeard S, Bennani S, Chassagnon G, Revel M-P. COVID-19 pneumonia: a review of typical CT findings and differential diagnosis. *Diagnostic and Interventional Imaging.* 2020;101(5):263–268.

127. Jalaber C, Lapotre T, Morcet-Delattre T, Ribet F, Jouneau S, Lederlin M. Chest CT in COVID-19 pneumonia: a review of current knowledge. *Diagnostic and Interventional Imaging.* 2020;101(7-8):431–437.

128. Lomoro P, Verde F, Zerboni F, Simonetti I, Borghi C, Fachinetti C, Natalizi A, Martegani A. COVID-19 pneumonia manifestations at the admission on chest ultrasound, radiographs, and CT: single-center study and comprehensive

radiologic literature review. *European Journal of Radiology Open*. 2020;7:100231.

129. Kanne JP, Bai H, Bernheim A, Chung M, Haramati LB, Kallmes DF, Little BP, Rubin G, Sverzellati N. COVID-19 imaging: What we know now and what remains unknown. *Radiology*. 2021;299(3):E262–E279.

130. Lang M, Som A, Carey D, Reid N, Mendoza DP, Flores EJ, Li MD, Shepard J-AO, Little BP. Pulmonary vascular manifestations of COVID-19 pneumonia. *Radiology: Cardiothoracic Imaging*. 2020;2(3):e200277.

131. Zheng Y, Wang L, Ben S. Meta-analysis of chest CT features of patients with COVID-19 pneumonia. *Journal of Medical Virology*. 2021;93(1):241–249.

132. Zantah M, Castillo ED, Townsend R, Dikengil F, Criner GJ. Pneumothorax in COVID-19 disease-incidence and clinical characteristics. *Respiratory Research*. 2020;21(1):1–9.

133. Alharthy A, Bakirova GH, Bakheet H, Balhamar A, Brindley PG, Alqahtani SA, Memish ZA, Karakitsos D. COVID-19 with spontaneous pneumothorax, pneumomediastinum, and subcutaneous emphysema in the intensive care unit: two case reports. *Journal of Infection and Public Health*. 2021;14(3):290–292.

134. Belletti A, Palumbo D, Zangrillo A, Fominskiy EV, Franchini S, Dell'Acqua A, Marinosci A, Monti G, Vitali G, Colombo S. Predictors of pneumothorax/pneumomediastinum in mechanically ventilated COVID-19 patients. *Journal of Cardiothoracic and Vascular Anesthesia*. 2021;35(12):3642–3651.

135. Ekanem E, Podder S, Donthi N, Bakhshi H, Stodghill J, Khandhar S, Mahajan A, Desai M. Spontaneous pneumothorax: an emerging complication of COVID-19 pneumonia. *Heart & Lung*. 2021;50(3):437–440.

136. Geraci TC, Williams D, Chen S, Grossi E, Chang S, Cerfolio RJ, Bizekis C, Zervos M. Incidence, management, and outcomes of patients with COVID-19 and pneumothorax. *The Annals of Thoracic Surgery*. 2021;s0003-4975(21):01545–01549.

137. Marciniak SJ, Farrell J, Rostron A, Smith I, Openshaw PJ, Baillie JK, Docherty A, Semple MG. COVID-19 Pneumothorax in the United Kingdom: a prospective observational study using the ISARIC WHO clinical characterisation protocol. *European Respiratory Journal*. 2021;58(3):2100929.

138. Martinelli AW, Ingle T, Newman J, Nadeem I, Jackson K, Lane ND, Melhorn J, Davies HE, Rostron AJ. Adeni A: COVID-19 and pneumothorax: a multicentre retrospective case series. *European Respiratory Journal*. 2020;56(5):2002697.

139. Wang XH, Duan J, Han X, Liu X, Zhou J, Wang X, Zhu L, Mou H, Guo S. High incidence and mortality of pneumothorax in critically Ill patients with COVID-19. *Heart & Lung*. 2021;50(1):37–43.

140. Cut TG, Tudoran C, Lazureanu VE, Marinescu AR, Dumache R, Tudoran M. Spontaneous Pneumomediastinum, Pneumothorax, Pneumopericardium and Subcutaneous Emphysema—Not So Uncommon Complications in Patients with COVID-19 Pulmonary Infection—A Series of Cases. *Journal of clinical medicine*. 2021;10(7):1346.

141. Elhakim TS, Abdul HS, Romero CP, Rodriguez-Fuentes Y. Spontaneous pneumomediastinum, pneumothorax and subcutaneous emphysema in COVID-19 pneumonia: a rare case and literature review. *BMJ Case Reports CP*. 2020;13(12):e239489.

142. Eperjesiova B, Hart E, Shokr M, Sinha P, Ferguson GT. Spontaneous pneumomediastinum/pneumothorax in patients with COVID-19. *Cureus*. 2020;12(7):e8996.

143. Lal A, Mishra AK, Akhtar J, Nabzdyk C. Pneumothorax and pneumomediastinum in COVID-19 acute respiratory distress syndrome. *Monaldi Archives for Chest Disease*. 2021;91(2).

144. Protrka MR, Ivanac G, Đudarić L, Vujević F, Brkljačić B. Spontaneous pneumomediastinum, pneumothorax and subcutaneous emphysema: radiological aspects of rare COVID-19 complications in 3 patients. *Radiology Case Reports*. 2021;16(11):3237–3243.

145. Chong WH, Saha BK, Hu K, Chopra A. The incidence, clinical characteristics, and outcomes of pneumothorax in hospitalized COVID-19 patients: a systematic review. *Heart & Lung*. 2021;50(5):599–608.

146. Capaccione KM, D'souza B, Leb J, Luk L, Duong J, Tsai W-Y, Navot B, Dumeer S, Mohammed A, Salvatore MM. Pneumothorax rate in intubated patients with COVID-19. *Acute and Critical Care*. 2021;36(1):81.

147. Xie Y, Wang X, Yang P, Zhang S. COVID-19 complicated by acute pulmonary embolism. *Radiology: Cardiothoracic Imaging*. 2020;2(2):e200067.

148. Poissy J, Goutay J, Caplan M, Parmentier E, Duburcq T, Lassalle F, Jeanpierre E, Rauch A, Labreuche J, Susen S. Pulmonary embolism in patients with COVID-19: awareness of an increased prevalence. *Circulation*. 2020;142(2):184–186.

149. Poyiadji N, Cormier P, Patel PY, Hadied MO, Bhargava P, Khanna K, Nadig J, Keimig T, Spizarny D, Reeser N. Acute pulmonary embolism and COVID-19. *Radiology*. 2020;297(3):E335–E338.

150. Ameri P, Inciardi RM, Di Pasquale M, Agostoni P, Bellasi A, Camporotondo R, Canale C, Carubelli V, Carugo S, Catagnano F. Pulmonary embolism in patients with COVID-19: characteristics and outcomes in the Cardio-COVID Italy multicenter study. *Clinical Research in Cardiology*. 2021;110(7):1020–1028.

151. Badr OI, Alwafi H, Elrefaey WA, Naser AY, Shabrawishi M, Alsairafi Z, Alsaleh FM. Incidence and outcomes of pulmonary embolism among hospitalized COVID-19 patients. *International Journal of Environmental Research and Public Health*. 2021;18(14):7645.

152. García-Ortega A, Oscullo G, Calvillo P, López-Reyes R, Méndez R, Gómez-Olivas JD, Bekki A, Fonfría C, Trilles-Olaso L, Zaldívar E. Incidence, risk factors, and thrombotic load of pulmonary embolism in patients hospitalized for COVID-19 infection. *Journal of Infection*. 2021;82(2):261–269.

153. Hauguel-Moreau M, Hajjam ME, De Baynast Q, Vieillard-Baron A, Lot A-S, Chinet T, Mustafic H, Bégué C, Carlier RY, Geri G. Occurrence of pulmonary embolism related to COVID-19. *Journal of Thrombosis and Thrombolysis*. 2021;52(1):69–75.

154. Mestre-Gómez B, Lorente-Ramos R, Rogado J, Franco-Moreno A, Obispo B, Salazar-Chiriboga D, Saez-Vaquero T, Torres-Macho J. Abad-Motos A, Cortina-Camarero C: Incidence of pulmonary embolism in non-critically ill COVID-19 patients. Predicting factors for a challenging diagnosis. *Journal of Thrombosis and Thrombolysis*. 2021;51(1):40–46.

155. Miró Ò, Jiménez S, Mebazaa A, Freund Y, Burillo-Putze G, Martín A, Martín-Sánchez FJ, García-Lamberechts EJ, Alquézar-Arbé A, Jacob J. Pulmonary embolism in patients with COVID-19: incidence, risk factors, clinical

characteristics, and outcome. *European Heart Journal.* 2021;42(33):3127–3142.

156. Scudiero F, Silverio A, Di Maio M, Russo V, Citro R, Personeni D, Cafro A, D'Andrea A, Attena E, Pezzullo S. Pulmonary embolism in COVID-19 patients: prevalence, predictors and clinical outcome. *Thrombosis Research.* 2021;198:34–39.

157. Suh YJ, Hong H, Ohana M, Bompard F, Revel M-P, Valle C, Gervaise A, Poissy J, Susen S, Hékimian G. Pulmonary embolism and deep vein thrombosis in COVID-19: a systematic review and meta-analysis. *Radiology.* 2021;298(2):E70–E80.

158. Planquette B, Le Berre A, Khider L, Yannoutsos A, Gendron N, de Torcy M, Mohamedi N, Jouveshomme S, Smadja DM, Lazareth I. Prevalence and characteristics of pulmonary embolism in 1042 COVID-19 patients with respiratory symptoms: a nested case-control study. *Thrombosis Research.* 2021;197:94–99.

159. Thachil J, Srivastava A. SARS-2 Coronavirus–Associated Hemostatic Lung Abnormality in COVID-19: Is It Pulmonary Thrombosis or Pulmonary Embolism? *Seminars in thrombosis and hemostasis.* Stuttgart, Germany: Thieme Medical Publishers; 2020:777–780.

160. Chong WH, Saha BK, Ramani A, Chopra A. State-of-the-art review of secondary pulmonary infections in patients with COVID-19 pneumonia. *Infection.* 2021:1–15.

161. Paramythiotou E, Dimopoulos G, Koliakos N, Siopi M, Vourli S, Pournaras S, Meletiadis J. Epidemiology and incidence of COVID-19-associated pulmonary aspergillosis (CAPA) in a Greek tertiary care academic reference hospital. *Infectious Diseases and Therapy.* 2021;10(3):1779–1792.

162. Blanco J-R, Cobos-Ceballos M-J, Navarro F, Sanjoaquin I, de Las Revillas FA, Bernal E, Buzon-Martin L, Viribay M, Romero L, Espejo-Perez S. Pulmonary long-term consequences of COVID-19 infections after hospital discharge. *Clinical Microbiology and Infection.* 2021;27(6):892–896.

163. Hayes JP. Considering the long-term respiratory effects of Covid-19. *Occupational Medicine (Oxford, England).* 2021;71(8):325–327.

164. Higgins V, Sohaei D, Diamandis EP, Prassas I. COVID-19: from an acute to chronic disease? Potential long-term health consequences. *Critical Reviews in Clinical Laboratory Sciences.* 2021;58(5):297–310.

165. Piazza C, Filauro M, Dikkers FG, Nouraei SR, Sandu K, Sittel C, Amin MR, Campos G, Eckel HE, Peretti G. Long-term intubation and high rate of tracheostomy in COVID-19 patients might determine an unprecedented increase of airway stenoses: a call to action from the European Laryngological Society. *European Archives of Oto-Rhino-Laryngology.* 2021;278:1–7.

166. Salehi S, Reddy S, Gholamrezanezhad A. Long-term pulmonary consequences of coronavirus disease 2019 (COVID-19): what we know and what to expect. *Journal of Thoracic Imaging.* 2020;35(4):W87–W89.

167. Song W-J, Hui CKM, Hull JH, Birring SS, McGarvey L, Mazzone SB, Chung KF. Confronting COVID-19-associated cough and the post-COVID syndrome: role of viral neurotropism, neuroinflammation, and neuroimmune responses. *The Lancet Respiratory Medicine.* 2021;9(5):533–544.

168. Wu X, Liu X, Zhou Y, Yu H, Li R, Zhan Q, Ni F, Fang S, Lu Y, Ding X, et al. 3-month, 6-month, 9-month, and 12-month respiratory outcomes in patients following COVID-19-related hospitalisation: a prospective study. *The Lancet Respiratory Medicine.* 2021;9(7):747–754.

169. SeyedAlinaghi S, Afsahi AM, MohsseniPour M, Behnezhad F, Salehi MA, Barzegary A, Mirzapour P, Mehraeen E, Dadras O: Late complications of COVID-19: a systematic review of current evidence. Archives of Academic Emergency Medicine 2021, 9(1):e14.

170. Wild JM, Porter JC, Molyneaux PL, George PM, Stewart I, Allen RJ, Aul R, Baillie JK, Barratt SL, Beirne P. Understanding the burden of interstitial lung disease post-COVID-19: the UK Interstitial Lung Disease-Long COVID Study (UKILD-Long COVID). *BMJ Open Respiratory Research.* 2021;8(1):e001049.

171. Fernández-de-Las-Peñas C, Guijarro C, Plaza-Canteli S, Hernández-Barrera V, Torres-Macho J. Prevalence of post-COVID-19 cough one year after SARS-CoV-2 infection: a multicenter study. *Lung.* 2021;199(3):249–253.

172. Cares-Marambio K, Montenegro-Jiménez Y, Torres-Castro R, Vera-Uribe R, Torralba Y, Alsina-Restoy X, Vasconcello-Castillo L, Vilaró J. Prevalence of potential respiratory symptoms in survivors of hospital admission after coronavirus disease 2019 (COVID-19): a systematic review and meta-analysis. *Chronic Respiratory Disease.* 2021;18:14799731211002240.

173. McDonald LT. Healing after COVID-19: are survivors at risk for pulmonary fibrosis?. *American Journal of Physiology-Lung Cellular and Molecular Physiology.* 2021;320(2):L257–L265.

174. Zhang C, Wu Z, Li JW, Tan K, Yang W, Zhao H, Wang GQ. Discharge may not be the end of treatment: Pay attention to pulmonary fibrosis caused by severe COVID-19. *Journal of Medical Virology.* 2021;93(3):1378–1386.

175. Vasarmidi E, Tsitoura E, Spandidos DA, Tzanakis N, Antoniou KM: Pulmonary fibrosis in the aftermath of the COVID-19 era. Experimental and Therapeutic Medicine 2020, 20(3):2557–2560.

176. George PM, Wells AU, Jenkins RG. Pulmonary fibrosis and COVID-19: the potential role for antifibrotic therapy. *The Lancet Respiratory Medicine.* 2020;8(8):807–815.

177. Spagnolo P, Balestro E, Aliberti S, Cocconcelli E, Biondini D, Della Casa G, Sverzellati N, Maher TM. Pulmonary fibrosis secondary to COVID-19: a call to arms?. *The Lancet Respiratory Medicine.* 2020;8(8):750–752.

178. Wigén J, Löfdahl A, Bjermer L, Elowsson-Rendin L, Westergren-Thorsson G. Converging pathways in pulmonary fibrosis and Covid-19: the fibrotic link to disease severity. *Respiratory Medicine: X: X.* 2020;2:100023.

179. Ojo AS, Balogun SA, Williams OT, Ojo OS. Pulmonary fibrosis in COVID-19 survivors: predictive factors and risk reduction strategies. *Pulmonary Medicine.* 2020:6175964.

180. Ambardar SR, Hightower SL, Huprikar NA, Chung KK, Singhal A, Collen JF. Post-COVID-19 pulmonary fibrosis: novel sequelae of the current pandemic. *Journal of Clinical Medicine.* 2021;10(11):2452.

181. Tanni SE, Fabro AT, de Albuquerque A, Ferreira EVM, Verrastro CGY, Sawamura MVY, Ribeiro SM, Baldi BG. Pulmonary fibrosis secondary to COVID-19: a narrative review. *Expert Review of Respiratory Medicine.* 2021:1–13.

182. Huang W, Wu Q, Chen Z, Xiong Z, Wang K, Tian J, Zhang S. The potential indicators for pulmonary fibrosis in survivors of severe COVID-19. *Journal of Infection.* 2021;82(2):e5–e7.

183. Yu M, Liu Y, Xu D, Zhang R, Lan L, Xu H. Prediction of the development of pulmonary fibrosis using serial thin-section CT and clinical features in patients discharged after treatment for COVID-19 pneumonia. *Korean Journal of Radiology*. 2020;21(6):746–755.

184. Li Y, Wu J, Wang S, Li X, Zhou J, Huang B, Luo D, Cao Q, Chen Y, Chen S. Progression to fibrosing diffuse alveolar damage in a series of 30 minimally invasive autopsies with COVID-19 pneumonia in Wuhan. *China. Histopathology*. 2021;78(4):542–555.

185. Ray A, Chaudhry R, Rai S, Mitra S, Pradhan S, Sunder A, Nag DS. Prolonged oxygen therapy post COVID-19 infection: factors leading to the risk of poor outcome. *Cureus*. 2021;13(2):e13357.

186. Wang Y, Jin C, Wu CC, Zhao H, Liang T, Liu Z, Jian Z, Li R, Wang Z, Li F. Organizing pneumonia of COVID-19: Time-dependent evolution and outcome in CT findings. *PloS One*. 2020;15(11):e0240347.

187. Barrot L, Asfar P, Mauny F, Winiszewski H, Montini F, Badie J, Quenot J-P, Pili-Floury S, Bouhemad B, Louis G. Liberal or conservative oxygen therapy for acute respiratory distress syndrome. *New England Journal of Medicine*. 2020;382(11):999–1008.

188. Guérin C, Reignier J, Richard J-C, Beuret P, Gacouin A, Boulain T, Mercier E, Badet M, Mercat A, Baudin O. Prone positioning in severe acute respiratory distress syndrome. *New England Journal of Medicine*. 2013;368(23):2159–2168.

189. Nishimura M. High-flow nasal cannula oxygen therapy in adults. *Journal of Intensive Care*. 2015;3(1):1–8.

190. Lodeserto FJ, Lettich TM, Rezaie SR. High-flow nasal cannula: mechanisms of action and adult and pediatric indications. *Cureus*. 2018;10(11):e3639.

191. Helviz Y, Einav S. A systematic review of the high-flow nasal cannula for adult patients. *Annual Update in Intensive Care and Emergency Medicine*. 2018;2018:177–191.

192. Demoule A, Vieillard Baron A, Darmon M, Beurton A, Géri G, Voiriot G, Dupont T, Zafrani L, Girodias L, Labbé V. High-flow nasal cannula in critically Ill patients with severe COVID-19. *American Journal of Respiratory and Critical Care Medicine*. 2020;202(7):1039–1042.

193. Calligaro GL, Lalla U, Audley G, Gina P, Miller MG, Mendelson M, Dlamini S, Wasserman S, Meintjes G, Peter J. The utility of high-flow nasal oxygen for severe COVID-19 pneumonia in a resource-constrained setting: a multi-centre prospective observational study. *EClinicalMedicine*. 2020;28:100570.

194. Xia J, Zhang Y, Ni L, Chen L, Zhou C, Gao C, Wu X, Duan J, Xie J, Guo Q. High-flow nasal oxygen in coronavirus disease 2019 patients with acute hypoxemic respiratory failure: a multicenter, retrospective cohort study. *Critical Care Medicine*. 2020;48(11):e1079.

195. Roca O, Messika J, Caralt B, García-de-Acilu M, Sztrymf B, Ricard J-D, Masclans JR. Predicting success of high-flow nasal cannula in pneumonia patients with hypoxemic respiratory failure: the utility of the ROX index. *Journal of Critical Care*. 2016;35:200–205.

196. Girou E, Schortgen F, Delclaux C, Brun-Buisson C, Blot F, Lefort Y, Lemaire F, Brochard L. Association of noninvasive ventilation with nosocomial infections and survival in critically ill patients. *JAMA*. 2000;284(18):2361–2367.

197. Nava S, Hill N. Non-invasive ventilation in acute respiratory failure. *The Lancet*. 2009;374(9685):250–259.

198. Carter C, Aedy H, Notter J. COVID-19 disease: non-invasive ventilation and high frequency nasal oxygenation. *Clin Integr Care*. 2020;1(100006).

199. Arulkumaran N, Brealey D, Howell D, Singer M. Use of non-invasive ventilation for patients with COVID-19: a cause for concern?. *The Lancet Respiratory Medicine*. 2020;8(6):e45.

200. Galiatsou E, Kostanti E, Svarna E, Kitsakos A, Koulouras V, Efremidis SC, Nakos G. Prone position augments recruitment and prevents alveolar overinflation in acute lung injury. *American Journal of Respiratory and Critical Care Medicine*. 2006;174(2):187–197.

201. Thompson AE, Ranard BL, Wei Y, Jelic S. Prone positioning in awake, nonintubated patients with COVID-19 hypoxemic respiratory failure. *JAMA Internal Medicine*. 2020;180(11):1537–1539.

202. Shelhamer MC, Wesson PD, Solari IL, Jensen DL, Steele WA, Dimitrov VG, Kelly JD, Aziz S, Gutierrez VP, Vittinghoff E. Prone positioning in moderate to severe acute respiratory distress syndrome due to COVID-19: a cohort study and analysis of physiology. *Journal of Intensive Care Medicine*. 2021;36(2):241–252.

203. Ehrmann S, Li J, Ibarra-Estrada M, Perez Y, Pavlov I, McNicholas B, Roca O, Mirza S, Vines D, Garcia-Salcido R. Awake prone positioning for COVID-19 acute hypoxaemic respiratory failure: a randomised, controlled, multinational, open-label meta-trial. *The Lancet Respiratory Medicine*. 2021;9(12):1387–1395.

204. Guan W-j, Ni Z-y, Hu Y, Liang W-h, Ou C-q, He J-x, Liu L, Shan H, Lei C-l, Hui DS. Clinical characteristics of coronavirus disease 2019 in China. *New England Journal of Medicine*. 2020;382(18):1708–1720.

205. Pulse. Differentiating viral Covid-19 pneumonia from bacterial pneumonia [https://www.pulsetoday.co.uk/covid-19-primary-care-resources/guides/differentiating-viral-covid-19-pneumonia-from-bacterial-pneumonia/]

206. Attaway AH, Scheraga RG, Bhimraj A, Biehl M, Hatipoğlu U. Severe COVID-19 pneumonia: pathogenesis and clinical management. *BMJ*. 2021;372:n436.

207. Widemann HP, National Heart L. Blood institute acute respiratory distress syndrome clinical trials network: comparison of two fluid-management strategies in acute lung injury. *New England Journal of Medicine*. 2006;354(24):2564–2575.

208. Frat J-P, Thille AW, Mercat A, Girault C, Ragot S, Perbet S, Prat G, Boulain T, Morawiec E, Cottereau A. High-flow oxygen through nasal cannula in acute hypoxemic respiratory failure. *New England Journal of Medicine*. 2015;372(23):2185–2196.

209. Amato MB, Meade MO, Slutsky AS, Brochard L, Costa EL, Schoenfeld DA, Stewart TE, Briel M, Talmor D, Mercat A. Driving pressure and survival in the acute respiratory distress syndrome. *New England Journal of Medicine*. 2015;372(8):747–755.

210. Li Z, Niu S, Guo B, Gao T, Wang L, Wang Y, Wang L, Tan Y, Wu J, Hao J. Stem cell therapy for COVID-19, ARDS and pulmonary fibrosis. *Cell Proliferation*. 2020;53(12):e12939.

211. Zanirati G, Provenzi L, Libermann LL, Bizotto SC, Ghilardi IM, Marinowic DR, Shetty AK, Da Costa JC. Stem cell-based therapy for COVID-19 and ARDS: a systematic review. *NPJ Regenerative Medicine*. 2021;6(1):1–15.

212. Shetty AK, Shetty PA, Zanirati G, Jin K. Further validation of the efficacy of mesenchymal stem cell infusions for

reducing mortality in COVID-19 patients with ARDS. *NPJ Regenerative Medicine*. 2021;6(1):1–3.

213. Lanzoni G, Linetsky E, Correa D, Messinger Cayetano S, Alvarez RA, Kouroupis D, Alvarez Gil A, Poggioli R, Ruiz P, Marttos AC. Umbilical cord mesenchymal stem cells for COVID-19 acute respiratory distress syndrome: a double-blind, phase 1/2a, randomized controlled trial. *Stem Cells Translational Medicine*. 2021;10(5):660–673.

214. Rajdev K, Spanel AJ, McMillan S, Lahan S, Boer B, Birge J, Thi M. Pulmonary barotrauma in COVID-19 patients with ARDS on invasive and non-invasive positive pressure ventilation. *Journal of Intensive Care Medicine*. 2021:08850666211019719.

215. Kangas-Dick A, Gazivoda V, Ibrahim M, Sun A, Shaw JP, Brichkov I, Wiesel O. Clinical characteristics and outcome of pneumomediastinum in patients with COVID-19 pneumonia. *Journal of Laparoendoscopic & Advanced Surgical Techniques*. 2021;31(3):273–278.

216. Ramalingam S, Arora H, Gunasekaran K, Muruganandam M, Nagaraju S. A unique case of spontaneous pneumomediastinum in a patient with COVID-19 and influenza coinfection. *Journal of Investigative Medicine High Impact Case Reports*. 2021;9:23247096211016228.

217. Cuker A, Tseng EK, Nieuwlaat R, Angchaisuksiri P, Blair C, Dane K, Davila J, DeSancho MT, Diuguid D, Griffin DO. American Society of Hematology 2021 guidelines on the use of anticoagulation for thromboprophylaxis in patients with COVID-19. *Blood Advances*. 2021;5(3):872–888.

218. Matli K, Farah R, Maalouf M, Chamoun N, Costanian C, Ghanem G. Role of combining anticoagulant and antiplatelet agents in COVID-19 treatment: a rapid review. *Open Heart*. 2021;8(1):e001628.

219. Canna SW, Behrens EM. Making sense of the cytokine storm: a conceptual framework for understanding, diagnosing, and treating hemophagocytic syndromes. *Pediatric Clinics*. 2012;59(2):329–344.

220. Melo AKG, Milby KM, Caparroz ALM, Pinto ACP, Santos RR, Rocha AP, Ferreira GA, Souza VA, Valadares LD, Vieira RM. Biomarkers of cytokine storm as red flags for severe and fatal COVID-19 cases: a living systematic review and meta-analysis. *PloS One*. 2021;16(6):e0253894.

221. Martínez-Sanz J, Muriel A, Ron R, Herrera S, Pérez-Molina JA, Moreno S, Serrano-Villar S. Effects of tocilizumab on mortality in hospitalized patients with COVID-19: a multicentre cohort study. *Clinical Microbiology and Infection*. 2021;27(2):238–243.

222. Gupta S, Wang W, Hayek SS, Chan L, Mathews KS, Melamed ML, Brenner SK, Leonberg-Yoo A, Schenck EJ, Radbel J. Association between early treatment with tocilizumab and mortality among critically ill patients with COVID-19. *JAMA Internal Medicine*. 2021;181(1):41–51.

223. Salama C, Han J, Yau L, Reiss WG, Kramer B, Neidhart JD, Criner GJ, Kaplan-Lewis E, Baden R, Pandit L. Tocilizumab in patients hospitalized with Covid-19 pneumonia. *New England Journal of Medicine*. 2021;384(1):20–30.

224. Horby P, Group RC. Dexamethasone in hospitalized patients with Covid-19. *New England Journal of Medicine*. 2021;384(8):693–704.

225. Dexamethasone and Oxygen Support Strategies in ICU Patients With Covid-19 Pneumonia (COVIDICUS) [https://clinicaltrials.gov/ct2/show/NCT04344730]

226. Singh AK, Singh R, Joshi SR, Misra A. Mucormycosis in COVID-19: a systematic review of cases reported worldwide and in India. *Diabetes & Metabolic Syndrome: Clinical Research & Reviews*. 2021;15(4):102146.

227. Beigel JH, Tomashek KM, Dodd LE, Mehta AK, Zingman BS, Kalil AC, Hohmann E, Chu HY, Luetkemeyer A, Kline S. Remdesivir for the treatment of Covid-19. *New England Journal of Medicine*. 2020;383(19):1813–1826.

228. Mariette X, Hermine O, Tharaux P-L, Resche-Rigon M, Steg PG, Porcher R, Ravaud P. Effectiveness of tocilizumab in patients hospitalized with COVID-19: a follow-up of the CORIMUNO-TOCI-1 randomized clinical trial. *JAMA Internal Medicine*. 2021;181(9):1241–1243.

229. Goletti D, Cantini F. Baricitinib therapy in Covid-19 pneumonia: an unmet need fulfilled. *New England Journal of Medicine*. 2021;384(9):867–869.

230. National Institutes of Health. Therapeutic Management of Nonhospitalized and Hospitalized Patients with Confirmed Coronavirus Disease (COVID-19) [https://www.covid19treatmentguidelines.nih.gov/management/clinical-management/hospitalized-adults-therapeutic-management/]

231. Clancy CJ, Schwartz IS, Kula B, Nguyen MH: Bacterial superinfections among persons with coronavirus disease 2019: a comprehensive review of data from postmortem studies. In: Open Forum Infectious Diseases: 2021. New York: Oxford University Press US: ofab065.

232. Beović B, Doušak M, Ferreira-Coimbra J, Nadrah K, Rubulotta F, Belliato M, Berger-Estilita J, Ayoade F, Rello J, Erdem H. Antibiotic use in patients with COVID-19: a 'snapshot' Infectious Diseases International Research Initiative (ID-IRI) survey. *Journal of Antimicrobial Chemotherapy*. 2020;75(11):3386–3390.

233. Pettit NN, Nguyen CT, Lew AK, Bhagat PH, Nelson A, Olson G, Ridgway JP, Pho MT, Pagkas-Bather J. Reducing the use of empiric antibiotic therapy in COVID-19 on hospital admission. *BMC Infectious Diseases*. 2021;21(1):1–7.

COVID-19 and the Cardiovascular System

6

Subramani Mani, MBBS, PhD, and Mark E. Garcia, MD

The heart, like the brain and liver, is a solitary vital organ. Anatomically and physiologically the heart plays a central role by pumping blood to various organs and tissues of the body, keeping them perfused and oxygenated and thereby maintaining their critical and life-sustaining functions. Disease processes involving the heart and causing cardiac injury are a matter of grave concern because of the potential for increased mortality and morbidity.

Epidemiology of Cardiac Injury From COVID-19

Precise estimates of the extent of cardiac injury and their ramifications in hospitalized patients with coronavirus disease 2019 (COVID-19) are difficult to determine. Thus the prevalence and clinical impact reported by various investigators vary depending on study sample characteristics and geography. Many of the early studies are reports from Wuhan and other regions of China because the initial outbreak occurred in the city of Wuhan and subsequently spread to different parts of Hubei and other provinces of China. Moreover, many of the patients hospitalized with COVID-19 had comorbidities of high blood pressure (BP) and cardiovascular disease (CVD) confounding precise estimates of new cardiac injury resulting from COVID-19. A study of 138 hospitalized patients with COVID-19 in Wuhan reported that 41 (31%) had high BP and 20 (15%) had CVD.[1] During the course of hospitalization, 23 (17%) developed arrhythmia and 10 (7%) manifested acute cardiac injury.[1] Another multicenter cohort study of 191 hospitalized patients with COVID-19 (135 from Jinyintan hospital and 56 from Wuhan pulmonary hospital) reported cardiovascular comorbidities of high BP in 58 patients (30%) and coronary artery disease (CAD) in 15 patients (8%).[2] The study also reported acute cardiac injury in 33 patients (17%).[2] Guo et al.[3] in a study of 187 patients hospitalized with COVID-19 in Wuhan city reported comorbidities of high BP in 61 patients (33%), CAD in 21 patients (11%), and cardiomyopathy in 8 patients (4%).[3] The study reported that 52 (28%) patients showed acute myocardial injury based on elevated troponin T level measurements.[3] A multicenter study of 5700 patients with COVID-19 admitted to hospitals in New York City and nearby regions reported comorbidities of high BP in 3026 patients (57%), CAD in 595 patients (11%), and congestive heart failure (CHF) in 371 patients (7%).[4] Based on elevated troponin levels, 801 patients (23%) showed evidence of acute myocardial injury.[4]

In a study of 2736 patients admitted to the Mount Sinai Health Systems Hospitals in New York City with COVID-19, Lala et al.[5] reported comorbidities of atrial fibrillation in 206 patients (8%), CAD in 453 patients (17%), heart failure (HF) in 276 patients (10%), and high BP in 1065 patients (39%).[5] Based on elevated troponin concentrations, a total of 985 patients (36%) demonstrated the presence of cardiac injury.[5]

From a meta-analysis of 20 studies with a pooled total of 6130 patients (range 21–2736), Fu et al.[6] reported a prevalence of 22% for cardiac injury (95% confidence interval [CI], 16%–28%). In their review of 26 studies involving a large patient population of 11,685, Bavishi et al.[7] reported a prevalence of 20% (range 5%–38%) for acute myocardial injury.

These studies provide a broad estimate in the range of 20% to 35% for acute myocardial injury in patients hospitalized with COVID-19.

History of Cardiovascular Effects From SARS-CoV-1 and MERS-CoV

The first SARS-CoV outbreak occurred in late 2002 and soon became a pandemic in early 2003, resulting in the death of more than 700 people, with a large cluster of fatalities reported from Hong Kong. This SARS-CoV-1 virus is thought to have originated in a single or multiple species of bats.[8] A more recent coronavirus pathogen is the Middle Eastern respiratory syndrome (MERS) coronavirus (MERS-CoV), which first emerged in 2012 in Saudi Arabia and spread to many countries in the region. By 2018, MERS-CoV had infected more than 2000 people, causing 803 deaths, the majority of them in Saudi Arabia. Camels and bats are considered to be reservoirs of this pathogen.[9]

Before the emergence of SARS, human coronaviruses typically caused only mild upper respiratory tract infections, resulting in the common cold. All this changed with the emergence of SARS-CoV, MERS-CoV, and the newest member SARS-CoV-2, the causative agent of the COVID-19 pandemic. Because the SARS-CoV-2 pandemic is still evolving, and there is considerable variance in testing protocols among the different countries, a precise mortality rate is hard to determine. Moreover, a majority of SARS-CoV-2 infections are thought to be asymptomatic or quite mild. Based on reported confirmed cases and deaths the world over, the mortality rate appears to be in the range of 2% to 3%.[10] In comparison, the mortality rate for SARS-CoV-1 was 10% and that of MERS-CoV 37%.[11]

A variety of thrombotic and hematological manifestations were reported with SARS-CoV-1 infection. They include pulmonary embolism (PE), deep vein thrombosis, venous thromboembolism (VTE), and pulmonary artery thrombosis.[12]

MERS-CoV disease is also associated with thrombotic and hematological manifestations. Thrombocytopenia was reported in about a third of laboratory-confirmed MERS-CoV patients and MERS-CoV–induced disseminated intravascular coagulation (DIC) was also reported.[12] Different types of cardiac manifestations

such as acute myocarditis, acute myocardial infarction (AMI), and HF were described in patients hospitalized with SARS-CoV-1 and MERS-CoV.[13] However, acute myocardial injury, including myocarditis, was not widespread with SARS-CoV-1 infections.[14]

SARS-CoV-1 can infect different types of immune cells, including monocytes, macrophages, and activated T lymphocytes, but can undergo replication only in alveolar epithelial cells. MERS-CoV is more aggressive; it infects the immune cells and alveolar epithelial cells and replicates inside these host cell types and lyses them.[15]

Pathophysiology and Potential Mechanisms of Cardiovascular Injury From COVID-19

SARS-CoV-2 is primarily a respiratory virus, and its predominant target is the lung. Like any major extrapulmonary organ, the heart and the general vasculature are also broadly susceptible in two ways: (1) direct infection of the cardiac tissue by the virus; and (2) indirect or systemic effects resulting from the host inflammatory response, endothelial activation, thrombotic changes, and coagulation dysfunction.[7,16–26] Fig. 6.1 provides an overview of these mechanisms of cardiac injury. The pathophysiology of cardiovascular injury is largely dependent on the renin-angiotensin system (RAS), which plays a key role in cardiovascular homeostasis.

Renin-Angiotensin System

The local RAS[27,28] plays a key role in mediating and channeling the mechanistic forces responsible for cardiovascular injury.[29] The RAS system and more specifically the hormone angiotensin is responsible for the maintenance of the cardiovascular homeostasis. The classic and counterregulatory renin-angiotensin (RA) pathways play key regulatory roles in this modulation of cardiovascular physiology. The key components of the *classic* RA pathway are (1) angiotensinogen is converted to angiotensin-1 by renin and (2) angiotensin-1 is further processed by the angiotensin-converting enzyme (ACE) to angiotensin-2. Angiotensin-2 induces vasoconstriction by binding to angiotensin-1 receptors (AT1Rs) on the vascular smooth muscle cells and also by the release of aldosterone from the adrenal cortex. In addition to vasoconstriction, activation of AT1R results in sympathetic stimulation, cardiac hypertrophy, fibrosis, and inflammation.[29]

The *counterregulatory* RA pathway has two salient components: (1) Angiotensin-1 is cleaved by angiotensin-converting enzyme 2 (ACE2) to generate angiotensin 1-9; (2) angiotensin 1-7 is formed by cleavage of

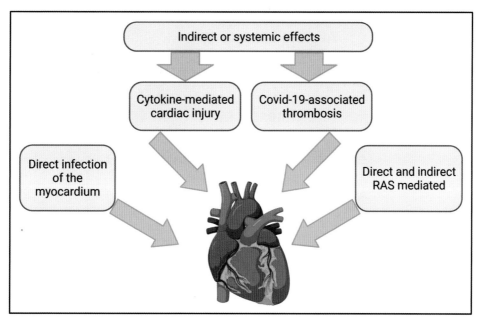

Fig. 6.1 Direct and Indirect Mechanisms of Cardiac Injury in COVID-19. There are two direct causes of cardiac injury—direct infection of the myocardium by the SARS-CoV-2 virus and direct renin-angiotensin system (RAS)–mediated injury, which is caused by the local cardiac RAS. The three indirect mechanisms are the cytokine-mediated cardiac injury, COVID-19 associated coagulation (thrombosis), and the injury resulting from systemic RAS. (Created with Biorender.)

angiotensin-2 by ACE2. Angiotensin 1-9 activates angiotensin-2 receptors (AT2R) to trigger nitric oxide production resulting in vasodilatation and concomitant lowering of BP. Angiotensin 1-7 binds to the proto-oncogene Mas receptor (MasR) causing dilatation of blood vessels and a reduction in BP. Both angiotensin 1-9 and angiotensin 1-7 peptides are cardioprotective and reduce inflammation, cardiac hypertrophy, and fibrosis.[29] Both receptors AT1R and AT2R are expressed in the heart and blood vessels.[27] Fig. 6.2 shows the regulatory and counterregulatory arms of the RAS.

ACE2 is a key element of the counterregulatory arm of RAS and is an essential regulator of heart function.[30] ACE2 is also the functional receptor for SARS-CoV-2; the SARS-CoV-2 spike protein binds to ACE2 for cellular entry of the virus. ACE2 has been shown to be upregulated in HF[31] and ACE2 mRNA levels are elevated in myocardial infarction (MI).[32] Inflammatory processes play a key role in the pathogenesis and natural history of many CVDs, including atherosclerosis, hypertension, cardiomyopathy, MI, and cardiac failure.[29,33–36] SARS-CoV-2 infection causes a functional depletion of ACE2 as the virus binds to ACE2 receptors for cellular entry. This causes downregulation of the counterregulatory arm of RAS and accumulation of angiotensin-2. Angiotensin-2 in turn binds to AT1R, triggering cardiac injury.

Direct Infection of the Myocardium

Direct entry of SARS-CoV-2 into cells is facilitated by the affinity of the viral spike protein S to the host cell ACE2 receptor, with the host protease transmembrane

protease serine 2 (TMPRSS2), acting as the enabler.[37,38] Many organs and tissues of the body express both ACE2 and TMPRSS2, including the lungs, heart, gut, liver, kidney, neurons, joints, and eye,[39–42] and this explains the tropism and potential of the virus to cause injury to these organs and tissues. Moreover, Chen et al.[39] showed that although the expression levels of ACE2 are lower in the heart compared with the gut and kidney, the levels were higher in the heart than in the lungs, which act as the primary targets for SARS-CoV-2.[39] Fig. 6.3 presents the ACE2 receptor expression profile in the cardiovascular system.

Different studies and case reports have demonstrated the presence of SARS-CoV-2 genomic RNA or viral particles morphologically identified as SARS-CoV-2 in myocardial tissue obtained from biopsy-confirmed myocarditis patients.[20,43,44] Tavazzi et al.[43] reported one of the earliest cases of biopsy-proven myocardial localization of viral particles with the morphology of a coronavirus in a COVID-19 patient who presented with cardiogenic shock. Escher et al.[44] identified SARS-CoV-2 genomic RNA in 5 of 104 endomyocardial biopsy (EMB) samples of patients with suspected myocarditis or unexplained HF.[44] A more recent study by Bearse et al.[20] looked at 41 consecutive autopsies of patients who died from COVID-19 to understand the relationship of myocardial injury to SARS-CoV-2 infection. Based on in situ hybridization (ISH) and NanoString transcriptomic (NST) profiling, the researchers determined that endomyocardial infection by SARS-CoV-2 was present in 30 of 41 cases (73%).[20] Cellular targets for SARS-CoV-2 include cardiomyocytes, pericytes, fibroblasts, and

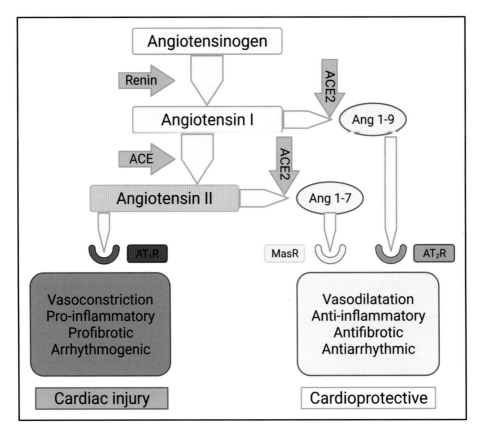

Fig. 6.2 Renin-Angiotensin System (RAS). Both the classic regulatory RAS pathway (Angiotensinogen → Angiotensin-1 → Angiotensin-2) and the counterregulatory pathway (Angiotensin-1 → Angiotensin 1-9, Angiotensin-2 → Angiotensin 1-7) are shown. The classic RAS arm can induce cardiac injury when excessive angiotensin-2 binds to AT1R. When SARS-CoV-2 saturates angiotensin-converting enzyme-2 (ACE2), which the virus binds for cellular entry, the counterregulatory arm is downregulated as less ACE2 is available. The counterregulatory RAS arm is cardioprotective. *AT1R,* Angiotensin type 1 receptor; *AT2R,* angiotensin-2 receptor angiotensin-2 receptor, *MasR,* MAS receptor. (Created with Biorender.)

resident macrophages of the heart.[14] Fig. 6.4 provides additional details of the mechanism of SARS-CoV-2 entry into the heart and blood vessels.

Based on ISH, NST profiling for virus positivity and histopathological findings of inflammatory infiltrates characteristic of myocyte injury for defining myocarditis, the researchers partitioned their study sample (n = 41) in three groups—virus-positive with myocarditis (n = 4), virus-positive without myocarditis (n = 26), and virus-negative without myocarditis (n = 11) to study the relationship between cardiac pathological changes and cardiac infection by the SARS-CoV-2 virus.[20] Table 6.1 presents the details of the pathological findings in the various groups. Electrocardiographic (ECG) abnormalities in the form of atrial fibrillation, premature atrial complexes, prolongation of QTc, and nonspecific ST segment and T wave alterations were observed disproportionately in patients whose hearts were infected with SARS-CoV-2.[20]

Pellegrini et al.[45] in their histopathological study of 40 patients hospitalized with COVID-19 who subsequently died, report that SARS-CoV-2 RNA was much more prevalent in the lung tissue (34/40 [85%]) compared with cardiac tissue (8/40 [20%])[45]

Cytokine-Mediated Cardiac Injury

The systemic inflammatory response, and the resulting concomitant cytokine storm, is a major contributor to cardiac injury from SARS-CoV-2 infection.[2,7,14,19,46–51] The aggravated inflammatory reaction resulting in increased cytokine production and release occurring in critically ill patients leads to the development of disseminated intravascular coagulopathy (DIC). In a study of 183 hospitalized patients with COVID-19 pneumonia, Tang et al.[52] reported that DIC was observed in most of the 21 patients who did not survive.[52] DIC could lead to microvascular thrombosis in coronary vessels resulting in myocardial injury.[14,53] Fig. 6.5 provides a summary of the cytokine storm phenomenon and its salient characteristics.

COVID-19–Associated Thrombosis

Critically ill hospitalized patients are at a high risk for thromboembolic complications.[12,54] In a cohort of 170 COVID-19 patients in intensive care in Boston area hospitals, more than 35% developed arterial or venous thromboemblism.[55] COVID-19–associated coagulopathy (CAC) has been postulated as a distinct condition separate from DIC and coagulation abnormalities resulting

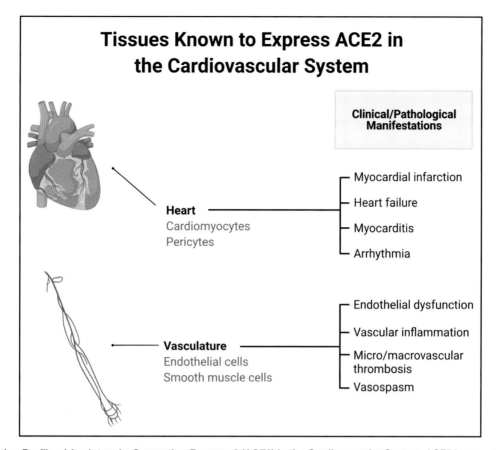

Fig. 6.3 Expression Profile of Angiotensin-Converting Enzyme-2 (ACE2) in the Cardiovascular System. ACE2 is expressed in the cardiomyocytes and pericytes of the heart and the endothelial and smooth muscle cells of the vasculature. The clinical and pathological manifestations resulting from SARS-CoV-2 infection of the heart and the vasculature are also enumerated. (Created with Biorender.)

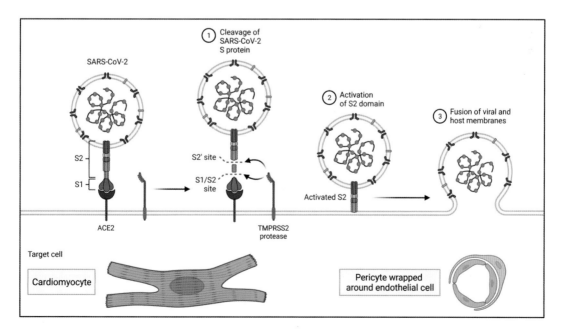

Fig. 6.4 SARS-CoV-2 Viral Entry. The virus enters the target cells—cardiomyocytes and pericytes—by binding to the angiotensin-converting enzyme-2 receptor. The viral entry and activation are facilitated by the cleavage of the SARS-CoV-2 S glycoprotein by TMPRSS2. Activation of the S2 domain of the S protein results in the fusion of the viral and host cell membrane, enabling entry of viral RNA into the host cell. *TMPRSS2,* Transmembrane protease serine 2. (Created with Biorender.)

Table 6.1 Findings of Cardiac Pathological Changes With SARS-CoV-2 Infection of the Heart (n = 41)

Description of Observed Pathological Conditions	Virus(+) With Myocarditis (n = 4)	Virus(+) Without Myocarditis (n = 26)	Virus(−) Without Myocarditis (n = 11)
SARS-CoV-2+ (cells/cm³)	1.2	1.2	0.2
Microthrombi present	1 (25%)	4 (15%)	0 (0%)
CD68+ CD3+ CD4+ density	High	Low	Low
Focal pericarditis	2 (50%)	6 (23%)	1 (9%)
Heart weight (grams)	593	449	480
Severe coronary artery disease	1 (25%)	5 (19%)	3 (27%)

Data from Bearse M, Hung YP, Krauson AJ, et al. Factors associated with myocardial SARS-CoV-2 infection, myocarditis, and cardiac inflammation in patients with COVID-19. *Mod Pathol.* 2021;1-13.

from acute respiratory distress syndrome (ARDS).[54,56,57] In the natural history of COVID-19, dysregulated coagulation has been documented in various studies as contributing to increased disease severity and higher mortality.[2,58,59] The causative mechanisms of CAC are multifactorial. Direct invasion of the vascular endothelium by SARS-CoV-2, inflammatory cytokines such as interleukin-6 (IL-6), IL-8, and tumor necrosis factor-alpha, and coagulation factors such as factor VIII, von Willebrand factor, and angiopoietin-2 are all significant contributors to the prothrombotic state, resulting in thrombus formation in COVID-19.[60,61]

DIC is characterized by a marked elevation in D-dimer and prothrombin time (PT) with concomitant reduction in fibrinogen and significant thrombocytopenia.[60] In CAC, D-dimer and fibrinogen are elevated and the PT is not markedly increased. Thrombocytopenia is also not a characteristic feature of CAC.[60] However, the CAC can evolve into a decompensated coagulopathy in critically ill COVID-19 patients.[60] Fibrinolysis suppression leading to fibrinolytic shutdown also has been observed in severe COVID-19 complicated by CAC.[60,62] There seems to be significant overlap in the pathophysiology of DIC and CAC. However, arterial thrombosis and vascular complications are characteristic of CAC[60] and microvascular thrombosis in coronary arteries is a distinct possibility.

Bois et al.[63] in their histopathological study of 15 COVID-19 patients found nonocclusive fibrin microthrombi without ischemic injury in 12 cases, but its clinical significance is not clear.[63] A larger histopathological study by Pellegrini et al.[45] that studied the hearts of 40 patients who died from COVID-19 reported that 14 of 40 subjects (35%) had evidence of cardiac injury in the form of myocyte necrosis. Most of them, 11 of 14 (79%), demonstrated focal myocyte necrosis; the major cause of myocyte necrosis was cardiac microthrombi, which were observed in 9 of 14 (64%) hearts with myocyte necrosis.[45] Both of these studies demonstrate the significance of microvascular thrombosis as a cause of cardiac injury in hospitalized patients with COVID-19.

Another potential pathophysiological mechanism of cardiac injury is the downregulation of ACE2 in SARS-CoV-2 infection. This was demonstrated in the mouse model by Oudit et al.[64] As mentioned earlier, ACE2 has been shown to have a protective effect on the heart and blood vessels based on its antiinflammatory,

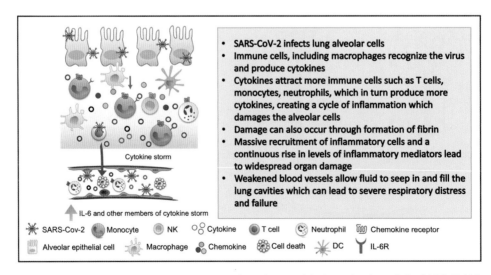

Fig. 6.5 Cytokine Storm. The immune response goes into overdrive after infection of the lung alveolar cells by SARS-CoV-2, resulting in cytokine release. The cytokines attract more immune cells, creating a vicious cycle causing large amounts of cytokines and chemokines to be released. Apart from local organ damage, a prolonged systemic elevation of large quantities of inflammatory cytokines and chemokines occurs, leading to damage to other vital organs such as the heart, liver, kidneys, and the brain. *DC,* Dendritic cell; *IL-6R,* interleukin-6 receptor; *NK,* natural killer (cell). (Modified from Lu L, Zhang H, Zhan M, et al. Preventing mortality in COVID-19 patients: which cytokine to target in a raging storm? *Front Cell Dev Biol.* 2020;8:677, with permission (creative common license. Created with Biorender.)

antifibrotic, antioxidative, and vasodilatory properties.[65] ACE2 converts angiotensin-2 to angiotensin 1-7, which reduces vasoconstriction mediated by the RAS. The downregulation of ACE2 causes angiotensin-2 to be upregulated, which results in an increased production of inflammatory cytokines[61,66] (see Fig. 6.2).

Clinical Manifestations and Complications

A spectrum of cardiovascular manifestations has been reported with SARS-CoV-2 infection.[3,6,18,20,24,40,42,67–93] The CVD presentations of COVID-19 include myocarditis,[20,94–96] acute coronary syndrome,[14,69,97–100] HF,[90,95,101–104] cardiac arrhythmias,[24,48,105–111] and various types of vascular complications and thromboembolic events.[12,16,17,21,22,26,52,54–60,62,63,75,112–123] Fig. 6.6 depicts the spectrum of cardiovascular clinical manifestations and complications of COVID-19.

Myocarditis

Myocarditis can result from direct viral myocardial invasion or consequent to systemic inflammation. A clinical diagnosis of myocarditis is arrived at based on laboratory and imaging markers of myocyte involvement such as elevated troponin levels and cardiac magnetic resonance (CMR) imaging features.[73,94,124] It is important to

exclude CAD, and when CMR is not feasible, it is recommended that cardiac CT angiography may be performed.[125] The clinical presentation of myocarditis can be variable from mild disease to fulminant myocarditis complicated by arrhythmias, HF, and cardiogenic shock.[126,127] Atrial and ventricular arrhythmias are quite common in the setting of myocarditis.[128,129] Various pathophysiological mechanisms have been postulated for the observed arrhythmicity in myocarditis.[125,129] Fig. 6.7 provides an illustration of these mechanisms leading to various types of arrhythmias in myocarditis. Myocarditis is an uncommon pathological diagnosis occurring in 5% to 10% of highly selected cases undergoing autopsy or EMB.[20,44,94] Elevated troponin levels have been shown to be associated with higher mortality in the setting of COVID-19.[2,3] The sequelae of myocarditis such as low-grade inflammation and fibrosis play a major role in disease progression leading to HF.[95]

It is important to distinguish fulminant myocarditis from sepsis; other differential diagnoses include acute coronary syndrome and sepsis-related cardiomyopathy.[125] Echocardiography, CMR, and cardiac computed tomography (CT) are useful in resolving the differential diagnosis; for a definitive diagnosis, EMB may be required.[125]

Acute Coronary Syndrome

Severe systemic inflammation, increased levels of circulating cytokines, and a hypercoagulable state observed

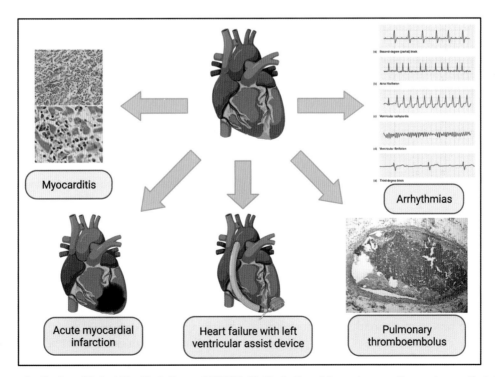

Fig. 6.6 Cardiovascular System Clinical Manifestations of COVID-19. Illustration of the various cardiovascular manifestations and complications such as myocarditis, acute myocardial infarction, heart failure, arrhythmias, and pulmonary embolism. (Created with Wikimedia image icons under creative commons license and Biorender.)

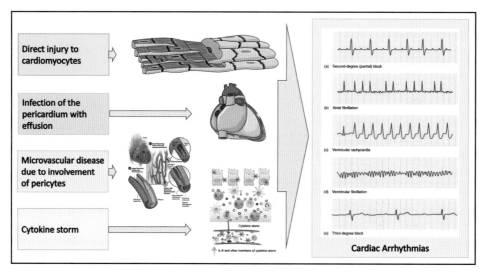

Fig. 6.7 Pathophysiological Mechanisms of Arrhythmias in Myocarditis. The figure illustrates four postulated mechanisms of arrhythmia generation in the setting of myocarditis: (1) direct injury to the cardiac muscle cells, (2) viral pericarditis with effusion, (3) microvascular disease due to infection of the pericytes by SARS-CoV-2, and (4) the systemic mechanism of cytokine storm. (Created with Wikimedia and Servier medical art icons under creative commons license.)

in COVID-19 have the potential for increased risk for AMI.[130] Based on a study of 28 COVID-19 patients with ST-elevation myocardial infarction (STEMI) from the Lombardy region of Italy, Stefanini et al.[100] reported that the first clinical manifestation of COVID-19 could be STEMI. Coronary angiography revealed a culprit lesion requiring revascularization in only 17 patients (61%), whereas the remaining 11 patients (39%) did not have obstructive CAD.[100] Diaz-Arocutipa et al.[99] performed a systematic review of 42 studies covering 161 COVID-19 patients with STEMI, which found obstructive CAD as the cause for ST elevation in 133 patients (83%). However, the mortality rate in the two groups, obstructive CAD, and nonobstructive CAD were similar ($\approx$ 30%).

The causes of acute myocardial injury in patients without CAD in the context of COVID-19 include myocarditis, cytokine storm and stress cardiomyopathy; hypoxemia, microvascular dysfunction resulting from small vessel thrombosis, and endotheliitis also have been postulated as potential causes in this setting.[14,123]

Heart Failure

HF occurs commonly in patients hospitalized with COVID-19. The prevalence is 25% among patients hospitalized with COVID-19 and about a third in patients whose condition is critical.[2,101] SARS-CoV-2 infection can also worsen preexisting cardiac failure, leading to a decompensated heart.[71] Based on a retrospective study of more than 132,000 hospitalized patients with a history of HF over a period of 6 months, the mortality rate among the three categories of hospitalized patients were as follows: (1) Non-COVID non-HF, 4512 deaths (4.5%); (2) non-COVID acute HF, 617 deaths (2.6%); and (3) COVID-19, 2026 deaths (24.2%).[131] Among hospitalized COVID-19 patients with a history of HF, with

a high risk for complications, 1 in 4 patients died during the course of hospitalization. As discussed earlier, SARS-CoV-2 uses the ACE2 receptor for cellular entry. The ACE2 receptor is known to be upregulated in the failing heart,[31] and this makes patients with a history of HF more susceptible to SARS-CoV-2 and potentially a more severe form of COVID-19.[131] Fig. 6.8 illustrates the pathophysiological mechanisms contributing to severe disease in COVID-19 patients presenting with a history of HF.[131–133]

Cardiac Arrhythmias

Early reports of the incidence of arrhythmias occurring in hospitalized patients with COVID-19 in Wuhan varied from 6% for ventricular arrhythmias[3] to 17% for all types of arrhythmias.[1] Based on their study of 700 patients hospitalized with COVID-19 at the University of Pennsylvania Hospital, Bhatla et al.[105] reported 53 arrhythmic events: 9 cardiac arrests, 25 atrial fibrillations, 9 clinically significant bradyarrhythmias, and 10 nonsustaining ventricular tachycardias. The cardiac arrests were independently associated with acute mortality whereas the other three types of arrhythmias did not independently contribute to increased mortality.

Based on a retrospective study of 4526 hospitalized patients worldwide with COVID-19, Coromilas et al.[134] reported an incidence of arrhythmias in 827 (18%) patients, most without a history of arrhythmias. Atrial fibrillation, atrial flutter, and supraventricular tachycardia were observed in 82% of the patients, ventricular arrhythmias were seen in 21%, and 23% developed bradyarrhythmias. Presence of arrhythmias resulted in an adverse prognosis; approximately 40% had to be mechanically ventilated, and the mortality in the arrhythmia group was 50%.

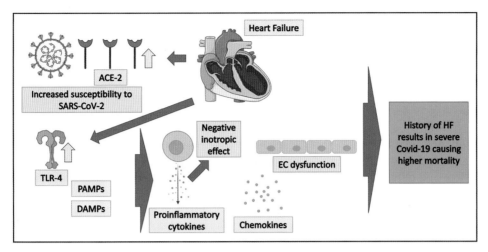

Fig. 6.8 Adverse COVID-19 Outcomes in Patients With History of Heart Failure *(HF)*. Angiotensin-converting enzyme-2 (ACE2) receptor is upregulated in individuals with a history of HF, making them more susceptible to SARS-CoV-2 and a severe disease course of COVID-19. In HF, Toll-like receptor-4 *(TLR-4)* is upregulated, and both the innate and adaptive immune systems are also activated with release of cytokines and chemokines. The activation of the innate immune response is mediated through PAMPs (derived from SARS-CoV-2) and DAMPs (released from compromised myocytes) binding to TLR-4. The proinflammatory cytokines that are released produce a negative inotropic effect. The negative inotropic effect causing reduced myocardial contractility, combined with the release of chemokines and endothelial cell dysfunction, result in further aggravation of HF, causing more severe disease and adverse outcomes. *DAMPs,* Damage-associated molecular patterns; *PAMPs,* pathogen-associated molecular patterns. (Created with Servier medical art icon under creative commons license and Biorender.)

Thromboembolic Events

VTE is common in hospitalized patients with COVID-19.[16] Wichmann et al.,[26] in their postmortem study of 12 consecutive deceased patients who had been hospitalized with COVID-19, found a high incidence of VTE (7/12 [58%]). Piazza et al.[55] observed an incidence of major arterial or venous thromboembolic event in in 60 of 170 (35%) patients with COVID-19 admitted to the intensive care unit (ICU), and in 6 of 229 (3%) in patients undergoing nonintensive care; DVT in 39 of 170 (23%) in the ICU setting and none in the non-ICU setting; PE in 3 of 170 (2%) in the ICU setting and 5 of 229 (2%) in the non-ICU setting.[55] Ribes et al.[135] in their review of thromboembolic events in COVID-19 reported a range of 25% to 69% for VTE in ICU setting, 15% to 53% for DVT in the non-ICU setting, 23% to 86% for DVT in the ICU setting, and an incidence of ≈ 20% for PE. In a multicenter cohort study of 1240 hospitalized patients with COVID-19, Fauvel et al.[136] reported an incidence of PE in 103 cases (8.3%).

Although D-dimer is a nonspecific marker of inflammation, a high level of D-dimer has been shown to be associated with adverse outcomes of severe and critical illness and higher mortality in hospitalized patients with COVID-19.[16,52,137] Prolonged PT also has been well-documented in hospitalized patients with COVID-19,[1,46] with worse prognosis and higher mortality associated with increase in PT.[2,52] The reduction in platelet count in hospitalized patients with COVID-19 has been mild to moderate but not clearly associated with severity of the disease.[16] However, Zhou et al.[2] reported that moderate thrombocytopenia was more frequent in nonsurvivors than among survivors.

Cardiovascular Comorbidities and COVID-19

The impact of cardiovascular comorbidities on COVID-19 resulting in adverse outcomes such as severe disease and increased mortality has been reported by various researchers.[4,89,138–143] Nashiry et al.[144] looked into the interactions of COVID-19 and cardiovascular comorbidities using a bioinformatics approach.[144] The two major cardiovascular comorbidities resulting in adverse outcomes in patients hospitalized with COVID-19 are CAD and hypertension.

Coronary Artery Disease

Based on their study of 8438 patients hospitalized with COVID-19 in the New York City area, of whom 9% had CAD, Kuno et al.[139] reported that patients with CAD had significantly higher rates of mechanical ventilation and mortality.[139] The relative risk for CAD was markedly higher for both mechanical ventilation and death in patients 50 years and younger.[139] Phelps et al.,[140] in their study of 4090 COVID-19–positive patients in Denmark, found that among patients who had severe disease or who died within 30 days of COVID-19 diagnosis, 20% had a history of CAD, and the representation of patients with a history of CAD in the nonsevere disease manifestation group was only 10%.[140]

Hypertension

Although the risk for infection with SARS-CoV-2 remains the same for hypertensive and normotensive individuals, patients with hypertension are at higher risk for developing a more severe disease and increased mortality.[77] However, Savoia et al.[145] and Kreutz et al.[146] argued that a direct role for hypertension as an independent risk factor for higher mortality in COVID-19 has not been clearly established. Because the prevalence of hypertension is higher in the older population, who have disproportionately suffered severe manifestations of COVID-19 resulting in increased mortality, the reported association between hypertension and severity of COVID-19 could be confounded by age and other comorbidities.[146]

Management of COVID-19–Related Cardiac Complications

The available evidence needed to guide management is mostly limited given the relative brief experience since the onset of SARS-CoV-2. This has left the medical community with little high-quality evidence on management of this disease. This holds especially true for the wide range of cardiovascular manifestations and complications. Most of the cardiovascular management strategies are from published regional experiences and extrapolations from prior well-established experiences.[14]

Myocardial Injury and Acute Coronary Syndromes

The assessment of troponin elevations with coexisting COVID-19 infection can be difficult in eliciting the cause. Myocardial injury defined as any cardiac troponin elevation is associated with significant morbidity and mortality.[23,147] Myocardial injury from COVID-19 is potentially from plaque rupture MI, inflammation, hypoxic injury, myocarditis, stress cardiomyopathy, microthrombi, or endothelial injury.[14,24,43] Management of troponin elevations in association with COVID-19 is mostly extrapolated from pre–COVID-19 existing recommendations.[14,147] Acute myocardial injury should initially be assessed for clinical deterioration, hemodynamic instability, and arrhythmias.[14] Imaging modalities should initially be performed with echocardiography and then consideration given for CMR imaging or CT scan based on clinical suspicion of the cause.[14,147] The majority of care is supportive in those with non–acute coronary syndrome troponin elevation. In general, supportive measures, including mechanical support, should be considered on a case-by-case basis.[14]

Troponin elevations in COVID-19 patients can be related to plaque rupture that is consistent with an AMI. During the COVID-19 pandemic, patients presenting with an AMI should be treated as probable or possible COVID-19 positive. Those presenting with a probable STEMI should be treated with a primary percutaneous coronary intervention (PCI) strategy in the standard of care fashion.[147,148] In those with ST elevations on electrocardiography and unclear diagnosis of STEMI, additional testing, including point-of-care ultrasound to evaluate for regional wall motion abnormality or coronary CT angiography (CCTA) in cases with conflicting information, may have to be considered.[148] The likelihood of having acute coronary syndromes versus nonacute coronary syndrome–associated troponin elevations should be weighed to help guide appropriate treatments.[147] Non–ST-elevation myocardial infarct (NSTEMI) management should be guided by risk stratification and identification of high-risk features.[147] A NSTEMI due to plaque rupture with high-risk features should be managed with an early invasive strategy with the intention of performing PCI; those without high-risk features should be carefully evaluated for alternative diagnoses. This should be undertaken along with management recommendations according to existing guidelines for noninvasive studies such as echocardiography or CCTA.[147,148]

Myocarditis

COVID-19 is associated with myocarditis, which can range from mild disease to fulminant myocarditis. The mechanism, risk factors, and prevalence are not well understood.[94,126,147] Myocarditis has a wide range of presentations but should be considered with new-onset HF, cardiogenic shock, and arrhythmias.[125,126] Troponin levels will be elevated and suggestive of myocardial injury but given the wide range of presentations, ischemia will often need to be ruled out first.[126] The troponin elevation associated with COVID-19 infections can be difficult to discern, creating a challenging diagnostic dilemma. Fig. 6.9 is useful in the approach to this management issue.[101]

Cardiac imaging plays an important role in diagnosis and prognosis in suspected COVID-19 myocarditis.[65,149] CMR imaging is the key imaging component to the diagnosis and prognosis in myocarditis.[65,88] CMR should use the Lake Louise consensus criteria for myocarditis evaluation.[125,150] If CMR is unavailable or cannot be performed, a cardiac CT scan with contrast and ECG gating should be considered.[125] Fig. 6.10 shows typical CMR features of myocarditis.[65] Fig. 6.11 shows CT scan features of COVID-19 pneumonia and myocarditis, and the CCTA study shows normal coronary arteries and can be used to rule out CAD.[149] EMB can be diagnostic for myocarditis but has the potential for yielding nondiagnostic results and causing significant complications. This has led to recommendations against routine EMB for suspected COVID-19–related myocarditis.[94,127,147,150]

The management of myocarditis associated with COVID-19 is extrapolated from existing evidence of viral myocarditis.[125] The mainstay of therapy is supportive care while managing potential hemodynamic instability/cardiogenic shock, HF, and tachyarrhythmias or bradyarrhythmias. An extremely severe form

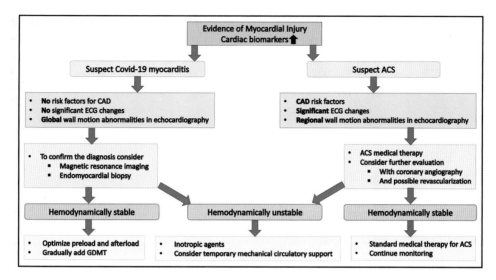

Fig. 6.9 Approach to the Management of COVID-19 Patients With Evidence of Myocardial Injury. An algorithm to manage cardiac injury based on a broad differentiation into viral myocarditis or acute coronary syndrome *(ACS)*, primarily a consequence of coronary artery disease *(CAD)*, and treat accordingly. The management converges into a common pathway if hemodynamic instability develops when inotropic agents and mechanical circulatory support devices would be needed. *ECG,* Electrocardiogram; *GDMT,* Guideline-directed medical therapy. (Figure redrawn from Bader F, Manla Y, Atallah B, Starling RC. Heart failure and COVID-19. *Heart Fail Rev.* 2021;26[1]:1-10.)

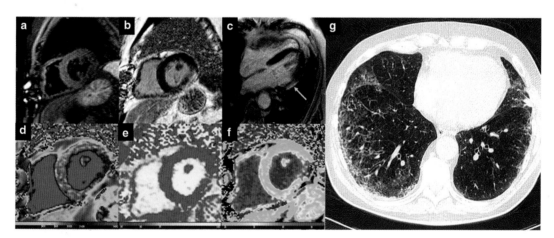

Fig. 6.10 COVID-19 Myocarditis. Patient with COVID-19 myocarditis. *(a)* Late gadolinium enhancement (LGE) of the inferolateral segments of the basal-midplanes with subepicardial pattern of distribution. *(b* and *c) Arrows* showing native T1 was increased on LGE-positive segments. *(d)* T2 mapping sequences revealed the presence of edema in the inferolateral segments of midventricular planes. *(e)* Extracellular volume (ECV) confirming presence of edema. *(g)* Chest computed tomography image showing ground-glass opacities in the inferior lobes with a peripheral distribution. (From Catapano F, Marchitelli L, Cundari G, et al. Role of advanced imaging in COVID-19 cardiovascular complications. *Insights Imaging.* 2021;12[1]:1-13, under creative commons license.)

of myocarditis, referred to as fulminant myocarditis, is associated with a rapid decline in cardiac function leading to cardiogenic shock. Hemodynamic support measures include inotropes and vasopressors along with mechanical circulatory support such as ventricular assist devices and extracorporeal membrane oxygenation.[125,126,150] The risk of using immunosuppressive agents in COVID-19 myocarditis is unknown, and it is reasonable to avoid these agents, especially during the active viral replication phase.[125] There is little evidence to support immunosuppression in suspected viral myocarditis and given the lack of data on guiding these therapies, there are no clear treatment recommendations.[125,147]

Heart Failure

HF in patients with COVID-19 infection is associated with increased morbidity and mortality.[2] COVID-19 and HF create a complex physiological cascade of multiple systemic and direct cardiac insults as described in Fig. 6.12.[101] The effects of these sequences of insults lead to the hemodynamic consequences resulting in decompensated HF. This can manifest as new-onset HF or an exacerbation or worsening of existing HF.[101,102]

Early in the pandemic, ACE inhibitors and angiotensin receptor blockers (ARBs) were thought to possibly increase COVID-19 infections. This was a cause for major concern, but multiple studies have now concluded that ACE inhibitors and ARBs are safe in COVID-19 infections

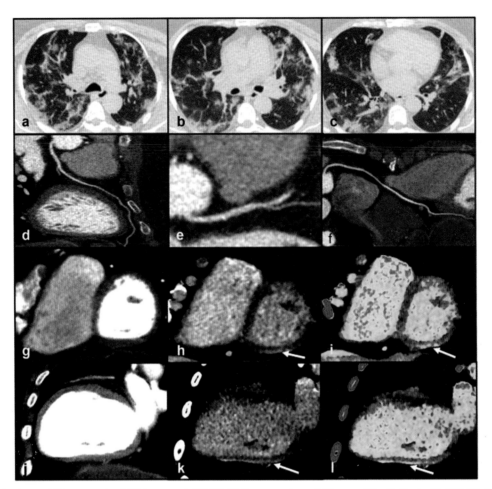

Fig. 6.11 Chest Computed Tomography (CT) Image of COVID-19 Pneumonia and Myocarditis. Patient with COVID-19 pneumonia with chest CT scan suggestive of myocarditis. (a, b, c) Bilateral ground-glass opacities with areas of consolidation. (d, e, f) Coronary CT tomography angiography (CCTA) excluding coronary artery disease in the left anterior descending artery (d), left circumflex (e) and right coronary artery (f). (g, j) CCTA excluding perfusion defects in the left ventricular myocardium. (h, k, i, l) Delayed postcontrast scan (h, k) and corresponding color-maps (i, l) with subepicardial area of hyperdensity in the basal, inferolateral wall of the left ventricle. (From Pontone G, Scafuri S, Mancini ME, et al. Role of computed tomography in COVID-19. J Cardiovasc Comput Tomogr. 2020;15[1]:27-36.)

and do not lead to increased COVID-19 test positivity.[151,152] ACE inhibitors and ARBs are a mainstay of treatment in HF, and these drugs should not be stopped in those with coexisting COVID-19 infections.[101,102,147,151,152] The same holds true for beta-blockers and mineralocorticoid receptor antagonists in chronic HF.[147]

Occurrence of HF in COVID-19 is common and is likely due to coexisting cardiovascular risk factors and the association with advanced age.[2,47] HF treatment should follow standards of care in accordance with guideline-directed medical therapy. Given the complexity of the HF management protocol, services of a multidisciplinary team that includes a HF expert should be availed in treating these complex patients.[101,147]

Hypertension

The association between hypertension and RAS inhibitors (ACE inhibitor and ARB) in COVID-19 infections is not clear and likely confounded by age and other comorbidities.[145,146] ACE inhibitors and ARBs are the cornerstones of therapy for hypertension and HF. They

are considered safe in COVID-19 patients with no evidence to support increased infectivity and should not be discontinued in patients with COVID-19.[138,145,146]

Cardiac Arrhythmias

In a large cohort study by Coromilas et al.,[134] the majority of arrhythmias in patients with COVID-19 were atrial arrhythmias (atrial fibrillation, atrial flutter, and supraventricular tachycardia). Ventricular arrhythmias, including ventricular tachycardia, nonsustained ventricular tachycardia, and ventricular fibrillation, were associated with significant mortality.[1] Arrhythmias were most common in patients in the ICU setting and corresponded to COVID-19 disease severity.[105,106,134] Mechanisms of arrhythmogenicity include myocardial injury, hypoxia, inflammation, autonomic system imbalances, electrolyte abnormalities, QT prolonging drugs, and cardiovascular comorbidities such as hypertension, CAD, and cardiomyopathies.[107] Many drug therapies, including hydroxychloroquine, azithromycin, tocilizumab, ritonavir, and many others, have been used in

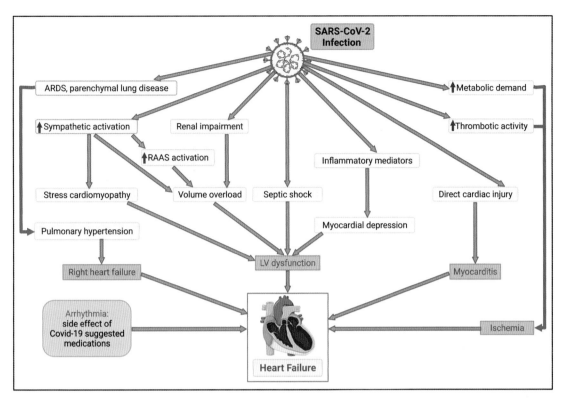

Fig. 6.12 Heart Failure (HF) and COVID-19. The physiological cascade of events resulting in HF through multiple mechanisms are shown. The intermediate stages of right heart failure, LV dysfunction, Myocarditis and ischemia are also illustrated. Both new HF and exacerbation of pre-existing HF occur in COVID-19. *ARDS,* Acute respiratory distress syndrome; *LV,* left ventricle; *RAAS,* renin-angiotensin-aldosterone system. (Redrawn from Bader F, Manla Y, Atallah B, Starling RC. Heart failure and COVID-19. *Heart Fail Rev.* 2021;26[1]:1-10.)

the treatment of COVID-19 infections and may prolong the QT interval and lead to polymorphic ventricular tachycardia (torsades de pointes).[107] In the study by Coromilas et al.,[134] the majority of the COVID-19–positive patients were treated with QTc prolonging medications but there were no differences in the type of arrhythmias based on drug therapy.

Specific treatment strategies on the management of COVID-19 patients with arrhythmias are limited by the lack of evidence, but mostly the treatment strategies will be similar to those in patients with infection-related arrhythmias and severe illnesses.[153] The management of arrhythmias needs to focus on awareness and continued emphasis of potential drug-drug interactions because many cardiac drugs (antiarrhythmic drugs, calcium channel blockers, beta-blockers, digoxin, and oral anticoagulants) can have significant interactions with COVID-19–specific therapies. These patients will need close observation and follow-up for development of arrhythmias using telemetry, routine electrocardiograms, and persistent monitoring for QTc prolongation.[107,153]

Thromboembolic Syndromes

COVID-19 disease severity is associated with higher risk for thromboembolic complications that increase mortality.[116] CAC is a fundamentally distinct process from DIC or other coagulopathies with a complex pathophysiological mechanism that is not fully understood. Although elevated D-dimer, fibrinogen, platelet counts, along with prolongation of prothrombin and proinflammatory states are key clinical features of CAC, the endothelial dysfunction component plays a unique and pivotal role in in this process.[52] Some of the more common clinical complications include microvascular thrombosis and venous and arterial thrombosis.[56]

Anticoagulation therapy in severe COVID-19 disease may be associated with decreased mortality.[154] Current treatment strategies are based on limited available data and experience to guide treatments, and most recommendations are formulations of professional bodies or expert opinions. This has provided the opportunity for institution-specific protocols.[56] Management strategies have varied based on COVID-19 disease severity, disease-specific conditions, and prevention versus treatment of thrombotic complications.[56,113,120] For VTE prophylaxis in hospitalized patients, there is consensus among leading societies to use prophylactic dose anticoagulation for hospitalized patients and data are insufficient to use higher than prophylactic dosing of anticoagulation for VTE prophylaxis.[113,155] Low-molecular-weight heparin and unfractionated heparin are preferred over oral anticoagulants because they have fewer drug-drug interactions. There are multiple drug-drug interactions with antiplatelet and oral anticoagulant medications involving the investigational COVID-19 treatments.[113,120,155]

Case Reports

Following our discussion of COVID-19–related clinical manifestations, complications, and their management, three case reports are presented that highlight and illustrate the impact on the heart and vasculature resulting from SARS-CoV-2 infection. These cases were selected from the pool of patients admitted to a tertiary care hospital attached to an academic medical center.

■ Case Report 6.1 COVID-19–Associated Myocarditis

This 52-year-old Hispanic man with no significant medical history had class I obesity with a body mass index (the weight in kilograms divided by the square of the height in meters) of 30. He was noted to have progressive cough, shortness of breath, and fevers of 40°C (104°F) for the past 5 days. He then developed acute-onset substernal chest pain prompting evaluation in the emergency department.

On presentation, he was febrile with a temperature of 40.2°C (104.4°F), heart rate of 137 beats/min, BP of 121/70 mm Hg, respiratory rate of 30 breaths/min, and an electrocardiogram showing sinus tachycardia with nonspecific ST/T waves in the anterior and inferior leads. Initial laboratory tests showed normal white blood cell count, normal hemoglobin, and mild thrombocytopenia. The kidney function and liver function were within normal ranges. He was confirmed positive for COVID-19 with a polymerase chain reaction test.

Given the initial presentation of chest pain and troponin elevation, the patient was treated for possible acute coronary syndrome with heparin infusion and aspirin. It was unclear if this was a myocardial infarction, pulmonary embolus, or myocarditis. A chest CT angiogram was performed, demonstrating likely reactive mediastinal lymph nodes and no PE. The transthoracic echocardiogram had a moderate to severely reduced left ventricular ejection fraction with normal chamber size, mildly dilated right ventricle with a mildly reduced systolic function, normal valve function, and Doppler findings not suggestive of pulmonary hypertension. The initial troponin I was 0.2 ng/mL and on day 2 peaked at 1.8 ng/mL. The N-terminal pro-brain natriuretic peptide (NT-proBNP) initially was 361 pg/mL and increased to 19,518 pg/mL.

On day 2, the patient continued to have chest pain and a cardiac catheterization was performed that showed mild nonobstructive CAD. A right heart catherization was done that had normal left- and right-sided filling pressures, normal pulmonary artery pressure, and normal cardiac output. Inflammatory markers were obtained that were significantly elevated with an erythrocyte sedimentation rate (ESR) at greater than 120 mm/hr, C-reactive protein (CRP) of 24 mg/dL, and elevated ferritin level of 3769 ng/mL. Cardiac magnetic resonance (CMR) imaging was performed for confirmation of myocarditis; it demonstrated findings consistent with myocarditis (Fig. 6.13). This involved mostly the anteroseptum with a left ventricular ejection fraction of 31% with normal chamber size and associated hypokinesis of the anteroseptal walls. This presentation was consistent with COVID-19–associated myocarditis.

Initially the patient did not have respiratory distress or concerns for pneumonia. However, the patient did have transient episodes of hypotension requiring a short intensive care unit stay. This was consistent with sepsis because of the viral infection and treated with supportive care. On day 4 of the hospitalization the patient developed decompensated HF; he had mild respiratory distress requiring up to 4 L/min of supplemental oxygen, which improved with intravenous diuretics. Empiric HF medications were slowly initiated after the sepsis had improved. He was treated for HF with reduced ejection fraction according to guideline medical therapy and was started on an angiotensin-converting enzyme inhibitor and appropriate beta-blocker before discharge. The patient was hospitalized for a total of 9 days.

This case demonstrates a typical manifestation of COVID-19–associated myocarditis causing a new-onset decompensated HF. This is an example of the virus causing myocardial injury by direct infection of the myocardium. Initially, a viral myocarditis was suspected, but given the need to rule out ischemia a cardiac catheterization was performed and then followed by

CMR to help confirm the diagnosis. He was treated in a similar manner according to the protocol for the management of COVID-19 patients with evidence of myocardial injury guideline shown in Fig. 6.9. The patient was administered supportive care using temporary hemodynamic support and followed with a gradual induction of guideline-directed medical therapy once the patient became stable. After 3 months of recovery and medical therapy, his left ventricular ejection fraction has improved to 45% and he has been without further heart failure episodes.

Case 1: Cardiac Magnetic Resonance Images of Covid-19 Myocarditis

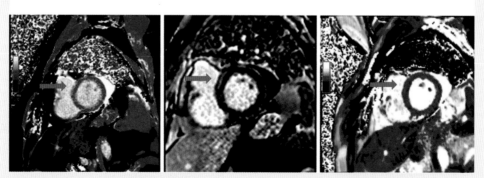

Fig. 6.13 Cardiac Magnetic Resonance (CMR) Images of COVID-19 Myocarditis. In the CMR images the *red arrows* point to the anteroseptal areas of involvement. The *left* image is precontrast T1-mapping, the *middle* image is postcontrast phase sensitive inversion recovery image. The *right* image is T2-mapping sequence. (Courtesy Dr. Jonathan Revels, DO.)

■ Case Report 6.2 COVID-19–Associated Coagulopathy With Stent Thrombosis

This 54-year-old Native American man had a history of type 2 diabetes, hypertension, hyperlipidemia, end-stage renal disease requiring hemodialysis, and coronary artery disease with prior distal right coronary artery (RCA) stent and developed severe COVID-19 infection. This patient had several days of progressive shortness of breath, fever, cough, and fatigue, with multiple family members in his household becoming COVID-19 positive. The patient initially presented to a small rural hospital and quickly decompensated, needing intubation, vasopressors for hemodynamic support, and transfer to a higher level of care facility. The patient developed acute respiratory distress syndrome (ARDS) as his hypoxia continued to worsen despite mechanical ventilation and

eventually was placed in the prone position. On day 8 and while in the prone position, the patient was noted to have ST elevations on monitor. A 12-lead ECG was obtained, confirming the ST elevations in the inferior leads consistent with an ST-segment elevation myocardial infarct (STEMI) (Fig. 6.14). The patient was emergently taken to the cardiac catheterization unit for primary percutaneous coronary intervention (PCI). The patient was noted to have stent thrombosis at the prior RCA stent (as seen in the coronary angiogram depicted in Fig. 6.15 and was successfully treated with a drug-eluting stent and initiation of dual-antiplatelet therapy. By this time, the patient was thought to be in the cytokine storm phase of the infection. He was continued on a heparin

Case 2: Covid-19-Associated Coagulopathy Causing STEMI—ECG

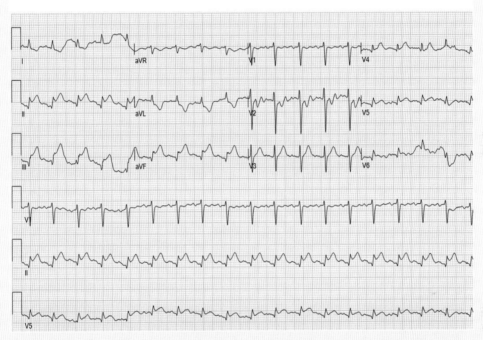

Fig. 6.14 COVID-19–Associated Coagulopathy Causing ST Elevation Myocardial Infarction *(STEMI)*—Electrocardiogram *(ECG).* The ECG shows inferior and lateral ST-segment elevations with 1-mm ST elevations in leads V5 and V6 and 2- to 3-mm ST elevations in leads II, III, and aVF.

Case 2: Covid-19-Associated Coagulopathy Causing Stent Thrombus—Coronary Angiogram

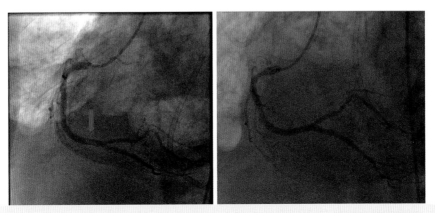

Fig. 6.15 COVID-19–Associated Coagulopathy Causing Stent Thrombosis—Coronary Angiogram. These images were obtained by cardiac catheterization of the right coronary artery (RCA). The *red arrows* show the near occlusive stent thrombus of the distal RCA. The second image is after stent placement, which shows a fully patent distal RCA.

infusion to help prevent other thromboembolic events and the patient met criteria for tocilizumab therapy, which was initiated. The patient had a prolonged complicated hospital course lasting 35 days and was discharged to a rehabilitation hospital.

This case showed evidence of direct myocardial injury given the ST segment elevations on electrocardiogram and a rapid rise of troponin I and was found to be a very late stent thrombosis causing a STEMI. The patient was treated in standard fashion with emergent primary PCI. Although this was not a case of plaque rupture leading to an AMI, the CAC and sepsis-related platelet dysfunction are thought to have played a role in this patient with late stent thrombosis.

■ **Case Report 6.3** COVID-19–Associated Coagulopathy With Large Right Ventricular Thrombus

A 56-year-old White man with no significant medical history presented to a small community hospital after 7 days of progressive shortness of breath and body aches. On presentation, he was confirmed to be COVID-19 positive and a chest radiograph demonstrated multifocal pneumonia consistent with COVID-19 pneumonia. He was initially treated with high-flow oxygen, dexamethasone, remdesivir, azithromycin, ceftriaxone, and enoxaparin injections for venous thromboembolism (VTE) prophylaxis. On day 3, despite medical therapy, he developed septic shock requiring vasopressors for hemodynamic support and progressive worsening of his hypoxia requiring intubation, for which empiric enoxaparin therapy was started because of concern for possible pulmonary embolism (PE). He was then transferred to a higher-level care hospital. On arrival, his white blood cell count was elevated at 32,000 cells/μL, hemoglobin was 16.9 g/dL, and platelet count was of 317,000/μL. His renal function and liver function tests were consistent with shock states with an initial creatinine value of 2.7 mg/dL that continued to increase and an aspartate transaminase and alanine transaminase of 5000 U/L and 3000 U/L, with a total bilirubin of 1.7 mg/dL. He was also noted to have significantly increased inflammatory markers with a C-reactive protein of 10.9 mg/dL and ferritin of 841 ng/mL.

A point-of-care echocardiogram was performed to assess cardiac function, which was of limited quality. Bedside transesophageal echocardiography was then performed that revealed a large right ventricular mass consistent with thrombus as seen in Fig. 6.16. The left and right ventricles had normal systolic function, and the wall motion was normal with no significant valve dysfunction. This result prompted a lower extremity Doppler ultrasound, which demonstrated large bilateral deep vein thrombosis. An unfractionated heparin infusion was started, and the blood cultures that were obtained had no bacterial growth.

This case illustrates an example of COVID-19–associated coagulopathy. The platelets were within a normal range, fibrinogen and lactate dehydrogenase were elevated at 661 mg/dL and 853 U/L, prothrombin time was elevated at 19 seconds, and the D-dimer was significantly elevated at greater than 35 mg/L. There was a large thrombus burden, including thrombus formation in a normal functioning right ventricle. These thrombi had developed and progressed despite the patient being on low-molecular-weight heparin for VTE prophylaxis and then put on therapeutic doses for high suspicion of PE. Because of the instability of the patient and not being able to safely transport, a CT angiogram to evaluate PE was not performed. Direct thrombolytic therapy and systemic thrombolytic therapy were also not reasonable options. The patient died from the COVID-19 infection–related complications 7 days after presentation from a PE, severe viral pneumonia, and septic shock.

Case 3: Covid-19-Associated Coagulopathy Causing Large RV Thrombus—Echocardiogram

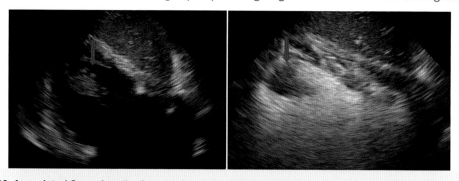

Fig. 6.16 COVID-19–Associated Coagulopathy Causing Large Right Ventricular Thrombus. Transesophageal echocardiogram images without contrast *(right)* and with contrast *(left)* of the right ventricle with *red arrows* showing the large apical thrombus. (Images courtesy of Trenton C Wray, MD.)

COVID-19–Induced Cardiac Complications and Long-Term Sequelae

The long-term direct consequences of COVID-19–related myocardial injury, endothelial dysfunction, and thrombosis are not known. Likewise, the long-term effects on preexisting CVDs after SARS-CoV-2 infection are also not known. Most of the insight comes from existing information on diseases not related to COVID-19. The current management of disease-specific long-term therapy is mostly derived from existing standards of care for conditions such as heart failure, arrhythmias, and myocardial infarctions.[126]

Rajpal et al.[156] performed CMR on 26 college athletes representing varying competitive sports who tested positive for SARS-CoV-2 and were asymptomatic or mildly symptomatic. CMR evaluation done 2 to 8 weeks after the positive test revealed findings consistent with myocarditis in 4 (15%) and 8 additional athletes (31%) showed radiological features of myocardial injury.[156]

In COVID-19–related myocardial injury (myocarditis or inflammation-related myocardial injury), imaging modalities such as CMR are demonstrating utility in the evaluation of continued myocardial involvement.[73,88,95] Early detection of persistent myocardial involvement despite recovery from COVID-19 can possibly help identify those at risk for cardiovascular complications from myocarditis, including arrhythmias and HF.[95] In a small retrospective study, Huang et al.[73] performed CMR on 26 patients who recovered from COVID-19 but had cardiovascular issues and demonstrated that 58% of patients had an abnormal CMR along with compromised right ventricular function that was statistically significant when compared with healthy controls.

Because very little is known about the long-term COVID-19 sequalae, it is suggested that patient registries will be of vital importance to develop an understanding of long-term post–COVID-19 complications and formulate management strategies. To achieve standardization of disease-specific care recommendations, there is a critical need for the establishment of long-term care with continued surveillance and screening for disease-specific complications.[82] In addition, given the paucity of guidance on post–COVID-19 long-term effects, it is important to collaborate with experts in various medical specialties and develop a multidisciplinary approach for the continued evaluation and care of these patients.[68]

Conclusion

Cardiac injury is common in SARS-CoV-2 infection, and patients can present with features of myocarditis, acute coronary syndromes, HF, or cardiac arrhythmias. Moreover, COVID-19 can exacerbate preexisting CVD, resulting in severe disease manifestations and complications leading to adverse outcomes. The COVID-19 pandemic is still evolving; the health care community and recovered patients are urged to stay tuned to the long-term sequelae of COVID-19.

REFERENCES

1. Wang D, Hu B, Hu C, Zhu F, Liu X, Zhang J, Wang B, Xiang H, Cheng Z, Xiong Y. Clinical characteristics of 138 hospitalized patients with 2019 novel coronavirus–infected pneumonia in Wuhan, China. *Jama.* 2020;323(11):1061–1069.
2. Zhou F, Yu T, Du R, Fan G, Liu Y, Liu Z, Xiang J, Wang Y, Song B, Gu X. Clinical course and risk factors for mortality of adult inpatients with COVID-19 in Wuhan, China: a retrospective cohort study. *The Lancet.* 2020;395(10229):1054–1062.
3. Guo T, Fan Y, Chen M, Wu X, Zhang L, He T, Wang H, Wan J, Wang X, Lu Z. Cardiovascular implications of fatal outcomes of patients with coronavirus disease 2019 (COVID-19). *JAMA cardiology.* 2020;5(7):811–818.
4. Richardson S, Hirsch JS, Narasimhan M, Crawford JM, McGinn T, Davidson KW, Barnaby DP, Becker LB, Chelico JD, Cohen SL. Presenting characteristics, comorbidities, and outcomes among 5700 patients hospitalized with COVID-19 in the New York City area. *Jama.* 2020;323(20):2052–2059.
5. Lala A, Johnson KW, Januzzi JL, Russak AJ, Paranjpe I, Richter F, Zhao S, Somani S, Van Vleck T, Vaid A. Prevalence and impact of myocardial injury in patients hospitalized with COVID-19 infection. *Journal of the American college of cardiology.* 2020;76(5):533–546.
6. Fu L, Liu X, Su Y, Ma J, Hong K. Prevalence and impact of cardiac injury on COVID-19: A systematic review and meta-analysis. *Clinical cardiology.* 2021;44(2):276–283.
7. Bavishi C, Bonow RO, Trivedi V, Abbott JD, Messerli FH, Bhatt DL. Acute myocardial injury in patients hospitalized with COV3ID-19 infection: a review. *Progress in cardiovascular diseases.* 2020;63(5):682–689.
8. Froude S, Hughes H. Newly discovered viruses. In: *Oxford textbook of medicine. 6th ed.* Edited by Firth J, Conlon C, Cox T; Oxford, UK: Oxford University Press; 2020.
9. Al Mutair A, Ambani Z. Narrative review of Middle East respiratory syndrome coronavirus (MERS-CoV) infection: updates and implications for practice. *Journal of International Medical Research.* 2020;48(1):0300060519858030.
10. Worldometers.info: COVID-19 Coronavirus Pandemic: [https://ns.worldometers.info/coronavirus/]. 2021.
11. Tsai P-H, Lai W-Y, Lin Y-Y, Luo Y-H, Lin Y-T, Chen H-K, Chen Y-M, Lai Y-C, Kuo L-C, Chen S-D, et al. Clinical manifestation and disease progression in COVID-19 infection. *Journal of the Chinese Medical Association.* 2021;84(1):3–8.
12. Giannis D, Ziogas IA, Gianni P. Coagulation disorders in coronavirus infected patients: COVID-19, SARS-CoV-1, MERS-CoV and lessons from the past. *Journal of Clinical Virology.* 2020;127:104362.
13. Liu Y, Wu S, Qin M, Jiang W, Liu X. The prevalence of cardiovascular comorbidities in COVID-19, SARS and MERS: pooled analysis of published data. *Journal of the American Heart Association.* 2020:e016812.
14. Hendren NS, Drazner MH, Bozkurt B, Cooper Jr LT. Description and proposed management of the acute COVID-19 cardiovascular syndrome. *Circulation.* 2020;141(23):1903–1914.
15. Liang Y, Wang M-L, Chien C-S, Yarmishyn AA, Yang Y-P, Lai W-Y, Luo Y-H, Lin Y-T, Chen Y-J, Chang P-C. Highlight of immune pathogenic response and hematopathologic effect in SARS-CoV, MERS-CoV, and SARS-Cov-2 infection. *Frontiers in Immunology.* 2020;11:1022.
16. Al-Ani F, Chehade S, Lazo-Langner A. Thrombosis risk associated with COVID-19 infection. A scoping review. *Thrombosis Research.* 2020;192:152–160.
17. Al-Samkari H, Karp Leaf RS, Dzik WH, Carlson JCT, Fogerty AE, Waheed A, Goodarzi K, Bendapudi PK, Bornikova L, Gupta S, et al. COVID-19 and coagulation: bleeding and thrombotic manifestations of SARS-CoV-2 infection. *Blood.* 2020;136(4):489–500.
18. Atri D, Siddiqi HK, Lang J, Nauffal V, Morrow DA, Bohula EA. COVID-19 for the cardiologist: a current review of the virology, clinical epidemiology, cardiac and other clinical

manifestations and potential therapeutic strategies. *JACC: Basic to Translational Science*. 2020.

19. Babapoor-Farrokhran S, Gill D, Walker J, Rasekhi RT, Bozorgnia B, Amanullah A. Myocardial injury and COVID-19: possible mechanisms. *Life Sciences*. 2020:117723.

20. Bearse M, Hung YP, Krauson AJ, Bonanno L, Boyraz B, Harris CK, Helland TL, Hilburn CF, Hutchison B, Jobbagy S. Factors associated with myocardial SARS-CoV-2 infection, myocarditis, and cardiac inflammation in patients with COVID-19. *Modern Pathology*. 2021:1–13.

21. Chan NC, Weitz JI. COVID-19 coagulopathy, thrombosis, and bleeding. *Blood*. 2020;136(4):381–383.

22. Chen L, Hu W, Guo X, Zhao P, Tang J, Gu Y, Huang N, Wang C, Cui A, Zhang D. Association of coagulation dysfunction with cardiac injury among hospitalized patients with COVID-19. *Scientific Reports*. 2021;11(1):1–12.

23. Giustino G, Croft LB, Stefanini GG, Bragato R, Silbiger JJ, Vicenzi M, Danilov T, Kukar N, Shaban N, Kini A, et al. Characterization of myocardial injury in patients with COVID-19. *Journal of the American College of Cardiology*. 2020;76(18):2043–2055.

24. Giustino G, Pinney SP, Lala A, Reddy VY, Johnston-Cox HA, Mechanick JI, Halperin JL, Fuster V. Coronavirus and cardiovascular disease, myocardial injury, and arrhythmia: JACC Focus seminar. *Journal of the American College of Cardiology*. 2020;76(17):2011–2023.

25. Basso C, Leone O, Rizzo S, De Gaspari M, van der Wal AC, Aubry M-C, Bois MC, Lin PT, Maleszewski JJ, Stone JR. Pathological features of COVID-19-associated myocardial injury: a multicentre cardiovascular pathology study. *European Heart Journal*. 2020;41(39):3827–3835.

26. Wichmann D, Sperhake J-P, Lütgehetmann M, Steurer S, Edler C, Heinemann A, Heinrich F, Mushumba H, Kniep I, Schröder AS. Autopsy findings and venous thromboembolism in patients with COVID-19: a prospective cohort study. *Annals of Internal Medicine*. 2020;173(4):268–277.

27. Paul M, Poyan Mehr A, Kreutz R. Physiology of local renin-angiotensin systems. *Physiological Reviews*. 2006;86(3):747–803.

28. De Mello WC. Local renin angiotensin aldosterone systems and cardiovascular diseases. *Medical Clinics*. 2017;101(1):117–127.

29. Ocaranza MP, Riquelme JA, García L, Jalil JE, Chiong M, Santos RA, Lavandero S. Counter-regulatory renin–angiotensin system in cardiovascular disease. *Nature Reviews Cardiology*. 2020;17(2):116–129.

30. Crackower MA, Sarao R, Oudit GY, Yagil C, Kozieradzki I, Scanga SE, Oliveira-dos-Santos AJ, da Costa J, Zhang L, Pei Y. Angiotensin-converting enzyme 2 is an essential regulator of heart function. *Nature*. 2002;417(6891):822–828.

31. Goulter AB, Goddard MJ, Allen JC, Clark KL. ACE2 gene expression is up-regulated in the human failing heart. *BMC Medicine*. 2004;2(1):1–7.

32. Kubota E, Dean RG, MacDonald PS, et al. Myocardial infarction increases ACE2 expression in rat and humans. *European heart Journal*. 2005;26(4):369–375.

33. Ruparelia N, Chai JT, Fisher EA, Choudhury RP. Inflammatory processes in cardiovascular disease: a route to targeted therapies. *Nature Reviews Cardiology*. 2017;14(3):133–144.

34. Oparil S, Acelajado MC, Bakris GL, Berlowitz DR, Cífková R, Dominiczak AF, Grassi G, Jordan J, Poulter NR, Rodgers A, et al. Hypertension. *Nat Rev Dis Primers*. 2018;4:18014.

35. Shirazi LF, Bissett J, Romeo F, Mehta JL. Role of inflammation in heart failure. *Current Atherosclerosis Reports*. 2017;19(6):27.

36. Imanaka-Yoshida K. Inflammation in myocardial disease: From myocarditis to dilated cardiomyopathy. *Pathology International*. 2020;70(1):1–11.

37. Hoffmann M, Kleine-Weber H, Schroeder S, Krüger N, Herrler T, Erichsen S, Schiergens TS, Herrler G, Wu N-H, Nitsche A. SARS-CoV-2 cell entry depends on ACE2 and TMPRSS2 and is blocked by a clinically proven protease inhibitor. *Cell*. 2020;181(2):271–280.

38. Lan J, Ge J, Yu J, Shan S, Zhou H, Fan S, Zhang Q, Shi X, Wang Q, Zhang L. Structure of the SARS-CoV-2 spike receptor-binding domain bound to the ACE2 receptor. *Nature*. 2020:1–6.

39. Chen L, Li X, Chen M, Feng Y, Xiong C. The ACE2 expression in human heart indicates new potential mechanism of heart injury among patients infected with SARS-CoV-2. *Cardiovascular Research*. 2020;116(6):1097–1100.

40. Clerkin KJ, Fried JA, Raikhelkar J, Sayer G, Griffin JM, Masoumi A, Jain SS, Burkhoff D, Kumaraiah D, Rabbani L. Coronavirus Disease 2019 (COVID-19) and Cardiovascular Disease. *Circulation*. 2020;141(20):1648–1655.

41. Zhou L, Xu Z, Castiglione GM, Soiberman US, Eberhart CG, Duh EJ. ACE2 and TMPRSS2 are expressed on the human ocular surface, suggesting susceptibility to SARS-CoV-2 infection. *The Ocular Surface*. 2020;18(4):537–544.

42. Liu PP, Blet A, Smyth D, Li H. The science underlying COVID-19: implications for the cardiovascular system. *Circulation*. 2020;142(1):68–78.

43. Tavazzi G, Pellegrini C, Maurelli M, Belliato M, Sciutti F, Bottazzi A, Sepe PA, Resasco T, Camporotondo R, Bruno R, et al. Myocardial localization of coronavirus in COVID-19 cardiogenic shock. *European Journal of Heart Failure*. 2020;22(5):911–915.

44. Escher F, Pietsch H, Aleshcheva G, Bock T, Baumeier C, Elsaesser A, Wenzel P, Hamm C, Westenfeld R, Schultheiss M. Detection of viral SARS-CoV-2 genomes and histopathological changes in endomyocardial biopsies. *ESC heart failure*. 2020;7(5):2440–2447.

45. Pellegrini D, Kawakami R, Guagliumi G, Sakamoto A, Kawai K, Gianatti A, Nasr A, Kutys R, Guo L, Cornelissen A. Microthrombi as a major cause of cardiac injury in COVID-19: a pathologic study. *Circulation*. 2021;143(10):1031–1042.

46. Huang C, Wang Y, Li X, Ren L, Zhao J, Hu Y, Zhang L, Fan G, Xu J, Gu X, et al. Clinical features of patients infected with 2019 novel coronavirus in Wuhan, China. *The Lancet*. 2020;395(10223):497–506.

47. Shi S, Qin M, Shen B, Cai Y, Liu T, Yang F, Gong W, Liu X, Liang J, Zhao Q. Association of cardiac injury with mortality in hospitalized patients with COVID-19 in Wuhan, China. *JAMA cardiology*. 2020.

48. Lazzerini PE, Boutjdir M, Capecchi PL. COVID-19, arrhythmic risk, and inflammation: mind the gap!. *Circulation*. 2020;142(1):7–9.

49. Moore JB, June CH. Cytokine release syndrome in severe COVID-19. *Science*. 2020;368(6490):473–474.

50. Zhyvotovska A, Yusupov D, Foronjy R, Nakeshbandi M, McFarlane SI, Salifu M. Insights into Potential Mechanisms

of Injury and Treatment Targets in COVID-19, SARS-Cov-2 Infection. *International journal of clinical research & trials.* 2020;5(1).

51. Gao YM, Xu G, Wang B, Liu BC. Cytokine storm syndrome in coronavirus disease 2019: a narrative review. *Journal of internal medicine.* 2021;289(2):147–161.

52. Tang N, Li D, Wang X, Sun Z. Abnormal coagulation parameters are associated with poor prognosis in patients with novel coronavirus pneumonia. *Journal of thrombosis and haemostasis.* 2020;18(4):844–847.

53. Adelborg K, Larsen JB, Hvas AM. Disseminated intravascular coagulation: epidemiology, biomarkers, and management. *British Journal of Haematology.* 2021;192(5):803–818.

54. Becker RC. COVID-19 update: Covid-19-associated coagulopathy. *Journal of thrombosis and thrombolysis.* 2020;50: 54–67.

55. Piazza G, Campia U, Hurwitz S, Snyder JE, Rizzo SM, Pfeferman MB, Morrison RB, Leiva O, Fanikos J, Nauffal V, et al. Registry of Arterial and Venous Thromboembolic Complications in Patients With COVID-19. *Journal of the American College of Cardiology.* 2020;76(18):2060–2072.

56. Salabei JK, Fishman TJ, Asnake ZT, Ali A, Iyer UG. COVID-19 Coagulopathy: Current knowledge and guidelines on anticoagulation. *Heart & Lung.* 2021;50(2):357–360.

57. Iba T, Levy JH, Levi M, Thachil J. Coagulopathy in COVID-19. *Journal of Thrombosis and Haemostasis.* 2020;18(9):2103–2109.

58. Cui S, Chen S, Li X, Liu S, Wang F. Prevalence of venous thromboembolism in patients with severe novel coronavirus pneumonia. *Journal of Thrombosis and Haemostasis.* 2020;18(6):1421–1424.

59. Liao D, Zhou F, Luo L, Xu M, Wang H, Xia J, Gao Y, Cai L, Wang Z, Yin P. Haematological characteristics and risk factors in the classification and prognosis evaluation of COVID-19: a retrospective cohort studyThe Lancet Haematology7; 2020:e671–e678.

60. Iba T, Levy JH, Connors JM, Warkentin TE, Thachil J, Levi M. Managing thrombosis and cardiovascular complications of COVID-19: Answering the questions in COVID-19-associated coagulopathy. *Expert review of respiratory medicine.* 2021;15(8):1003–1011.

61. Du F, Liu B, Zhang S. COVID-19: the role of excessive cytokine release and potential ACE2 down-regulation in promoting hypercoagulable state associated with severe illness. *Journal of thrombosis and thrombolysis.* 2020:1–17.

62. Wright FL, Vogler TO, Moore EE, Moore HB, Wohlauer MV, Urban S, Nydam TL, Moore PK, McIntyre Jr RC. Fibrinolysis shutdown correlation with thromboembolic events in severe COVID-19 infection. *Journal of the American College of Surgeons.* 2020;231(2):193–203. e191.

63. Bois MC, Boire NA, Layman AJ, Aubry M-C, Alexander MP, Roden AC, Hagen CE, Quinton RA, Larsen C, Erben Y. COVID-19–associated nonocclusive fibrin microthrombi in the heart. *Circulation.* 2021;143(3):230–243.

64. Oudit G, Kassiri Z, Jiang C, Liu P, Poutanen S, Penninger J, Butany J. SARS-coronavirus modulation of myocardial ACE2 expression and inflammation in patients with SARS. *European journal of clinical investigation.* 2009;39(7):618–625.

65. Catapano F, Marchitelli L, Cundari G, Cilia F, Mancuso G, Pambianchi G, Galea N, Ricci P, Catalano C, Francone M. Role of advanced imaging in COVID-19 cardiovascular complications. *Insights into Imaging.* 2021;12(1):1–13.

66. Banu N, Panikar SS, Leal LR, Leal AR. Protective role of ACE2 and its downregulation in SARS-CoV-2 infection leading to Macrophage Activation Syndrome: Therapeutic implications. *Life sciences.* 2020:117905.

67. Akhmerov A, Marbán E. COVID-19 and the Heart. *Circulation research.* 2020;126(10):1443–1455.

68. Becker RC. Anticipating the long-term cardiovascular effects of COVID-19. *J Thromb Thrombolysis.* 2020;50(3):512–524.

69. Becker RC. Toward understanding the 2019 Coronavirus and its impact on the heart. *J Thromb Thrombolysis.* 2020;50(1):33–42.

70. Fox SE, Akmatbekov A, Harbert JL, Li G, Brown JQ, Vander Heide RS: Pulmonary and cardiac pathology in African American patients with COVID-19: an autopsy series from New Orleans. *The Lancet Respiratory Medicine* 2020, 8(7):681-686.

71. Fried JA, Ramasubbu K, Bhatt R, Topkara VK, Clerkin KJ, Horn E, Rabbani L, Brodie D, Jain SS, Kirtane A. The variety of cardiovascular presentations of COVID-19. *Circulation.* 2020;141(23):1930–1936.

72. Guzik TJ, Mohiddin SA, Dimarco A, Patel V, Savvatis K, Marelli-Berg FM, Madhur MS, Tomaszewski M, Maffia P, D'Acquisto F, et al. COVID-19 and the cardiovascular system: implications for risk assessment, diagnosis, and treatment options. *Cardiovascular Research.* 2020;116(10): 1666–1687.

73. Huang L, Zhao P, Tang D, Zhu T, Han R, Zhan C, Liu W, Zeng H, Tao Q, Xia L. Cardiac involvement in patients recovered from COVID-2019 identified using magnetic resonance imaging. *Cardiovascular Imaging.* 2020;13(11): 2330–2339.

74. Huang Z, Huang P, Du B, Kong L, Zhang W, Zhang Y, Dong J. Prevalence and clinical outcomes of cardiac injury in patients with COVID-19: A systematic review and meta-analysis. *Nutrition, Metabolism and Cardiovascular Diseases.* 2021;31(1):2–13.

75. Kadosh BS, Garshick MS, Gaztanaga J, Moore KJ, Newman JD, Pillinger M, Ramasamy R, Reynolds HR, Shah B, Hochman J. COVID-19 and the Heart and Vasculature: Novel Approaches to Reduce Virus-Induced Inflammation in Patients With Cardiovascular Disease. *Arteriosclerosis, Thrombosis, and Vascular Biology.* 2020;40(9):2045–2053.

76. Kang Y, Chen T, Mui D, Ferrari V, Jagasia D, Scherrer-Crosbie M, Chen Y, Han Y. Cardiovascular manifestations and treatment considerations in covid-19. *Heart.* 2020;106(15): 1132–1141.

77. Kaye AD, Spence AL, Mayerle M, Sardana N, Clay CM, Eng MR, Luedi MM, Turpin MAC, Urman RD, Cornett EM. The impact of COVID-19 infection on the cardiovascular system: an evidence-based analysis of risk factors and outcomes. *Best Practice & Research Clinical Anaesthesiology.* 2021;35(3):437–448.

78. Manji H, Carr AS, Brownlee WJ, Lunn MP. Neurology in the time of covid-19. *J Neurol Neurosurg Psychiatry.* 2020;91(6):568–570.

79. Luo J, Zhu X, Jian J, Chen X, Yin K. Cardiovascular disease in patients with COVID-19: evidence from cardiovascular pathology to treatment. *Acta biochimica et biophysica Sinica.* 2021;53(3):273–282.

80. Madjid M, Safavi-Naeini P, Solomon SD, Vardeny O. Potential effects of coronaviruses on the cardiovascular system: a review. *JAMA cardiology.* 2020;5(7):831–840.

81. Mehra MR, Desai SS, Kuy S, Henry TD, Patel AN. Cardio-vascular Disease, Drug Therapy, and Mortality in Covid-19. *New England Journal of Medicine*. 2020;382(25):e102.

82. Mitrani RD, Dabas N, Goldberger JJ. COVID-19 cardiac injury: Implications for long-term surveillance and out-comes in survivors. *Heart rhythm*. 2020;17(11):1984–1990.

83. Nishiga M, Wang DW, Han Y, Lewis DB, Wu JC. COVID-19 and cardiovascular disease: from basic mechanisms to clin-ical perspectives. *Nature Reviews Cardiology*. 2020:1–16.

84. Sattar Y, Ullah W, Rauf H. COVID-19 cardiovascular epi-demiology, cellular pathogenesis, clinical manifestations and management. *International Journal of Cardiology Heart & Vasculature*. 2020;29:100589.

85. Soumya R, Unni TG, Raghu K. Impact of COVID-19 on the Cardiovascular System: A Review of Available Reports. *Cardiovascular drugs and therapy*. 2020:1–15.

86. Szekely Y, Lichter Y, Taieb P, Banai A, Hochstadt A, Merdler I, Gal Oz A, Rothschild E, Baruch G, Peri Y. The Spectrum of Cardiac Manifestations in Coronavirus Disease 2019 (COVID-19)-a Systematic Echocardiographic Study. *Circulation*. 2020;142(4):342–353.

87. Topol EJ. COVID-19 can affect the heart. *Science*. 2020;370(6515):408–409.

88. Wang H, Li R, Zhou Z, Jiang H, Yan Z, Tao X, Li H, Xu L. Cardiac involvement in COVID-19 patients: mid-term follow up by cardiovascular magnetic resonance. *Journal of Cardiovascular Magnetic Resonance*. 2021;23(1):1–12.

89. Xu H, Hou K, Xu R, Li Z, Fu H, Wen L, Xie L, Liu H, Selva-nayagam JB, Zhang N. Clinical Characteristics and Risk Factors of Cardiac Involvement in COVID-19. *Journal of the American Heart Association*. 2020;9(18):e016807.

90. Yancy CW, Fonarow GC. Coronavirus disease 2019 (COVID-19) and the heart—Is heart failure the next chapter? *JAMA cardiology*. 2020;5(11):1216–1217.

91. Zheng Y-Y, Ma Y-T, Zhang J-Y, Xie X. COVID-19 and the cardiovascular system. *Nature Reviews Cardiology*. 2020:1–2.

92. Zhou M, Wong C-K, Un K-C, Lau Y-M, Lee JC-Y, Tam FC-C, Lau Y-M, Lai W-H, Tam AR, Lam Y-Y, et al. Cardiovascular sequalae in uncomplicated COVID-19 survivors. *PLOS ONE*. 2021;16(2):e0246732.

93. Zhu H, Rhee J-W, Cheng P, Waliany S, Chang A, Witteles RM, Maecker H, Davis MM, Nguyen PK, Wu SM. Cardio-vascular complications in patients with COVID-19: conse-quences of viral toxicities and host immune response. *Current cardiology reports*. 2020;22(5):1–9.

94. Kawakami R, Sakamoto A, Kawai K, Gianatti A, Pellegrini D, Nasr A, Kutys B, Guo L, Cornelissen A, Mori M. Patho-logical evidence for SARS-CoV-2 as a cause of myocarditis: JACC review topic of the week. *Journal of the American College of Cardiology*. 2021;77(3):314–325.

95. Shchendrygina A, Nagel E, Puntmann VO, Valbuena-Lopez S. COVID-19 myocarditis and prospective heart failure burden. *Expert review of cardiovascular therapy*. 2021;19(1):5–14.

96. Tucker NR, Chaffin M, Bedi Jr KC, Papangeli I, Akkad A-D, Arduini A, Hayat S, Eraslan G, Muus C, Bhattacharyya RP. Myocyte-Specific Upregulation of ACE2 in Cardiovascular Disease: Implications for SARS-CoV-2–Mediated Myocar-ditis. *Circulation*. 2020;142(7):708–710.

97. Bangalore S, Sharma A, Slotwiner A, Yatskar L, Harari R, Shah B, Ibrahim H, Friedman GH, Thompson C, Alviar CL, et al. ST-Segment Elevation in Patients with Covid-19 — A Case Series. *New England Journal of Medicine*. 2020;382(25):2478–2480.

98. Dewey M, Siebes M, Kachelrieß M, Kofoed KF, Mau-rovich-Horvat P, Nikolaou K, Bai W, Kofler A, Manka R, Kozerke S, et al. Clinical quantitative cardiac imaging for the assessment of myocardial ischaemia. *Nature Reviews Cardiology*. 2020;17(7):427–450.

99. Diaz-Arocutipa C, Torres-Valencia J, Saucedo-Chinchay J, Cuevas C. ST-segment elevation in patients with COVID-19: a systematic review. *Journal of Thrombosis and Thromboly-sis*. 2021;52(3):738–745.

100. Stefanini GG, Montorfano M, Trabattoni D, Andreini D, Ferrante G, Ancona M, Metra M, Curello S, Maffeo D, Pero G, et al. ST-Elevation Myocardial Infarction in Patients With COVID-19. *Circulation*. 2020;141(25):2113–2116.

101. Bader F, Manla Y, Atallah B, Starling RC. Heart failure and COVID-19. *Heart Failure Reviews*. 2021;26(1):1–10.

102. DeFilippis EM, Reza N, Donald E, Givertz MM, Lindenfeld J, Jessup M. Considerations for heart failure care during the coronavirus disease 2019 (COVID-19) pandemic. *JACC: Heart Failure*. 2020;8(8):681–691.

103. Freaney PM, Shah SJ, Khan SS. COVID-19 and heart failure with preserved ejection fraction. *Jama*. 2020;324(15):1499–1500.

104. Unudurthi SD, Luthra P, Bose RJ, McCarthy J, Kontaridis MI. Cardiac inflammation in COVID-19: Lessons from heart failure. *Life Sciences*. 2020:118482.

105. Bhatla A, Mayer MM, Adusumalli S, Hyman MC, Oh E, Tierney A, Moss J, Chahal AA, Anesi G, Denduluri S. COVID-19 and cardiac arrhythmias. *Heart Rhythm*. 2020;17(9):1439–1444.

106. Colon CM, Barrios JG, Chiles JW, McElwee SK, Russell DW, Maddox WR, Kay GN. Atrial arrhythmias in COVID-19 patients. *Clinical Electrophysiology*. 2020;6(9):1189–1190.

107. Manolis AS, Manolis AA, Manolis TA, Apostolopoulos EJ, Papatheou D, Melita H. COVID-19 infection and cardiac arrhythmias. *Trends in cardiovascular medicine*. 2020;30(8):451–460.

108. O'Shea CJ, Thomas G, Middeldorp ME, Harper C, Elliott AD, Ray N, Lau DH, Campbell K, Sanders P. Ventricular arrhythmia burden during the coronavirus disease 2019 (COVID-19) pandemic. *European Heart Journal*. 2020;42(5):520–528.

109. Kochav SM, Coromilas E, Nalbandian A, Ranard LS, Gupta A, Chung MK, Gopinathannair R, Biviano AB, Garan H, Wan EY. Cardiac arrhythmias in COVID-19 infection. *Circulation: Arrhythmia and Electrophysiology*. 2020;13(6):e008719.

110. Lazzerini PE, Laghi-Pasini F, Boutjdir M, Capecchi PL. Car-dioimmunology of arrhythmias: the role of autoimmune and inflammatory cardiac channelopathies. *Nature Reviews Immunology*. 2019;19(1):63–64.

111. Peltzer B, Manocha KK, Ying X, Kirzner J, Ip JE, Thomas G, Liu CF, Markowitz SM, Lerman BB, Safford MM. Out-comes and mortality associated with atrial arrhythmias among patients hospitalized with COVID-19. *Journal of Cardiovascular Electrophysiology*. 2020;31(12):3077–3085.

112. Asakura H, Ogawa H. COVID-19-associated coagulopathy and disseminated intravascular coagulation. *International Journal of Hematology*. 2020:1–13.

113. Bikdeli B, Madhavan MV, Jimenez D, Chuich T, Dreyfus I, Driggin E, Nigoghossian CD, Ageno W, Madjid M, Guo Y, et al. COVID-19 and Thrombotic or Thromboembolic

Disease: Implications for Prevention, Antithrombotic Therapy, and Follow-Up: JACC State-of-the-Art Review. *Journal of the American College of Cardiology.* 2020;75(23):2950–2973.

114. Helms J, Tacquard C, Severac F, Leonard-Lorant I, Ohana M, Delabranche X, Merdji H, Clere-Jehl R, Schenck M, Gandet FF. High risk of thrombosis in patients with severe SARS-CoV-2 infection: a multicenter prospective cohort study. *Intensive care medicine.* 2020;46(6):1089–1098.

115. Klok F, Kruip M, Van der Meer N, Arbous M, Gommers D, Kant K, Kaptein F, van Paassen J, Stals M, Huisman M. Incidence of thrombotic complications in critically ill ICU patients with COVID-19. *Thrombosis research.* 2020;191:145–147.

116. Kunutsor SK, Laukkanen JA. Incidence of venous and arterial thromboembolic complications in COVID-19: a systematic review and meta-analysis. *Thrombosis research.* 2020;196:27–30.

117. Lo MW, Kemper C, Woodruff TM. COVID-19: Complement, Coagulation, and Collateral Damage. *The Journal of Immunology.* 2020;205(6):1488–1495.

118. Luo H-c, You C-y, Lu S-w, Fu Y-q. Characteristics of coagulation alteration in patients with COVID-19. *Annals of Hematology.* 2021;100(1):45–52.

119. Mucha SR, Dugar S, McCrae K, Joseph DE, Bartholomew J, Sacha G, Militello M. Coagulopathy in COVID-19. *Cleve Clin J Med.* 2020;87(8):461–468.

120. Ortega-Paz L, Capodanno D, Montalescot G, Angiolillo D. COVID-19 Associated Thrombosis and Coagulopathy: Review of the Pathophysiology and Implications for Antithrombotic Management. *Journal of the American Heart Association.* 2021;10(3):e019650.

121. Tan CW, Tan JY, Wong WH, Cheong MA, Ng IM, Conceicao EP, Low JGH, Ng HJ, Lee LH. Clinical and laboratory features of hypercoagulability in COVID-19 and other respiratory viral infections amongst predominantly younger adults with few comorbidities. *Scientific Reports.* 2021;11(1):1793.

122. Terpos E, Ntanasis-Stathopoulos I, Elalamy I, Kastritis E, Sergentanis TN, Politou M, Psaltopoulou T, Gerotziafas G, Dimopoulos MA. Hematological findings and complications of COVID-19. *American journal of hematology.* 2020;95(7):834–847.

123. Varga Z, Flammer AJ, Steiger P, Haberecker M, Andermatt R, Zinkernagel AS, Mehra MR, Schuepbach RA, Ruschitzka F, Moch H. Endothelial cell infection and endotheliitis in COVID-19. *The Lancet.* 2020;395(10234):1417–1418.

124. Luetkens JA, Isaak A, Öztürk C, Mesropyan N, Monin M, Schlabe S, Reinert M, Faron A, Heine A, Velten M. Cardiac MRI in Suspected Acute COVID-19 Myocarditis. *Radiology: Cardiothoracic Imaging.* 2021;3(2):e200628.

125. Siripanthong B, Nazarian S, Muser D, Deo R, Santangeli P, Khanji MY, Cooper Jr LT, Chahal CAA. Recognizing COVID-19–related myocarditis: The possible pathophysiology and proposed guideline for diagnosis and management. *Heart rhythm.* 2020;17(9):1463–1471.

126. Liu J, Deswal A, Khalid U. COVID-19 myocarditis and long-term heart failure sequelae. *Current opinion in cardiology.* 2021;36(2):234–240.

127. Kociol RD, Cooper LT, Fang JC, Moslehi JJ, Pang PS, Sabe MA, Shah RV, Sims DB, Thiene G, Vardeny O. Recognition and initial management of fulminant myocarditis: a

scientific statement from the. *Circulation.* 2020;141(6):e69–e92.

128. Peretto G, Sala S, Rizzo S, Palmisano A, Esposito A, De Cobelli F, Campochiaro C, De Luca G, Foppoli L, Dagna L. Ventricular arrhythmias in myocarditis: characterization and relationships with myocardial inflammation. *Journal of the American College of Cardiology.* 2020;75(9):1046–1057.

129. Peretto G, Sala S, Rizzo S, De Luca G, Campochiaro C, Sartorelli S, Benedetti G, Palmisano A, Esposito A, Tresoldi M. Arrhythmias in myocarditis: state of the art. *Heart Rhythm.* 2019;16(5):793–801.

130. Long B, Brady WJ, Koyfman A, Gottlieb M. Cardiovascular complications in COVID-19. *The American journal of emergency medicine.* 2020;38(7):1504–1507.

131. Bhatt AS, Jering KS, Vaduganathan M, Claggett BL, Cunningham JW, Rosenthal N, Signorovitch J, Thune JJ, Vardeny O, Solomon SD. Clinical Outcomes in Patients With Heart Failure Hospitalized With COVID-19. *Heart Failure.* 2021;9(1):65–73.

132. Murphy SP, Kakkar R, McCarthy CP, Januzzi Jr JL. Inflammation in heart failure: JACC state-of-the-art review. *Journal of the American College of Cardiology.* 2020;75(11):1324–1340.

133. Adamo L, Rocha-Resende C, Prabhu SD, Mann DL. Reappraising the role of inflammation in heart failure. *Nature Reviews Cardiology.* 2020;17(5):269–285.

134. Coromilas EJ, Kochav S, Goldenthal I, Biviano A, Garan H, Goldbarg S, Kim J-H, Yeo I, Tracy C, Ayanian S. Worldwide survey of COVID-19 associated arrhythmias. *Circulation: Arrhythmia and Electrophysiology.* 2021;14(3):e009548.

135. Ribes A, Vardon-Bounes F, Mémier V, Poette M, Au-Duong J, Garcia C, Minville V, Sié P, Bura-Rivière A, Voisin S. Thromboembolic events and Covid-19. *Advances in Biological Regulation.* 2020;77:100735.

136. Fauvel C, Weizman O, Trimaille A, Mika D, Pommier T, Pace N, Douair A, Barbin E, Fraix A, Bouchot O. Pulmonary embolism in COVID-19 patients: a French multicentre cohort study. *European heart journal.* 2020;41(32):3058–3068.

137. Guan W-j, Ni Z-y, Hu Y, Liang W-h, Ou C-q, He J-x, Liu L, Shan H, Lei C-l, Hui DS. Clinical characteristics of coronavirus disease 2019 in China. *New Englund Journal of Medicine.* 2020;382(18):1708–1720.

138. Desai A, Voza G, Paiardi S, Teofilo FI, Caltagirone G, Pons MR, Aloise M, Kogan M, Tommasini T, Savevski V. The role of anti-hypertensive treatment, comorbidities and early introduction of LMWH in the setting of COVID-19: A retrospective, observational study in Northern Italy. *International Journal of Cardiology.* 2021;324:249–254.

139. Kuno T, Takahashi M, Obata R, Maeda T. Cardiovascular comorbidities, cardiac injury, and prognosis of COVID-19 in New York City. *American heart journal.* 2020;226:24–25.

140. Phelps M, Christensen DM, Gerds T, Fosbøl E, Torp-Pedersen C, Schou M, Køber L, Kragholm K, Andersson C. Biering-Sørensen T: Cardiovascular comorbidities as predictors for severe COVID-19 infection or death. *European Heart Journal-Quality of Care and Clinical Outcomes.* 2021;7(2):172–180.

141. Hu L, Chen S, Fu Y, Gao Z, Long H, Ren H-w, Zuo Y, Wang J, Li H, Xu Q-b. Risk factors associated with clinical outcomes in 323 coronavirus disease 2019 (COVID-19) hospitalized patients in Wuhan, China. *Clinical infectious diseases.* 2020;71(16):2089–2098.

142. Ssentongo P, Ssentongo AE, Heilbrunn ES, Ba DM, Chinchilli VM. Association of cardiovascular disease and 10 other pre-existing comorbidities with COVID-19 mortality: A systematic review and meta-analysis. *PloS one.* 2020;15(8):e0238215.

143. Sabatino J, De Rosa S, Di Salvo G, Indolfi C. Impact of cardiovascular risk profile on COVID-19 outcome. A meta-analysis. *PloS one.* 2020;15(8):e0237131.

144. Nashiry A, Sarmin Sumi S, Islam S, Quinn JM, Moni MA: Bioinformatics and system biology approach to identify the influences of COVID-19 on cardiovascular and hypertensive comorbidities. *Briefings in bioinformatics* 2021, 22(2):1387–1401.

145. Savoia C, Volpe M, Kreutz R. Hypertension, a Moving Target in COVID-19: Current Views and Perspectives. *Circulation Research.* 2021;128(7):1062–1079.

146. Kreutz R, Algharably EAE-H, Azizi M, Dobrowolski P, Guzik T, Januszewicz A, Persu A, Prejbisz A, Riemer TG, Wang J-G. Hypertension, the renin–angiotensin system, and the risk of lower respiratory tract infections and lung injury: implications for COVID-19: European Society of Hypertension COVID-19 Task Force Review of Evidence. *Cardiovascular research.* 2020;116(10):1688–1699.

147. ESC ESoC. ESC guidance for the diagnosis and management of CV disease during the COVID-19 pandemic. *Eur Heart J.* 2020:1–115.

148. Mahmud E, Dauerman HL, Welt FG, Messenger JC, Rao SV, Grines C, Mattu A, Kirtane AJ, Jauhar R, Meraj P. Management of acute myocardial infarction during the COVID-19 pandemic. *Journal of the American College of Cardiology.* 2020;76(11):1375–1384.

149. Pontone G, Scafuri S, Mancini ME, Agalbato C, Guglielmo M, Baggiano A, Muscogiuri G, Fusini L, Andreini D, Mushtaq S. Role of computed tomography in COVID-19. *Journal of cardiovascular computed tomography.* 2020;15(1):27–36.

150. Friedrich MG, Sechtem U, Schulz-Menger J, Holmvang G, Alakija P, Cooper LT, White JA, Abdel-Aty H, Gutberlet M, Prasad S. Cardiovascular magnetic resonance in myocarditis: A JACC White Paper. *Journal of the American College of Cardiology.* 2009;53(17):1475–1487.

151. Reynolds HR, Adhikari S, Pulgarin C, Troxel AB, Iturrate E, Johnson SB, Hausvater A, Newman JD, Berger JS, Bangalore S. Renin–angiotensin–aldosterone system inhibitors and risk of Covid-19. *New England Journal of Medicine.* 2020;382(25):2441–2448.

152. Mehta N, Kalra A, Nowacki AS, Anjewierden S, Han Z, Bhat P, Carmona-Rubio AE, Jacob M, Procop GW, Harrington S. Association of use of angiotensin-converting enzyme inhibitors and angiotensin II receptor blockers with testing positive for coronavirus disease 2019 (COVID-19). *JAMA cardiology.* 2020;5(9):1020–1026.

153. Dherange P, Lang J, Qian P, Oberfeld B, Sauer WH, Koplan B, Tedrow U. Arrhythmias and COVID-19: A review. *JACC: Clinical Electrophysiology.* 2020;6(9):1193–1204.

154. Tang N, Bai H, Chen X, Gong J, Li D, Sun Z. Anticoagulant treatment is associated with decreased mortality in severe coronavirus disease 2019 patients with coagulopathy. *Journal of Thrombosis and Haemostasis.* 2020;18(5):1094–1099.

155. National Institutes of Health. Antithrombotic Therapy in Patients with COVID-19 [https://www.covid19treatment-guidelines.nih.gov]

156. Rajpal S, Tong MS, Borchers J, Zareba KM, Obarski TP, Simonetti OP, Daniels CJ. Cardiovascular magnetic resonance findings in competitive athletes recovering from COVID-19 infection. *JAMA cardiology.* 2021;6(1):116–118.

Neurological Manifestations of COVID-19

7

Madihah Hepburn, MD, Christopher Newey, DO, MS, FNCS, and Pravin George, DO

Epidemiology of Neurological Manifestations of COVID-19

SARS-CoV-2, the causative virus of coronavirus 2019 (COVID-19) disease, initially emerged in the Wuhan region of China and rapidly spread worldwide. The exact origins of SARS-CoV-2 are unknown, but a non-human origin similar to that of the other human coronaviruses, that is, the Middle East respiratory syndrome coronavirus (MERS-CoV) and severe acute respiratory syndrome coronavirus-1 (SARS-CoV-1), is considered to be the most likely scenario. The index cases in Wuhan were all associated with the Huanan Seafood Wholesale Market, which is a place where live animals and seafood are sold. Animal-to-human and human-to-human spread by respiratory droplet is thought to be the most likely cause and transmission route.

SARS-CoV-2 is an RNA virus belonging to the family Coronaviridae, which is classified into four genera: α-coronavirus, β-coronavirus, γ-coronavirus, and δ-coronavirus. The α-coronavirus and β-coronavirus genera only infect mammals. The β-coronavirus group includes several human pathogenic viruses previously associated with smaller outbreaks in the years preceding 2019. Before December 2019, there were six coronaviruses known to infect humans with varying severity ranging from mild upper respiratory tract symptoms to more pathogenic strains (MERS-CoV and SARS-CoV-1) that have caused pandemics, albeit on a smaller scale

compared with SARS-CoV-2 over the last two decades.[1-3] As of May 2022, the World Health Organization (WHO) has reported more than 500 million cases of SARS-CoV-2 globally and more than 6 million COVID-19 related deaths.[5] Human coronaviruses have been historically associated with respiratory symptoms and fever related to pneumonia or upper respiratory tract infection. Less frequently reported symptoms include gastrointestinal and cardiovascular symptoms, but this family of viruses can also have direct and indirect effects on the central and peripheral nervous systems leading to neurological sequelae.[4,5]

COVID-19 first gained attention as a pulmonary illness featuring mild to moderate cough, fever, and malaise. The initial reports of the incubation period of SARS-CoV-2 varied between 3 and 7 days, and best estimates now have suggested a range from 2 to 14 days for the viral incubation period.[2,4]

In some patients there is a rapid immunogenic response that leads to worsening hypoxemic respiratory failure that in mild to moderate cases requires the support of low-flow oxygen therapy and non-invasive ventilatory support. In about 10% of cases the severity progresses to acute respiratory distress syndrome (ARDS) requiring intensive care unit (ICU) admission, invasive mechanical ventilation and advanced therapies for respiratory support, including prone positioning and extracorporeal membrane oxygenation (ECMO) as well as immunomodulatory therapy.[5a] The most severe cases of COVID-19 were also complicated by hypercoagula-bility leading to venous thromboembolism and dissem-inated intravascular coagulation (DIC) and multiorgan failure; including acute renal and liver failure. Patients at higher risk for this increased severity of disease were noted to be of older age and male sex.[6] A population study based on public health data in a Chinese popula-tion noted that the risk for symptomatic infection increased with age, and patients above 59 years of age were 5.1 times more likely to die after developing symp-toms compared with those patients between 30 and 59 years of age.[6,7] A prospective observational study of European patients with COVID-19 in early 2020 during the peak of the pandemic found that the average age of patients admitted to the intensive care unit (ICU) was 63 years and the average age of the ICU nonsurvi-vors was 71 years. Overall, in this cohort the patients with more severe disease were older, men, and had at least one co-morbid medical illness including essential hypertension, diabetes mellitus, ischemic heart disease and/or chronic pulmonary illness.[8] Additional demo-graphic groups that have shown a trend toward increased severity of disease include those who were obese, immunosuppressed, or pregnant.[8–10]

As COVID-19 cases accumulated worldwide, reports of associated neurological symptoms emerged from several centers around the world. A retrospective case series from Wuhan, China reported 45.5% of patients with severe COVID-19 disease had neurological symp-toms, including acute cerebrovascular disease, acute encephalopathy, and skeletal muscle symptoms.[11-13] An analysis of nearly 4000 hospitalized COVID-19 patients from both the United States and Europe found that approximately 80% experienced some form of neuro-logical symptom, most commonly encephalopathy, headache, ageusia, anosmia, coma, and/or stroke.[14] Additional neurological symptoms, including delirium, dizziness, and headaches, have been reported with other coronavirus infections prior to the SARS-CoV-2 outbreak.[15,16]

The neurological manifestations associated with SARS-CoV-2 infection range in severity. A few of the symptoms, such as myopathy, delirium, and encephalopathy, are the consequence of critical illness; however, some short- and longer-term peripheral and CNS manifestations may be related to the effect of the virus on the endothelium, direct neuronal invasion, and cytokine storming. A nar-rative review of neurological symptoms associated with SARS-CoV-2 infection delineated a prevalence ranging from 4.3% to 73% in a total of 2533 hospitalized patients with COVID-19. The most common neurological symp-toms were myalgia (32.4%), headache (20.4%), and impaired consciousness or encephalopathy (21.3%).[4] A cohort study of 3744 patients in two large global con-sortia reported that approximately 80% of patients hos-pitalized with COVID-19 were documented to have neurological symptoms with headache and anosmia

being the most common self-reported symptoms.[16a] Nearly 40% of the central nervous system (CNS) condi-tions were described as nonspecific encephalopathies, with a smaller proportion of postinfectious and parain-fectious syndromes, including encephalitis, acute necro-tizing encephalopathy, acute transverse myelitis, and acute demyelinating encephalomyelitis. Cerebrovascular diseases, including both ischemic and hemorrhagic strokes, cerebral venous thrombosis, and posterior revers-ible encephalopathy (PRES), were another category of common CNS conditions described in hospitalized patients with COVID-19. Peripheral nervous system syn-dromes included classic sensorimotor Guillain-Barré syn-drome (GBS) and associated variants including Miller-Fischer syndrome, axonal, pure motor or sensory and pharyngeal-cervical-brachial forms.[4,16b] Critical illness neuropathy and myopathy have also been described as neurological symptoms of SARS-CoV-2 infec-tion however they are related to prolonged ICU hospi-talization and mechanical ventilation rather than a direct viral neurotropic effect. Anosmia and ageusia are among the most commonly reported peripheral nervous symp-toms. These symptoms have been previously described in other human coronavirus infections, typically as part of their symptomatic phase or as postacute sequelae, but in SARS-CoV-2 infection these symptoms were prominent in otherwise asymptomatic persons or as the initial man-ifestation of COVID-19 disease.[4,15,17,16b]

The end result is that the neurological symptoms of COVID-19 can have both acute consequences affecting morbidity and mortality and chronic consequences for patients who are recovering, which ultimately affects their quality of life.

Historical Background of Neurological Effects of the Coronavirus Family

Human coronaviruses are a family of single-stranded, non-segmented, enveloped RNA viruses that contains seven unique strains, including SARS-CoV, MERS-CoV, and SARS-CoV-2.[17a] Human coronaviruses have demon-strated CNS tropism in vitro (cell cultures) and in vivo (animal) studies. In vitro studies have shown that human coronavirus strains can infect multiple types of neural cell cultures, including neuroblastoma, neuro-glioma, and astrocytoma and microglial and oligoden-drocytic cell lines. The potential for neuroinvasion by human coronaviruses has been demonstrated inciden-tally in brain autopsy samples from multiple sclerosis patients which showed a higher prevalence of corona-virus compared with other diseases and normal controls. Additionally, the detection of viral RNA in human brain autopsy samples from patients with human coronavirus supports their neurotropic and neuroinvasive proper-ties.[16–19] Postmortem studies of SARS-CoV-1 patients demonstrated viral particles within multiple regions of the brain—thalamus, cerebrum, brainstem, hypothalamus; however, in both animal and human studies, viral particles were not found in cerebellar tissue.[19a] MERS-CoV invasion into neuronal tissue was noted to be highest in the brainstem and thalamus. MERS-CoV patients had less direct evidence of neuroinvasion; however, several patients with severe disease manifestations developed altered consciousness, encephalopathy, seizures, ataxia, and focal neurological deficits with radiological changes on both computed tomography (CT) and brain magnetic resonance imaging (MRI) involving small vessels, including lacunar infarcts.[18,19a,19b]

In vivo studies of SARS-CoV-1 describe the proliferation of proinflammatory cytokines that are active in promoting blood–brain barrier breakdown, namely interleukin-8 (IL-8) and monocyte chemoattractant protein-1 (MCP1).[20,21]

MCP1 is a proinflammatory mediator that is expressed in CNS cells, including astrocytes, neurons, and microglia. MCP1 may be upregulated in conditions that target and degrade the blood–brain barrier and can recruit additional inflammatory cells.[20,21] The proinflammatory effects of the human coronaviruses were also initially described in autopsy reports, including one that describes high serum levels of monokine induced by gamma interferon (Mig), also kown as CXCL-9 chemokine, in SARS-CoV-1 patients that was associated with neural invasion. SARS-CoV-1 neural invasion induced expression of Mig chemokine in gliocytes, leading to attraction of CD68 monocytes and CD3 + T-lymphocytes to sites of virus infection. The resultant systemic

inflammatory cascade is one of the contributors to direct brain tissue injury.[20,21] This neuronal injury is then manifested in acute and ultimately chronic neurological symptoms known to be associated with human coronavirus infections.

Headache, dizziness, encephalopathy, meningoencephalitis, stroke, seizures, and neuromuscular weaknesses have been described extensively in the literature as both acute and at times as prodromal symptoms associated with SARS-CoV-2 infection. Many of these symptoms were also reported in the postinfectious period, with some symptoms such as headache, dizziness, encephalopathy, and neuropathy persisting for weeks to months after acute illness.[4,13,15,22–29] Neurological symptoms associated with SARS-CoV-2 were initially described in the acute period of infection and illness. However, as more time has elapsed the neurological symptoms in the postacute and recovery periods have been described as persisting months after resolution of the acute illness; this is now referred to as postacute sequelae of SARS-CoV-2 infection—neuro-PASC.[30]

Pathophysiology, Pathogenesis, and Proposed Mechanisms of the SARS-CoV-2 Virus and the Nervous System

Neuropathological findings were noted in SARS-CoV-2 patients in the latter part of 2020 once autopsy studies were made available. Findings in some of these studies substantiated the potential for a direct neurotropic and

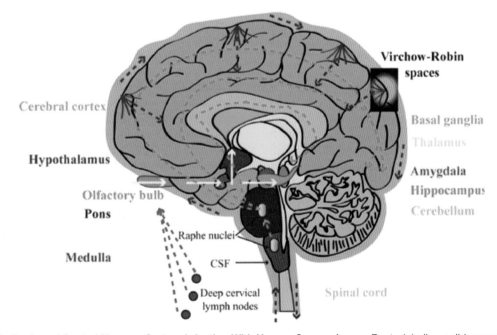

Fig. 7.1 Possible Routes of Central Nervous System Infection With Human Coronaviruses. Route 1 *(yellow solid arrows):* olfactory nerve to olfactory cortex of temporal lobe to hippocampus to amygdala, or to hypothalamus. Route 2 *(green dot arrows):* via serotonergic dorsal raphe system. Route 3 *(red dot arrows):* via hematogenous route and Virchow-Robin spaces. Route 4 *(gray dot arrows):* via lymphatic system. Dissemination routes with empiric data are indicated by *solid arrows,* and speculative ones are indicated by *dot arrows.* (from Cheng Q et al. doi:10.1016/j.ebiom.2020.102799).[18] *CSF,* Cerebrospinal fluid.

neuroinvasive mechanism of action to the disease process. The spike (S) protein on the cell membrane of SARS-CoV-2 is considered to be a key to the virus's ability to invade and modulate the nervous system.[18,24,31–33] Several routes of viral entry into the CNS were theorized, mainly through hematogenous and transneuronal spread.[24,31] A unique mechanism for SARS-CoV-2 neuronal transmission proposed that the acquisition of the viral particles through the olfactory receptor neurons was possible by the olfactory nerve, which acted as a conduit to allow movement across the cribriform plate of the ethmoid bone after initial infection in the nasal passages and upper respiratory tract epithelium, leading to the initial symptoms of anosmia and ageusia. The direct invasion by the olfactory nerve was theorized to lead to cerebral invasion and hippocampal and brainstem spread.[31,34]

The hematogenous route is another mechanism of direct neuronal invasion that has been described in SARS-CoV-2 infection. SARS-CoV-2, similar to other human coronaviruses, uses the S-protein on the viral cell membrane to bind angiotensin-converting enzyme-2 (ACE2) receptors located in various organs in order to access and enter host cells.[18,19] The ACE2 receptors are most notable in the respiratory epithelium of humans, but is also expressed strongly throughout the body, including in brain, heart, and adipose tissue, as well as throughout the vascular endothelium.[19] Once bound, the virus undergoes fusion and endocytosis and then sheds its coat within the cell. Viral RNA is then translated, and viral particles are released from the host cells.[22] In the CNS, ACE2 receptors are ubiquitous, especially in astrocytes, microglia, and oligodendrocytes. There are a number of neurons that also contain ACE2 receptors along the motor cortex, temporal regions, substantia nigra, thalamus, and olfactory bulb.[24] Using the ACE2 receptors is one of the hypothesized mechanisms of direct neuronal effect by SARS-CoV-2. Additionally, it was postulated that SARS-CoV-2 could spread to the CNS in a manner similar to that of the human immunodeficiency virus (HIV), in which infected immune cells pass from the blood through the blood–brain barrier to infect the CNS.[24] Once CNS penetration occurs, SARS-CoV-2 is thought to harm brain tissue directly by entering neuronal tissue using ACE2 entry and viral replication, or indirectly through immunogenic response.

Along with the direct neurotropic effects of SARS-CoV-2, the indirect effects of the virus leading to neuronal damage also have been described. These indirect effects on the nervous system are typically related to hypoxic brain injury, blood pressure dysregulation, severe metabolic disturbances, coagulopathy, and immune-mediated neurological damage.[13,15,17,23,24,34,35,35a] Hypoxic-ischemic brain injury occurs as a consequence of the viral replication within pneumocytes, which leads to diffuse alveolar and interstitial inflammatory exudate and ultimately impairment of gas exchange; this is clinically manifested as pneumonia and in severe cases

progression to ARDS. In addition to the severe clinical hypoxemic manifestations, COVID-19 patients have been reported to experience silent hypoxia at a prevalence as high as 20% to 40%.[34,36] The indirect effect of systemic hypoxemia in COVID-19 patients on the CNS have been described in both autopsy and radiological studies. A case series of postmortems performed on patients with COVID-19 who died of respiratory failure describes the presence of ischemic red neurons within the hippocampus and parahippocampal and cerebellar regions that are consistent with global ischemic injury. The brainstem of these patients also demonstrated reactive gliosis and microglia, which are reflective of hypoxic-ischemic injury that occurred directly before death.[35,36,37] Although autopsy reports of hypoxic ischemic brain injury in COVID-19 patients are limited, additional information can be found in neuroimaging reports of MRI and CT patterns found in acutely ill COVID-19 patients, especially ones with prolonged ICU hospitalizations. Diffuse leukoencephalopathy has been described as symmetrical confluent white matter hyperintensities on T2-weighted sequences, as well as restricted diffusion on diffusion-weighted imaging. The observed pattern of leukoencephalopathy in these patients seem to spare the infratentorial and juxtacortical white matter and has been reported as both an acute phenomenon and a delayed posthypoxic event. Additional hypoxic-ischemic radiographic patterns on MRI have included symmetrical involvement of the basal ganglia.[38,39]

Another indirect effect of SARS CoV-2 on the nervous system is mediated through the immunogenicity of the SARS-CoV-2 virus, which can cause a cytokine storm in a small percentage of individuals. This leads to the activation of a number of immune-mediated inflammatory pathways that eventually cause complement and coagulation cascade stimulation, disseminated intravascular coagulation, and ultimately multiorgan dysfunction.[23] Additionally, the effect of SARS-CoV-2 on the vascular system through ACE2 receptors leads to blood pressure dysregulation, which may be manifested as hypertension and in addition to the coagulopathy increases the risk for both spontaneous intracerebral hemorrhage and ischemic stroke.[34]

COVID-19 and the Peripheral Nervous System

Anosmia and Dysgeusia

During the early phase of the SARS-CoV-2 pandemic, in addition to respiratory symptoms, there were frequent reports of olfactory dysfunction with loss of smell (anosmia/hyposmia) or altered sensations of taste (dysgeusia). These anecdotal reports included both published and unpublished data in the early days of the pandemic.[40-42] The reports became so common that the

Centers for Disease Control and Prevention listed anosmia and ageusia/dysgeusia as a prodromal symptom of COVID-19. The British Association of Otorhinolaryngology and the American Academy of Otolaryngology-Head and Neck Surgery in 2020 both proposed that symptoms of olfactory and gustatory dysfunction be added to the screening lists for possible COVID-19 infection.[43,44] A systematic review and meta-analysis of patients with confirmed SARS-CoV-2 infection found that about 41% and 38% had olfactory or gustatory dysfunction, respectively, as their initial manifesting symptom.[44] The onset was usually sudden and may precede other typical COVID-19 symptoms, and the olfactory or gustatory dysfunction lasted an average of 1 to 3 weeks, unlike other forms of postviral olfactory or gustatory dysfunction, caused by direct damage to the olfactory sensory neurons and therefore leading to a more common recovery timeline of months.[45,46]

The mechanism leading to olfactory or gustatory dysfunction in COVID-19 is not fully elucidated; however, olfactory dysfunction is not uncommon as a postviral phenomenon of many other upper respiratory tract infections. Overall, postviral olfactory dysfunction occurs in at least 40% of patients with upper respiratory tract infections and approximately 10% to 15% of these olfactory or gustatory dysfunctions are caused by coronaviruses.[47,48] The olfactory or gustatory dysfunction symptoms in COVID-19 commonly arise in otherwise asymptomatic persons or as the prodromal symptom of COVID-19 rather than in conjunction with other typical upper respiratory tract symptoms (nasal congestion, sore throat), unlike other respiratory infections that cause olfactory or gustatory dysfunction. As discussed earlier, SARS-CoV-2 infects cells by binding its spike (S) protein with the ACE2 protein on the targeted cells. Based on this, the mechanism for olfactory or gustatory dysfunction in COVID-19 has been postulated to be related to the potential neurotrophic properties of SARS-CoV-2 leading to transneuronal spread through the olfactory nerve. However, these ACE2 receptors are expressed by nonneuronal supporting cells of the olfactory epithelium rather than directly within the olfactory neurons, casting doubt on the putative neurotropic mechanism of olfactory or gustatory dysfunction.[44-46,49] Although other neurotropic virus models have been able to demonstrate direct neuronal invasion by the olfactory nerve, pathological evidence to support this mechanism in SARS-CoV-2 infection is lacking.

Autopsies of patients with COVID-19 have found that the brain contains the lowest levels of SARS-CoV-2 compared with other organs. Animal models to investigate the mechanism of olfactory or gustatory dysfunction in SARS-CoV-2 have revealed variable results; one study of intranasal inoculation of SARS-CoV-2 in mouse models expressing human ACE2 receptors resulted in identification of the virus within the brain.[46] Other models have demonstrated the presence of SARS-CoV-2

in the olfactory sensory support cells rather than the olfactory bulb, suggesting that the mechanism of olfactory or gustatory dysfunction is more of an inflammatory nature, which leads to faster recovery compared with other postviral olfactory or gustatory dysfunction.[45,46]

MRI of the olfactory nerves can provide more details regarding the cause of olfactory dysfunction and predict recovery of olfactory function. A study using dedicated MRI of the olfactory nerves in patients with persistent olfactory or gustatory dysfunction related to COVID-19 after resolution of other symptoms was used to evaluate parameters, including olfactory cleft opacification, olfactory bulb volume, morphology, signal intensity, the architecture of olfactory nerve filia, and any signal abnormalities of the primary olfactory cortex. The majority of patients had opacification of the olfactory cleft (73.9%), and there were also changes in the morphology and T2 signal abnormalities of the olfactory bulb, along with decrease in the amount of olfactory nerve filia and objective reduction in olfactory bulb volume. The decreased amount of olfactory nerve filia resulting from clumping or loss of nerves suggest both inflammatory and degenerative loss as a result of SARS-CoV-2 infection.[45] These structural changes potentially result in olfactory dysfunction from injury to the supporting cells of the olfactory epithelium. Another mechanism of olfactory or gustatory dysfunction is seen in the secondary inflammatory changes of the olfactory clefts that manifest as opacification on MRI of the olfactory nerves. Inflammatory changes are related to invasion of SARS-CoV-2 leading to mucosal edema and narrowing of the olfactory cleft; this hypothesis was supported in an imaging review showing olfactory cleft opacification in the majority of patients with COVID-19–related anosmia.[45]

Although the mechanism of olfactory and gustatory dysfunction in patients with COVID-19 remains largely hypothetical, there has been overwhelming evidence using objective tests of smell and taste that anosmia/hyposmia and dysgeusia/ageusia are reliable prodromal symptoms of infection with SARS-CoV-2.

Guillain-Barré Syndrome and Associated Variants

Acute inflammatory demyelinating polyneuropathy (AIDP), more commonly known by its eponym Guillain-Barré syndrome (GBS), is an autoimmune disease in which an inciting event such as an infection (commonly bacterial or viral) or vaccination incites the production of autoantibodies by molecular mimicry leading to demyelination of peripheral nerves with subsequent ascending paresis/paralysis, sensory disturbances, and ophthalmoparesis and in severe cases diaphragmatic weakness and bulbar dysfunction requiring mechanical ventilation.

The mechanism of GBS as a parainfectious or postinfectious phenomenon of SARS-CoV-2 infection is

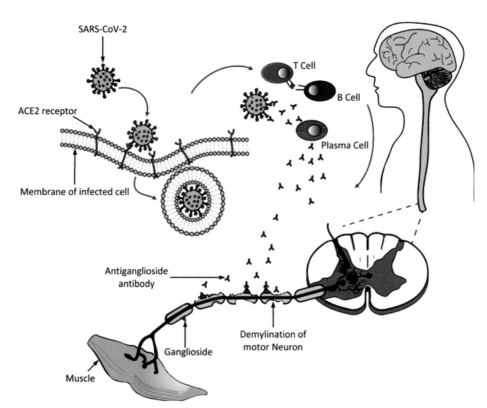

Fig. 7.2 Schematic Representation of the Likely Pathophysiology of COVID-19–Associated Guillain-Barré Syndrome.[52] SARS-COV-2 has a high affinity for the angiotensin-converting enzyme-2 (ACE2) receptor, which is located throughout the nasopharynx, the central nervous system, and on blood vessels. SARS-COV-2 binds this receptor and is endocytosed. Because of molecular mimicry, antibodies are formed against the virus through the T-cell–B-cell interactions and may bind the gangliosides located on the peripheral neurons. This may result in an autoimmune response that destroys the myelin and/or axons. The demyelination or axonal damage disrupts neural transmission, which causes the GBS symptoms such as muscle weakness, paralysis, coordination problems, breathing difficulties, and autonomic dysfunction. *ACE2,* Angiotensin-converting enzyme-2.

postulated to be one of molecular mimicry. The production of autoantibodies through exposure of antigen epitopes and molecular mimicry in GBS may be related to the initial SARS-CoV-2 viral infection and resultant inflammatory cascade. SARS-CoV-2 epitopes have demonstrated cross-reactivity with autoantigens including heat shock proteins and proteins within the brainstem associated with GBS and respiratory failure respectively.[50] In general, the increased proportion of serum inflammatory markers, including CRP, IL-6, IL-1, and tumor necrosis factor-alpha, in cases with GBS and COVID-19 seem to support the dysimmune theory.[50,51]

As illustrated in Fig. 7.2, antibodies are formed against SARS-CoV-2 and/or pathogens bind to gangliosides on the surface membranes of peripheral motor and sensory neurons and cause immune-mediated damage to the myelin sheath and/or axons. The SARS-CoV-2 infection is postulated then to trigger an adaptive immune response in which T-cell–B-cell interactions result in the production of SARS-CoV-2–specific antibodies, but a similarity in viral and ganglioside peptide sequences or structure can result in the development of autoimmunity.[52] The Schwann cell ganglioside peptide sequences located on the myelin sheath of axons and membranes of neurons may act as receptors for these antiganglioside antibodies, which neutralizes the neurons' complement

inhibitory activity and turns them into targets for an autoimmune-mediated destruction of myelin sheaths or axons. Depending on the nature of the damage, an individual may experience either the demyelinating or axonal GBS subtype, which differ not only in symptom manifestations but also in likelihood of recovery.[52]

The difficulty in distinguishing causality from association during a novel pandemic is a feature of the case reports and case series reported during the early part of the pandemic. GBS is not an uncommon illness and is the leading cause of flaccid paralysis globally, with an estimated incidence of 2.66 cases per 100,000 person-years across all age groups worldwide.[53] The initial reports of GBS associated with COVID-19 seemed to center mainly on adults; however, as the pandemic progressed, reports of GBS precipitated by SARS-CoV-2 infection also surfaced in pediatric age groups.[51,53] During the initial peak of the pandemic, reports of cases of ascending paralysis and respiratory failure surfaced in temporal association with COVID-19 symptoms. One review estimated that the mean time to onset of neurological symptoms, which were typically limb paresthesias or pain and weakness, was approximately 11 days, and another study of 37 patients reported that the timing of symptom onset ranged between 3 and 28 days.[54,55] Another series including patients from China,

Italy, and the United States noted that the majority of COVID-19 patients with GBS symptoms presented in the parainfectious period; therefore the typical GBS symptoms of weakness, bulbar dysfunction, facial paresis, and respiratory failure occurred concomitantly with their COVID-19 symptoms. There were also rare cases of post-COVID GBS in which symptoms followed up to 4 weeks after their initial COVID-19 illness.[55,56] A larger systematic review of GBS cases associated with COVID-19 described the common clinical manifestations in 72 patients in whom sensory symptoms (72.2%) alone or with limb paresis (65.2%) associated with areflexia were also the most common symptoms at the time of onset. Cranial nerve involvement, including facial nerve paresis or ophthalmoparesis, were rare at onset, but nearly 25% of the patients developed these symptoms along with bulbar dysfunction as the disease progressed. Within this review, autonomic symptoms were uncommon; however, other reviews have reported an increased risk for autonomic dysfunction in patients with COVID-19–associated GBS.[51,52] Additionally, nearly a third of the patients in this systematic review developed respiratory symptoms.[51,56] These symptoms also concomitantly evolved with active SARS-CoV-2 infection, and therefore it would be difficult to differentiate association from causation—that is, whether GBS causes respiratory failure in this setting.

Another difficulty in establishing a link between SARS-CoV-2 infection and GBS is the heterogeneity of diagnostic testing, especially in the early days of the pandemic. The majority of patients in the various series did have elevated inflammatory markers, including D-dimer, C-reactive protein (CRP), and erythrocyte sedimentation rate, as would be expected in a parainfectious manifestation. Additionally, more neuron-/myelin-specific antibodies were found in some series, including ganglioside antibodies. One of the largest systematic reviews reported only a small proportion of their cases being tested for antiganglioside antibodies (33/73), and of these cases anti-GD1b and anti-GM antibodies were positive in only one patient with Miller-Fisher syndrome and one with classical GBS. A multicenter series of studies in the United States found that the majority of patients who underwent a lumbar puncture for evaluation showed albuminocytological dissociation with elevated protein and low cell counts; however, as previous publications have reported, SARS-CoV-2 could not be isolated in any of the CSF samples tested.[51,54-56] In an earlier study of GBS case reports related to COVID-19, the authors note that no antiganglioside antibodies were identified for the majority of the cases, except for four patients, the first who had anti-GM2 immunoglobulin G (IgG)/IgM; a second with anti-GM2 IgM, anti-GD3 IgM, and anti-GT1b IgG; one patient with Miller-Fischer syndrome and GD1b-IgG; and one patient with acute motor axonal neuropathy (AMAN) subtype with GD1b-IgG.[52] These data suggest a nonimmunological

mechanism of GBS; however, they point out that elevated anti-GM2 IgG/IgM is a rare occurrence in GBS but has been reported in different subtypes with clinical heterogeneity of IgM, whereas IgG is predominantly associated with cranial GBS variants, especially in patients presenting with oculomotor and vestibular dysfunction, characterized by dizziness.[57] In their study, irrespective of their anti-GM2 IgG/IgM positivity, none of their studied patients had signs of cranial neuropathy, but they all experienced autonomic dysfunction and received mechanical ventilation. Additionally, the presence of these antibodies is consistent with known neuroimmunological responses to infection, especially molecular mimicry. They point out that improvement in response to immunoglobulin therapy also provides further support for the immune-mediated neuropathogenesis of COVID-19–related GBS. Alternatively, they also suggest that the absence of antiganglioside antibodies in a majority of the tested patients could mean that nonimmunological mechanisms such as direct infection of the nervous system could also be involved in the onset of GBS symptoms. As with some of the other neuromanifestations of COVID-19, viral neurotropism may play a role in mediating GBS symptoms. Lack of an abundance in cases of SARS-CoV-2 polymerase chain reaction (PCR) and RNA positivity in the CSF and brain points away from this theory. However, absence of SARS-CoV-2 samples in the CSF and CNS tissue samples should not rule out the possibility for direct viral involvement in the cause of GBS and other neurological disorders because by the time neurological symptoms are noted the viral load may have dropped to undetectable levels.

Systematic reviews of manifestations of GBS with COVID-19 that are drawn from centers worldwide found that when electrodiagnostic testing could be performed the most common diagnosis was demyelinating polyradiculopathy consistent with GBS. A smaller proportion of cases demonstrated axonal damage that met diagnostic criteria for acute motor and sensory axonal neuropathy (AMSAN), and these cases were often characterized by cranial neuropathies along with areflexic weakness. Miller-Fisher syndrome and acute motor axonal neuropathy (AMAN) were rarer variants.[51,55,56]

Regardless of the mechanism of GBS associated with COVID-19, the treatment approaches have not differed from treatment of classic GBS. Immune-modulating strategies using either intravenous immunoglobulin or plasma exchange alongside supportive care for respiratory symptoms and hemodynamics constitute the standard therapeutic approach. Vaccines that are effective against SARS-CoV-2 are now available globally, and some concern has arisen that GBS cases may be seen as a postvaccination phenomenon similar to GBS associated with influenza vaccine. Only a few case reports exist, and the current guidelines emphasize the lack of clear evidence linking GBS to SARS-CoV-2 vaccines and recommendations to continue with the SARS-CoV-2 vaccine for persons who previously have had GBS related to vaccination remain. At present, despite many millions of SARS-CoV-2 doses administered in countries with extensive vaccination programs such as the United Kingdom and the United States, no causal link between the vaccine and GBS has been identified. The risk for death or long-term complications from COVID-19 in adults still far exceeds any possible risk for GBS by several orders of magnitude.

COVID-19 and the Central Nervous System

Encephalopathy and Encephalitis

Encephalopathy has consistently been associated with COVID-19. In a multicenter study of 3055 patients from 28 centers in 13 countries, encephalopathy was found to be common (49%).[25] Unfortunately, it is not clear if the encephalopathy results directly from the proposed neurotropic effects of the infection, indirectly such as from fever or the sequelae of secondary brain injury, such as ischemic stroke, intracerebral hemorrhage, PRES, and prolonged seizures, or by some other not yet described mechanism. Additionally, encephalopathy in critically ill patients tends to be multifactorial, and factors such as use of sedatives, reversed sleep-wake cycle, and metabolic derangements (acute kidney injury, transaminitis, hypernatremia), are also additive effects to the development of acute encephalopathy. Many institutions are establishing postacute COVID-19 clinics to follow the trajectory of these encephalopathic COVID patients to document the natural history of this illness. Case example 7.1 describes the multifactoral contributors to acute encephalopathy in SARS-CoV-2 infection with abnormal neuroimaging (Figures 7.3 and 7.4), elevated opening pressure on initial spinal tap, mild CSF pleocytosis and markedly elevated CSF protein as well as seizures.

Transverse Myelitis

An underappreciated neurological manifestation of SARS-CoV-2 is transverse myelitis. Transverse myelitis is likely underappreciated and underreported given the difficulties in obtaining appropriate imaging in these patients, who are often severely critically ill. The following case report (7.2) highlights transverse myelitis occurring in a patient with SARS-CoV-2 infection.

Seizures

Throughout the pandemic, findings of new-onset seizures related to COVID-19 were reported, but few were able to decisively show causation as a result of direct CNS involvement. Seizures are likely a result of the accumulation of inflammatory markers, causing local cortical irritation that precipitates seizures related to COVID-19 infection.[11] Initially, breakthrough seizures in epileptic patients were more commonly seen. Although CSF may contain markers of inflammation, the treatment of this infection is largely supportive, and with the additional risk for coagulopathy precipitated by SARS-CoV-2, a lumbar puncture may not be justifiable unless there is an alternative diagnosis to be sought. A limitation of our case series is that CSF was not typically obtained because of patient factors that made lumbar puncture a relative contraindication and a CSF PCR test for SARS-CoV-2 was not yet commercially available. As this disease continues to spread, we will learn more about its direct and/or indirect epileptogenesis.[11]

Early in the pandemic, the connection of seizure risk and COVID-19 infection was not clear. As centers collaborated and shared data, we learned more. A recent multicenter research collaborative project has shed light on the incidence of seizures in patients with COVID-19.[58] This article from nine centers that included 197 patients hospitalized with COVID-19 reported seizures in 9.6% of patients, with 5.6% being nonconvulsive. Interestingly, epileptiform abnormalities were present in 48.7% of this population. COVID-19 patients with preexisting structural injury were found to have a higher risk for seizure (14.3% vs. 3.7%; odds ratio, 4.33).[58]

Cerebrovascular Disease

Stroke in patients with COVID-19 was studied quite extensively throughout the initial waves of the pandemic because there was an association with systemic illness and younger age.[59,60] There have been several proposed mechanisms of an increased risk for ischemic stroke with COVID-19. SARS-CoV-2 infection has been hypothesized to cause a secondary coagulopathy, possibly through the formation of antiphospholipid antibodies.[61,62] It remains unknown whether these antibodies are acute phase reactants that reflect disease severity or truly pathogenic by increasing thrombotic complications. Similarly, it is unclear, but speculated, that SARS-CoV-2 can cause a virus-induced vasculitis. An autopsy study of three COVID-19 patients revealed evidence of direct viral infection of endothelial cells and diffuse endothelialitis involving multiple organ systems.[63] It is most likely that the increased risk for stroke seen in patients with COVID is related to the severe acute illness and procoagulant state, the related systemic inflammatory response.

The cause of hemorrhagic stroke in COVID-19 patients is less understood. Among COVID-19 cases with respiratory failure and mechanical ventilation, microhemorrhages have been reported.[64,65]

■ Case Example: 7.1 Encephalitis

A 37-year-old woman without significant medical history presented with acute altered mental status and flexor posturing. She was vaccinated with the two-injection series of mRNA-1273. She was 8 months out from her second shot and had not received a booster shot. She developed a sore throat 5 days before hospitalization and chills and fevers about 2 days after initial symptoms. Home testing was positive for SARS-CoV-2 by antigen testing. A day later, her husband noticed that she was having difficulty setting up a zoom call, then later she abruptly left her house for no particular reason with the television remote and her 4-year-old daughter. She was later found by police parked at a construction site parking lot in her car covered in emesis. On arrival to the emergency department, her temperature was 97.1°F, her blood pressure was 100/59 mm Hg, and she was minimally reactive and disoriented. Naloxone 0.2 mg was given, with no improvement in mental status.

A head CT revealed some hypoattenuation in the bilateral thalami (Fig. 7.3). CT angiography of the head and neck did not show any evidence of large vessel occlusion, vasculitis, or venous or sinus thrombosis.

Her laboratory test results were notable for positive SARS-CoV-2 status by PCR; urine toxicology screen was positive for benzodiazepine (received lorazepam [Ativan]) and negative for salicylate and acetaminophen. She had mild anemia, no leukocytosis, and no overt evidence of metabolic derangement. Her ammonia concentration was within normal limits at 11 μ/dL, and both serum thyroid-stimulating hormone (TSH) and thyroxine (T_4) were low at 0.19 mIU/ml and 0.91 ng/dL, respectively.

She had multiple episodes of "seizure-like activity" for which she received a total of 16 mg of lorazepam and 4 mg of midazolam and was given loading doses of intravenous anti-seizure medications (ASM) including fosphenytoin, levetiracetam, and phenobarbital. She was intubated for airway protection. Lumbar puncture was performed, and CSF analysis revealed a glucose value of 111 mg/dl, protein 197 mg/dl, but no CSF pleocytosis. Ceftriaxone, vancomycin, and acyclovir were initiated for empiric coverage of meningitis.

In the neurological ICU, her vital signs were within normal limits. Her neurological examination was significant for inability to respond to verbal or painful stimuli, bilateral small but sluggishly reactive pupils, bilateral extensor posturing, and hyperreflexia in both lower extremities.

Brain MRI revealed markedly abnormal appearance of the bilateral caudate, thalami, midbrain, and pons, with additional abnormality involving the medial aspect of both temporal lobes (Fig. 7.4). Her antimicrobial regimen was discontinued, and remdesivir was initiated.

A lumbar puncture was repeated, which revealed a raised intracranial pressure (ICP) (opening pressure 38 cm H_2O). CSF analysis revealed 0 red blood cells (RBCs), 3 white blood cells (WBCs) (16% polymorphonuclear neutrophils, 42% lymphocytes, and 42% macrophages), normal glucose, and elevated protein of 315 mg/dL. Ganglioside and encephalitis panels including herpes simplex virus PCR, Epstein-Barr virus PCR, cytomegalovirus PCR, varicella-zoster virus PCR, thyroglobulin antibody, and thyroid peroxidase antibodies were ordered, and results were negative. A brain tissue

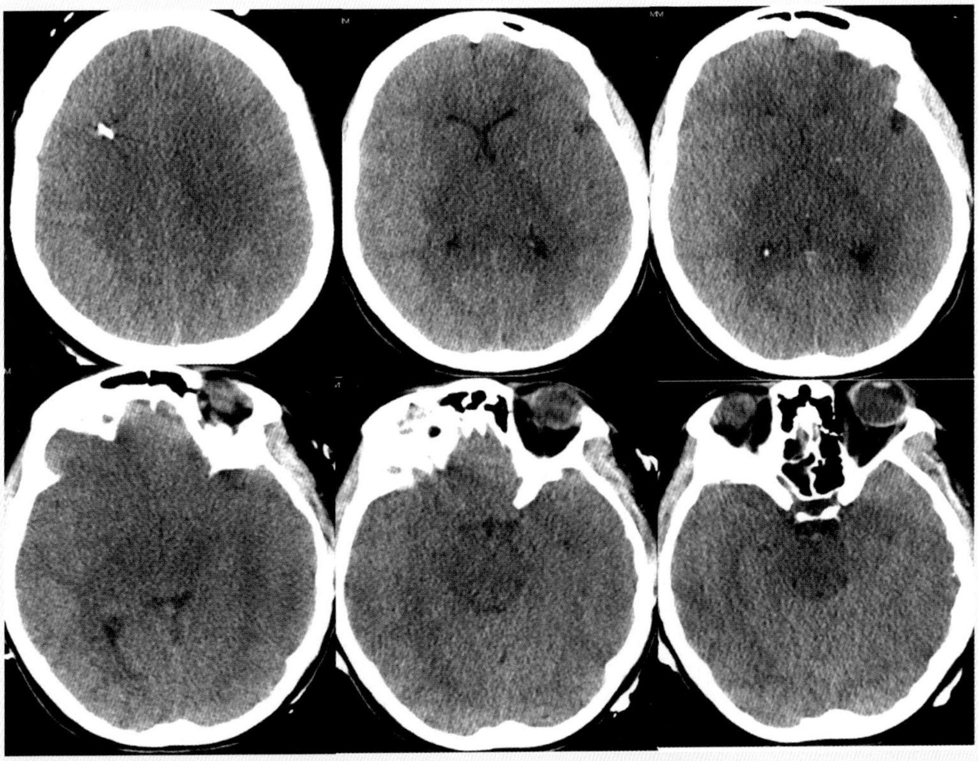

Fig. 7.3 Non-contrast head computed tomography revealed progressive diffuse cerebral edema with diffuse sulcal effacement involving the supratentorium and infratentorium and confluent hypoattenuation within the basal ganglia and brainstem.

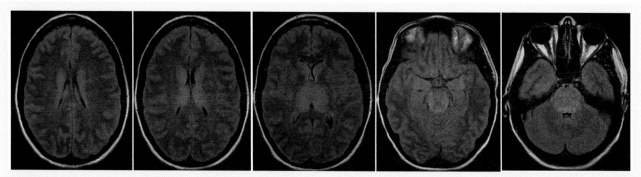

Fig. 7.4 Brain T2-weighted fluid attenuated inversion recovery (FLAIR) axial image revealing hyperintense, rather symmetrical, signals in the bilateral caudate, thalami, midbrain, and pons, with additional abnormality involving the medial aspect of both temporal lobe.

oxygenation/intracerebral pressure monitor was placed, and repeat head CT showed progressive diffuse cerebral edema with diffuse sulcal effacement involving the supratentorium and infratentorium and confluent hypoattenuation within the basal ganglia and brainstem (see Fig. 7.2), as well as increased ICP (>25 cm H_2O), for which she received several doses of 23.4% NaCl over the next few days.

She was started on intravenous pulse steroids and five sessions of plasmapheresis. Her mental status drastically improved by plasmapheresis day 1, and completely normalized by postoperative day 5.

■ Case Example: 7.2 Transverse Myelitis

A 43-year-old woman with no medical history presented to the emergency department with progressive bilateral lower extremity weakness and paresthesias that began 2 days earlier. She described a sharp pain in her mid-back between her shoulders along her "bra strap area." Her weakness progressed symmetrically, from her feet to her thighs. She described having decreased sensation from her nipple line to her feet, including arms and hands. She tested positive for SARS-CoV-2 12 days before presentation and recovered at home. Her CRP was 1.1 mmol/L (normal 0.5–2.2 mmol/L). Her basic metabolic panel and complete blood count were unremarkable. An MRI of the spine was obtained (Fig. 7.5A). It was significant for a diffusely abnormal signal in the central cord of the majority of the spinal cord extending from C5/C6 to T11/T12 with ill-defined enhancement. She was started on high-dose intravenous methylprednisolone (Solu-Medrol) and remdesivir. Within a few hours of admission, she went into respiratory distress and required intubation. A lumbar puncture was obtained and contained 949 cells/μL white blood cells (WBCs; normal 0–5 cells/μL), 276 cells/μL red blood cells (RBCs; normal 0–5 cells/μL), 201 mg/dL protein (normal

15–45 mg/dL), and 157 mg/dL glucose (normal 40–70 mg/dL). The IgG index was elevated at 1.09, and myelin basic protein was elevated at greater than 112 (normal <5.5). The remainder of the inflammatory, autoimmune, and infectious workup was unremarkable. She was treated with plasma exchange and completed a course of methylprednisolone. Despite this, her weakness progressed to flaccid quadriplegia. She had episodes of dysautonomia, including bradyarrhythmias and hypotension, requiring treatment. Repeat MRI (see Fig. 7.5B) of the neuraxis showed worsening T2 hyperintensity with mild contrast enhancement involving the medulla, cerebellar tonsils, and inferior pons. She was treated with intravenous immunoglobulin (IVIG). Repeat lumbar puncture had improved to WBCs 5 cells/μL, RBCs 5 cells/μL, protein 31 mg/dL, and glucose 123 mg/dL. A third MRI (see Fig. 7.5C) showed marked improvement in the T2 hyperintensity. Given the likely monophasic nature of the transverse myelitis, she did not require an immunomodulator. She was, however, continued on prednisone with a plan to slowly taper over a course of weeks. She was transferred to a long-term acute care facility.

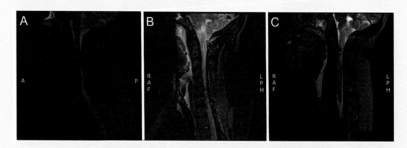

Fig. 7.5 Initial magnetic resonance image (MRI) (A) showing diffusely abnormal signal in the central cord of the majority of the spinal cord extending from C5/C6 to T11/T12 with ill-defined enhancement followed by a second MRI (B) showing worsening despite treatment with methylprednisolone and plasmapheresis. A third MRI (C) after all therapies (steroids, plasmapheresis, and intravenous immunoglobulin) administered shows marked improvement in the T2 hyperintensity.

Hemorrhages may reflect the underlying microangiopathic process, with microhemorrhages seen in moderate to severe COVID-19 cases. Proangiopathic mechanisms also may be related to the overall systemic inflammatory response.

Cerebral venous thrombosis has been reported with increased incidence in COVID-19 cases. Viral infections are associated with coagulopathy.[66] Similar to cases of hemorrhage and ischemic stroke, direct or indirect activation of endothelial cells by viruses may impair coagulation and fibrinolytic systems leading to cerebral venous thrombosis. Antiphospholipid antibody presence and D-dimer elevations related to COVID-19 are also implicated in the incidence of cerebral venous thrombosis.[67]

Long COVID and Neurological Postacute Sequelae of SARS-CoV-2 Infection

People diagnosed with COVID-19 have frequently reported long-term sequelae of the disease, especially related to cognitive function. The reported "brain fog" or cognitive dysfunction that many experience remains somewhat in its initial evaluation phase at the time of this writing. Regardless of the severity of the disease, many patients report symptoms of mental slowing or cloudiness during the acute phase of illness, their early convalescent period and as long as six months after the intial infection. Patients hospitalized with COVID-19 seem to have worsened cognitive impairment. Impairments in executive functioning, processing speed, category fluency, memory encoding, and recall were predominant among hospitalized patients versus outpatients.[27,68] These findings are not specific to COVID-19 because they have been reported in other viral illnesses such as influenza.[69] Future studies are needed to identify the risk factors and mechanisms underlying cognitive dysfunction and the treatment options for patients who experience these impairments.

COVID 19 and Challenges

COVID-19 presents unique challenges in the care of patients with neurological symptoms. At the beginning of the pandemic there were trends toward more delayed presentations to the hospital because of patients avoiding healthcare facilities because of the fear of becoming infected with SARS-CoV-2. As a result, patients with time-sensitive neurological illnesses, such as ischemic stroke, were often presenting outside of the time window for acute reperfusion therapies such as intravenous tissue plasminogen activator (tPA) and endovascular therapy.

Patients with COVID-19 who were critically ill often had coagulopathies (thrombocytopenia, prolonged partial thromboplastin time/international normalized ratio) or were under treatment for venous thromboembolic diseases that required therapeutic anticoagulation. These clinical challenges made a lumbar puncture to obtain CSF unsafe because of thrombocytopenia or inability to safely interrupt their anticoagulation.

Acute cerebrovascular complications may be underestimated in patients with COVID-19 because of increased usage of sedation and paralytics to manage respiratory failure that may mask neurological deficits. Additionally, because of concerns of exposure and transmission involved with transporting these patients, there may be underutilization of neurological consultation, neuroimaging, and electroencephalography, leading to confounding factors that prevent estimation of the true prevalence of cerebrovascular disease burden in these patients. The timing and mechanisms of cerebrovascular disease during the course of illness are not well known. In some patients, neurological symptoms may be the only disease manifestation.

Summary

In summary, neurological manifestations in COVID-19 infection are heterogenous, affecting both the central and peripheral nervous systems directly or indirectly as a consequence of critical and systemic illness. We are still early in understanding the apparent unique connection between SARS-CoV-2 and the nervous system.

REFERENCES

1. Khan M, Adil SF, Alkhathlan HZ, Tahir MN, Saif S, Khan M, Khan ST. COVID-19: a global challenge with old history, epidemiology and progress so far. *Molecules (Basel, Switzerland)*. 2020;26(1):39. doi:10.3390/molecules26010039.
2. Rabi FA, Zoubi Al, M. S, Kasasbeh GA, Salameh DM, Al-Nasser AD. SARS-CoV-2 and Coronavirus Disease 2019: what we know so far. *Pathogens (Basel, Switzerland)*. 2020;9(3):231. doi:10.3390/pathogens9030231.
3. Cui J, Li F, Shi ZL. Origin and evolution of pathogenic coronaviruses. *Nature reviews. Microbiology*. 2019;17(3):181–192. doi:10.1038/s41579-018-0118-9.
4. Maury A, Lyoubi A, Peiffer-Smadja N, de Broucker T, Meppiel E. Neurological manifestations associated with SARS-CoV-2 and other coronaviruses: A narrative review for clinicians. *Revue Neurologique*. 2021;177(1-2):51–64. doi:10.1016/j.neurol.2020.10.001.
5. World Health Organization. (2022, May 17) WHO Coronavirus (COVID-19) Dashboard. https://covid19.who.int/
5a. Ragab Dina, et al. The COVID-19 Cytokine Storm; What We Know So Far. *Frontiers in Immunology*. 2020;11. doi:10.3389/fimmu.2020.01446. In press.
6. Gao YD, Ding M, Dong X, Zhang JJ, Kursat Azkur A, Azkur D, Gan H, Sun YL, Fu W, Li W, Liang HL, Cao YY, Yan Q, Cao C, Gao HY, Brüggen MC, van de Veen W, Sokolowska M, Akdis M, Akdis CA. Risk factors for severe and critically ill COVID-19 patients: a review. *Allergy*. 2021;76(2):428–455. doi:10.1111/all.14657.

7. Wu JT, Leung K, Bushman M, Kishore N, Niehus R, de Salazar PM, Cowling BJ, Lipsitch M, Leung GM. Estimating clinical severity of COVID-19 from the transmission dynamics in Wuhan, China. *Nature Medicine*. 2020;26(4):506–510. doi:10.1038/s41591-020-0822-7.

8. Garcia Wendel, D. P, Fumeaux T, Guerci P, Heuberger DM, Montomoli J, Roche-Campo F, Schuephach RA, Hilty MPRISC-19-ICU Investigators. Prognostic factors associated with mortality risk and disease progression in 639 critically ill patients with COVID-19 in Europe: Initial report of the international RISC-19-ICU prospective observational cohort. *EClinicalMedicine*. 2020;25:100449. doi:10.1016/j.eclinm.2020.100449.

9. Kucirka LM, Norton A, Sheffield JS. Severity of COVID-19 in pregnancy: A review of current evidence. *American journal of reproductive immunology (New York, N.Y.: 1989)*. 2020;84(5):e13332. doi:10.1111/aji.1333.

10. Yang J, Hu J, Zhu C. Obesity aggravates COVID-19: A systematic review and meta-analysis. *Journal of medical virology*. 2021;93(1):257–261. doi:10.1002/jmv.26237.

11. Hepburn M, Mullaguri N, George P, Hantus S, Punia V, Bhimraj A, Newey CR. Acute Symptomatic Seizures in Critically Ill Patients with COVID-19: Is There an Association?. *Neurocritical care*. 2021;34(1):139–143. doi:10.1007/s12028-020-01006-1.

12. Shereen MA, Khan S, Kazmi A, Bashir N, Siddique R. COVID-19 infection: Origin, transmission, and characteristics of human coronaviruses. *Journal of advanced research*. 2020;24:91–98. doi:10.1016/j.jare.2020.03.005.

13. Mao L, Wang M, Chen S, et al. Neurological Manifestations of Hospitalized Patients with COVID-19 in Wuhan, China: A Retrospective Case Series Study. *SSRN Electronic Journal*. 2020;77(6):683–690.

14. Johansson MA, Quandelacy TM, Kada S, Prasad PV, Steele M, Brooks JT, Slayton RB, Biggerstaff M, Butler JC. SARS-CoV-2 Transmission From People Without COVID-19 Symptoms. *JAMA network open*. 2021;4(1):e2035057. doi:10.1001/jamanetworkopen.2020.35057.

15. Helms J, Kremer S, Merdji H, Clere-Jehl R, Schenck M, Kummerlen C, Collange O, Boulay C, Fafi-Kremer S, Ohana M, Anheim M, Meziani F. Neurologic Features in Severe SARS-CoV-2 Infection. *The New England journal of medicine*. 2020;382(23):2268–2270. doi:10.1056/NEJMc2008597.

16. Steardo L, Steardo Jr L, Zorec R, Verkhratsky A. Neuroinfection may contribute to pathophysiology and clinical manifestations of COVID-19. *Acta physiologica (Oxford, England)*. 2020;229(3):e13473. doi:10.1111/apha.13473.

16a. Chou SH, Beghi E, Helbok R, et al. Global Incidence of Neurological Manifestations Among Patients Hospitalized With COVID-19—A Report for the GCS-NeuroCOVID Consortium and the ENERGY Consortium. *JAMA Netw Open*. 2021;4(5):e2112131. doi:10.1001/jamanetworkopen.2021.12131.

16b. Andalib Sasan, et al. Peripheral Nervous System Manifestations Associated with COVID-19. *Current Neurol Neurosci Rep*. 2021;21. doi:10.1007/s11910-021-01102-5. In press.

17. Niazkar HR, Zibaee B, Nasimi A, Bahri N. The neurological manifestations of COVID-19: a review article. *Neurol Sci*. 2020 Jul;41(7):1667–1671. doi:10.1007/s10072-020-04486-3 PMID: 32483687; PMCID: PMC7262683.

17a. https://www.cdc.gov/coronavirus/types.html, 2020. [Accessed 22 May 2022].

18. Cheng Q, Yang Y, Gao J. Infectivity of human coronavirus in the brain. *EBioMedicine*. 2020;56:102799. doi:10.1016/j.ebiom.2020.102799.

19. Arbour N, Day R, Newcombe J, Talbot PJ. Neuroinvasion by human respiratory coronaviruses. *Journal of virology*. 2000;74(19):8913–8921. doi:10.1128/jvi.74.19.8913-8921.2000.

19a. Siddiqui Ruqaiyyah, et al. SARS-CoV-2 invasion of the central nervous: a brief review. Hospital Practice. 2021. doi:10.1080/21548331.2021.1887677.

19b. MacLean M.A, et al. The potential role of microvascular pathology in the neurological manifestations of coronavirus infection. Fluids and Barriers of the CNS. 2020. doi:10.1186/s12987-020-00216-1.

20. Xu J, Zhong S, Liu J, Li L, Li Y, Wu X, Li Z, Deng P, Zhang J, Zhong N, Ding Y, Jiang Y. Detection of severe acute respiratory syndrome coronavirus in the brain: potential role of the chemokine Mig in pathogenesis. *Clinical infectious diseases*. 2005;41(8):1089–1096. doi:10.1086/444461.

21. Yamashita M, Yamate M, Li GM, Ikuta K. Susceptibility of human and rat neural cell lines to infection by SARS-coronavirus. *Biochemical and biophysical research communications*. 2005;334(1):79–85. doi:10.1016/j.bbrc.2005.06.061.

22. Jin Y, Yang H, Ji W, Wu W, Chen S, Zhang W, Duan G. Virology, Epidemiology, Pathogenesis, and Control of COVID-19. *Viruses*. 2020;12(4):372. doi:10.3390/v12040372.

23. Ahmad I, Rathore FA. Neurological manifestations and complications of COVID-19: A literature review. *Journal of clinical neuroscience: official journal of the Neurosurgical Society of Australasia*. 2020;77:8–12. doi:10.1016/j.jocn.2020.05.017.

24. Zubair AS, McAlpine LS, Gardin T, Farhadian S, Kuruvilla DE, Spudich S. Neuropathogenesis and Neurologic Manifestations of the Coronaviruses in the Age of Coronavirus Disease 2019: A Review. *JAMA neurology*. 2020;77(8):1018–1027. doi:10.1001/jamaneurol.2020.2065.

25. Chou SHY, Beghi E, Helbok R, et al. Global Incidence of Neurological Manifestations Among Patients Hospitalized With COVID-19-A Report for the GCS-NeuroCOVID Consortium and the ENERGY Consortium. *JAMA Netw Open*. 2021;4:e2112131.

26. Rogers JP, Watson CJ, Badenoch J, et al. Neurology and neuropsychiatry of COVID-19: a systematic review and meta-analysis of the early literature reveals frequent CNS manifestations and key emerging narratives. *Journal of Neurology, Neurosurgery & Psychiatry*. 2021;92:932–941.

27. Frontera JA, Yang D, Lewis A, Patel P, Medicherla C, Arena V, Fang T, Andino A, Snyder T, Madhavan M. A prospective study of long-term outcomes among hospitalized COVID-19 patients with and without neurological complications. *Journal of the neurological sciences*. 2021;426:117486.

28. Al-Ramadan A, Rabab'h O, Shah J, Gharaibeh A. Acute and post-acute neurological complications of COVID-19. *Neurology International*. 2021;13(1):102–119.

29. Attal N, Martinez V, Bouhassira D. Potential for increased prevalence of neuropathic pain after the COVID-19 pandemic. *Pain reports*. 2021;6(1).

30. Moghimi N, Di Napoli M, Biller 3 J, Siegler JE, Shekhar R, McCullough LD, Harkins MS, Hong E, Alaouieh DA, Mansueto G, Divani AA. The Neurological Manifestations of

Post-Acute Sequelae of SARS-CoV-2 infection. *Current neurology and neuroscience reports.* 2021;21(9):44. doi:10.1007/s11910-021-01130-1.

31. Vonck K, Garrez I, De Herdt V, Hemelsoet D, Laureys G, Raedt R, Boon P. Neurological manifestations and neuro-invasive mechanisms of the severe acute respiratory syndrome coronavirus type 2. *European journal of neurology.* 2020;27(8):1578–1587. doi:10.1111/ene.14329.

32. Román GC, Spencer PS, Reis J, Buguet A, Faris MEA, Katrak SM, Láinez M, Medina MT, Meshram C, Mizusawa H, Öztürk S, Wasay MWFN Environmental Neurology Specialty Group. The neurology of COVID-19 revisited: A proposal from the Environmental Neurology Specialty Group of the World Federation of Neurology to implement international neurological registries. *J Neurol Sci.* 2020 Jul 15;414:116884.

33. von Weyhern CH, Kaufmann I, Neff F, Kremer M. Early evidence of pronounced brain involvement in fatal COVID-19 outcomes. *Lancet.* 2020;365(10241):e109.

34. Abboud H, Abboud FZ, Kharbouch H, Arkha Y, El Abbadi N, El Ouahabi A. COVID-19 and SARS-Cov-2 Infection: Pathophysiology and Clinical Effects on the Nervous System. *World neurosurgery.* 2020;140:49–53. doi:10.1016/j.wneu.2020.05.193.

35. Kantonen J, Mahzabin S, Mäyränpää MI, Tynninen O, Paetau A, Andersson N, Sajantila A, Vapalahti O, Carpén O, Kekäläinen E, Kantele A, Myllykangas L. Neuropathologic features of four autopsied COVID-19 patients. *Brain Pathol.* 2020;30(6):1012–1016 Nov.

35a. Iadecola Constantino Effects of COVID-19 on the Nervous System. Cell. 2020. doi:10.1016/j.cell.2020.08.028. In this issue.

36. Rahman A, Tabassum T, Araf Y, Al Nahid A, Ullah MA, Hosen MJ. Silent hypoxia in COVID-19: pathomechanism and possible management strategy. *Molecular biology reports.* 2021;48(4):3863–3869. doi:10.1007/s11033-021-06358-1.

37. Fabbri VP, Foschini MP, Lazzarotto T, Gabrielli L, Cenacchi G, Gallo C, Aspide R, Frascaroli G, Cortelli P, Riefolo M, Giannini C, D'Errico A. Brain ischemic injury in COVID-19-infected patients: a series of 10 post-mortem cases. *Brain pathology (Zurich, Switzerland).* 2021;31(1):205–210. doi:10.1111/bpa.12901.

38. Moonis G, Filippi CG, Kirsch C, Mohan S, Stein EG, Hirsch JA, Mahajan A. The Spectrum of Neuroimaging Findings on CT and MRI in Adults With COVID-19. *AJR. American journal of roentgenology.* 2021;217(4):959–974. doi:10.2214/AJR.20.24839.

39. Bhinder KK, Siddiqi AR, Tahir MJ, Maqsood H, Ullah I, Yousaf Z. Bilateral basal ganglia ischemia associated with COVID-19: a case report and review of the literature. *Journal of medical case reports.* 2021;15(1):563. doi:10.1186/s13256-021-03165-x.

40. Science Daily. (2021, January 6). Patient-reported loss of smell in 86 percent of mild COVID-19 cases, study finds. https://www.sciencedaily.com/releases/2021/01/210106082713.htm

41. American Academy of Otolaryngology- Head and Neck Surgery. (2020, March 22). Anosmia. https://www.entnet.org/covid-19/anosmia/

42. Kaye R, Chang C, Kazahaya K, Brereton J, Denneny 3rd JC. COVID-19 Anosmia Reporting Tool: Initial Findings. *Otolaryngology–head and neck surgery: official journal of American Academy of Otolaryngology-Head and Neck Surgery.* 2020;163(1):132–134. doi:10.1177/0194599820922992.

43. Meng X, Deng Y, Dai Z, Meng Z. COVID-19 and anosmia: A review based on up-to-date knowledge. *American journal of otolaryngology.* 2020;41(5):102581. doi:10.1016/j.amjoto.2020.102581.

44. Agyeman AA, Chin KL, Landersdorfer CB, Liew D, Ofori-Asenso R. Smell and Taste Dysfunction in Patients With COVID-19: A Systematic Review and Meta-analysis. *Mayo Clinic proceedings.* 2020;95(8):1621–1631. doi:10.1016/j.mayocp.2020.05.030.

45. Kandemirli SG, Altundag A, Yildirim D, Tekcan Sanli DE, Saatci O. Olfactory Bulb MRI and Paranasal Sinus CT Findings in Persistent COVID-19 Anosmia. *Academic radiology.* 2021;28(1):28–35. doi:10.1016/j.acra.2020.10.006.

46. Brann DH, Tsukahara T, Weinreb C, Lipovsek M, Van den Berge K, Gong B, Chance R, Macaulay IC, Chou HJ, Fletcher RB, Das D, Street K, de Bezieux HR, Choi YG, Risso D, Dudoit S, Purdom E, Mill J, Hachem RA, Matsunami H..., Datta SR. Non-neuronal expression of SARS-CoV-2 entry genes in the olfactory system suggests mechanisms underlying COVID-19-associated anosmia. *Science advances.* 2020;6(31):eabc5801. doi:10.1126/sciadv.abc5801.

47. Matschke J, Lütgehetmann M, Hagel C, Sperhake JP, Schröder AS, Edler C, Mushumba H, Fitzek A, Allweiss L, Dandri M, Dottermusch M, Heinemann A, Pfefferle S, Schwabenland M, Sumner Magruder D, Bonn S, Prinz M, Gerloff C, Püschel K, Krasemann S, Aepfelbacher M, Glatzel M. Neuropathology of patients with COVID-19 in Germany: a post-mortem case series. *Lancet Neurol.* 2020;19:919–929. doi:10.1016/s1474-4422(20)30308-2.

48. Hopkins C, Surda P, Kumar N. Presentation of new onset anosmia during the COVID-19 pandemic. *Rhinology.* 2020;58:295–298.

49. Schaller T, Hirschbühl K, Burkhardt K, Braun G, Trepel M, Märkl B, Claus R. Postmortem examination of patients with COVID-19. *J Am Med Assoc.* 2020;323:2518–2520.

50. Solomon IH, Normandin E, Bhattacharyya S, Mukerji SS, Keller K, Ali AS, et al. Neuropathological features of COVID-19. *N Engl J Med.* Sep; 2020;383:989–99256. GBS/CIDP Foundation. COVID-19 vaccines and the GBS/CIDP community. https://www.gbs-cidp.org/covid-19-vaccines-and-the-gbscidp-community/.

51. Abu-Rumeileh S, Abdelhak A, Foschi M, Tumani H, Otto M. Guillain-Barré syndrome spectrum associated with COVID-19: an up-to-date systematic review of 73 cases. *Journal of neurology.* 2021;268(4):1133–1170. doi:10.1007/s00415-020-10124-x.

52. Kajumba MM, Kolls BJ, Koltai DC, Kaddumukasa M, Kaddumukasa M, Laskowitz DT. COVID-19-Associated Guillain-Barré Syndrome: Atypical Para-infectious Profile, Symptom Overlap, and Increased Risk of Severe Neurological Complications. SN Compr. *Clin. Med.*. 2020;2:2702–2714. doi:10.1007/s42399-020-00646-w.

53. Sejvar JJ, Baughman AL, Wise M, Morgan OW. Population incidence of Guillain-Barré syndrome: a systematic review and meta-analysis. *Neuroepidemiology.* 2011;36(2):123–133. doi:10.1159/000324710.

54. Trujillo Gittermann LM, Valenzuela Feris SN, von Oetinger Giacoman A. Relation between COVID-19 and Guillain-Barré syndrome in adults. Systematic review.

Relación entre COVID-19 y síndrome de Guillain-Barré en adultos. Revisión sistemática. *Neurologia (Barcelona, Spain)*. 2020;35(9):646–654. doi:10.1016/j.nrl.2020.07.004.

55. Caress JB, Castoro RJ, Simmons Z, Scelsa SN, Lewis RA, Ahlawat A, Narayanaswami P. COVID-19-associated Guillain-Barré syndrome: the early pandemic experience. *Muscle & Nerve*. 2020;62(4):485–491. doi:10.1002/mus.27024.

56. Paliwal VK, Garg RK, Gupta A, Tejan N. Neuromuscular presentations in patients with COVID-19. Neurological Sciences: Official Journal of the Italian Neurological Society and of the Italian Society of. *Clinical Neurophysiology*. 2020;41(11):3039–3056. doi:10.1007/s10072-020-04708-8.

57. Kim JK, Kim YH, Yoon BA, Cho JY, Oh SY, Shin HY, Kim JS, Park KH, Kim SY, Suh BC, Seok HY, Yoo JH, Bae JS. Clinical heterogeneity of anti-GM2-ganglioside-antibody syndrome. *J Clin Neurol*. 2018;14(3):401–406.

58. Lin L, Al-Faraj A, Ayub N, et al. Electroencephalographic abnormalities are common in COVID-19 and are associated with outcomes. *Annals of Neurology*. 2021;89(5):872–883.

59. Bowles L, Platton S, Yartey N, et al. Lupus anticoagulant and abnormal coagulation tests in patients with covid-19. *N Engl J Med*. 2020;383(3):288–290.

60. Avula A, Nalleballe K, Narula N, et al. COVID-19 presenting as stroke. *Brain Behav Immun*. 2020;87:115–119.

61. Zhang Y, Xiao M, Zhang S, et al. Coagulopathy and antiphospholipid antibodies in patients with covid-19. *N Engl J Med*. 2020;382(17):e38.

62. Shoskes A, Migdady I, Fernandez A, Ruggieri P, Rae-Grant A. Cerebral microhemorrhage and purpuric rash in COVID-19: the case for a secondary microangiopathy. *J Stroke Cerebrovasc Dis*. 2020;29(10):105111.

63. Varga Z, Flammer AJ, Steiger P, et al. Endothelial cell infection and endotheliitis in COVID-19. *Lancet*. 2020;395(10234):1417–1418.

64. Radmanesh A, Derman A, Lui YW, et al. COVID-19–associated diffuse leukoencephalopathy and microhemorrhages. *Radiology*. 2020;297(1):E223–E227.

65. Fitsiori A, Pugin D, Thieffry C, Lalive P, Vargas MI. Unusual microbleeds in brain MRI of Covid-19 patients. *J Neuroimaging*. 2020;30(5):593–597 Jon.12755.

66. Goeijenbier M, van Wissen M, van de Weg C, Jong E, Gerdes VE, Meijers JC, Brandjes DP, van Gorp ECJ. Review: viral infections and mechanisms of thrombosis and bleeding. *Med Virol*. 2012 Oct; 84(10):1680–1696.

67. Yang J, Zheng Y, Gou X, Pu K, Chen Z, Guo Q, Ji R, Wang H, Wang Y, Zhou Y. Prevalence of comorbidities and its effects in patients infected with SARS-CoV-2: a systematic review and meta-analysis. *Int J Infect Dis*. 2020 May;94:91–95.

68. Varga Z, Flammer AJ, Steiger P, et al. Endothelial cell infection and endotheliitis in COVID-19. *Lancet*. 2020;395(10234):1417–1418.

69. Beraki S, Aronsson F, Karlsson H, Ogren SO. Kristensson K. Influenza A virus infection causes alterations in expression of synaptic regulatory genes combined with changes in cognitive and emotional behaviors in mice. *Mol Psychiatry*. 2005;10(3):299–308.

Oral Cavity and COVID-19: Clinical Manifestations, Pathology, and Dental Profession

Mythily Srinivasan, MDS, PhD, and Thankam Thyvalikakath, MDS, DMD, PhD

OUTLINE

The Oral Cavity and Viral Infections

The oral cavity is home to a vast microbial flora that also include a robust community of viruses. Although the viruses that infect bacteria or bacteriophages constitute the majority, viruses that infect human cells form a significant component of the oral microbiome.[1,2] Much like bacteria, viral communities are also site-specific alterations that can lead to disease. Indeed, one of the earliest associations of biofilm virome with human disease is the increased membership of lytic bacteriophages in subgingival plaque in periodontal disease.[3] Although the evidence for oral virome and the contributions to oral health and disease is still emerging, the proclivity for specific viruses to affect the oral cavity is well recognized.[4,5] Furthermore, direct communication between the oropharynx and the nasopharynx makes the highly vascularized oral tissues more vulnerable to viruses harboring the respiratory or gastrointestinal (GI) tract. Consequently, many of these viruses have been implicated in the cause of chronic oral mucosal lesions.[5,6] In the sections that follow, we briefly review the oral manifestations of major DNA and RNA viruses, discuss the SARS-CoV-2 infection with particular focus on the pathology of oral symptoms, debate the scope of salivary diagnostics for SARS-CoV-2 infections, and, finally, the potential of SARS-CoV-2 transmission through saliva, including the spread in dental offices.

Viral Infections With Significant Orofacial Manifestations

DNA Viruses

The human herpesvirus (HHV) family constitute the most common viral infections of the oral cavity. They are relatively large, enveloped, double-stranded DNA viruses with icosahedral symmetry. Of the eight members in the family, the herpes simplex virus-1 (HSV-1) infection is the most common and is characterized by painful mucosal ulcers affecting the attached gingiva, such as the hard palate and the gum tissues surrounding the teeth and the portions of the jawbones encasing them. Following primary infection, the HSV typically remains latent in sensory nerve ganglia, and a recurrence occurs when the virus is reactivated, often seen clinically as herpes labialis characterized by periodic appearance of cold sores or ulcers in the lip.[7–9] Infections by varicella zoster virus (VZV) and Epstein Barr virus (EBV) viruses are the next common HHV infections. VZ causes chickenpox that could manifest with blue Koplik spots in the oral mucosa, and the EB virus causes infectious mononucleosis (the kissing disease). Human papillomavirus (HPV) is a small, nonenveloped, double-stranded DNA virus with icosahedral symmetry and more than 70 genotypes. HPV 16 and 18 are often associated with benign papillomatous lesions of the oral mucosa. In addition, focal epithelial hyperplasia, or Heck disease, and condyloma constitute oral HPV infections.[6,10,11] A significant finding is that HHVs are established risk factors for oral cancers and precancerous lesions. This role has been variably attributed to the virus-induced dysbiosis, increased inflammation, and production of carcinogenic metabolites.[12]

RNA Viruses

Among the retroviruses, the human immunodeficiency virus (HIV) is the most common to cause infection of the oral cavity. Other RNA viruses causing oral infections include Ebola; enteroviruses causing hand, foot, and mouth disease (HFMD); influenza B and C viruses; and coronaviruses. HIV is an enveloped retrovirus transmitted through sexual contact or by infected body fluids. This virus primarily infects the lymphocytes, resulting in immunodeficiency with consequent clinical manifestations of increased opportunistic infections affecting the lungs and other organs, including the oral mucosa. Interestingly, infectious HIV virions have been shown to be internalized by oral epithelial cells and retained in vesicular compartments for several days. Subsequent contact with lymphocytes or dendritic cells is thought to direct the clinical presentation and potentially promote the viral spread.[13,14] Ebola virus is a nonsegmented, negative-stranded RNA virus surrounded by an outer viral envelope studded with viral glycoprotein spikes. The virus primarily causes hemorrhagic fever, and gingival bleeding that is typically associated with other forms of hemorrhage such as epistaxis and bleeding at injection sites. Oral mucosal ulcers, inflammation, and painful red and white patches are other symptoms reported in Ebola virus infections.[15] HFMD is caused by the Picornaviridae family of viruses in the genus enterovirus. Outbreaks of HFMD have more often been caused by two types of enterovirus A species, coxsackievirus A16 (CVA16), or enterovirus 71 (EV71). Oral manifestations are vesicular lesions much like those observed on the skin of hand and feet.[16,17]

Zoonotic Viruses

Influenza and severe acute respiratory syndrome (SARS) heralded the surge of zoonotic virus outbreaks. Globally, influenza epidemics cause major health and economic concerns. These viruses cause self-limiting upper respiratory tract infections in immunocompetent individuals and cause lower respiratory tract infections in immunocompromised subjects and the elderly.[15] Although the primary symptoms are due to respiratory tract infection, the oral cavity could be a major site for the initiation, progression, and pathological processes of the influenza virus–induced infections. Dry mouth, vesiculobullous lesions, aphthous-like lesions, dysgeusia, and anosmia are common oral manifestations. Coinfection with oral bacteria is thought to aggravate the severity of the lung pathological conditions with increasing morbidity and mortality.[18,19]

Coronaviruses are enveloped, positive-sense, single-stranded RNA ($+$ssRNA) viruses with a size varying between 26 and 32 kilobases (kb), the largest genome of known RNA viruses. The four subgroups of this family are alpha (α), beta (β), gamma (γ), and delta (δ) coronaviruses. All coronaviruses are zoonotic pathogens, although the mechanisms and routes of transmission from animal to human remain unknown.[20–22] The primary transmission is thought to be mediated by direct contact with the intermediary host animals, and consumption of milk or uncooked meat have been suggested as potential sources of infection.[21]

This century has seen the emergence of three novel β coronaviruses; namely the SARS-CoV (SARS-CoV-1), the Middle Eastern respiratory syndrome (MERS-CoV), and most recently the novel SARS-CoV-2 that cause severe human diseases and death. The first SARS-CoV-1 outbreak was reported in 2002 in Guangdong, China. The outbreak resulted in more than 8000 infections, with a devastating effect on local and regional economies.[23] The second coronavirus outbreak occurred in 2012 when a few Saudi Arabian nationals were diagnosed with the MERS-CoV infection, which later spread to 27 countries with an approximately 20% to 35% mortality rate.[24–26]

The third and the most recent outbreak is the infection by the SARS-CoV-2 virus that caused COVID-19. This virus, first reported in the city of Wuhan in China, spread rapidly constituting a global pandemic affecting individuals in all continents.[20,24,27] As of June 2021, globally over 163 million individuals were infected with SARS-CoV-2 and nearly 3.4 million individuals had died.[28] A critical feature of COVID-19 was the wide variance in clinical severity among infected people and high mortality. In this chapter, we focus on oral manifestations, mechanisms, and significance of oral fluids in SARS-CoV-2 infection.

SARS-CoV-2 and the Oral Cavity
Oral Manifestations of SARS-CoV-2 Infection

SARS-CoV-2–infected individuals present a multitude of oral lesions, including ulcers, petechiae, vesiculobullous lesions, and dysgeusia or ageusia.[29–33] However, there are considerable inconsistencies in the literature as to the time of oral manifestations with respect to the status of SARS-CoV-2 infection and the stage of COVID-19. Given the large population of SARS-CoV-2–infected individuals globally, some studies have speculated that the oral manifestations could be coincidental or could represent adverse drug-induced responses. Some of the erosive and ulcerative lesions on the oropharynx, palate, and posterior tongue have been suggested as lesions secondary to mechanical intubations. Thus it is not clear whether the oral lesions are true manifestations of the viral infection

■ **Box 8.1** Rationale That Supports Oral Manifestations as Truly Representing SARS-CoV-2 Infection

■ **Box 8.1** Rationale That Supports Oral Manifestations as Truly Representing SARS-CoV-2 Infection

- Much like the nasopharynx, the oral mucosa being exposed to the environment could be the site of first encounter with SARS-CoV-2, and hence oral symptoms could be the first sign of COVID-19.
- Inflammatory reactions, in particular vascular inflammation, have been associated with the multiorgan involvement of COVID-19.[4-6] The highly vascularized oral mucosa is likely to be vulnerable, and the reports of oral ulcers, loss of taste, and petechiae in COVID-19 could be attributed to such inflammatory reactions.
- Histopathological similarities were observed between the thrombotic vessels in oral lesions and in the pulmonary diffuse thrombotic disease in COVID-19.[10,11]
- Specific entry receptors for SARS-CoV-2 are expressed in oral mucosa.[12-15]
- Oral lesions have been observed in other viral lesions such as the herpes simplex virus, herpes zoster virus, and Epstein-Barr virus infections.[16-22]
- Concurrent or coinfection of SARS-CoV-2 infected lung with oral pathogens have been frequently observed.[26]

■ **Box 8.2** Classification of Oral Manifestations of COVID-19

1. Chemosensory perception
   a. Dysgeusia
   b. Ageusia
2. Oral mucosal lesions
   a. Apthous ulcer
   b. Herpertiform ulcer
   c. Vesiculobullous lesions
   d. White lesions, plaques
   e. Mucositis, mucosal erosions
3. Salivary gland symptoms
   a. Xerostomia
   b. Sialadenitis
4. Periodontal and bone symptoms
   a. Bleeding gums, Swelling
   b. Bone pain
5. Other:
   a. Lesions due to trauma associated with intubation
   b. Drug induced ulcers.
   c. Secondary opportunistic infections such as oral candidiasis

or a secondary phenomenon resulting from opportunistic infections or adverse effects of treatment.[32]

The rationalr for oral manifestations as true effects of SARS-CoV-2 infection are listed in Box 8.1. It is well recognized that are SARS-CoV-2 infection is transmitted by aerosols and the oral mucosa, much like the nasopharynx, could be the initial site of contact with the virus. The presence of entry factors for the SARS-CoV-2 in oral tissues suggests susceptibility to infection (discussed later).[43,53,55,56] Further, much of the oral soft tissues are highly vascular and in a state of inflammation supporting increased vulnerability to SARS-CoV-2 infection, as the virus exhibited strong association with vascular inflammation in other organs.[4,5] Significantly, a few studies have reported the presence of oral pathogens in the bronchoalveolar lavage fluid from SARS-CoV-2–infected diseased lungs, suggesting coinfection or superinfection.

Clinical observations during the initial period of the pandemic may not have recorded oral manifestations, particularly in the context of the unexpected severity and mortality associated with COVID-19. As the testing for SARS-CoV-2 infection increased, the emphasis was on identifying early clinical manifestations to prevent and eliminate the rapid spread of infection. Several case reports and a few case series identified variable oral symptoms in SARS-CoV-2–positive individuals, and there was evidence that the oral manifestations could even constitute manifesting clinical features of COVID-19.[29-31,34,35]

In general, taste dysfunction, or dysgeusia, is the most reported oral symptom, with a prevalence rate ranging between 37% and 63% and occasional reports of loss of taste in more than 90% of the case series.[30,36,37]

The initial symptom could be inflamed painful fungiform papillae of short duration of about a day, which then gives rise to an irregular asymptomatic ulcer that often heals completely without scar formation in about a week.[36,37] In addition, glossitis and plaque-like lesions on the dorsum of the tongue have been reported in COIVD-19 patients.[30,34,38].

A broad classification of oral manifestations of SARS-CoV-2 infection is given in Box 8.2. Chen et al.[39] first reported xerostomia as a symptom in COVID-19 patients with an equal sex distribution and a prevalence of 46.3% in their study cohort. Subsequent studies also reported xerostomia as an early symptom in asymptomatic health care professionals or mildly symptomatic SARS-CoV-2–positive individuals. The hyposalivation not only results in decreased antimicrobial proteins and peptides but also reduces the efficacy of oral mucosal surface as a physical barrier. In addition, the reduction of saliva secretion may be linked to gustatory dysfunction.[29,40] Meta-analysis of available information identified additional oral symptoms such as, aphthous ulcers and vesiculobullous lesions in COVID-19 patients positive individuals. Pooled prevalence of oral manifestations derived from the strength of the observations in the number of infected individuals are listed in Table 8.1. (Box 8.3 and Box 8.4)

Mechanisms of Oral Manifestations of SARS-CoV-2

SARS-CoV-2 Entry Into Host Cells: A Brief Review

To cause infection, the virus must enter the host cells and replicate. The entry of SARS-CoVs in target cells is

Table 8.1 Pooled Prevalence of Oral Manifestations in COVID-19

Symptom	Number of Studies (Total No. Patients)	Number of Patients (%)	Reference
Dysgeusia	40 (10,228)	10,220 (99%)	40
	59 (29,349)	13,615 (46%)	44
	140	67 (47.9%)	49
	111	66 (59.5%)	47
	1 (573)	318 (55.5%)	48
	3	2 (66.6%)	50
Oral mucosal lesions	7 (case reports)	8	51
	140	29 (tongue plaque) (20.7%) 6 (lesions on other oral mucosal sites) (4.3%)	49
	? (304 nonhospitalized)	75 (tongue) (24.7%) 3 (other oral mucosal sites) (<1%)	52
	74	23 (tongue) (31%) 35 (other oral mucosal lesions) (47.3%)	53
	1 (573)	117 (oral ulcers) (20.4%)	48
	1 (1237)	21 (<1%) 3 (tongue) (<1%) 18 (other mucosal regions) (<1%)	54
Salivary gland: Xerostomia	1 (573)	273 (47.6%)	48
	140	72 (51.4%)	49
	111	51 (45.9%)	47

■ **Box 8.3** Potential Mechanisms by Which Poor Oral Health Contribute to COVID-19 Susceptibility

1. Chronic periodontitis is associated with elevated salivary cytokines and harmful enzymes. Aspiration of salivary cytokines injures the alveolar epithelium, making it more susceptible for viral infection.[93,94]
2. The SARS-CoV-2 spike protein has been shown to interact with the lipid A component of lipopolysaccharide, the cell wall structure of gram-negative bacteria. Because poor oral hygiene is often associated with higher gram-negative content of oral microbiome, preexisting gram-negative bacterial infection, and the associated presence of lipopolysaccharide might exacerbate local lung inflammation. This is a consequence of SARS-CoV-2 spike protein binding by enhanced nuclear factor-κB activation.[108,109] This shows that poor oral hygiene is contributing to the increased susceptibility of individuals in nursing care facilities to SARS-CoV-2 infection.

Potential mechanisms by which oral bacteria contribute to the COVID-19 pathogenesis:

1. Oral bacterial migration or transport causing ventilator-associated pneumonia.[90]
2. Oral bacterial infection or superinfection of the lower respiratory tract.[89,91]
3. Oral soft and hard tissue surfaces as reservoirs of respiratory pathogens and as sources of lung reinfection through microaspiration.[95,108]

■ **Box 8.4** Advantages and Limitations of Saliva for Diagnosis of SARS-CoV-2

Advantages
- Easy access and feasibility for frequent collection.
- Higher compliance to test for SARS-CoV-2 under reduced direct contact.
- Positive salivary detection of SARS-CoV-2 in patients with a negative nasopharyngeal swab consistent with true infection.[1-3]

Limitations
- Many studies evaluated saliva admixed with oropharyngeal fluid.[7-9]
- A potential limitation is detection of RNA in levels near the sensitivity limits.
- A negative result is not a guarantee of the absence of SARS-CoV-2 infection.

facilitated by the interaction between the spike proteins protruding from the surface of the virus and the host cell surface receptors. In silico, molecular and functional assays have identified a metallopeptidase cell surface receptor named angiotensin-converting enzyme-2 (ACE2) on host cells as a common entry receptor for all coronaviruses. The spike (S) protein of SARS-CoV-2 is composed of two subunits, S1 and S2. The S1 subunit contains a receptor-binding domain that recognizes and binds to the host receptor ACE2, whereas the S2 subunit mediates viral cell membrane fusion by forming a six-helical bundle by the two-heptad repeat domain.[41] SARS-CoV-2 has been shown to bind ACE2 with higher affinity than SARS-CoV-1.[42] Other host cell proteases that facilitate or promote the viral entry include furin and the transmembrane protease serine (TMPRSS). Furin, ACE2, desintegrin, and metalloproteinase domain 17 (ADAM17) or tumor necrosis factor-alpha (TNF-α)–converting enzyme (TACE) are proteases that cleave the viral spike protein between S1 and S2. Whereas the S1 domain potentially facilitates receptor binding, the S2 domain regulates the fusion of the virus with the host cell.[43,44] The TMPRSS belongs to a family of 17 members, divided into four subfamilies (HAT/DESC, epsin/TMPRSS, matriptase, and Corin).[45] The TMPRSS2 of the epsin subfamily has been shown to participate in mediating SARS-CoV-2 entry. Much like furin, the TMPRSS2 also cleaves the spike protein between the S1 and the S2 subunits. The S2 subunit then undergoes conformational changes to complete the fusion of the viral envelope with the host cell membrane, mediating receptor internalization and facilitating viral entry.[46] Replication within the target cells establishes the SARS-CoV-2 infection, leading to subsequent tissue damage.[44,47]

Pathogenesis of Oral Mucosal Lesions in COVID-19

In humans, ACE2 is predominantly observed in epithelial cells in contact with the environment, although expression also has been reported in internal organs, including the kidney and the heart.[44,47,48] The oral cavity in direct contact with the external environment is at an increased risk for viral invasion. Although one of the primary functions of the oral mucosa is to provide a barrier against microbial invasion, the surface epithelial cells often express receptors that would allow attachment and penetration of the cell membrane by the microbes.[49–52] Based on the analyses of two public RNA sequence databases, Xu et al.[53] first reported that ACE2 was differentially expressed in the oral mucosa in different sites, with the highest expression in the tongue and floor of the mouth. They confirmed the high expression of ACE2 in oral epithelial cells by single cell transcriptome analysis of normal oral mucosal biopsy samples.[53] Subsequently, we and others also showed that ACE2 is abundantly expressed in the lining mucosa of the oral cavity and the dorsum of the tongue (Fig. 8.1). In addition, the oral epithelial cells also express furin and TMPRSS2, supporting the potential for viral spike protein cleavage and SARS-CoV-2 internalization. The expression of TMPRSS2 is also observed in the acinar, myoepithelial and the epithelial cells lining the ducts in the salivary glands.[43,54,55] SARS-CoV-2 transcripts have been identified in oral mucosal tissue autopsies from COVID-19 patients.[56]

Emerging evidence suggests that in addition to ACE2, the SARS-CoV-2 also uses other pattern recognition receptors such as Toll-like receptors (TLRs) for host cell entry[57] (see Fig. 8.1B). In particular, the observations of TLR upregulation by damage-associated molecular patterns in clinical samples and the proposed models of direct binding of spike protein with TLRs 1, 4, and 6 suggest specific roles for these TLRs in facilitating the viral entry and/or in mediating the clinical symptoms of COVID-19.[57–59] It has been suggested that the dysbiosis secondary to the invading SARS-CoV-2 increases the prevalence of pathogenic bacteria, which in turn modulates the innate host responses resulting in the release of cytokines and inflammation.[60,61] Such inflammatory reactions secondary to viral entry in mucosal and vascular cells has been used to explain the oral erosion, ulcers, and lingual pain in COVID-19.[62–65] Collectively, these observations suggest that SARS-CoV-2 can infect a wide variety of oral tissues and cells and provide the scientific rationale for the oral symptoms in infected individuals.

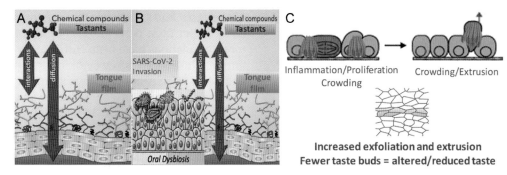

Fig. 8.1 Schematic Representation of the Mechanisms of Oral Manifestations of COVID-19. Following SARS-CoV-2 exposure, the virus could infect the oral mucosa. (A) The epithelial cells lining the oral mucosa express cell surface angiotensin-converting enzyme-2 (ACE2). (B) Upon binding the ACE2 on the host cell surface, the spike protein of the SARS-CoV-2 activates the host proteases such as tumor necrosis-α converting enzyme (TACE) that cleaves both the spike protein and the ACE2 at the transmembrane region. The virus then enters the cell, and the ACE2 ectodomain is released as soluble ACE2 (sACE2). Toll-like receptor-4 (TLR-4) on oral epithelial cells potentially upregulated by the local dysbiosis secondary to viral trigger could facilitate viral entry by itself or assist the interaction of the viral spike protein with the ACE2. (C) Activation of TLR signal transduction induces inflammatory cell infiltration, macrophage activation, and facilitation of further viral invasion. (D) These changes lead to oral manifestations such as mucosal erosion and ulcer formation.

Pathogenesis of Hyposalivation in COVID-19

SARS-CoV-2 Entry Factors in Salivary Gland Tissues

Xerostomia is a common complaint in COVID-19, suggesting that the virus potentially infects the salivary glands. Substantiting the clinical symptom are the molecular characteristics of oral tissues exhibiting abundant expression of ACE2, the host cell receptor of SARS-CoV-2 entry, in the parotid gland acinar cells and in the epithelial cells lining the salivary gland ducts as determined by single-cell RNA-sequencing atlases and clustering analyses.[33] A high expression of ACE2 has been reported in the granular cells and the ductal epithelial cells of the salivary glands.[54,66] Further, genotype-tissue expression studies have shown that TMPRSS2 is moderately expressed in the salivary glands. In particular, the relative expressions of ACE2 and TMPRSS2 in the salivary glands was similar to that in the respiratory and GI epithelia that are prone to SARS-CoV-2 infection.[45] The presence of ACE2 and TMPRSS2 at both the genetic and the protein levels have been futher confirmed by in situ hybridization and immunohistochemistry.[45,54] A high expression of ACE2 has been reported in the granular cells and the ductal epithelial cells of the salivary glands.[54,66]

SARS-CoV-2 Infection and Replication in Salivary Gland Tissues

SARS-CoV-2 transcripts have been detected in postmortem salivary gland tissues of COVID-19 patients.[56,67] The viral RNA was detected by quantitative PCR (qPCR) in the parotid and submandibular salivary gland tissues and in the minor salivary gland tissues.[56] Histological examination showed that the ductal epithelial cells of the salivary glands exhibited morphological changes consistent with viral infection, including cytoplasmic and nuclear vacuolization and nuclear polymorphism. The glandular acinar cells exhibited enlarged nuclei and degenerating zymogen granules. Electron microscopy showed that the acinal cells and the epithelial cells lining the salivary gland ducts exhibited spherical 70- to 100-nm viral particles, consistent in size and shape with the Coronaviridae family. These cells also exhibited degeneration of organelles in infected cells and the presence of a cluster of nucleocapsids suggestive of viral replication.[56,67] Interestingly, the SARS-CoV-2 viral load was observed to be higher in minor salivary gland tissues as compared to that in the parotid tissues. In situ hybridization and immunohistochemistry showed increased presence of the viral transcripts in the minor gland ductal epithelial cells and in the acinar cells expressing ACE2, although significant variability was observed in the extent of individual cell infection. Significantly, these observations in postmortem salivary gland tissues were also observed in minor salivary gland tissues from acutely infected individuals with COVID-19.[56,67]

Collectively, based on the expression and distribution of SARS-CoV-2 entry factors in the salivary gland tissues and the potential infectivity, it is suggested that the SARS-CoV-2 enters the epithelial cells and replicates, causing acute sialadenitis and destruction of acinar cells. Resolution of the acinar cell inflammation by fibroblast proliferation and connective tissue fibrosis, could lead to hyposalivation and the consequent symptom of dry mouth. Sialadenitis and dry mouth are frequently reported as common symptoms of COVID-19.[29,34,40,68]

Pathogenesis of Loss of Taste in COVID-19

As discussed earlier, systematic analyses showed that the gustatory dysfunction is one of the most common symptoms of COVID-19.[30,36,63,69,70] The epithelial cells of the dorsum of the tongue, including the taste bud cells, have been shown to coexpress the viral entry receptors ACE2 and TMPRSS2.[53,64,71] Indeed, the density of ACE2 receptor expression has been observed to be higher in tongue tissues than that in the buccal mucosa or gingiva.[59,62,65] Sakaguchi et al.[72] showed by immunohistochemisry that ACE2 and TMPRSS2 are localized in human fungiform papillae taste cells. Significantly, Han et al.[73] showed by single cell profile analysis of tongue tissues that the distribution of ACE2-positive cells correlated with typical the gene markers of taste buds, including TAS1R3, TAS2R4, TAS2R14, SNAP25, and NCAM1.[73] Furthermore, taste bud cells have been shown to express TLRs more abundantly than the nongustatory lingual epithelium. Specifically, TLRs-2, -3, and -4 are highly observed in the gustducin-expressing type II taste bud cells.[74,75] Thus the expression of multiple viral entry receptors makes taste bud cells highly susceptible for SARS-CoV-2 infections.[57,74] Pertinently, human taste bud cells have also been shown to support SARS-CoV-2 replication.[71] Biopsies of the dorsum of the tongue from COVID-19 patients showed transcripts of the SARS-CoV-2 by real-time polymerase chain reaction (PCR).[56] Direct infection of the taste bud cells promotes inflammation and this could affect taste perception.[65,76,77] Consistently, gustatory dysfunctions have been correlated with high serum interleukin-6 (IL-6), a key cytokine upregulated in acute and persistent SARS-CoV-2 infection.[62]

Taken together, a conceptual framework for the pathogenesis of dysgeusia in long-COVID could be proposed (Fig. 8.2). SARS-COV-2 infection of the tongue epithelial cells, including the taste buds, modulates the host responses, and prolonged exposure will precipitate an exaggerated inflammatory reaction. Mucosal inflammation increases the epithelial cell exfoliation, a source of viral shedding in saliva and a potential cause for invasion of bystander epithelial cells. The lag in replenishment of the lost cells together with the reduced stem cell turnover could result in fewer taste buds. The reduced sensory perception precipitate dysgeusia. It will

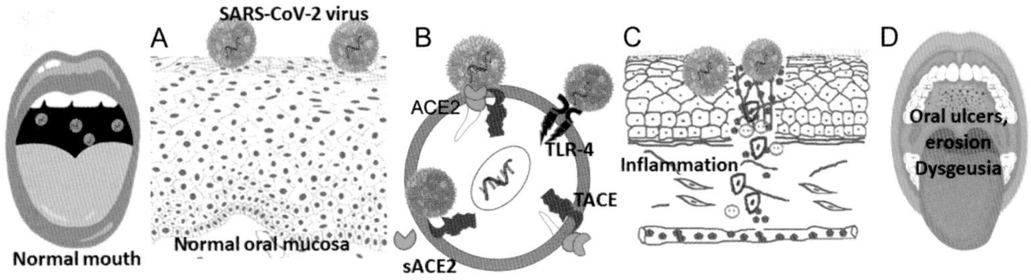

Fig. 8.2 Schematic Representation of Potential Mechanisms for Taste Dysfunction in Long-COVID. (A) The lingual epithelium covered by a tongue film that includes extruded/exfoliated cells, microbiota, and residual saliva. The concentration of microbial metabolization products and the proportion of epithelial cells, including the taste cells, in the tongue film module taste sensitivity. The tastants diffuse the tongue film either unaltered or modulated by the metabolization products and reach taste receptor cells through the apical opening of the taste buds. Each taste bud includes tightly packed taste receptor cells, supporting (basal) cells and stem cells that replenish the continuously replacing taste receptor cells. (B) Dysbiosis secondary to viral invasion disrupts the commensal homeostasis (abundance of pathogenic or opportunistic oral microbes) and induce innate inflammatory responses. Persistent irritation induces host responses and increases epithelial proliferation, extrusion, and exfoliation. (C) Pressure on replenishment of taste receptor cells places increased demand on stem cells and thereby compromises taste bud homeostasis, affecting taste perception. *ACE2,* Angiotensin-converting enzyme-2; *sACE2,* soluble ACE2; *TACE,* tumor necrosis-α converting enzyme; *TLR4,* Toll-like receptor-4.

be interesting to investigate whether salivary epithelial cell analyses could reveal specific markers of dysgeusia in individuals with long-COVID.[64]

The Oral Microbiome and COVID-19

The Oral Flora and Lung Microbiome in Health

A healthy human inhales 12 to 15 times per minute at rest, on average, with approximately 20% of the air in the lungs being exchanged during each breath. The popular belief that the healthy lungs are sterile has been dismantled by a large body of evidence that supports the presence of a healthy lung microbiome, which when disturbed can contribute to many lung pathological conditions.[78] Multiple theories have been proposed for the development of the lung microbiome.[79,80] The logical topological community theory proposes that the initial seeding of the lung microbiome occurs from the nearby anatomical sites based on the species similarity between the oropharyngeal and the nasopharyngeal microbiome with that of the lung microbiome.[81,82] The proximity and the anatomical continuity of the oral cavity and the lower respiratory tract suggests that the oropharyngeal microbiota could be a major contributor to the lung microbiome. Indeed, compositionally, bacterial communities from the lung are observed to be indistinguishable from the upper airways, albeit about 2 to 4 logs lower in biomass.[81] The air passing through the oropharynx is admixed with saliva laden with inhaled microbes, oral microbes, and trapped particulates.[82] The movement of the air not only assists in the development of the aerodigestive mucosal biofilm but also plays a role in the frequent modulation of the microbiome secondary to the flow and the composition of salivary microbiota.[83,84] Further movement of the epiglottis that diverts the solid contents to the esophagus and the air

to the respiratory tract creates biologically significant number of aerosols. Microaspiration of these aerosols contributes to the vast majority of the constant microbial seeding of the lower airways from the oral cavity during health.[79,84,85] Thus, in general, the healthy lung does not contain a constant or distinct microbiome, but instead contains low levels of bacterial sequences largely similar to those of the upper respiratory tract flora.[81,86] Analysis of 16S rDNA and deep sequencing suggest that the lung-specific sequences are not shared among individuals. The biogeography theory posits that the spatiotemporal variability of the lung is influenced by the continual stream of immigrant bacterial species by microaspiration and selective replication of specific bacteria taxa.[86,87] Hence, this theory provides a rational explanation for the observations that despite the close resemblance of the lung microbiome to the oral microbiome, certain bacteria are represented in higher abundance in the lung microbiome than expected from the corresponding oral microbiomes. This is likely due to a selective advantage in replication among those bacteria taxa in the lung microenvironment as opposed to the oral microenvironment.[84]

The Role of Oral Bacteria in Lung Microbiome Dysbiosis

As stated previously, the balance of three factors determines and shapes the lung microbiome: (1) microbial immigration into the airways, (2) elimination of microbes from the airways, and (3) the relative reproduction rates of the microbes found in the airways as influenced by the local environment for microbial growth.[81] Acute and chronic lung diseases can dramatically change the ecological determinants of the lung microbiome, resulting in markedly different microbial communities.[88] Inflammation alters the lung microbiome by affecting the regional growth conditions as a result of changes imposed in nutrient availability, temperature, pH, and oxygen tension.[16,80] A shift in the microbiome composition away from the *Prevotella, Veillonella,* and *Streptococcus* spp. that dominate the healthy lung microbiome toward Gammaproteobacteria, the class that contains many common gram-negative "pathogens" associated with lung diseases, has been observed in inflammatory pathological lung conditions.[78]

Epidemiological studies support the notion that the oral flora is of relevance to acute and chronic lung disease.[16,79,89] An increase in bacterial immigration from the oropharynx occurs, and several oral anaerobes and facultative species have been cultured from infected lung fluids. These include *Porphyromonas gingivalis, Bacteroides gracilis, Bacteroides oralis, Bacteroides buccae, Eikenella corrodens, Fusobacterium nucleatum, Fusobacterium necrophorum, Actinobacillus actinomycetemcomitans,* peptostreptococci, *Clostridium,* and *Actinomyces.*[16,79,90–93] Although poor oral health has been associated with an increased risk for respiratory disease, improving oral health resulted in a reduction of respiratory events among patients in nursing homes and intensive care units (ICUs).[79,93]

Several mechanisms have been postulated for the role of oral bacteria in the pathogenesis of respiratory infection. Aspiration of oral pathogens into the lower respiratory tract can precipitate lung infection.[79] Cytokines originating from periodontal tissues may alter respiratory epithelium promoting invasion and infection by bacterial pathogens.[93,94] Alternatively, periodontal disease–associated enzymes in saliva may modify the mucosal surfaces to promote adhesion and colonization by respiratory pathogens.[95] Furthermore, backward mucus flow by the ciliary epithelium of the bronchial mucosa toward the oropharynx permit bidirectional movement of the microbiome during the coughing reflex.[79,84,86] The oral mucosa thus could act as a reservoir of respiratory pathogens, which are then aspirated into the lung with salivary droplets.[79,90,93]

Coronavirus Infections, Bacterial Coinfections, Pathological Lung Conditions, and the Role of the Oral Microbiome

The Triad of Coronavirus Infections, Bacterial Coinfections, and Pathological Lung Conditions

Considerable evidence suggests that the influenza and other respiratory viral infections predispose patients to secondary bacterial coinfection or superinfections, often leading to severe clinical disease.[96–98] During the 1918 Spanish flu pandemic by H1N1 influenza virus, secondary pneumonia resulting from bacterial superinfection had a major role in the high mortality rates experienced globally. High mortality secondary to bacterial

coinfection was also detected in approximately 30% of cases in the 2009 H1N1 pandemic despite administration of appropriate antibiotics.[99,100]

Clinical symptoms of COVID-19 infections range from mild or moderate flu-like symptoms to severe pneumonia requiring oxygen support.[27,101] Meta-analysis, systematic reviews, and clinical data show that the predominant causes of mortality in COVID-19 are pathological conditions of the respiratory system, including pneumonia, chronic lower respiratory tract disease, respiratory distress syndrome, respiratory failure, and multiorgan failure secondary to suppurative pulmonary infection. Many of these symptoms and pathological conditions in COVID-19 patients are attributed to bacterial or fungal coinfections and are associated with poor clinical outcome, especially in critically ill patients.[27,101,102]

Interestingly, it has been suggested that as opposed to two other beta coronaviruses, SARS-CoV-1 and MERS-CoV, the SARS-CoV-2 infection facilitated/promoted increased secondary bacterial and/or fungal coinfections or superinfections.[103] The difficulty in obtaining site-specific samples without cross-contamination with oropharynx and saliva is a hurdle in characterizing the upper and lower respiratory tract microbiome. However, few available reports on the analysis of bronchoalveolar lavage samples suggest that the lower respiratory tract or the lung microbiota of deceased COVID-19 patients included complex colonization by bacterial and fungal opportunistic species.[85,104] Although the alpha diversity of the lung microbiome did not differ between the COVID-19–positive and COVID-19–negative patients, significant changes in the microbial composition and relative abundance of specific bacteria have been observed in COVID-19 lung tissues as compared with that in the healthy lungs. Indeed, investigating the lung and the blood microbiome of COVID-19 patients by high-throughput RNA sequencing, Dereschuk et al.[104] observed that 91 bacterial and 14 fungal species were differentially abundant in lung biopsy samples, 13 bacteria and 9 fungal species were differentially abundant in the blood mononuclear cells, and 12 bacteria and 57 fungal species were differentially abundant in bronchoalveolar lavage fluid.

The Role of Oral Microbiome in COVID-19 Lung Disease

The mechanisms of bacterial coinfection or superinfection during or after viral infections consist of complex multifactorial processes mediated by interactions among the viruses, the bacteria, and the host immune system (Box 8.3). Direct mucosal/epithelial damage by the virus could modulate microbial colonization, causing dysbiosis of the respiratory mucosa, and the consequent dysregulations of the immune responses increase the susceptibility to secondary bacterial coinfections.[98] Alternatively, bacterial pneumonia can develop secondary to aspiration of pathogenic oral/oropharyngeal bacteria into the lower respiratory tract.[93,96,105] Pertinently, the *Bacteroides* spp. identified as abundant in the lung tissues, in the bronchoalveolar lavage fluid, and the blood of COVID-19 patients are common colonizers of oral flora. At the phylum level, the Proteobacteria, Firmicutes, Bacteroidetes, and Actinobacteria reported in COVID-19 are also abundant in the normal oral microbiome.[106,107] Interestingly, a similar specific oral bacterial preponderance that influenced pneumonia development was previously reported in influenza infections.[108] Although these studies have not correlated the lung microbiome with the oral flora, the observations support translocation of oral bacteria into the respiratory tract, with aspiration of saliva the primary mode. The salivary microbiota is a "conglomerate of bacteria shed from oral surfaces" and could serve as a reservoir of multiple pathogens.[83] Significantly, it has been suggested that not only the microbial translocation but also that of bacterial components from saliva could contribute to the disease aggravation in COVID-19. The SARS-CoV-2 spike protein has been shown to bind the lipopolysaccharide (LPS), and the interaction is mediated between the lipid A component of the LPS and the S1/S2 furin cleavage site in the spike protein.[108] In silico docking studies showed that the interaction of LPS with the spike protein is structurally very similar to the binding orientation of LPS with its coreceptors, CD14 or MD2.[108] Functionally, the LPS potentiated the proinflammatory effects of the SARS-CoV-2 spike protein, as shown by upregulated nuclear factor-kappa B (NF-κB) activity in cells exposed to both LPS and the spike protein.[108,109] Pertinently, mass spectrometric characterization of salivary LPS suggested that the saliva of patients with chronic periodontitis possessed hyperacylated and phosphorylated lipid A isoforms that are highly immunogenic.[110] In this context, it is tempting to speculate that the aspiration of saliva with the chemically active form of LPS could potentiate further the inflammatory responses of SARS-CoV-2 infection and aggravate the lung pathological condition.

As the name suggests, severe acute respiratory distress is the most common cause for hospitalization in COVID-19.[27,101] Hypoxemia is common in hospitalized patients, and mechanical ventilation is the mainstay of management. Ventilator-associated pneumonia remains a frequent serious complication of these treatment modalities and is often associated with increased mortality.[111] Pathologically, the ventilator-associated pneumonia has been attributed to the dysbiosis in the lower respiratory tract. Microbial modifications in the oropharyngeal regions and bacterial migration to the respiratory tract has been suggested as the nidus for transcolonization and the dysbiosis.[112] The source of the microbial shift in oropharynx could be from either the gut flora or the respiratory tract. It is suggested that the oral epithelium provides niche surfaces for adherence of the bacteria from the respiratory tract that potentially

act as reservoirs.[95,113] Retranslocation to the respiratory tract by microaspiration is suggested as yet another cause for ventilator-associated pneumonia. Immunoinflammatory responses to the altered microflora leads to pneumonia, tissue loss, and consequent death.[83,113]

The Role of Oral Microbiome in Causing Taste Dysfunction in COVID-19

As stated earlier, the lingual epithelial cells, including the taste receptor cells, express multiple entry factors for SARS-CoV-2 virus. Indeed, the SARS-CoV-2 has been shown to replicate in human taste bud cells supporting infective potential.[71] Furthermore, the SARS-CoV-2 invasion could promote a favorable environment for coinfections and contribue to the variable symptoms of ageusia or dysgeusia that either exist for short duration or persist for longer periods.[60] Analyzing oropharyngeal swabs from hospitalized COVID-19 patients, Iebba et al.[114] reported that a select panel of oral bacteria and cytokines is predictive of neurological symptoms, including hyposmia and dysgeusia in SARS-CoV-2–infected individuals. Specifically, the bacterial genera of *Streptococcus, Veillonella, Prevotella, Lactobacillus, Capnocytophaga, Porphyromonas, Abiotrophia, Aggregatibacter,* and *Atopobium* were increased in swabs from COVID-19 patients compared to that from with healthy (SARS-CoV-2 non infected) controls, whereas the genera of *Rothia, Haemophilus, Parvimonas, Fusobacterium,* and *Gemella* were decreased in oral samples in COVID-19 patients.[114,115] In this context it is interesting to note that a previous study reported that the relative abundance of the *Fusobacterium* and *Rothia* on the dorsum of the tongue correlated positively with the perception of sweet and salt taste, respectively.[116] However, only few studies have addressed the role of the oral microbiome in taste perception. Although it is tempting to speculate that the changes in the bacterial genera observed in COVID-19 patients could be at least partially related to the symptom of dysgeusia, more data are needed to resolve the pathogenesis of the condition. Furthermore, in COVID-19, it is not known whether oral dysbiosis is the cause or effect of SARS-CoV-2 infection and whether it could be related to postviral complications.

Salivary Diagnostics, Transmission, and Biomarkers for COVID-19

Saliva for Diagnosis of SARS-CoV-2 Infection

The COVID-19 diagnosis is based on the detection of SARS-CoV-2 RNA by real-time PCR.[117] Molecular diagnostic tests for quantitating the viral RNA include the traditional bench real-time qPCR system, a high-throughput real-time qPCR system (automated from RNA extraction to reporting of results), and direct rapid RNA extraction-free real-time qPCR kits have been widely used globally (3). Additional methods include reverse transcription–loop-mediated isothermal amplification and a rapid antigen test that combines immunochromatography with an enzyme immunoassay to detect the viral nucleocapsid (N) protein, for potential use as point-of-care tests.[118]

Although SARS-CoV-2 RNA detection in the nasopharyngeal swab is considered the gold standard method for COVID-19 diagnosis, demand for swabs early in the pandemic drove a rapid collapse of supply chains, with shortages of personal protective equipment required by health care workers for sample collection.[119–121] Further, the sample acquisition involved close contact of health care workers with the infected or suspected SARS-COV-2–positive individuals, increasing the risk for transmission. In addition, the specimen collection procedure was invasive and uncomfortable for patients. These shortcomings fostered search for use of alternative sampling methods for detecting the virus. More importantly, the rapid spread of the virus necessitated urgent development of methods for repeated sampling and mass testing.

Alternative samples assessed for SARS-CoV-2 detection include pooled nasal mid-turbinate swabs, throat swabs, oropharyngeal wash, and saliva.[119–125] Each of the sample collection methods and the validity of the specimen with respect to SARS-CoV-2 detection has merits and drawbacks. Although all alternative methods were attempted as self-collected specimens with no contact with health care workers to minimize the risk for transmission, saliva collection was easier, less invasive, and more acceptable. Mishra et al.[124] conducted a retrospective analysis of the validity of nonrespiratory samples for detecting the coronaviruses responsible for the previous three pandemics of the 21st century. Assessing data from a total of 3274 that included 802 SARS-CoV-1 samples and 2347 SARS-CoV-2 samples, they found that the sensitivity of nonrespiratory specimens for detection of SARS-CoV-2 was lower at 57.5% (95% CI, -1.2%–116.2%) than that for SARS-CoV-1 at 96.7% (95% CI, 87.6%–100.0%).[124]

Previously, during the SARS-CoV-1 pandemic, a high concordance was observed between the saliva and the nasopharyngeal swabs as diagnostic specimens.[126] Use of saliva for detection of SARS-CoV-2 was first reported by To et al.,[127] during the initial outbreak. They assessed the saliva of 12 nasopharyngeal swab–confirmed COVID-19 patients between 0 and 7 days of hospitalization. They reported a median viral load in saliva at 3.3×10^6 copies/mL, with a range of 9.9×10^2 and 1.2×10^8 copies/mL.[127,128] Subsequent studies testing saliva alone or testing both saliva and paired nasopharyngeal swab samples suggested that the SARS-CoV-2 titer in saliva was equivalent or even higher than that in the nasopharyngeal swab. The sensitivity of SARS-CoV-2 RNA detection in saliva ranged between 81.6% and 100%, and the specificity ranged between 88.4% and 100%.[117,121,129] Indeed, the virus was detected in

the saliva of asymptomatic individuals, albeit at lower titers (10^4–10^5 copies/mL) when the nasopharyngeal swabs were negative. Because the real-time PCR is based on well-characterized and validated primers, detection of SARS-CoV-2 RNA in saliva is not classified as false positive but rather as false negative or misclassification of nasopharyngeal samples. Further, in contrast to the inconsistent nasopharyngeal swab results, the viral titer in saliva decreased progressively in severely ill COVID-19 patients during recovery. In this context, the temporal analysis of SARS-CoV-2 viral load in saliva could serve a pivotal role for the translation of salivary tests in the clinic.[130] Furthermore, glandular saliva from the parotid gland duct yielded high titers of the virus suggesting that SARS-CoV-2 targets the ductal and/or glandular epithelial cells.[126,128] Interestingly, fecal-oral transmission has been suggested as a source of the virus in saliva in COVID-19 patients presenting with GI symptoms with fecal shedding of SARS-CoV-2.[131,132]

Encouraged by the data from early studies, the use of saliva as a specimen for detecting SARS-CoV-2 increased globally. Several systematic reviews and met-analytic studies conducted comparative analyses of the sensitivity of saliva and that of the gold standard nasopharyngeal swabs as biospecimens for detecting SARS-CoV-2[119,120,125,133–135] (Table 8.2). Collectively, there is evidence that the saliva as specimen exhibits high sensitivity and specificity for detecting SARS-CoV-2 (Box 8.4). Further, the feasibility of frequent and self-collection of saliva are distinct advantages in infections with rapid spread and transmission such as SARS-CoV-2. Indeed, Eduardo evaluated 55 self-collected unstimulated saliva samples from hospitalized COVID-19 patients and demonstrated that the saliva samples were 87.3% in agreement with the nasopharyngeal swab for the detection of SARS-CoV-2 virus.[123] In contrast, in studies comparing paired nasopharyngeal swabs and self-collected saliva obtained simultaneously, saliva samples exhibited lower sensitivity ranging from 16% to of 24.4%.[136–138] Nagura-Ikeda et al.[139] reported that the viral RNA was detected at significantly higher percentages (65.6%–93.4%) in saliva specimens self-collected within 9 days of symptom onset. However, the virus detection was lower as the time passed after at least 10 days of symptoms (22.2%–66.7%) and in specimens collected from asymptomatic patients (40.0%–66.7%).[139] In asymptomatic individuals, random saliva samples (92.3%) were superior or equivalent to the pooled nasopharyngeal and oropharyngeal samples (73.2%) for detecting the SARS-CoV-2 virus by amplification of the open reading frame 1a (ORF1a) and nucleocapsid (N) genes.[8] Reanalysis of SARS-CoV-2–positive frozen saliva samples by immunochromatographic assay and chemiluminescent enzyme immunoassay detected SARS-CoV-2 in 41% by the former method and in 91% of samples by the latter method.[135]

Table 8.2 Comparison of Saliva and Other Specimens for Detecting SARS-CoV-2

	Sample						
	Nasopharyngeal Swab	Nasal Midturbinate Swab	Oro pharyngeal swab	Pooled nasal and Oral Swabs	Throat Swab	Saliva	Reference
1	97%	86% (CI, 77–93)		95% (CI, 93–100)	68% (CI, (35–94)	85% (CI, 75–93)	125
2	85.8% (CI, 80–97.6)					87.3% (CI, 81.3–91.6)	134
3	94% (CI, 90–98)	82% (CI, 73–90)	84% (CI, 57–100)	97% (CI, 90–100)		88% (CI, 81–93)	133
4	87% (CI, 77-95)		44% (CI, 35–52)	95% (CI: 80-99)	82% (CI, 76-88)	83% (CI, 77–89)	120
5	84.8% (CI, 76.8–92.4)					83.2% (CI, 74.7–91.4)	119
6	98% (CI, 89–100)					91% (CI, 80–99)	139

Note: A nonexhaustive compilation of studies reporting the sensitivity of SARS-CoV-2 detection in the indicated sample type.
CI, Confidence interval.

Despite these observations, considerable skepticism surrounds the use of saliva as a specimen for infectious diseases (Box 8.4). The nonstandard methods of specimen acquisition and the contaminations from food are potential confounding factors. The wide range in detection also could be due to the nature of the saliva sample—for example, the viscosity interfering with the detection methods, which also have been variable. An additional significant confounder that precludes complete validation of saliva as a biospecimen for viral detection, is the inconsistency in the time of collection with respect to the start of infection. Whereas some studies were based on saliva collected from hospitalized individuals at varying days after testing positive, others have reported results of saliva samples collected at the same time as the nasopharyngeal sample collection.[136–140] Furthermore, the differential expression of the receptor for the virus in the oral mucosa could contribute to the variation in the sensitivity of detection from studies around the globe.[43,48,141]

SARS-CoV-2 Transmission by Saliva

Chen et al.[39] reported high titers of SARS-CoV-2 in pure saliva collected from salivary gland ducts of severely ill COVID-19 patients. A potential source is the release of the viral particles from the infected and necrosed salivary gland tissues.[67] Another source is release of viral particles from the infected oral epithelial cells.[56,71] Pertinently, autopsy tissues from COVID-19 patients showed that the epithelial cells on the dorsum of the tongue exhibited detectable levels of SARS-COV-2 by real-time PCR, suggesting viral infection.[56] Interestingly, the exfoliated epithelial cells in saliva as well as the epithelial cells lining the salivary gland ducts have been

shown to exhibit viral particles by in situ hybridization.[56,67] Additional sources of SARS-COV-2 in saliva are from the infected oropharyngeal tissues and lungs. Therefore saliva-associated droplets are significant sources of transmission of SARS-CoV-2 between humans.[142–144] Saliva droplets are generated as particles of moisture and droplets consisting of microorganisms during breathing, talking, coughing, or sneezing. The distance the droplets travel depends on the size, with larger droplets tending to settle quickly. Very small droplets (<5 µM) may evaporate, become droplet nuclei or aerosol, and could contribute to the airborne transmission of infections.[145,146] Positive airborne transmission depends on the duration of stability of the infectious agent in aerosols and the susceptibility of the individual in the path of the aerosols. The observed stability of airborne SARS-CoV-1 and SARS-CoV-2 by real-time PCR and in viable cultures suggests transmission of coronaviruses by short- and long-range aerosols.[130,147]

Salivary Biomarkers for Coronavirus Infections

As stated earlier, SARS-CoV-2 has been consistently detected in saliva and at least one study suggests that the viral load is higher in saliva than in the nasopharyngeal swabs.[3] It has been suggested that the saliva with higher viral load could represent a better specimen for SARS-CoV-2 detection in asymptomatic carriers with lower false-negative rates than the widely used nasopharyngeal swab.[140,148]

Whole saliva is a mixture of secretions from salivary glands, blood, and cells lining the oral mucosa, and cellular components that include corpuscles, exfoliated epithelial cells, and microbiome. Hence, salivary proteome and transcriptome have been assessed for markers for oral and systemic diseases.[149,150] Identification of diagnostic and prognostic markers is particularly important for SARS-CoV-2 infection and variants because the clinical course is highly unpredictable with serious consequences. The source of the biomarkers could be systemic, derived from the circulation and the local sources within the oral cavity.

Several blood biomarkers have been assessed for COVID-19, including C-reactive protein, serum amyloid A, IL-6, lactate dehydrogenase, neutrophil-to-lymphocyte ratio, D-dimer, cardiac troponin, and renal-injury biomarkers.[151,152] Systematic analyses suggested that all of these markers showed significantly higher levels in patients with severe complications of COVID-19 infection compared with their nonsevere counterparts.[151,153,154] Because the proteomic profile of saliva shares many features of the plasma proteome, there is a likelihood of similar dysregulated expression within saliva. Many of these plasma proteins have been measured in saliva and assessed as potential biomarkers for oral and systemic diseases.[150,155,156] Interestingly, a positive correlation between the development of gustatory dysfunctions in COVID-19 and increase in serum IL-6 has been reported, suggesting its potential as a biomarker.[62] Because saliva is easily accessible for frequent collection, it is speculated that assessment of salivary IL-6 could be a marker to identify SARS-CoV-2–infected individuals likely to become symptomatic.

It is well recognized that the entry factor for SARs-CoV-2, the ACE2 receptor, is expressed widely in different cell types. Although predominantly present as bound to cell membranes, extracellular shedding gives rise to a soluble form, sACE2, that can be detected in the circulation.[41,47] ACE2 also plays a critical role in the renin-angiotensin pathway and contributes significantly to the regulation of blood pressure.[141] In health and in stable chronic diseases, the plasma sACE2 level probably reflects the balance between the expression and availability of ACE2 at the cellular level. Elevated levels of circulating sACE2 have been observed in patients with atrial fibrillation and heart failure.[157,158] Preexisting cardiovascular disease is a risk factor for SARS-CoV-2; therefore it is likely that the infection could trigger variations in ACE2 expression. Higher plasma level of sACE2 observed in a few case reports of COVID-19 patients could reflect a higher cellular expression of ACE2.[141,159–161] It has been suggested that the sACE2 could potentially sequester the coronavirus and prevent disease development.[162,163] However, persistent infection can lead to reduced membrane-bound ACE2 and thus contribute to disease development. Thus assessment for circulating sACE2 could be a marker for identification of asymptomatic or presymptomatic COVID-19.[161]

As reported by several studies, the observations of abundant expression of ACE2 and TMPRSS-2 in the oral mucosa, particularly in the surface epithelial cells of the tongue, suggest that the oral epithelial cells could represent potential sites of entry or reservoirs of SARS-CoV-2.[43,45,71–73] Thus sACE2 arising from the extracellular shedding could be measured in the saliva. The TNF-α and IL-6 often induced by the viral attachment and infection could not only increase ACE2 ectodomain shedding from oral epithelial cells, but also upregulate epithelial cell exfoliation.[164] In addition to the extracellular shedding, glandular saliva and passive diffusion from circulation are other potential sources of sACE2 in saliva. Interestingly, the sACE2 activity was lower in the saliva of hospitalized COVID-19 patients.[165] It is likely that much like the circulating sACE2, variations in salivary sACE2 could reflect the stage of SARS-CoV-2 infection and COVID-19.

Alternatively, because longitudinal observations in a few SARS-CoV-2–positive cases showed that the viral load in saliva is consistently higher during the symptomatic phase, it is likely that the sACE2 in saliva is sequestered by the higher viral load.[121,125,130] Taken together, it is likely that the sACE2 levels in saliva will parallel the viral load in CoV-2–infected individuals and represent a biomarker underscoring the transition from asymptomatic to symptomatic COVID-19. Further, in the context of a recent suggestion that the influenza virus upregulates ACE2 expression and potentially enhances the risk for SARS-CoV-2 infection, assessment of ACE2 alone could be of greater significance in early identification of future outbreaks with SARS-CoV variants.[39,166]

SARS-CoV-2 and the Dental Office

Risk for Direct Transmission

As discussed previously, direct contact by respiratory droplets or aerosols is widely thought to be the most common mode of COVID-19 transmission. Rotary or surgical instruments, including handpieces, ultrasonic scalers, or air-water syringes, used in routine dental practice generate visible spatter and droplets of saliva admixed with blood. The number and size of saliva droplets generated not only vary with the dental procedure but also among people, suggesting heterogeneous transmission potential. Contamination on the clinical gowns and inner surface of the masks of dental hygienists with saliva droplets has been reported after ultrasonic cleaning. Although the surgical masks protect the mucous membrane of the mouth and nose from the spatter, they do not provide complete protection from airborne infections.[144,145,167]

Positive airborne transmission depends on the duration of stability of the infectious agent in aerosols and the susceptibility of the individual in the path of the aerosols. A study from the University of Nebraska Medical Center demonstrated that the SARS-CoV-2 genome was detectable not only in air samples from rooms of COVID-19 patients but also in 66.7% of air samples obtained from hallways outside patient rooms.[168] Using a Bayesian regression model, van Doremalen et al.[147] compared the stability of SARS-CoV-2 and SARS-CoV-1 in aerosols. They found that much like the SARS-CoV-1, the SARS-CoV-2 pathogen also remained viable in aerosols throughout the 3-hour period of experimental duration. Taken together, these observations substantiate the high risk for direct airborne transmission of the COVID-19 virus to dental health care professionals.

Indirect Contact Transmission

Clusters of COVID-19 infection in meat processing plants and church attendees, as well as the success of social distancing in reducing the infection, suggest additional modes of transmission of the airborne virus.[169] Respiratory droplets are generated by talking, breathing, sneezing, and coughing. Often large droplets with infectious agents get deposited on hard surfaces and become sources of transmission. Indeed, during the previous outbreaks, the SARS-CoV-1 and the MERS-CoV pathogens were shown to survive on dry metal, ceramic, or plastic surfaces for unusually long periods (4–6 days) at room temperature.[170] Further, SARS-CoV-1 exhibited a dose–response relationship, being stable on disposable plastic for a short period of 1 hour after low-dose inoculation (10^4 dose/mL) but surviving for 2 days at higher inoculation concentration (10^6 dose/mL).[171] SARS-CoV-2 is expected to share features of stability similar to those of SARS-CoV-1 and MERS-CoV.[170,171] Recently Liu et al.[143] analyzed 35 aerosol samples from patient areas and medical staff areas in two hospitals in Wuhan, China for SARS-CoV-2 by digital PCR. They observed that the droplets deposited on the surfaces of ICU workstations tested positive for the virus. The stability of SARS-CoV-2 assessed in a more controlled environment was found to be much like SARS-CoV-1 as shown by the stability of the laboratory-created SARS-CoV-2 aerosols for 72 hours on stainless steel and plastic surfaces.[147] In clinical dental settings, contamination by hands soiled with saliva that repeatedly touch dental operatory equipment and return to the patient's mouth during treatments can easily increase the area of contaminated surfaces. This will in turn increase the chances of transmission to all personnel with access to the operatory and enhance the risk for cross-contamination between patients for extended periods. Therefore it is imperative that dentists are aware of updated knowledge about the modes of transmission of SARS-CoV-2 and follow the recommended infection control measures in dental settings.

Conclusion

Although SARS-CoV-2 was detected in saliva early in the course of the COVID-19 pandemic and taste dysfunction was recognized as one of the early symptoms, comprehensive understanding of oral manifestations is still evolving. Emerging concerns include complaints of persistent symptoms for extended periods in recovered individuals. Significantly, loss of taste is consistently reported as a common symptom of long-COVID, defined as persistence of symptoms 4 weeks after infection.[69] The expression of the entry factors of SARS-CoV-2, including ACE2 in oral epithelial cells and taste receptor cells, viral invasion–induced dysbiosis, localized inflammatory responses, immune dysfunctions, and drug-induced adverse reactions have all been suggested as potential mechanisms for the oral manifestations in COVID-19. Interesting results from preliminary microbiome studies have raised research questions and opportunities for understanding the complex relationship between the oral microbiome and the coronavirus infections. This is particularly significant in the continued emergence of SARS-CoV-2 variants and their unknown clinical effects. The emerging data on salivary biomarkers has also stimulated interest in early recognition of asymptomatic carriers. Furthermore, because convincing evidence supports airborne transmission, the importance of personal protection and precautionary measures to prevent transmission at the dental offices are emphasized.

REFERENCES

1. Abeles SR, Robles-Sikisaka R, Ly M, et al. Human oral viruses are personal, persistent and gender-consistent. *ISME J.* 2014;8(9):1753–1767.
2. Li N, Ma W-T, Fan Q-L, Hua J-L, et al. The commensal microbiota and viral infection: a comprehensive review. *Front Immunol.* 2019;10:1551.
3. Ly M, Abeles SR, Boehn TK, et al. Altered oral viral ecology in association with periodontal disease. *mBio.* 2014;5(3) e01133-14.
4. Robles-Sikisaka R, Ly M, Boehn T, et al. Association between living environment and human oral viral ecology. *ISME J.* 2013;7(9):1710–1724.
5. Scully C, Samaranayake LP. Emerging and changing viral diseases in the new millennium. *Oral Dis.* 2016;22(3):171–179.
6. Scully C, Epstein J, Cox PM. Viruses and chronic disorders involving the human oral mucosa. *Oral Surg Oral Med Oral Pathol.* 1991;72(5):537–544.
7. Crimi S, Fiorillo L, Bianchi A, et al. Herpes Virus, Oral Clinical Signs and QoL: Systematic Review of Recent Data. *Viruses.* 2019;11(5).
8. Hairston BR, Bruce AJ, Rogers 3rd RS. Viral diseases of the oral mucosa. *Dermatol Clin.* 2003;21(1):17–32.
9. Stoopler ET. Oral herpetic infections (HSV 1-8). *Dent Clin North Am.* 2005;49(1):15–29 vii.
10. Syrjanen S. Oral manifestations of human papillomavirus infections. *Eur J Oral Sci.* 2018;126(Suppl 1):49–66.
11. Wong MCS, Vlantis AC, Liang M, et al. Persistence and clearance of oral human papillomavirus infections: A prospective population-based cohort study. *J Med Virol.* 2020:jmv26130.
12. Shillitoe EJ. The Microbiome of Oral Cancer. *Crit Rev Oncog.* 2018;23(3-4):153–160.

13. Askinyte D, Matulionyte R, Rimkevicius A. Oral manifestations of HIV disease: A review. *Stomatologija*. 2015;**17**(1):21–28.

14. Heron SE, Elahi S. HIV infection and compromised mucosal immunity: oral manifestations and systemic inflammation. *Front Immunol*. 2017;**8**:241.

15. Samaranayake L, Scully C, Nair RG, Petti S. Viral haemorrhagic fevers with emphasis on Ebola virus disease and oro-dental healthcare. *Oral Dis*. 2015;**21**(1):1–6.

16. Segal LN, Clemente JC, Tsay J-C J, et al. Enrichment of the lung microbiome with oral taxa is associated with lung inflammation of a Th17 phenotype. *Nat Microbiol*. 2016;**1**:16031.

17. Wang C, Zhou S, Xue W, et al. Comprehensive virome analysis reveals the complexity and diversity of the viral spectrum in pediatric patients diagnosed with severe and mild hand-foot-and-mouth disease. *Virology*. 2018;**518**:116–125.

18. Henkin RI, Larson AL, Powell RD. Hypogeusia, dysgeusia, hyposmia, and dysosmia following influenza-like infection. *Ann Otol Rhinol Laryngol*. 1975;**84**(5 Pt 1):672–682.

19. Henkin RI, Martin BM, Agarwal RP. Decreased parotid saliva gustin/carbonic anhydrase VI secretion: an enzyme disorder manifested by gustatory and olfactory dysfunction. *Am J Med Sci*. 1999;**318**(6):380–391.

20. Alanagreh L., Alzoughool F., Atoum M. The human coronavirus disease COVID-19: its origin, characteristics, and insights into potential drugs and its mechanisms. Pathogens. 2020;**9**(5):331.

21. Cascella, M., Rajnik M, Aleem A, et al., Features, Evaluation, and Treatment of Coronavirus (COVID-19), in StatPearls. 2021: Treasure Island (FL).

22. Singla R, Mishra A, Joshi R, et al. Human animal interface of SARS-CoV-2 (COVID-19) transmission: a critical appraisal of scientific evidence. *Vet Res Commun*. 2020;**44**(3-4):119–130.

23. Cherry JD, Krogstad P. SARS: the first pandemic of the 21st century. *Pediatr Res*. 2004;**56**(1):1–5.

24. Meo SA, Alhowikan AM, Al-Khaliwi T, al. t. Novel coronavirus 2019-nCoV: prevalence, biological and clinical characteristics comparison with SARS-CoV and MERS-CoV. *Eur Rev Med Pharmacol Sci*. 2020;**24**(4):2012–2019.

25. Rahman, A. and Sarkar A, Risk factors for fatal middle east respiratory syndrome coronavirus infections in Saudi Arabia: analysis of the WHO Line List, 2013–2018. 2019. **109**(9): p. 1288-1293.

26. Shereen MA, Kahn S, Kazmi A, et al. COVID-19 infection: Origin, transmission, and characteristics of human coronaviruses. *J Adv Res*. 2020;**24**:91–98.

27. Adhikari SP, Meng S, Wu Y-J, et al. Epidemiology, causes, clinical manifestation and diagnosis, prevention and control of coronavirus disease (COVID-19) during the early outbreak period: a scoping review. *Infect Dis Poverty*. 2020;**9**(1):29.

28. Centers for Disease Control and Prevention. *COVID Data Tracker*.. 2020. [cited April 2020; Available from. https://covid.cdc.gov/covid-data-tracker/#datatracker-home.

29. Abubakr N, Salem ZA, Kamel AHM. Oral manifestations in mild-to-moderate cases of COVID-19 viral infection in the adult population. *Dent Med Probl*. 2021;**58**(1):7–15.

30. Amorim Dos Santos J, AGC Normando, Carvalho da Silva RL, et al. Oral Manifestations in Patients with COVID-19: A Living Systematic Review. *J Dent Res*. 2021;**100**(2):141–154.

31. Diaz Rodriguez M, Jimenez Romera A, Villarroel M. Oral manifestations associated with COVID-19. *Oral Dis*. 2020. doi:10.1111/odi.13555.

32. Etemad-Moghadam S, Alaeddini M. Is SARS-CoV-2 an Etiologic Agent or Predisposing Factor for Oral Lesions in COVID-19 Patients? A Concise Review of Reported Cases in the Literature. *Int J Dent*. 2021;**2021**:6648082.

33. Huang N, Pérez P, Byrd KM. SARS-CoV-2 infection of the oral cavity and saliva. *Nat Med*. 2021;**27**(5):892–903.

34. Cruz Tapia RO, Peraza Labrador AJ, Guimaraes DM, Matos Valdez LH. Oral mucosal lesions in patients with SARS-CoV-2 infection. Report of four cases. Are they a true sign of COVID-19 disease? *Spec Care Dentist*. 2020;**40**(6):555–560.

35. Fidan V, Koyuncu H, Akin O. Oral lesions in Covid 19 positive patients. *Am J Otolaryngol*. 2021;**42**(3):102905.

36. Agyeman AA, Chin KL, Landersdorfer CB, et al. Smell and Taste Dysfunction in Patients With COVID-19: A Systematic Review and Meta-analysis. *Mayo Clin Proc*. 2020;**95**(8):1621–1631.

37. Schwab J, Jensen CD, Fjaeldstad AW. Sustained Chemosensory Dysfunction during the COVID-19 Pandemic. *ORL J Otorhinolaryngol Relat Spec*. 2021:1–10.

38. Saniasiaya J, Islam MA, Abdullah B. Prevalence and Characteristics of Taste Disorders in Cases of COVID-19: A Meta-analysis of 29,349 Patients. *Otolaryngol Head Neck Surg*. 2021;**165**(1):33–42.

39. Chen L, Zhao J, Peng J, et al. Detection of SARS-CoV-2 in saliva and characterization of oral symptoms in COVID-19 patients. *Cell Prolif*. 2020;**53**(12):e12923.

40. Fantozzi PJ, Pampena E, Di Vanna D, et al. Xerostomia, gustatory and olfactory dysfunctions in patients with COVID-19. *Am J Otolaryngol*. 2020;**41**(6):102721.

41. Li W, Moore MJ, Vasilieva N, et al. Angiotensin-converting enzyme 2 is a functional receptor for the SARS coronavirus. *Nature*. 2003;**426**(6965):450–454.

42. Lan J, Ge J, Yu J, et al. Structure of the SARS-CoV-2 spike receptor-binding domain bound to the ACE2 receptor. *Nature*. 2020;**581**(7807):215–220.

43. Zhong M, Lin B, Pathak JL, et al. ACE2 and Furin Expressions in Oral Epithelial Cells Possibly Facilitate COVID-19 Infection via Respiratory and Fecal-Oral Routes. *Front Med (Lausanne)*. 2020;**7**:580796.

44. Zipeto D, da Fonesca Palmeira J, Argañaraz GA, Argañaraz ER. ACE2/ADAM17/TMPRSS2 Interplay May Be the Main Risk Factor for COVID-19. *Front Immunol*. 2020;**11**:576745.

45. Pascolo L, Zupin L, Melato M, et al. TMPRSS2 and ACE2 Coexpression in SARS-CoV-2 Salivary Glands Infection. *J Dent Res*. 2020;**99**(10):1120–1121.

46. Hoffmann M, Klein-Weber H, Schroeder S, et al. SARS-CoV-2 Cell Entry Depends on ACE2 and TMPRSS2 and Is Blocked by a Clinically Proven Protease Inhibitor. *Cell*,. 2020;**181**(2):271-280 e8.

47. Devaux CA, Rolain JM, Raoult D. ACE2 receptor polymorphism: Susceptibility to SARS-CoV-2, hypertension, multi-organ failure, and COVID-19 disease outcome. *J Microbiol Immunol Infect*. 2020;**53**(3):425–435.

48. Hamming I, Timens W, Bulthuis MLC, et al. Tissue distribution of ACE2 protein, the functional receptor for SARS coronavirus. A first step in understanding SARS pathogenesis. *J Pathol*. 2004;**203**(2):631–637.

49. Groeger S, Meyle J. *Oral Mucosal Epithelial Cells. Front Immunol*. 2019;**10**:208.

50. Swidergall M, Solis NV, Lionakis MS, Filler SG. EphA2 is an epithelial cell pattern recognition receptor for fungal beta-glucans. *Nat Microbiol*. 2018;**3**(1):53–61.

51. Swidergall M, Solis NV, Millet N, et al. Activation of EphA2-EGFR signaling in oral epithelial cells by *Candida albicans* virulence factors. *PLoS Pathog.* 2021;**17**(1):e1009221.

52. Uehara A, Suguwara Y, Kurata S, et al. Chemically synthesized pathogen-associated molecular patterns increase the expression of peptidoglycan recognition proteins via toll-like receptors, NOD1 and NOD2 in human oral epithelial cells. *Cell Microbiol.* 2005;**7**(5):675–686.

53. Xu H, Zhong L, Deng J, et al. High expression of ACE2 receptor of 2019-nCoV on the epithelial cells of oral mucosa. *Int J Oral Sci.* 2020;**12**(1):8.

54. Song J, Li Y, Huang X, et al. Systematic analysis of ACE2 and TMPRSS2 expression in salivary glands reveals underlying transmission mechanism caused by SARS-CoV-2. *J Med Virol.* 2020;**92**(11):2556–2566.

55. Srinivasan M, Zunt SL, Goldblatt LI. Oral epithelial expression of angiotensin converting enzyme-2: Implications for COVID-19 diagnosis and prognosis. *bioRxiv.* 2020:2020.06.22.165035.

56. Salas Orozco MF, Niño-Martínez N, Martínez-Castañón G-A, et al. Presence of SARS-CoV-2 and Its Entry Factors in Oral Tissues and Cells: A Systematic Review. *Medicina (Kaunas).* 2021;**57**(6):523.

57. Gadanec LK, McSweeny KR, Qaradakhi T, et al. Can SARS-CoV-2 Virus Use Multiple Receptors to Enter Host Cells?. *Int J Mol Sci.* 2021;**22**(3):992.

58. Choudhury A, Mukherjee S. In silico studies on the comparative characterization of the interactions of SARS-CoV-2 spike glycoprotein with ACE-2 receptor homologs and human TLRs. *J Med Virol.* 2020;**92**(10):2105–2113.

59. Sohn KM, Lee SG, Kim HJ, et al. COVID-19 Patients Upregulate Toll-like Receptor 4-mediated Inflammatory Signaling That Mimics Bacterial Sepsis. *J Korean Med Sci.* 2020;**35**(38):e343.

60. Cox MJ, Loman N, Bogaert D, O'Grady J. Co-infections: potentially lethal and unexplored in COVID-19. *Lancet Microbe.* 2020;**1**(1):e11.

61. Ngo VL, Gewirtz AT. Microbiota as a potentially-modifiable factor influencing COVID-19. *Curr Opin Virol.* 2021;**49**:21–26.

62. Cazzolla AP, Lovero R, Lo Muzio L, et al. Taste and Smell Disorders in COVID-19 Patients: Role of Interleukin-6. *ACS Chem Neurosci.* 2020;**11**(17):2774–2781.

63. Mastrangelo A, Bonato M, Cinque P. Smell and taste disorders in COVID-19: From pathogenesis to clinical features and outcomes. *Neurosci Lett.* 2021;**748**:135694.

64. Srinivasan M. Taste Dysfunction and Long COVID-19. *Frontiers in Cellular and Infection Microbiology.* 2021;**11**(647):716563.

65. Wang H, Zhou M, Brand J, Huang L, et al. Inflammation and taste disorders: mechanisms in taste buds. *Ann N Y Acad Sci.* 2009;**1170**:596–603.

66. Liu L, Wei K, Alvarez X, et al. Epithelial cells lining salivary gland ducts are early target cells of severe acute respiratory syndrome coronavirus infection in the upper respiratory tracts of rhesus macaques. *J Virol.* 2011;**85**(8):4025–4030.

67. Matuck BF, Dohlnikoff M, Nunes Duarte-Neto A, et al. Salivary glands are a target for SARS-CoV-2: a source for saliva contamination. *J Pathol.* 2021;**254**(3):239–243.

68. Favia G, Tempesta A, Barile G, et al. Covid-19 Symptomatic Patients with Oral Lesions: Clinical and Histopathological Study on 123 Cases of the University Hospital Policlinic of Bari with a Purpose of a New Classification. *J Clin Med.* 2021;**10**(4):757.

69. Biadsee A, Dagan O, Ormianer Z, et al. Eight-month follow-up of olfactory and gustatory dysfunctions in recovered COVID-19 patients. *Am J Otolaryngol.* 2021;**42**(4):103065.

70. Cooper KW, Brann DH, Farruggia MC, et al. COVID-19 and the Chemical Senses: Supporting Players Take Center Stage. *Neuron.* 2020;**107**(2):219–233.

71. Doyle ME, Appleton A, Liu QR, et al. Human Type II Taste Cells Express Angiotensin-Converting Enzyme 2 and Are Infected by Severe Acute Respiratory Syndrome Coronavirus 2 (SARS-CoV-2). *Am J Pathol.* 2021;**191**(9):1511–1519.

72. Sakaguchi W, Kubota N, Shimizu T, et al. Existence of SARS-CoV-2 Entry Molecules in the Oral Cavity. *Int J Mol Sci.* 2020;**21**(17):6000.

73. Han Q, Peng J, Xu H, et al. Taste Cell Is Abundant in the Expression of ACE2 Receptor of 2019-nCoV. *Preprints.* 2020 (2020040424).

74. Meunier N, Briand L, Jacquin-Piques A, et al. COVID 19-Induced Smell and Taste Impairments: Putative Impact on. *Physiology. Front Physiol.* 2020;**11**:625110.

75. Wang H, Zhou M, Brand J, Huang L. Inflammation activates the interferon signaling pathways in taste bud cells. *J Neurosci.* 2007;**27**(40):10703–10713.

76. Ambaldhage V, Puttabuddi JH, Nunsavath PN, et al. Taste disorders: A review. *Journal of Indian Academy of Oral Medicine and Radiology.* 2014;**26**(1):69–76.

77. Risso D, Drayna D, Morini G. Alteration, Reduction and Taste Loss: Main Causes and Potential Implications on Dietary Habits. *Nutrients.* 2020;**12**(11):3284.

78. Moffatt MF, Cookson WO. The lung microbiome in health and disease. *Clin Med (Lond).* 2017;**17**(6):525–529.

79. Gaeckle NT, Pragman AA, Pendleton KM, et al. The Oral-Lung Axis: The Impact of Oral Health on Lung Health. *Respir Care.* 2020;**65**(8):1211–1220.

80. Huffnagle GB, Dickson RP, Lukacs NW. The respiratory tract microbiome and lung inflammation: a two-way street. *Mucosal Immunol.* 2017;**10**(2):299–306.

81. Charlson ES, Bittinger K, Haas AR, et al. Topographical continuity of bacterial populations in the healthy human respiratory tract. *Am J Respir Crit Care Med.* 2011;**184**(8):957–963.

82. Scannapieco FA. Role of oral bacteria in respiratory infection. *J Periodontol.* 1999;**70**(7):793–802.

83. Belstrom D. The salivary microbiota in health and disease. *J Oral Microbiol.* 2020;**12**(1):1723975.

84. Dickson RP, Erb-Downward JR, Freeman CM, et al. Spatial Variation in the Healthy Human Lung Microbiome and the Adapted Island Model of Lung Biogeography. *Ann Am Thorac Soc.* 2015;**12**(6):821–830.

85. Gaibani P, Viciani E, Bartoletti M, et al. The lower respiratory tract microbiome of critically ill patients with COVID-19. *Sci Rep.* 2021;**11**(1):10103.

86. Dickson RP, Huffnagle GB. The Lung Microbiome: New Principles for Respiratory Bacteriology in Health and Disease. *PLoS Pathog.* 2015;**11**(7):e1004923.

87. Whiteson KL, Bailey B, Bergkessel M, et al. The upper respiratory tract as a microbial source for pulmonary infections in cystic fibrosis. Parallels from island biogeography. *Am J Respir Crit Care Med.* 2014;**189**(11):1309–1315.

88. Dickson RP, Huang YJ, Martinez FJ, Huffnagle GB. The lung microbiome and viral-induced exacerbations of chronic obstructive pulmonary disease: new observations, novel approaches. *Am J Respir Crit Care Med.* 2013;**188**(10):1185–1186.

89. Gomes-Filho IS, Passos JS, Seixas da Cruz S. Respiratory disease and the role of oral bacteria. *J Oral Microbiol.* 2010;**2**.

90. Bao L, Zhang C, Dong J, et al. Oral Microbiome and SARS-CoV-2: Beware of Lung Co-infection. *Front Microbiol.* 2020;**11**:1840.

91. Chen X, Liao B, Cheng L, et al. The microbial coinfection in COVID-19. *Appl Microbiol Biotechnol.* 2020;**104**(18):7777–7785.

92. Kageyama S, Takeshita T, Furuta M, et al. Relationships of Variations in the Tongue Microbiota and Pneumonia Mortality in Nursing Home Residents. *J Gerontol A Biol Sci Med Sci.* 2018;**73**(8):1097–1102.

93. Mammen MJ, Scannapieco FA, Sethi S. Oral-lung microbiome interactions in lung diseases. *Periodontol.* 2000;**83**(1):234–241.

94. Sampson V, Kamona N, Sampson A. Could there be a link between oral hygiene and the severity of SARS-CoV-2 infections?. *Br Dent J.* 2020;**228**(12):971–975.

95. Scannapieco FA, Wang B, Shiau HJ. Oral bacteria and respiratory infection: effects on respiratory pathogen adhesion and epithelial cell proinflammatory cytokine production. *Ann Periodontol.* 2001;**6**(1):78–86.

96. Jia L, Xie J, Zhao J, et al. Mechanisms of Severe Mortality-Associated Bacterial Co-infections Following Influenza Virus Infection. *Front Cell Infect Microbiol.* 2017;**7**:338.

97. Peteranderl C, Herold S, Schmoldt C. Human Influenza Virus Infections. *Semin Respir Crit Care Med.* 2016;**37**(4):487–500.

98. Rynda-Apple A, Robinson KM, Alcorn JF. Influenza and Bacterial Superinfection: Illuminating the Immunologic Mechanisms of Disease. *Infect Immun.* 2015;**83**(10):3764–3770.

99. Morris DE, Cleary DW, Clarke SC. Secondary Bacterial Infections Associated with Influenza Pandemics. *Front Microbiol.* 2017;**8**:1041.

100. Sheng ZM, Chertow DS, Ambroggio X, et al. Autopsy series of 68 cases dying before and during the 1918 influenza pandemic peak. *Proc Natl Acad Sci U S A,.* 2011;**108**(39):16416–16421.

101. Zhou F, Yu T, Du R, et al. Clinical course and risk factors for mortality of adult inpatients with COVID-19 in Wuhan, China: a retrospective cohort study. *Lancet.* 2020;**395**(10229):1054–1062.

102. Elezkurtaj S, Greuel S, Ihlow J, et al. Causes of death and comorbidities in hospitalized patients with COVID-19. *Sci Rep.* 2021;**11**(1):4263.

103. Lansbury L, Lim B, Baskaran V, Lim WS. Co-infections in people with COVID-19: a systematic review and meta-analysis. *J Infect.* 2020;**81**(2):266–275.

104. Dereschuk K, Apostol L, Ranjan I, et al. Identification of Lung and Blood Microbiota Implicated in COVID-19 Prognosis. *Cells.* 2021;**10**(6):1452.

105. Hoque MN, Akter S, Mishu ID, et al. Microbial co-infections in COVID-19: Associated microbiota and underlying mechanisms of pathogenesis. *Microb Pathog.* 2021;**156**:104941.

106. Aas JA, Paster BJ, Stokes LN, et al. Defining the normal bacterial flora of the oral cavity. *J Clin Microbiol.* 2005;**43**(11):5721–5732.

107. Zhang Y, Wang X, Li H, et al. Human oral microbiota and its modulation for oral health. *Biomed Pharmacother.* 2018;**99**:883–893.

108. Petruk G, Puthia M, Petrlova J, et al. SARS-CoV-2 spike protein binds to bacterial lipopolysaccharide and boosts proinflammatory activity. *J Mol Cell Biol.* 2020;**12**(12):916–932.

109. Ouyang W, Xie T, Fang H, et al. Variable Induction of Pro-Inflammatory Cytokines by Commercial SARS CoV-2 Spike Protein Reagents: Potential Impacts of LPS on In Vitro Modeling and Pathogenic Mechanisms In Vivo. *Int J Mol Sci.* 2021;**22**(14):7549.

110. McIlwaine C, Strachan A, Harrington Z, et al. Comparative analysis of total salivary lipopolysaccharide chemical and biological properties with periodontal status. *Arch Oral Biol.* 2020;**110**:104633.

111. Lim ZJ, Subramaniam A, Ponnapa Reddy M, et al. Case Fatality Rates for Patients with COVID-19 Requiring Invasive Mechanical Ventilation. A Meta-analysis. *Am J Respir Crit Care Med.* 2021;**203**(1):54–66.

112. Bahrani-Mougeot FK, Paster BJ, Coleman S, et al. Molecular analysis of oral and respiratory bacterial species associated with ventilator-associated pneumonia. *J Clin Microbiol.* 2007;**45**(5):1588–1593.

113. Wu Y, Cheng X, Jiang G, et al. Altered oral and gut microbiota and its association with SARS-CoV-2 viral load in COVID-19 patients during hospitalization. *NPJ Biofilms Microbiomes.* 2021;**7**(1):61.

114. Iebba V, Zanotta N, Campisciano G, et al. Profiling of oral microbiota and cytokines in COVID-19 patients. *bioRxiv.* 2020:2020.12.13.422589.

115. Ma S, Zhang F, Zhou F, et al. Metagenomic analysis reveals oropharyngeal microbiota alterations in patients with COVID-19. *Signal Transduct Target Ther.* 2021;**6**(1):191.

116. Cattaneo C, Riso P, Laureati M, et al. Exploring Associations between Interindividual Differences in Taste Perception, Oral Microbiota Composition, and Reported Food Intake. *Nutrients.* 2019;**11**(5):1167.

117. Tsujimoto Y, Terada J, Kimura M, et al. Diagnostic accuracy of nasopharyngeal swab, nasal swab and saliva swab samples for the detection of SARS-CoV-2 using RT-PCR. *Infect Dis (Lond).* 2021;**53**(8):581–589.

118. Carter LJ, Garner LV, Smoot JW, et al. Assay Techniques and Test Development for COVID-19 Diagnosis. *ACS Cent Sci.* 2020;**6**(5):591–605.

119. Butler-Laporte G, Lawandi A, Schiller I, et al. Comparison of Saliva and Nasopharyngeal Swab Nucleic Acid Amplification Testing for Detection of SARS-CoV-2: A Systematic Review and Meta-analysis. *JAMA Intern Med.* 2021;**181**(3):353–360.

120. Khiabani K, Amirzade-Iranaq MH. Are saliva and deep throat sputum as reliable as common respiratory specimens for SARS-CoV-2 detection? A systematic review and meta-analysis. *Am J Infect Control.* 2021;**49**(9):1165–1176.

121. Wyllie AL, Fournier J, Casanovas-Massana A, et al. Saliva or Nasopharyngeal Swab Specimens for Detection of SARS-CoV-2. *N Engl J Med.* 2020;**383**(13):1283–1286.

122. Bwire GM, Majigo MV, Njiro BJ, Mawazo A. Detection profile of SARS-CoV-2 using RT-PCR in different types of clinical specimens: A systematic review and meta-analysis. *J Med Virol.* 2021;**93**(2):719–725.

123. de Paula Eduardo F, Bezinelli LM, Rodrigues de Araujo CA, et al. Self-collected unstimulated saliva, oral swab, and nasopharyngeal swab specimens in the detection of SARS-CoV-2. *Clin Oral Investig.* 2022;26920:1561–1567.

124. Mishra C, Meena S, Meena JK, et al. Detection of three pandemic causing coronaviruses from non-respiratory samples: systematic review and meta-analysis. *Sci Rep.* 2021;**11**(1):16131.

125. Tsang NNY, So HC, Ng KY, et al. Diagnostic performance of different sampling approaches for SARS-CoV-2 RT-PCR testing: a systematic review and meta-analysis. *Lancet Infect Dis.* 2021;**21**(9):1233–1245.

126. Wang WK, Chen SY, Liu I-J, et al. Detection of SARS-associated coronavirus in throat wash and saliva in early diagnosis. *Emerg Infect Dis.* 2004;**10**(7):1213–1219.

127. To KK, Tsang O T-Y, Yip C C-Y, et al. Consistent detection of 2019 novel coronavirus in saliva. *Clin Infect Dis.* 2020;**71**(15):841–843.

128. To KK, Tsang O T-Y, Leung W-S, et al. Temporal profiles of viral load in posterior oropharyngeal saliva samples and serum antibody responses during infection by SARS-CoV-2: an observational cohort study. *Lancet Infect Dis.* 2020;**20**(5):565–574.

129. Ota K, Yanagihara K, Sasaki D, et al. Detection of SARS-CoV-2 using qRT-PCR in saliva obtained from asymptomatic or mild COVID-19 patients, comparative analysis with matched nasopharyngeal samples. *PLoS One.* 2021;**16**(6):e0252964.

130. Ott IM, Strine MS, Watkins AE, et al. Stability of SARS-CoV-2 RNA in Nonsupplemented Saliva. *Emerg Infect Dis.* 2021;**27**(4):1146–1150.

131. Ding S, Liang TJ. Is SARS-CoV-2 Also an Enteric Pathogen With Potential Fecal-Oral Transmission? A COVID-19 Virological and Clinical Review. *Gastroenterology.* 2020;**159**(1):53–61.

132. Guo M, Tao W, Flavell RA, Zhu S. Potential intestinal infection and faecal-oral transmission of SARS-CoV-2. *Nat Rev Gastroenterol Hepatol.* 2021;**18**(4):269–283.

133. Bastos ML, Perlman-Arrow S, Menzies D, Campbell JR, et al. The Sensitivity and Costs of Testing for SARS-CoV-2 Infection With Saliva Versus Nasopharyngeal Swabs : A Systematic Review and Meta-analysis. *Ann Intern Med.* 2021;**174**(4):501–510.

134. Lee RA, Herigon JC, Benedetti A, et al. Performance of Saliva, Oropharyngeal Swabs, and Nasal Swabs for SARS-CoV-2 Molecular Detection: a Systematic Review and Meta-analysis. *J Clin Microbiol.* 2021;**59**(5) e02881-20.

135. Yokota I, Sakaurazawa T, Sugita J, et al. Performance of Qualitative and Quantitative Antigen Tests for SARS-CoV-2 Using Saliva. *Infect Dis Rep.* 2021;**13**(3):742–747.

136. Bidkar V, Mishra M, Gade N, Selvaraj K. Conventional Naso-Oropharyngeal Sampling Versus Self-Collected Saliva Samples in COVID-19 Testing. *Indian J Otolaryngol Head Neck Surg.* 2021:1–7.

137. Braz-Silva PH, Mamana AC, Romano CM, et al. Performance of at-home self-collected saliva and nasal-oropharyngeal swabs in the surveillance of COVID-19. *J Oral Microbiol.* 2020;**13**(1):1858002.

138. Ku CW, Shivani D, Kwan JQT, et al. Validation of self-collected buccal swab and saliva as a diagnostic tool for COVID-19. *Int J Infect Dis.* 2021;**104**:255–261.

139. Nagura-Ikeda M, Imai K, Tabada S, et al. Clinical Evaluation of Self-Collected Saliva by Quantitative Reverse Transcription-PCR (RT-qPCR), Direct RT-qPCR, Reverse Transcription-Loop-Mediated Isothermal Amplification, and a Rapid Antigen Test To Diagnose COVID-19. *J Clin Microbiol.* 2020;**58**(9) e01438-20.

140. Silva J, Lucas C, Sundaram M, et al. Saliva viral load is a dynamic unifying correlate of COVID-19 severity and mortality. *medRxiv.* 2021:01.04.2124923.

141. Osman IO, Melenotte C, al. Broqui Pet. Expression of ACE2, Soluble ACE2, Angiotensin I, Angiotensin II and Angiotensin-(1-7) Is Modulated in COVID-19 Patients. *Front Immunol.* 2021;**12**:625732.

142. Kutti-Sridharan G, Vegunta R, Vegunta R, et al. SARS-CoV2 in Different Body Fluids, Risks of Transmission, and Preventing COVID-19: A Comprehensive Evidence-Based Review. *Int J Prev Med.* 2020;**11**:97.

143. Liu Y, Ning Z, Chen Y, et al. Aerodynamic analysis of SARS-CoV-2 in two Wuhan hospitals. *Nature.* 2020;**582**(7813):557–560.

144. Peng X, Xu X, Li Y, et al. Transmission routes of 2019-nCoV and controls in dental practice. *Int J Oral Sci.* 2020;**12**(1):9.

145. Harrel SK, Molinari J. Aerosols and splatter in dentistry: a brief review of the literature and infection control implications. *J Am Dent Assoc.* 2004;**135**(4):429–437.

146. Innes N, Johnson IG, Al-Yaseen W, et al. A systematic review of droplet and aerosol generation in dentistry. *J Dent.* 2021;**105**:103556.

147. van Doremalen N, Bushmaker T, Morris DH, et al. Aerosol and Surface Stability of SARS-CoV-2 as Compared with SARS-CoV-1. *N Engl J Med.* 2020;**382**(16):1564–1567.

148. Williams E, Bond K, Zhang B, et al. Saliva as a Noninvasive Specimen for Detection of SARS-CoV-2. *J Clin Microbiol.* 2020;**58**(8) e00776-20.

149. Janardhanam SB, Zunt SL, Srinivasan M. Quality assessment of saliva bank samples. *Biopreserv Biobank.* 2012;**10**(3):282–287.

150. Srinivasan M, Blackburn C, Mohamed M, et al. Literature-based discovery of salivary biomarkers for type 2 diabetes mellitus. *Biomark Insights.* 2015;**10**:39–45.

151. Kermali M, Khalsa RK, Pillai K, et al. The role of biomarkers in diagnosis of COVID-19 - A systematic review. *Life Sci.* 2020;**254**:117788.

152. Samprathi M, Jayashree M. Biomarkers in COVID-19: An Up-To-Date Review. *Front Pediatr.* 2020;**8**;607647.

153. Moutchia J, Pokharel P, Kerri A, et al. Clinical laboratory parameters associated with severe or critical novel coronavirus disease 2019 (COVID-19): A systematic review and meta-analysis. *PLoS One.* 2020;**15**(10):e0239802.

154. Zhan H, Chen H, Liu C, et al. Diagnostic Value of D-Dimer in COVID-19: A Meta-Analysis and Meta-Regression. *Clin Appl Thromb Hemost.* 2021;**27**:10760296211010976.

155. Katsani KR, Sakellari D. Saliva proteomics updates in biomedicine. *J Biol Res (Thessalon).* 2019;**26**:17.

156. Lee YH, Zhou H, Reiss JK, et al. Direct saliva transcriptome analysis. *Clin Chem.* 2011;**57**(9):1295–1302.

157. Fernandez-Ruiz I. ACE2 level as a marker of CVD. *Nat Rev Cardiol.* 2020;**17**(12):759.

158. Sama IE, Voors AA. Circulating plasma angiotensin-converting enzyme 2 concentration is elevated in patients with kidney disease and diabetes. *Eur Heart J.* 2020;**41**(32):3099.

159. García-Ayllón MS, Moreno-Pérez O, García-Arriaza J, et al. Plasma ACE2 species are differentially altered in COVID-19 patients. *FASEB J.* 2021;**35**(8):e21745.

160. Kragstrup TW, Søgaard Singh H, Grundberg I, et al. Plasma ACE2 predicts outcome of COVID-19 in hospitalized patients. *PLoS One.* 2021;**16**(6):e0252799.

161. Wallentin L, Lindbäck J, Eriksson N, et al. Angiotensin-converting enzyme 2 (ACE2) levels in relation to risk factors for COVID-19 in two large cohorts of patients with atrial fibrillation. *Eur Heart J.* 2020;41(41):4037–4046.

162. Patel SK, Juno JA, Lee, et al. Plasma ACE2 activity is persistently elevated following SARS-CoV-2 infection: implications for COVID-19 pathogenesis and consequences. *Eur Respir J.* 2021;57(5):2003730.

163. Yeung ML, Teng JLL, Jia L, et al. Soluble ACE2-mediated cell entry of SARS-CoV-2 via interaction with proteins related to the renin-angiotensin system. *Cell.* 2021;184(8):2212–2228 e12.

164. Lundström A, Ziegler L, Havervall S, et al. Soluble angiotensin-converting enzyme 2 is transiently elevated in COVID-19 and correlates with specific inflammatory and endothelial markers. *J Med Virol.* 2021;93(10):5908–5916.

165. Ermel A, Thyvalikakath TP, Foroud T, et al. Can salivary innate immune molecules provide clue on taste dysfunction in COVID-19?. *Front Cell Infect Microbiol.* 2021;12:727430.

166. Gu S, Chen Y, Wu Z, et al. Alterations of the Gut Microbiota in Patients With Coronavirus Disease 2019 or H1N1 Influenza. *Clin Infect Dis.* 2020;71(10):2669–2678.

167. Eghbali Zarch R, Hosseinzadeh P. COVID-19 from the perspective of dentists: A case report and brief review of more than 170 cases. *Dermatol Ther.* 2021;34(1):e14717.

168. Santarpia JL, Rivera DN, Herrera V, et al. Aerosol and surface contamination of SARS-CoV-2 observed in quarantine and isolation care. *Sci Rep.* 2020;10(1):12732.

169. Azuma K, Yanagi U, Kagi N, et al. Environmental factors involved in SARS-CoV-2 transmission: effect and role of indoor environmental quality in the strategy for COVID-19 infection control. *Environ Health Prev Med.* 2020;25(1):66.

170. Kampf G, Todt D, Pfaender S, Steinmann E. Persistence of coronaviruses on inanimate surfaces and their inactivation with biocidal agents. *J Hosp Infect.* 2020;104(3):246–251.

171. Geller C, Varbanov M, Duval RE. Human coronaviruses: insights into environmental resistance and its influence on the development of new antiseptic strategies. *Viruses.* 2012;4(11):3044–3068.

Gastrointestinal Manifestations of COVID-19

Pooja Lal, MD, Dhyanesh A. Patel, MD, and Michael F. Vaezi, MD, PhD

Prevalence of Gastrointestinal Symptoms

The first reported case of severe acute respiratory syndrome coronavirus 2 (SARS-CoV-2) in the United States presented on January 19, 2020 with symptoms of cough and nausea and vomiting and diarrhea developed on day 2 of admission. Although the serum remained negative, both the stool and respiratory specimens tested positive by real-time reverse transcriptase polymerase chain reaction (rRT-PCR) for SARS-CoV-2.[1] Multiple studies have since been published reporting gastrointestinal (GI) manifestations of coronavirus disease 2019 (COVID-19).[2-7] The most common symptoms reported in the literature include diarrhea, nausea, vomiting, abdominal pain, anorexia, and dysgeusia/ageusia.[8-21] In a study by Han et al.,[22] 67 patients had diarrhea as their first symptom of COVID-19 infection and patients with enteric symptoms presented significantly later than those who had respiratory symptoms. More recently, gustatory dysfunction has been described in patients presenting with dysgeusia.[23] In a recent meta-analysis of 25,252 patients with COVID-19, 20.3% presented with GI symptoms and 26.7% had confirmed fecal viral shedding with positive fecal RNA RT-PCR test (Fig. 9.1).[6] Interestingly, SARS-CoV-2 virus has been shown to persist in stool samples even after respiratory tract specimens were found to be negative, which might suggest prolonged shedding.[24] However, it is important to acknowledge that GI symptoms have always been prevalent in patients with respiratory viral illnesses. In the 2009 H1N1 (swine flu) pandemic, pooled prevalence of GI symptoms was even higher compared with COVID-19 at 31% with confirmed fecal shedding in 20.6% (see Fig. 9.1).[25]

Implications of Gastrointestinal Symptoms in COVID-19

Few studies have suggested that the presence of GI symptoms is associated with worse outcomes in COVID-19 patients. Patients with primarily GI symptoms of COVID-19 have longer duration from illness onset to hospital admission.[26] They are also more likely to have fever (62.4%), have delayed virus clearance, and more likely to have a virus shedding in the stool.[22] A study by Jin et al.[27] compared complications of acute respiratory distress syndrome (ARDS), liver injury, and shock in COVID-19 patients with and without GI symptoms and found significantly higher percentages of ARDS (6.8% vs. 2.9%) and liver injury (17.6% vs. 8.9%) in those with GI symptoms (Fig. 9.2). They also reported a significantly higher number of patients who required mechanical ventilation and intensive care unit admission in patients with GI symptoms. In another multicenter study, patients without GI symptoms were more likely to be discharged early compared with patients

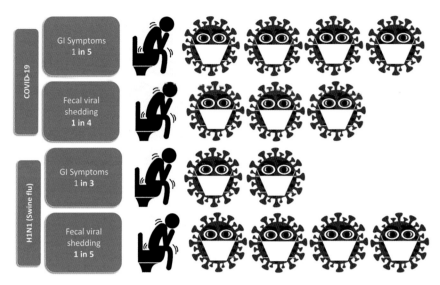

Fig. 9.1 Overall Prevalence of Gastrointestinal *(GI)* Symptoms and Fecal Viral Shedding in COVID-19 and H1N1 (Swine Flu).

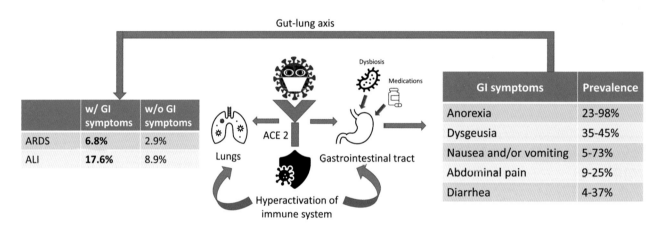

Fig. 9.2 Proposed Mechanism of How SARS-CoV-2 Affects Lung and Gastrointestinal (GI) Tract Through Angiotensin-Converting Enzyme-2 (ACE2) Receptor. Dysbiosis of the microbiome and acid suppressive medications might affect susceptibility of the gut and hyperactivation of the immune system. Patients with GI symptoms are at higher risk for acute respiratory distress syndrome (ARDS) and acute lung injury (ALI).

with GI symptoms (60% vs. 34%).[28] Hence, presence of GI symptoms in patients with COVID-19 might be a predictor for worse clinical outcomes.

Mechanism on How SARS-CoV-2 Affects Gut Health

Angiotensin-Converting Enzyme-2 Receptor Mechanism

SARS-CoV-2 has characteristic transmembrane trimeric proteins that enable the binding and fusion of the viral particle to the cellular membrane of the host cell. The virus enters the host cell by attaching to the angiotensin-converting enzyme-2 (ACE2) receptors, which have a high affinity for the spike (S) protein of the virus.[29] These ACE2 receptors are expressed in pulmonary, esophageal, small intestinal, and colonic epithelial cells.[30] GI manifestations of COVID-19 can be explained by the high expression of ACE2 receptors in the gut and extensive infection of the enterocytes.[31] After cell entry, virus-specific RNA and proteins are generated in the host cytoplasm to generate new virions, which are then released into the GI tract.[32] This explains the persistence of viral RNA in stool samples of infected patients.

Another mechanism by which COVID-19 can cause significant damage to the host is the cytokine storm, a hyperactivation of the immune system to evoke a substantial inflammatory response. T-helper cytokines, both Th1- and Th2-type responses, cause changes in contractility of inflamed intestinal smooth muscle.[33] Th1-type cytokines downregulate L-type Ca^{2+} channels and upregulate G protein signaling, which contributes to hypocontractility of inflamed intestinal smooth muscle. Conversely, Th2-type cytokines cause hypercontractilty by signal transducer and activator of transcription (STAT) 6 or mitogen-activated protein (MAP) kinase signaling pathways.[33] A cytokine profile characterized by increased interleukin-2 (IL-2), IL-7, granulocyte-colony stimulating factor, interferon-gamma (IFN-γ) inducible protein 10, monocyte chemoattractant protein 1, macrophage inflammatory protein 1-α, and tumor necrosis factor-alpha (TNF-α) has been associated with COVID-19 disease severity.[34] One study from Wuhan, China reported a significant association between elevated inflammatory markers and poor COVID-19 outcomes suggesting hyperinflammation as the main cause of decompensation.[35] For example, mean ferritin serum/plasma levels in nonsurvivors were 1297.6 ng/mL versus 614.0 ng/mL in survivors ($P < .001$) and mean IL-6 serum/plasma levels were 11.4 ng/mL in patients who did not survive versus 6.8 ng/mL in those who did ($P < .0001$).[35] IL-6 activation and secretion by infected cells causes hyperactivation of the innate immune system and increased vascular permeability as a result of activation of vascular endothelial growth factor (VEGF), which in turn causes shock and ARDS.[36] Tocilizumab, a humanized monoclonal antibody binding the IL-6 receptor (IL-6R), can effectively block IL-6 signal transduction in patients with severe COVID-19.[37] A meta-analysis of 2112 patients enrolled in the tocilizumab group and 6160 patients in the standard of care group found that tocilizumab use was associated with decreased all-cause mortality in patients with signs of hyperinflammation with C-reactive protein (CRP) levels of 100 mg/L or greater, but also with a longer hospital stay when CRP levels were less than 100 mg/L.[38]

Impact of SARS-CoV-2 on Gut Microbiota

Increasing evidence of viral RNA detection in stool samples of infected patients underscores the importance of fecal-oral transmission of SARS-CoV-2. Multiple investigators have reported the presence of ribonucleotides of SARS-CoV-2 in the feces of up to 50% of infected patients.[39–41] Furthermore, SARS-CoV-2 RNA has been found in specimens from the esophagus, stomach, duodenum, and rectum.[19]

The gut microbiota plays an important role in the GI tract and is responsible for a variety of physiological processes, including protection against infections, regulation of the immune system, and metabolism. A balance in the diversity of gut flora is critical to performing these functions. Interestingly, studies have shown a significantly decreased bacterial diversity in gut flora, increased proportions of opportunistic infections, and a relative low abundance of beneficial symbionts in patients infected with COVID-19 compared with healthy controls.[42] Some have suggested administration of probiotics or consideration of fecal microbiota

transplantation (FMT) to improve the microbial dysbiosis in patients with COVID-19, but efficacy is unclear and these treatments have not been rigorously studied.[43,44]

Gut microbiota might also modulate pulmonary immunity through effects on lung microbiota. Gut dysbiosis has been associated with functional disability of alveolar macrophages to perform necessary function, including reduction in reactive oxygen species–mediated killing of bacteria.[45] This association has been termed "gut-lung axis" and is reportedly bidirectional, where not only the microbial components such as endotoxins from the gut can change pulmonary immunity but lung infections also have a clinically significant impact on gut microbiota.[46] To further prove this connection, studies have shown a link between gut dysbiosis and respiratory infections. Gut dysbiosis has been linked to increased risk for respiratory infections, but has also been shown to play a key role in the pathogenesis of sepsis, ARDS, and multiorgan failure in a culture-independent manner.[47,48] This association can be explained by the phenomenon of the leaky gut.

An intact intestinal barrier prevents bacterial translocation of gut flora and its metabolic components into the bloodstream and other organs. This protective barrier is dysregulated by unfavorable changes in the gut microbiota. Furthermore, gut dysbiosis also causes decreased production of bacteria-derived short-chain fatty acids such as butyric acid and acetic acid, which are vital in regulating the immune and inflammatory responses.[49] This dysregulation facilitates the translocation of immunogenic bacterial components, including toxins and lipopolysaccharides, leading to uncontrolled immune activation and inflammation.[50] Toll-like receptor 4 (TLR4) activation has been shown to play a pivotal role in this immune system activation. Dysregulated TLR4 activation is involved in acute systemic sepsis, in chronic inflammatory diseases, and in viral infections, such as influenza infection.[51] Fig. 9.2 shows the proposed mechanism of how SARS-CoV-2 affects the lung and GI tract.

Impact of Gastric Acid Reduction on COVID-19 Outcomes

Proton Pump Inhibitors

Proton pump inhibitors (PPIs) are one of the most prescribed group of drugs for the treatment of various gastric acid–associated disorders. Although the impact of acid suppression on COVID-19 is unclear, theoretically, less acidic pH achieved with PPI therapy might not inactivate the virus.[52] Furthermore, SARS-CoV-2 uses ACE2 receptor as the primary target to enter the host cell. These receptors are expressed by the glandular cells of the GI tract, mainly in the stomach, duodenum, and rectum.[42] Activity of ACE2 also varies with pH and temperature. A pH of 7.5 seems optimal for its functioning.[53] Because PPIs decrease acid production, they can theoretically increase binding of the virus to enterocytes and increase GI tract inoculation.

Clinical studies done on the effect of PPIs on COVID-19 have revealed controversial results. One survey-based study enrolled 53,130 participants and revealed that individuals taking PPIs once or twice daily had significantly higher odds of reporting a positive COVID-19 test compared with individuals who did not take PPIs.[54] On the other hand, individuals taking histamine-2 receptor antagonists were not found to have an increased risk. This study was heavily criticized because of numerous methodological inconsistencies with concerns for selection bias and lack of ability to verify the responses in an online survey study. In addition, the number of participants tested for COVID-19 was not mentioned in the study, neither in the overall cohort nor in individual groups.[55,56] This raises the possibility of a bias resulting from a disproportionately higher number of people in the PPI cohort having been tested for COVID-19. The demographics of the COVID-19–positive group were also significantly different compared with those of the overall study participants. Patients in the PPI group were younger, and the study did not control of comorbid conditions.[57]

On the other hand, a Korean nationwide cohort study reported that PPI use did not increase susceptibility to COVID-19 infection, but patients currently taking PPIs had 79% greater risk for severe clinical outcomes.[58] More recently, a secondary analysis of a retrospective cohort study aiming to better characterize digestive manifestations in patients hospitalized with COVID-19 across 36 medical centers in North America found that after adjusting for measured baseline confounders, PPI use was not independently associated with the need for mechanical ventilation (odds ratio [OR], 1.02 [0.73–1.43]).[59] Hence, because of conflicting evidence and unclear clear association between PPI and COVID-19 outcomes, these medications, when used for appropriate proven indication, should be continued in the lowest effective dose.

Histamine Receptor Antagonists (H₂-Blockers)

Histamine and its role in diverse pathophysiological processes have been studied widely in the field of medicine.[60] It is found in a variety of cells and tissues, predominantly in mast cells and basophils. It is stored in cytoplasmic granules and is a part of the cascade of inflammatory markers released in response to immune or nonimmune stimuli, including viral infections.[61,62] Histamine performs multiple physiological functions by activating four types of G protein–coupled receptors, designated as H_1 to H_4.[60] These receptors have been

linked to various immune reactions, gastric acid secretion, and allergic reactions. This led to the development of histamine-2 receptor antagonists (H_2RAs) to treat various allergies and GI disorders.[60] COVID-19 has been associated with mast cell activation, causing histamine release in the early phase of inflammation, and late activation provoked the generation of proinflammatory IL-1 family members, including IL-1, IL-6, and IL-33.[63] Several studies have explored the antiinflammatory properties of antihistamines as a protective mechanism against hyperinflammation related to COVID-19.

Freedberg et al.[64] retrospectively studied 1620 patients admitted with COVID-19. Of those, 84 (5.1%) received famotidine within 24 hours of admission to hospital. The group taking famotidine had a reduced risk for clinical deterioration leading to intubation or death. This was an observational study with limited relevant prior data. Another retrospective, observational study demonstrated improved clinical outcomes, including lower in-hospital mortality, a lower composite of death and/or intubation, and lower levels of serum markers for serious disease in the famotidine group compared with nonusers.[65] In contrast, a territory-wide retrospective cohort study in all patients with COVID-19 from Hong Kong investigated the association between famotidine use and severity of COVID-19. They did not find any statistically significant correlation between famotidine and COVID-19 severity.[66] However, more recently a secondary analysis of a cohort involving more than 1800 patients across 36 medical centers in North America found that H_2RA use was actually associated with 1.5 higher odds of requiring mechanical ventilation relative to patients not exposed to H_2RA (confidence interval [CI], 1.11–2.19).[59] This finding persisted after both propensity scores matched analysis and sensitivity analyses and also showed an association between H_2RA exposure and higher in-hospital mortality (OR, 1.48; 95% CI, 1.04–2.12). It is important to recognize that studies showed a favorable effect of famotidine treatment during active disease, rather than preadmission exposure. The latter showed potential deleterious effects. Given these discrepancies, caution should be used regarding medications aimed at acid secretion in patients with COVID-19.

Impact of COVID-19 in Inflammatory Bowel Disease

Inflammatory bowel disease (IBD) is a chronic inflammatory disease of the GI tract. There is contradictory evidence regarding the impact on COVID-19 on patients with IBD. According to a study from northern California and the SECURE-IBD registry from France and Italy, IBD patients did not have a higher rates of SARS-CoV-2 positivity than that of the general population, despite 37% of the cohort receiving immunosuppressants and/or biologicals that may affect virus susceptibility.[67,68] In fact, data from China through the IBD Elite Union, which covers the seven largest IBD referral centers in China, indicated that patients with IBD had a decreased risk for severe COVID-19 compared with that of the general population.[69] The risk for COVID-19–associated mortality in IBD patients also has been found to be lower compared with that of the general population, with diarrhea being the only prominent symptom of active infection in some patients.[70] The relative risk for acquisition of COVID-19 was not different between ulcerative colitis (UC) and Crohn's disease (CD), but patients with UC might have higher rates of hospitalization (27.3% vs. 5.3%).[71]

Pathogenesis of COVID-19 in Inflammatory Bowel Disease

The pathogenesis of COVID-19 in IBD patients is complex and multifactorial, including altered immune responses, microbial dysbiosis, environmental stimulants, and malnutrition,[72] leading to dysregulated inflammatory cascades. Patients with active IBD generally present with symptoms of abdominal pain, nausea, vomiting, low appetite, and diarrhea, which overlap with the GI symptoms of COVID-19 infection, making it a diagnostic challenge. Moreover, inflammatory processes in IBD cause damaged mucosal barriers leading to increased permeability, adhesion, and translocation of intestinal microorganisms, dysregulated immune response, and release of proinflammatory cytokines. This allows the virus to enter the lamina propria through increased mucosal permeability, which results in an aggravated immune response. This immune response causes excessive release of cytokines, resulting in cytokine storm.[72]

Cytokines, such as IFN-γ, which are upregulated in IBD, have also been shown to induce ACE2 receptor expression.[73] SARS-CoV-2 relies on these ACE2 receptors for entry into the cytoplasm, and hence blocking the expression of these receptors can theoretically reduce the infectious burden by blocking cellular entry. Moreover, other proinflammatory cytokines such as TNF-α and IL-6 are upregulated in both IBD and COVID-19, and hence antiinflammatory therapies used in IBD can theoretically reduce the severity of COVID-19 by decreasing the risk for a cytokine release "storm." As a result, COVID-19 may have a milder course in patients with IBD.[74]

Impact of Inflammatory Bowel Disease Therapy on COVID-19 Outcomes

The most widely used IBD therapies include glucocorticoids, biologicals, or novel small molecule inhibitors to control intestinal inflammation. Corticosteroids have been shown to increase the risk for poor outcome for SARS,[75] Middle Eastern respiratory syndrome (MERS),[76] and influenza.[77] These patients were more likely to require mechanical ventilation, vasopressors, and renal replacement therapy.[76] In a study of 525 cases from 33 countries, risk factors for severe COVID-19 among patients with IBD included increasing age (adjusted OR [aOR], 1.04; 95% CI, 1.01–1.02), two or more comorbidities (aOR, 2.9; 95% CI, 1.1–7.8), systemic corticosteroids (aOR 6.9; 95% CI, 2.3–20.5), and sulfasalazine or 5-aminosalicylate use (aOR, 3.1; 95% CI, 1.3–7.7).[78] Due to the possible risk for worse clinical outcomes, the World Health Organization (WHO) recommends against the use of steroids in patients with IBD who are actively infected with COVID-19.[79] Patients with IBD should taper steroids to the lowest possible dose tolerated and discontinue it completely whenever possible. Locally acting steroids, such as budesonide and beclomethasone, have low systemic availability and are associated with significantly fewer side effects when compared with systemic steroids.[80–82]

Contrary to steroids in IBD, TNF antagonist (anti-TNF) treatment was not associated with severe COVID-19 (aOR, 0.9; 95% CI, 0.4–2.2) and even may be protective.[78] Similarly, a nationwide veterans administration cohort study of 37,857 patients with IBD found that neither immunomodulators (OR, 0.9; 95% CI, 0.23–4.03) nor anti-TNF (OR, 0.58; 95% CI, 0.17–1.9) was associated with an increased risk for severe COVID-19.[83] However, combination therapy of steroids and thiopurines with anti-TNF medications might increase risk for severe COVID-19.[84]

In the absence of robust data, reasonable strategies to minimize the burden of COVID-19 infection in the IBD population include early and careful detection of active infection in patients, restricting the use of corticosteroids, treatment with monotherapy, and continuity of care.[85] Fig. 9.3 shows the impact of COVID-19 in IBD.

Impact of Irritable Bowel Disease Therapies on COVID-19 Antibodies

Development of vaccination against COVID-19 has been a fundamental step to suppress viral transmission. Some medications, such as anti-TNF drugs are known to suppress protective immunity after vaccinations, such as pneumococcal,[86] influenza,[87] and hepatitis B.[88] A study by Kennedy et al.[89] showed that infliximab therapy was associated with impaired serological responses to SARS-CoV-2 infection. This impairment was more pronounced in patients who were treated with a combination therapy with infliximab and an immunomodulator. In contrast, another study assessing serological response to mRNA COVID-19 vaccines in patients with IBD found adequate antibody titers.[90] Based on this, expert

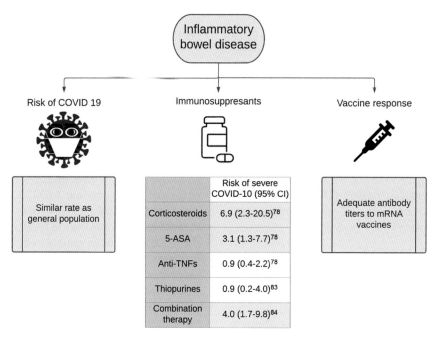

Fig. 9.3 Impact of COVID-19 in Inflammatory Bowel Disease Including Risk of Disease, Effect of Different Immunosuppressants, and Vaccine Response in This Population.

consensus advocates that patients with IBD should be vaccinated against SARS-COV-2.[91]

Impact of COVID-19 on Liver

Pathophysiology

Similar to intestinal mucosa, SARS-CoV-2 attaches itself to the liver target cell by interactions between the spike glycoprotein (S) and its receptor ACE2. After the initial attachment, SARS-CoV-2 undergoes processing by a plasma membrane–associated type II transmembrane serine protease (TMPRSS2) and is finally released into the host cell cytoplasm.[92] Liver organoids were found to have a dramatic increase of viral load at 24 hours after infection, which suggests that human liver ductal organoids are susceptible to SARS-CoV-2 and support robust viral replication.[93] SARS-CoV-2 also impairs the barrier and bile acid transporting functions of cholangiocytes through the dysregulation of genes involved in tight junction formation and bile acid transportation. Therefore it has been suggested that the liver damage in COVID-19 patients might be the result of direct cholangiocyte injury and consequent bile acid accumulation caused by SARS-CoV-2 infection.[93] Contradictory to that, postmortem liver biopsy in patients who died from COVID-19 showed only microvesicular steatosis, accompanied by hyperactivation of T cells, suggesting that liver injury is likely immune mediated rather than direct cytopathic damage.[94] It is postulated that the hepatocellular injury could be a result of nonviral damage, but the inability of liver parenchyma to regenerate by

cholangiocyte precursor cells might impair liver repair, leading to further deterioration of liver function.[94] The COVID-19–associated cytokine storm could also potentially cause direct hepatotoxicity by uncontrolled immune response against the hepatocytes. Significant elevation of proinflammatory markers, including CRP, serum ferritin, lactate dehydrogenase, IL-6, and IL-2 in patients with COVID-19, and liver injury supports this hypothesis.[94]

COVID-19 and Chronic Liver Disease

There is a paucity of data on the effects of CLD in patients with COVID-19. A study by Mantovani et al.[95] revealed that individuals with COVID-19 had significant liver enzyme elevations and coagulopathy, which is likely a result of the immune response to the virus. The presence of CLD did not alter the course of COVID-19 compared with patients without CLD. Similarly, Lippi et al.[96] showed that presence of CLD did not affect the severity or mortality related to COVID-19 infection. However, other studies have shown higher mortality in patients with cirrhosis with a relative risk of 4.6 compared with 3.0 in patients with no underlying liver disease. These patients were also found to have increased risk for hospitalization compared with patients without CLD. Another study evaluated 103 patients with cirrhosis and 49 with noncirrhotic CLD and found that deaths occurred in 12.2% of CLD without cirrhosis, 24% with Child-Turcotte-Pugh (CTP)-A cirrhosis, 43% with CTP-B cirrhosis, and 63.0% with CTP-C cirrhosis.[97] The cause of death included lung, cardiac, and liver disease related to COVID-19. A multicenter study by Bajaj et al.[98] compared outcomes of patients with liver cirrhosis plus COVID-19 compared age- and sex-matched patients with COVID-19 alone and cirrhosis alone. This study concluded that cirrhosis plus COVID-19 had mortality similar to that of patients with cirrhosis alone but higher mortality than patients with only COVID-19. Finally, a model of end-stage liver disease (MELD) score from the European Foundation for the Study of Chronic Liver Failure, Organ Failure, and Cirrhosis (CLIF-OF and CLIF-C) has been shown to predict mortality in cirrhotic patients with COVID-19.[99]

Similar to data for CLD, data are very limited on the effect of COVID-19 in patients with alcoholic liver disease or alcoholic hepatitis. The psychosocial stressors caused by the pandemic have resulted in increased consumption of alcohol and alcohol use–related disorders throughout the world. This has resulted in increased cases and severity of alcoholic hepatitis. Patients with alcohol use disorder tend to have other comorbidities, which increase the risk for severe COVID-19.[100] Although there are no treatment guidelines for the management of alcoholic hepatitis in patients with COVID-19, it is recommended to exercise caution regarding glucocorticoids.[100] Definitive recommendations also cannot be made regarding treatment of autoimmune liver disease in patients with COVID-19; however, preliminary guidance has been published by several different societies. These guidelines recommend no change in treatment for autoimmune hepatitis in the absence of severe COVID-19, lymphopenia, or superinfections.[101–103]

There is also limited experience regarding treatment options for COVID-19 in patients with preexisting liver disease. Commonly used medications, including remdesivir, hydroxychloroquine, tocilizumab, and steroids, have not been associated with worsening liver disease.[94] Patients with a history of hepatitis B should be monitored for reactivation during active COVID-19 treatment.[104]

Impact of COVID-19 on Pancreatic Disorders

Data are limited on the association between COVID-19 and pancreatic disorders. Some case reports describe acute pancreatitis as the initial manifesting sign of COVID-19.[105,106] Inamdar et al.[107] performed a retrospective, observational study including patients 18 years old and older admitted to 12 hospitals in New York during the COVID-19 pandemic. They compared patients with acute pancreatitis and COVID-19 to a group of patients with acute pancreatitis but without COVID-19. Their findings revealed that a significantly higher number of patients with COVID-19 had an undetermined cause of pancreatitis, indicating that COVID-19 might play a causative role. They also found that

length of stay and the need for mechanical ventilation were significantly higher in the acute pancreatitis group with COVID-19 compared with patients without COVID-19. In contrast, a retrospective, multicenter study by Miró et al.[108] investigated the potential relationship between COVID-19 and five different clinical conditions, including acute pancreatitis, that could be influenced by SARS-CoV-2 infection. Their findings revealed that the prevalence of acute pancreatitis in the COVID-19 group was less than in the non–COVID-19 group (OR, 0.44 [0.33–0.60]). Given these contradictory findings, more studies are needed to define the association between pancreatic disorders and COVID-19 to formulate the treatment plan accordingly for these patients.

Association Between Angiotensin-Converting Enzyme Inhibitor and Angiotensin Receptor Blocker Use and Gastrointestinal Symptoms in COVID-19

A significant number of COVID-19 patients have associated GI symptoms or liver abnormalities. As mentioned earlier, the virus enters the host cell by attaching to ACE2 receptors. These receptors are highly expressed in the GI tract, explaining the prevalence of GI manifestations in COVID-19 infection. Interestingly, some studies have explored the effects of ACE inhibitors and angiotensin receptor blockers (ARBs) on clinical outcomes of COVID-19. A study by Zhang et al.[109] determined the association between in-hospital ACE inhibitor/ARB use and all-cause mortality in patients with hypertension who were hospitalized for COVID-19. They reported an overall lower risk for all-cause mortality in patients using ACE inhibitors/ARBs compared with nonusers. A similar study by Tan et al.[110] reported the protective effect of ACE inhibitors/ARBs on pulmonary symptoms and interestingly found that the ACE inhibitor/ARB group had a significantly lower risk for developing GI symptoms and liver function abnormalities throughout the disease course. GI symptoms such as diarrhea, nausea/vomiting and abdominal pain were more prevalent in the non–ACE inhibitors/ARB group. Theoretically, use of an ACE inhibitor or ARB can upregulate ACE2 expression, which is responsible for viral entry into the host cell. This mechanism can increase SARS-CoV-2 uptake and result in increased disease severity. Contrarily, increased ACE2 expression downregulates the renin-angiotensin system and serves as a counterbalance to ACE function.[109] In addition, increased ACE2 activity can potentially result in increased conversion of ACE2 to angiotensin, which has protective antiinflammatory properties. Despite these theoretical associations, there are no clear data regarding the net effect of ACE inhibitors/ARBs on clinical outcomes in COVID-19. Cardiovascular societies recommended continuing the use of ACE inhibitors/ARBs in patients with preexisting hypertension and COVID-19.[111]

Postinfectious Gastrointestinal Symptoms

The long-term effects of COVID-19 on various organ systems remain largely unclear. A recent study revealed that patients affected with COVID-19 had postinfectious symptoms that persisted 6-months after acute infection. The main symptoms described in this study included fatigue or muscle weakness, sleep difficulties, anxiety, depression, and impaired pulmonary diffusion capacities and abnormal chest imaging in patients who were more severely ill.[112] Given these findings, it is not unreasonable to assume that some fraction of patients might develop postinfectious GI disorders.

Clinical entities such as postinfectious irritable bowel syndrome (IBS) or functional dyspepsia have been well-defined in the literature. Postinfectious IBS (PI-IBS) resembles IBS diarrhea-type illness that has an acute onset after an episode of infectious gastroenteritis.[113] The incidence of PI-IBS varies from 4% to 36%[114] based on different studies from different regions. Similarly, the prevalence of functional dyspepsia after an episode of acute gastroenteritis ranges from 2.8% to 42.4%.[115]

To investigate the long-term GI health consequences of COVID-19, Weng et al.[116] interviewed 117 patients with COVID-19 90 days after discharge to determine the prevalence of GI symptoms that were not present within the month before onset of COVID-19. They found a that 44% of patients had GI symptoms after discharge. The most common GI sequelae were loss of appetite (24%), nausea (18%), acid reflux (18%), and diarrhea (15%). Less common symptoms included abdominal distention (14%), belching (10%), vomiting (9%), abdominal pain (7%), and bloody stools (2%). Hence, despite recovery from acute COVID-19, gastroenterologists might see a higher prevalence of postinfectious symptoms related to dyspepsia and PI-IBS. These may be long-lasting disturbances of the brain-gut axis and/or the gut microbiome.

Conclusion

Although SARS-CoV-2 is primarily a respiratory virus, it can lead to various systemic diseases involving the GI tract, including the liver and pancreaticobiliary systems. The main mechanism of entry into the cells involves ACE2 receptors, which are highly expressed in the GI tract, causing symptoms such as diarrhea, nausea, vomiting, and abdominal pain. There are also reports of acute liver and pancreatic injury in a subset of patients. Patients with IBD do not appear to be at higher risk for COVID-19 or its complications despite use of immunosuppressive therapy. The persistence of viral RNA in stool samples indicates viral replication and subsequent shedding in the GI tract. Finally, as the pandemic resolves, gastroenterologists might see higher incidence of post–COVID-19 GI symptoms in their clinic.

REFERENCES

1. Holshue ML, DeBolt C, Lindquist S, et al. First case of 2019 novel coronavirus in the United States. *N Engl J Med.* 2020;382(10):929–936. doi:10.1056/nejmoa2001191.
2. Zhang L, Han C, Zhang S, et al. Diarrhea and altered inflammatory cytokine pattern in severe coronavirus disease 2019: Impact on disease course and in-hospital mortality. *J Gastroenterol Hepatol.* 2020;36(2) 431-429. doi:10.1111/jgh.15166.
3. Zheng T, Yang C, Wang HY, et al. Clinical characteristics and outcomes of COVID-19 patients with gastrointestinal symptoms admitted to Jianghan Fangcang Shelter Hospital in Wuhan, China. *J Med Virol.* 2020;92(11):2735–2741. doi:10.1002/jmv.26146.
4. Wong SH, Lui RNS, Sung JJY. Covid-19 and the digestive system. *J Gastroenterol Hepatol.* 2020;35(5):744–748. doi:10.1111/jgh.15047.
5. Tian Y, Rong L, Nian W, He Y. Review article: gastrointestinal features in COVID-19 and the possibility of faecal transmission. *Aliment Pharmacol Ther.* 2020;51(9):843–851. doi:10.1111/apt.15731.
6. Elshazli RM, Kline A, Elgaml A, et al. Gastroenterology manifestations and COVID-19 outcomes: A meta-analysis of 25,252 cohorts among the first and second waves. *J Med Virol.* 2021;93(5):2740–2768. doi:10.1002/jmv.26836.
7. Aghemo A, Piovani D, Parigi TL, et al. COVID-19 digestive system involvement and clinical outcomes in a large academic hospital in Milan, Italy. *Clin Gastroenterol Hepatol.* 2020;18(10):2366–2368.e3. doi:10.1016/j.cgh.2020.05.011.
8. Hajifathalian K, Krisko T, Mehta A, et al. Gastrointestinal and hepatic manifestations of 2019 novel coronavirus disease in a large cohort of infected patients from New York: clinical implications. *Gastroenterology.* 2020;159(3):1137–1140.e2. doi:10.1053/j.gastro.2020.05.010.
9. Cholankeril G, Podboy A, Aivaliotis VI, et al. High prevalence of concurrent gastrointestinal manifestations in patients with severe acute respiratory syndrome coronavirus 2: early experience from California. *Gastroenterology.* 2020;159(2):775–777. doi:10.1053/j.gastro.2020.04.008.
10. Xu X, Yu C, Qu J, et al. Imaging and clinical features of patients with 2019 novel coronavirus SARS-CoV-2. *Eur J Nucl Med Mol Imaging.* 2020;47(5):1275–1280. doi:10.1007/s00259-020-04735-9.
11. Yao N, Wang SN, Lian JQ, et al. Clinical characteristics and influencing factors of patients with novel coronavirus pneumonia combined with liver injury in Shaanxi region. *Zhonghua Gan Zang Bing Za Zhi.* 2020;28(3):234–239. doi:10.3760/cma.j.cn501113-20200226-00070.
12. Kong I, Park Y, Woo Y, et al. Early epidemiological and clinical characteristics of 28 cases of coronavirus disease in South Korea. *Osong Public Heal Res Perspect.* 2020;11(1):8–14. doi:10.24171/j.phrp.2020.11.1.03.
13. Liu L, Liu W, Zheng Y, et al. A preliminary study on serological assay for severe acute respiratory syndrome coronavirus 2 (SARS-CoV-2) in 238 admitted hospital patients. *Microbes Infect.* 2020;22(4-5):206–211. doi:10.1016/j.micinf.2020.05.008.

14. Chen Q, Quan B, Li X, et al. A report of clinical diagnosis and treatment of nine cases of coronavirus disease 2019. *J Med Virol*. 2020;92(6):683–687. doi:10.1002/jmv.25755.

15. jin Zhang J, X Dong, yuan Cao Y, et al. Clinical characteristics of 140 patients infected with SARS-CoV-2 in Wuhan, China. *Allergy Eur J Allergy Clin Immunol*. 2020;75(7):1730–1741. doi:10.1111/all.14238.

16. Zhao Z, Xie J, Yin M, et al. Clinical and laboratory profiles of 75 hospitalized patients with novel coronavirus disease 2019 in Hefei, China. *medRxiv*. March 2020:2020.03.01.20029785. doi:10.1101/2020.03.01.20029785

17. Zhou F, Yu T, Du R, et al. Clinical course and risk factors for mortality of adult inpatients with COVID-19 in Wuhan, China: a retrospective cohort study. *Lancet*. 2020;395(10229):1054–1062. doi:10.1016/S0140-6736(20)30566-3.

18. Luo S, Zhang X, Xu H. Don't Overlook Digestive Symptoms in Patients With 2019 Novel Coronavirus Disease (COVID-19). *Clin Gastroenterol Hepatol*. 2020;18(7):1636–1637. doi:10.1016/j.cgh.2020.03.043.

19. Lin L, Jiang X, Zhang Z, et al. Gastrointestinal symptoms of 95 cases with SARS-CoV-2 infection. *Gut*. 2020;69(6):997–1001. doi:10.1136/gutjnl-2020-321013.

20. Yan S, Song X, Lin F, et al. Clinical characteristics of coronavirus disease 2019 in Hainan, China. *medRxiv*. March 2020:2020.03.19.20038539. doi:10.1101/2020.03.19.20038539.

21. Pung R, Chiew CJ, Young BE, et al. Investigation of three clusters of COVID-19 in Singapore: implications for surveillance and response measures. *Lancet*. 2020;395(10229):1039–1046. doi:10.1016/S0140-6736(20)30528-6.

22. Han C, Duan C, Zhang S, et al. Digestive Symptoms in COVID-19 Patients with Mild Disease Severity: Clinical Presentation, Stool Viral RNA Testing, and Outcomes. *Am J Gastroenterol*. 2020;115(6):916–923. doi:10.14309/ajg.0000000000000664.

23. Tong JY, Wong A, Zhu D, Fastenberg JH, Tham T. The Prevalence of Olfactory and Gustatory Dysfunction in COVID-19 Patients: A Systematic Review and Meta-analysis. *Otolaryngol - Head Neck Surg (United States)*. 2020;163(1):3–11. doi:10.1177/0194599820926473.

24. Parasa S, Desai M, Thoguluva Chandrasekar V, et al. Prevalence of Gastrointestinal Symptoms and Fecal Viral Shedding in Patients With Coronavirus Disease 2019: A Systematic Review and Meta-analysis. *JAMA Netw open*. 2020;3(6):e2011335. doi:10.1001/jamanetworkopen.2020.11335.

25. Minodier L, Charrel RN, Ceccaldi PE, et al. Prevalence of gastrointestinal symptoms in patients with influenza, clinical significance, and pathophysiology of human influenza viruses in faecal samples: What do we know?. *Virol J*. 2015;12(1). doi:10.1186/s12985-015-0448-4.

26. Mao R, Qiu Y, He JS, et al. Manifestations and prognosis of gastrointestinal and liver involvement in patients with COVID-19: a systematic review and meta-analysis. *Lancet Gastroenterol Hepatol*. 2020;5(7):667–678. doi:10.1016/S2468-1253(20)30126-6.

27. Jin X, Lian JS, Hu JH, et al. Epidemiological, clinical and virological characteristics of 74 cases of coronavirus-infected disease 2019 (COVID-19) with gastrointestinal symptoms. *Gut*. 2020;69(6):1002–1009. doi:10.1136/gutjnl-2020-320926.

28. Pan L, Mu M, Yang P, et al. Clinical characteristics of COVID-19 patients with digestive symptoms in Hubei, China: A descriptive, cross-sectional, multicenter study. *Am J Gastroenterol*. 2020;115(5):766–773. doi:10.14309/ajg.0000000000000620.

29. Wan Y, Shang J, Graham R, Baric RS, Li F. Receptor Recognition by the Novel Coronavirus from Wuhan: an Analysis Based on Decade-Long Structural Studies of SARS Coronavirus. *J Virol*. 2020;94(7). doi:10.1128/jvi.00127-20 e00127-20.

30. Gui M, Song W, Zhou H, et al. Cryo-electron microscopy structures of the SARS-CoV spike glycoprotein reveal a prerequisite conformational state for receptor binding. *Cell Res*. 2017;27(1):119–129. doi:10.1038/cr.2016.152.

31. Hamming I, Timens W, Bulthuis MLC, Lely AT, Navis GJ, van Goor H. Tissue distribution of ACE2 protein, the functional receptor for SARS coronavirus. A first step in understanding SARS pathogenesis. *J Pathol*. 2004;203(2):631–637. doi:10.1002/path.1570.

32. Weiss SR, Navas-Martin S. Coronavirus Pathogenesis and the Emerging Pathogen Severe Acute Respiratory Syndrome Coronavirus. *Microbiol Mol Biol Rev*. 2005;69(4):635–664. doi:10.1128/mmbr.69.4.635-664.2005.

33. Akiho H. Cytokine-induced alterations of gastrointestinal motility in gastrointestinal disorders. *World J Gastrointest Pathophysiol*. 2011;2(5):72–81. doi:10.4291/wjgp.v2.i5.72.

34. Huang C, Wang Y, Li X, et al. Clinical features of patients infected with 2019 novel coronavirus in Wuhan, China. *Lancet*. 2020;395(10223):497–506. doi:10.1016/S0140-6736(20)30183-5.

35. Ruan Q, Yang K, Wang W, Jiang L, Song J. Clinical predictors of mortality due to COVID-19 based on an analysis of data of 150 patients from Wuhan, China. *Intensive Care Med*. 2020;46(5):846–848. doi:10.1007/s00134-020-05991-x.

36. Moore JB, June CH. Cytokine release syndrome in severe COVID-19. *Science (80-)*. 2020;368(6490):473-474. doi:10.1126/science.abb8925.

37. Zhang C, Wu Z, Li JW, Zhao H, Wang GQ. Cytokine release syndrome in severe COVID-19: interleukin-6 receptor antagonist tocilizumab may be the key to reduce mortality. *Int J Antimicrob Agents*. 2020;55(5):105954. doi:10.1016/j.ijantimicag.2020.105954.

38. Nugroho CW, Suryantoro SD, Yuliasih Y, et al. Optimal use of tocilizumab for severe and critical COVID-19: A systematic review and meta-analysis. *F1000Research*. 2021;10. doi:10.12688/f1000research.45046.1.

39. Young BE, Ong SWX, Kalimuddin S, et al. Epidemiologic Features and Clinical Course of Patients Infected with SARS-CoV-2 in Singapore. *JAMA - J Am Med Assoc*. 2020;323(15):1488–1494. doi:10.1001/jama.2020.3204.

40. Effenberger M, Grabherr F, Mayr L, et al. Faecal calprotectin indicates intestinal inflammation in COVID-19. *Gut*. 2020;69(8):1543–1544. doi:10.1136/gutjnl-2020-321388.

41. Xiao F, Tang M, Zheng X, Liu Y, Li X, Shan H. Evidence for Gastrointestinal Infection of SARS-CoV-2. *Gastroenterology*. 2020;158(6):1831–1833.e3. doi:10.1053/j.gastro.2020.02.055.

42. Gu S, Chen Y, Wu Z, et al. Alterations of the gut microbiota in patients with coronavirus disease 2019 or H1N1

influenza. *Clin Infect Dis.* 2020;71(10):2669–2678. doi:10.1093/cid/ciaa709.

43. Xu K, Cai H, Shen Y, et al. Management of COVID-19: the Zhejiang experience. *Zhejiang Da Xue Xue Bao Yi Xue Ban.* 2020;49(2):147-157. doi:10.3785/j.issn.1008-9292.2020.02.02

44. Liu F, Ye S, Zhu X, et al. Gastrointestinal disturbance and effect of fecal microbiota transplantation in discharged COVID 19 patients. *J Med Case Rep.* 2021;15(1). doi:10.1186/s13256-020-02583-7.

45. Clarke TB. Early innate immunity to bacterial infection in the lung is regulated systemically by the commensal microbiota via Nod-like receptor ligands. *Infect Immun.* 2014;82(11):4596–4606. doi:10.1128/IAI.02212-14.

46. Dumas A, Bernard L, Poquet Y, Lugo-Villarino G, Neyrolles O. The role of the lung microbiota and the gut–lung axis in respiratory infectious diseases. *Cell Microbiol.* 2018;20(12):e12966. doi:10.1111/cmi.12966.

47. Dickson RP. The microbiome and critical illness. *Lancet Respir Med.* 2016;4(1):59–72. doi:10.1016/S2213-2600(15)00427-0.

48. Groves HT, Higham SL, Moffatt MF, Cox MJ, Tregoning JS. Respiratory viral infection alters the gut microbiota by inducing inappetence. *MBio.* 2020;11(1) 03236-10. doi:10.1128/mBio.03236-19.

49. Gonçalves P, Araújo JR, Di Santo JP. A cross-talk between microbiota-derived short-chain fatty acids and the host mucosal immune system regulates intestinal homeostasis and inflammatory bowel disease. *Inflamm Bowel Dis.* 2018;24(3):558–572. doi:10.1093/ibd/izx029.

50. Fernandes R, Viana SD, Nunes S, Reis F. Diabetic gut microbiota dysbiosis as an inflammaging and immunosenescence condition that fosters progression of retinopathy and nephropathy. *Biochim Biophys Acta - Mol Basis Dis.* 2019;1865(7):1876–1897. doi:10.1016/j.bbadis.2018.09.032.

51. Perrin-Cocon L, Aublin-Gex A, Sestito SE, et al. TLR4 antagonist FP7 inhibits LPS-induced cytokine production and glycolytic reprogramming in dendritic cells, and protects mice from lethal influenza infection. *Sci Rep.* 2017;7:40791. doi:10.1038/srep40791.

52. Darnell MER, Subbarao K, Feinstone SM, Taylor DR. Inactivation of the coronavirus that induces severe acute respiratory syndrome, SARS-CoV. *J Virol Methods.* 2004;121(1):85–91. doi:10.1016/j.jviromet.2004.06.006.

53. Aragão DS, Cunha TS, Arita DY, et al. Purification and characterization of angiotensin converting enzyme 2 (ACE2) from murine model of mesangial cell in culture. *Int J Biol Macromol.* 2011;49(1):79–84. doi:10.1016/j.ijbiomac.2011.03.018.

54. Almario CV, Chey WD, Spiegel BMR. Increased Risk of COVID-19 Among Users of Proton Pump Inhibitors. *Am J Gastroenterol.* 2020;115(10):1707–1715. doi:10.14309/ajg.0000000000000798.

55. Hadi YB, Naqvi SF, Kupec JT. Risk of COVID-19 in Patients Taking Proton Pump Inhibitors. *Am J Gastroenterol.* 2020;115(11):1919–1920. doi:10.14309/ajg.0000000000000949.

56. Hajifathalian K, Katz PO. Regarding "Increased Risk of COVID-19 in Patients Taking Proton Pump Inhibitors. *Am J Gastroenterol.* 2020;115(11):1918–1919. doi:10.14309/ajg.0000000000000920.

57. Aby ES, Rodin H, Debes JD. Proton Pump Inhibitors and Mortality in Individuals With COVID-19. *Am J Gastroenterol.* 2020;115(11):1918. doi:10.14309/ajg.0000000000000992.

58. Lee SW, Ha EK, Yeniova AÖ, et al. Severe clinical outcomes of COVID-19 associated with proton pump inhibitors: A nationwide cohort study with propensity score matching. *Gut.* 2021;70(1):76–84. doi:10.1136/gutjnl-2020-322248.

59. Elmunzer BJ, Wolf BJ, Scheiman JM, et al. Association Between Preadmission Acid Suppressive Medication Exposure and Severity of Illness in Patients Hospitalized With COVID-19. *Gastroenterology.* 2021;160(4):1417–1422.e14. doi:10.1053/j.gastro.2020.11.007.

60. Tiligada E, Ennis M. Histamine pharmacology: from Sir Henry Dale to the 21st century. *Br J Pharmacol.* 2020;177(3):469–489. doi:10.1111/bph.14524.

61. Borriello F, Iannone R, Marone G. Histamine release from mast cells and basophils. In: *Handbook of Experimental Pharmacology* Vol 241: Springer New York LLC; 2017:1–19. doi:10.1007/164_2017_18.

62. Marshall JS, Portales-Cervantes L, Leong E. Mast cell responses to viruses and pathogen products. *Int J Mol Sci.* 2019;20(17). doi:10.3390/ijms20174241.

63. Kritas SK, Ronconi G, Caraffa A, Gallenga CE, Ross R, Conti P. Mast cells contribute to coronavirus-induced inflammation: New anti-inflammatory strategy. *J Biol Regul Homeost Agents.* 2020;34(1):9–14. doi:10.23812/20-Editorial-Kritas.

64. Freedberg DE, Conigliaro J, Wang TC, et al. Famotidine Use Is Associated With Improved Clinical Outcomes in Hospitalized COVID-19 Patients: A Propensity Score Matched Retrospective Cohort Study. *Gastroenterology.* 2020;159(3):1129–1131.e3. doi:10.1053/j.gastro.2020.05.053.

65. Mather JF, Seip RL, McKay RG. Impact of Famotidine Use on Clinical Outcomes of Hospitalized Patients With COVID-19. *Am J Gastroenterol.* 2020;115(10):1617–1623. doi:10.14309/ajg.0000000000000832.

66. Cheung KS, Hung IFN, Leung WK. Association Between Famotidine Use and COVID-19 Severity in Hong Kong: A Territory-wide Study. *Gastroenterology.* 2021;160(5):1898–1899. doi:10.1053/j.gastro.2020.05.098.

67. Gubatan J, Levitte S, Balabanis T, Patel A, Sharma A, Habtezion A. SARS-CoV-2 Testing, Prevalence, and Predictors of COVID-19 in Patients with Inflammatory Bowel Disease in Northern California. *Gastroenterology.* 2020;159(3):1141–1144.e2. doi:10.1053/j.gastro.2020.05.009.

68. Allocca M, Fiorino G, Zallot C, et al. Incidence and Patterns of COVID-19 Among Inflammatory Bowel Disease Patients From the Nancy and Milan Cohorts. *Clin Gastroenterol Hepatol.* 2020;18(9):2134–2135. doi:10.1016/j.cgh.2020.04.071.

69. Mao R, Liang J, Shen J, et al. Implications of COVID-19 for patients with pre-existing digestive diseases. *Lancet Gastroenterol Hepatol.* 2020;5(5):426–428. doi:10.1016/S2468-1253(20)30076-5.

70. Taxonera C, Sagastagoitia I, Alba C, Mañas N, Olivares D, Rey E. 2019 novel coronavirus disease (COVID-19) in patients with inflammatory bowel diseases. *Aliment Pharmacol Ther.* 2020;52(2):276–283. doi:10.1111/apt.15804.

71. Singh AK, Jena A, Kumar-M P, Sharma V, Sebastian S. Risk and outcomes of coronavirus disease (COVID-19) in

patients with inflammatory bowel disease: a systematic review and meta-analysis. *United Eur Gastroenterol J.* 2020;9(2). doi:10.1177/2050640620972602.

72. De Souza HSP, Fiocchi C. Immunopathogenesis of IBD: Current state of the art. *Nat Rev Gastroenterol Hepatol.* 2016;13(1):13–27. doi:10.1038/nrgastro.2015.186.

73. Neurath MF. COVID-19 and immunomodulation in IBD. *Gut.* 2020;69(7):1335–1342. doi:10.1136/gutjnl-2020-321269.

74. Papa A, Gasbarrini A, Tursi A. Epidemiology and the Impact of Therapies on the Outcome of COVID-19 in Patients With Inflammatory Bowel Disease. *Am J Gastroenterol.* 2020;115(10):1722–1724. doi:10.14309/ajg.000000000000830.

75. Stockman LJ, Bellamy R, Garner PSARS. Systematic review of treatment effects. *PLoS Med.* 2006;3(9):1525–1531. doi:10.1371/journal.pmed.0030343.

76. Arabi YM, Mandourah Y, Al-Hameed F, et al. Corticosteroid therapy for critically ill patients with middle east respiratory syndrome. *Am J Respir Crit Care Med.* 2018;197(6):757–767. doi:10.1164/rccm.201706-1172OC.

77. Ni YN, Chen G, Sun J, Liang BM, Liang ZA. The effect of corticosteroids on mortality of patients with influenza pneumonia: A systematic review and meta-analysis. *Crit Care.* 2019;23(1). doi:10.1186/s13054-019-2395-8.

78. Brenner EJ, Ungaro RC, Gearry RB, et al. Corticosteroids, But Not TNF Antagonists, Are Associated With Adverse COVID-19 Outcomes in Patients With Inflammatory Bowel Diseases: Results From an International Registry. *Gastroenterology.* 2020;159(2):481–491.e3. doi:10.1053/j.gastro.2020.05.032.

79. World Health Organization; 2020. Clinical Management of Severe Acute Respiratory Infection (SARI) When COVID-19 Disease Is Suspected; Interim Guidance, 13 March 2020.

80. Sherlock ME, Seow CH, Steinhart AH, Griffiths AM. Oral budesonide for induction of remission in ulcerative colitis*Cochrane Database of Systematic Reviews*: John Wiley & Sons, Ltd; 2010. doi:10.1002/14651858.cd007698.pub2.

81. Manguso F, Bennato R, Lombardi G, Riccio E, Costantino G, Fries W. Efficacy and safety of oral beclomethasone dipropionate in ulcerative colitis: A systematic review and meta-analysis. *PLoS One.* 2016;11(11):e0166455. doi:10.1371/journal.pone.0166455.

82. Van Assche G, Manguso F, Zibellini M, et al. Oral prolonged release beclomethasone dipropionate and prednisone in the treatment of active ulcerative colitis: Results from a double-blind, randomized, parallel group study. *Am J Gastroenterol.* 2015;110(5):708–715. doi:10.1038/ajg.2015.114.

83. Khan N, Patel D, Xie D, Lewis J, Trivedi C, Yang YX. Impact of Anti-Tumor Necrosis Factor and Thiopurine Medications on the Development of COVID-19 in Patients With Inflammatory Bowel Disease: A Nationwide Veterans Administration Cohort Study. *Gastroenterology.* 2020;159(4):1545–1546.e1. doi:10.1053/j.gastro.2020.05.065.

84. Ungaro RC, Brenner EJ, Gearry RB, et al. Effect of IBD medications on COVID-19 outcomes: Results from an international registry. *Gut.* 2021;70(4):725–732. doi:10.1136/gutjnl-2020-322539.

85. Brain O, Satsangi J. Therapeutic Decisions in Inflammatory Bowel Disease in the SARS-Cov-2 Pandemic.

Gastroenterology. 2020;160(5):1883–1884. doi:10.1053/j.gastro.2020.05.083.

86. Melmed GY, Agarwal N, Frenck RW, et al. Immunosuppression impairs response to pneumococcal polysaccharide vaccination in patients with inflammatory bowel disease. *Am J Gastroenterol.* 2010;105(1):148–154. doi:10.1038/ajg.2009.523.

87. Caldera F, Hillman L, Saha S, et al. Immunogenicity of High Dose Influenza Vaccine for Patients with Inflammatory Bowel Disease on Anti-TNF Monotherapy: A Randomized Clinical Trial. *Inflamm Bowel Dis.* 2020;26(4):593–602. doi:10.1093/ibd/izz164.

88. Pratt PK, David N, Weber HC, et al. Antibody Response to Hepatitis B Virus Vaccine is Impaired in Patients with Inflammatory Bowel Disease on Infliximab Therapy. *Inflamm Bowel Dis.* 2018;24(2):380–386. doi:10.1093/ibd/izx001.

89. Kennedy NA, Goodhand JR, Bewshea C, et al. Anti-SARS-CoV-2 antibody responses are attenuated in patients with IBD treated with infliximab. *Gut.* 2021;70(5):865–875. doi:10.1136/gutjnl-2021-324388.

90. Wong S-Y, Dixon R, Pazos VM, et al. Serological response to mRNA COVID-19 vaccines in IBD patients receiving biological therapies. *Gastroenterology.* April 2021. doi:10.1053/j.gastro.2021.04.025.

91. Siegel CA, Melmed GY, McGovern DPB, et al. SARS-CoV-2 vaccination for patients with inflammatory bowel diseases: Recommendations from an international consensus meeting. *Gut.* 2021;70(4):635–640. doi:10.1136/gutjnl-2020-324000.

92. Kuhn JH, Li W, Choe H, Farzan M. Angiotensin-converting enzyme 2: A functional receptor for SARS coronavirus. *Cell Mol Life Sci.* 2004;61(21):2738–2743. doi:10.1007/s00018-004-4242-5.

93. Zhao B, Ni C, Gao R, et al. Recapitulation of SARS-CoV-2 infection and cholangiocyte damage with human liver ductal organoids. *Protein Cell.* 2020;11(10):771–775. doi:10.1007/s13238-020-00718-6.

94. Praveen S, Ashish K, Anikhindi SHA, et al. Effect of COVID-19 on Pre-existing Liver disease: What Hepatologist Should Know?. *J Clin Exp Hepatol.* 2021. doi:10.1016/j.jceh.2020.12.006.

95. Mantovani A, Beatrice G, Dalbeni A. Coronavirus disease 2019 and prevalence of chronic liver disease: A meta-analysis. *Liver Int.* 2020;40(6):1316–1320. doi:10.1111/liv.14465.

96. Lippi G, De Oliveira MHS, Henry BM. Chronic liver disease is not associated with severity or mortality in Coronavirus disease 2019 (COVID-19): A pooled analysis. *Eur J Gastroenterol Hepatol.* 2020;33(1):114–115. doi:10.1097/MEG.0000000000001742.

97. Moon AM, Webb GJ, Aloman C, et al. High mortality rates for SARS-CoV-2 infection in patients with pre-existing chronic liver disease and cirrhosis: Preliminary results from an international registry. *J Hepatol.* 2020;73(3):705–708. doi:10.1016/j.jhep.2020.05.013.

98. Bajaj JS, Garcia-Tsao G, Biggins SW, et al. Comparison of mortality risk in patients with cirrhosis and COVID-19 compared with patients with cirrhosis alone and COVID-19 alone: Multicentre matched cohort. *Gut.* 2021;70(3):531–536. doi:10.1136/gutjnl-2020-322118.

99. Iavarone M, D'Ambrosio R, Soria A, et al. High rates of 30-day mortality in patients with cirrhosis and COVID-19. *J Hepatol.* 2020;73(5):1063–1071. doi:10.1016/j.jhep.2020.06.001.

100. Da BL, Im GY, Schiano TD. Coronavirus Disease 2019 Hangover: A Rising Tide of Alcohol Use Disorder and Alcohol-Associated Liver Disease. *Hepatology.* 2020;72(3):1102–1108. doi:10.1002/hep.31307.

101. Fix OK, Hameed B, Fontana RJ, et al. Clinical Best Practice Advice for Hepatology and Liver Transplant Providers During the COVID-19 Pandemic: AASLD Expert Panel Consensus Statement. *Hepatology.* 2020;72(1):287–304. doi:10.1002/hep.31281.

102. Boettler T, Newsome PN, Mondelli MU, et al. Care of patients with liver disease during the COVID-19 pandemic: EASL-ESCMID position paper. *JHEP Reports.* 2020;2(3):100113. doi:10.1016/j.jhepr.2020.100113.

103. Gregory C, Rino G, Richard G, et al. Clinical practice guidance for hepatology and liver transplant providers during the COVID-19 pandemic: APASL expert panel consensus recommendations. *Hepatol Int.* 2020;14(4):415–428. doi:10.1007/s12072-020-10054-w.

104. Zou X, Fang M, Huang J. Liver function should be monitored when treating COVID-19 in chronic HBV-infected patients. *Clin Gastroenterol Hepatol.* 2020;18(13):3056–3057. doi:10.1016/j.cgh.2020.07.062.

105. Aloysius MM, Thatti A, Gupta A, Sharma N, Bansal P, Goyal H. COVID-19 presenting as acute pancreatitis. *Pancreatology.* 2020;20(5):1026–1027. doi:10.1016/j.pan.2020.05.003.

106. Karimzadeh S, Manzuri A, Ebrahimi M, Huy NT. COVID-19 presenting as acute pancreatitis: lessons from a patient in Iran. *Pancreatology.* 2020;20(5):1024–1025. doi:10.1016/j.pan.2020.06.003.

107. Inamdar S, Benias PC, Liu Y, Sejpal DV, Satapathy SK, Prevalence Trindade AJ. Prevalence, risk factors, and outcomes of hospitalized patients with coronavirus disease 2019 presenting as acute pancreatitis. *Gastroenterology.* 2020;159(6):2226–2228.e2. doi:10.1053/j.gastro.2020.08.044.

108. Miró Ò, Llorens P, Jiménez S, et al. Frequency of five unusual presentations in patients with COVID-19: results of the UMC-19-S1. *Epidemiol Infect.* 2020;148:e189. doi:10.1017/S0950268820001910.

109. Zhang P, Zhu L, Cai J, et al. Association of inpatient use of angiotensin-converting enzyme inhibitors and angiotensin II receptor blockers with mortality among patients with hypertension hospitalized with COVID-19. *Circ Res.* 2020;126(12):1671–1681. doi:10.1161/CIRCRESAHA.120.317134.

110. Di Tan N, Qiu Y, Bin Xing X, Ghosh S, Chen MH, Mao R. Associations between angiotensin-converting enzyme inhibitors and angiotensin II receptor blocker use, gastrointestinal symptoms, and mortality among patients with COVID-19. *Gastroenterology.* 2020;159(3):1170–1172.e1. doi:10.1053/j.gastro.2020.05.034.

111. Bavishi C, Maddox TM, Messerli FH. Coronavirus disease 2019 (COVID-19) infection and renin angiotensin system blockers. *JAMA Cardiol.* 2020;5(7):745–747. doi:10.1001/jamacardio.2020.1282.

112. Huang C, Huang L, Wang Y, et al. 6-month consequences of COVID-19 in patients discharged from hospital: a cohort study. *Lancet.* 2021;397(10270):220–232. doi:10.1016/S0140-6736(20)32656-8.

113. Thabane M, Marshall JK. Post-infectious irritable bowel syndrome. *World J Gastroenterol.* 2009;15(29):3591–3596. doi:10.3748/wjg.15.3591.

114. Lee YY, Annamalai C, Rao SSC. Post-Infectious Irritable Bowel Syndrome. *Curr Gastroenterol Rep.* 2017;19(11):1–10. doi:10.1007/s11894-017-0595-4.

115. Futagami S, Itoh T, Sakamoto C. Systematic review with meta-analysis: Post-infectious functional dyspepsia. *Aliment Pharmacol Ther.* 2015;41(2):177–188. doi:10.1111/apt.13006.

116. Weng J, Li Y, Li J, et al. Gastrointestinal sequelae 90 days after discharge for COVID-19. *Lancet Gastroenterol Hepatol.* 2021;6(5):344–346. doi:10.1016/s2468-1253(21)00076-5.

Kidney Manifestations of COVID-19

Laura A. Binari, MD, Natalie N. McCall, MD, and Anna P. Burgner, MD, MEHP

Despite a few early reports during the COVID-19 pandemic that suggested no or minimal increased risk for acute kidney injury (AKI) from infection with SARS-CoV-2, we have learned through the course of the pandemic that this infection is associated with an increased risk for multiple types of AKI. AKI is defined as a sudden decrease in kidney function that occurs over hours. The Kidney Disease: Improving Global Outcomes (KDIGO) clinical practice guidelines stages AKI based on its severity.[1] Stage 1 AKI is the least severe, with a rise in creatinine of 1.5 to 1.9 times the baseline, increase of creatinine of greater than 0.3 mg/dL, or urine output less than 0.5 mL/kg per hour for 6 to 12 hours. Stage 2 AKI is defined as a rise in creatinine of 2 to 2.9 times the baseline creatinine or a urine output less than 0.5 mL/kg per hour for longer than 12 hours. Stage 3 AKI is the most severe, with an increase in creatinine greater than 3 times the baseline, initiation of renal replacement therapy (RRT), anuria for longer than 12 hours, or a urine output less than 0.3 mL/kg per hour for longer than 24 hours.

As will be discussed in this chapter, the pathogenesis of AKI in patients with COVID-19 is multifactorial, including direct viral effects, indirect effects (hypovolemia/hypervolemia, systemic inflammation, superinfection, rhabdomyolysis, microthrombi) or sequelae from disease management (nephrotoxins, lung-kidney crosstalk). In addition, this chapter will explore the management of AKI in patients with SARS-CoV-2 infection. This chapter will also discuss SARS-CoV-2 infection in patients with end-stage kidney disease and with kidney transplants.

Acute Kidney Injury Incidence and Mortality Associated With SARS-CoV-2 Infection

AKI incidence has varied based on the geographic location and clinical situation during the pandemic. A meta-analysis of over 13,000 patients reported an AKI prevalence of 17%, although the range from the individual studies that made up the meta-analysis was broad at 0.5% to 80%.[2] Critically ill patients are more likely to have AKI in the setting of COVID-19; they are also more likely to have stage 3 AKI and require renal replacement therapy (RRT).[3] Patients with COVID-19 appear to have a higher risk for AKI compared with other patients admitted to the hospital, and it is independent of severity of illness.[4] AKI is more common in patients with COVID-19 than in patients with influenza.[5] When compared with other members of the Coronaviridae family, AKI incidence appears to be the highest in patients with Middle East respiratory syndrome (MERS) but is similar between patients with COVID-19 and severe acute respiratory syndrome (SARS).[6]

Multiple studies have demonstrated that the COVID-19–associated AKI occurs soon after hospitalization and occurs temporally close to when respiratory failure occurs.[7,8] Risk factors identified for development of AKI include older age, male sex, history of diabetes mellitus, history of hypertension, presence of shock, and need for invasive ventilation.[7,9] Patients with worse inflammatory markers are also at higher risk for development of AKI.[10]

Mortality is high in AKI in the setting of COVID-19. AKI in the setting of COVID-19 appears to be associated with more mortality than patients with AKI from other viral pneumonias, AKI from all-comers in a historical cohort, and AKI occurring during the pandemic in patients without COVID-19.[10] A meta-analysis found that mortality in patients with AKI and COVID-19 was 52% compared with 11% for all-comers with COVID-19.[2] Patients with severe AKI requiring RRT have the highest mortality of patients with AKI. In addition, the more organ failures a critically ill patient with COVID-19–associated AKI has, the higher is the mortality.[11] Mortality of AKI associated with COVID-19, MERS, and SARS is similar on the basis of two meta-analyses.[6,12]

The need for RRT is higher in patients with COVID-19–associated AKI compared with other causes of AKI. The need for RRT has varied based on geographic region studied and the patient cohort. The more severely ill patients are as evidenced by being hospitalized in the critical care unit (CCU), the more likely they are to need RRT.[3] Overall, approximately 5% of patients with COVID-19 need RRT[2] whereas approximately 30% of patients admitted to CCUs with COVID-19 will need RRT.[3,13]

From the available data to date, there has been a suggestion that the incidence of AKI has decreased as the pandemic has progressed.[14,15] It is unknown why this has happened. This may reflect the evolution of improving clinical understanding and care over the course of the pandemic and the increasing availability of medications that can be used to treat COVID-19. It also may reflect that patients evaluated later in these studies had less hypoxia and fewer inflammatory markers that were less elevated.

In patients who survive COVID-19–associated AKI, persistent kidney function abnormalities often persist. In patients who require RRT, approximately 50% to 60% do not survive and 5% to 10% continue to need RRT at discharge from the hospital.[3,10,16] In one study, approximately two-thirds of patients with AKI during their COVID-19 hospitalization had recovered kidney function back to their baseline by posthospitalization follow-up.[3] However, in long-term follow-up, patients with COVID-19–associated AKI had more loss of glomerular filtration rate (GFR) after recovery than patients with AKI from other causes.[17]

Although at the time of publication, data are still being gathered and interpreted, it seems clear that AKI in the setting of COVID-19 occurs more frequently with other illnesses and is associated with a higher mortality. As the pandemic rages on, we may be getting better at treating COVID-19 and preventing the onset of AKI. It will be important for patients who survive COVID-19–associated AKI to continue to have their kidney function monitored after hospital discharge because of long-term risks for persistent kidney dysfunction.

The causes of AKI in COVID-19 are discussed in the following section and summarized in Table 10.1.

Table 10.1 Summary of the Causes of Acute Kidney Injury in COVID-19 Illness			
Kidney Injury	**Clinical Findings and Features**	**Proposed Mechanism of Injury**	**Occurrence**
[a]Patients can have multiple types of renal injury at the same time			
GLOMERULAR			
COVID-associated nephropathy (COVAN): Secondary collapsing FSGS	Nephrotic range-proteinuria ± nephrotic syndrome (hypoalbuminemia, edema) High-risk APOL1 genotype (G1/G1, G2/G1, or G2/G2) Increase in serum creatinine	COVID-19 infection serves as a "second hit" in individuals predisposed to glomerular injury as a result of high-risk APOL1 allele variants	Overall uncommon but most reported glomerular disease in COVID-19
Anti-GBM disease	Preceding COVID-19 infection Pulmonary-renal syndrome (rapidly progressive glomerulonephritis + alveolar hemorrhage) Proteinuria Microscopic hematuria Increase in serum creatinine Elevated Anti-GBM titer	COVID-19 infection promotes immune response to glomerular basement membrane (noncollagenous domain of α3-chain of collagen type IV)	Rare

Table 10.1 Summary of the Causes of Acute Kidney Injury in COVID-19 Illness—cont'd

Kidney Injury	Clinical Findings and Features	Proposed Mechanism of Injury	Occurrence
ANCA vasculitis	RPGN Alveolar hemorrhage Arthralgias Leukocytoclastic vasculitis Hematuria with RBC casts Proteinuria (both <3.5 g/day and nephrotic range reported) + c-ANCA and/or p-ANCA	Not yet well described. COVID-19 could be "second hit" in predisposed individuals	Rare
IgA vasculitis	Preceding COVID-19 infection Cutaneous vasculitis (purpuric rash) Abdominal pain Arthralgias Hypertension Hematuria with dysmorphic RBCs/RBC casts Variable amount of proteinuria Variable severity of AKI	Not yet well described. COVID-19 could be second hit in predisposed individuals, resulting in increase in circulating galactose-deficient IgA1 antibodies, production of antibodies and formation of immune complexes	Rare
Membranous nephropathy	Nephrotic syndrome Hematuria ± Increase in serum creatinine + anti-PLA2R	Not yet well described. COVID-19 could be second hit in predisposed individuals. Respiratory infection could illicit an anti-PLA2R autoimmune response	Rare
TUBULAR			
Acute tubular injury	Increase in serum creatinine Low-level proteinuria (<3.5 g/day) Proximal tubule dysfunction (impaired kidney handling of phosphate and uric acid)	Ischemic injury resulting from decreased kidney perfusion secondary to hemodynamic instability and/or volume depletion secondary to severe infection	Most common
Rhabdomyolysis (myoglobin cast nephropathy)	Dark urine Myalgias Muscle weakness Elevated CPK Increase in serum creatinine Myoglobin casts + blood detected by urine dipstick but minimal urine RBC	Induced by viral infection, drug-induced, or the result of electrolyte abnormalities	Rare reports in literature. Can be a cause of acute tubular injury
VASCULAR			
Thrombotic microangiopathy	Increase in serum creatinine Hemolytic anemia Thrombocytopenia Hypertension	Complement-mediated (Rule out other potential risk factors)	Rare

ANCA, Antineutrophil cytoplasmic antibodies; *APOL1*, apolipoprotein L1; *CPK*, creatinine phosphokinase; *FSGS*, focal segmental glomerulosclerosis; *GBM*, glomerular basement membrane; *IgA*, immunoglobulin A; *PLA2R*, phospholipase A2 receptor; *RPGN*, rapidly progressive glomerulonephritis; *RBC*, red blood cells.

Could Viral Tropism in Kidney Parenchyma Be Responsible for Acute Kidney Injury?

Evidence is mixed for viral tropism of SARS-CoV-2 in kidney parenchyma. Early autopsy studies suggest viral tropism with evidence of coronavirus-like particles in the cytoplasm of kidney proximal tubular epithelial cells and in the podocytes by electron microscopy and either immunofluorescent staining with an antibody targeting SARS-CoV-2 nucleoprotein or with in situ hybridization.[18,19]

There is a pathophysiological basis for possible tropism. The angiotensin-converting enzyme-2 (ACE2) receptor is the main cellular entry point for SARs-CoV-2 and is expressed on the brush border of proximal tubular cells and podocytes.

Subsequent studies have not shown viral inclusions at the light microscopic level or viral particles at the ultrastructural level.[20-22] This may be in part due to timing of biopsy, with some studies delaying kidney biopsy because detectable SARS-CoV-2 may wane with time. Other studies did not report timing between positive viral polymerase chain reaction (PCR) and kidney biopsy. One study suggested lower levels of SARS-CoV-2 organotropism outside of the lungs so viral titers and severity of illness may play a role in detection.[19]

Tubular Injury in COVID-19

Small autopsy, biopsy series, and case reports show that acute tubular injury (ATI) is the most common histopathological finding with patients who develop AKI during their COVID-19 illness. These studies have included a variety of patients across clinical contexts from severe COVID-19 that ultimately led to the patient's death to nonhospitalized patients presenting with abnormal kidney function and proteinuria and or hematuria.[18,20-23] By light microscopy, varying degrees of tubular injury have been reported with descriptions of diffuse loss of brush border, nonisometric vacuolar degeneration, frank epithelial necrosis, and cellular debris within the tubular lumens.

The largest study, an autopsy study of 42 postmortem kidneys, showed that ATI was the main pathological finding correlating with patients with AKI. This study found that the degree of ATI was mild compared with the elevation in serum creatinine.[20] A multicenter trial of 14 native kidney biopsies and 3 transplant kidney biopsies in patients who presented with confirmed SARS-CoV-2 infection, AKI, and proteinuria/hematuria, found the most common histological finding was ATI in (14/17, 82%). Of note, most patients in this cohort had mild COVID-19 symptoms. Only three patients had severe COVID-19, and most biopsies were performed after the individuals had negative status by reverse transcription (RT)-PCR.[22] Another single-center native kidney biopsy series of 10 hospitalized patients with AKI and COVID-19 found that all biopsy samples showed varying degrees of ATI. One patient in this series had myoglobin casts, serum creatine kinase levels greater than 92,000 and evidence of ATI, suggesting rhabdomyolysis contributing to AKI and ATI.[21]

It is likely that insults that drive ATI and AKI in patients with severe COVID-19 are multifactorial. Patients with COVID-19 often present with acute hypoxia but also may present with nausea, vomiting, and diarrhea. These hemodynamic alterations are likely drivers of prerenal or ischemic injury. In severe COVID-19 illness, the SARS-CoV-2 virus can induce a cytokine storm leading to massive release of granulocyte colony-stimulating factor, interleukins, and interferon and lead to overt septic shock.[24,25] These patients often require pressor support and are exposed to one or more nephrotoxic medications. In these cases, hemodynamic alterations, cytokine injury, or drug effects can directly or indirectly injure the kidney. As discussed earlier and reported in other series, rhabdomyolysis with pigmented casts can also contribute to ATI and AKI.[21,23]

In short, ATI is the most common cause of AKI in the setting of COVID-19. It is likely multifactorial from both ischemic and toxic injury. It may be seen even in the setting of mild COVID-19. Similarly, ATI is also the most common cause of AKI seen in past influenza pandemics.[26]

Glomerular Disease and COVID-19

Although the more common kidney injury found in patients with COVID-19 is ATI, patients also can present with proteinuria and/or microscopic hematuria. In the early phases of the pandemic, a retrospective cohort study from China of 333 patients admitted with COVID-19 pneumonia detected hematuria in 41.7% and proteinuria in 65.8%.[27] Although low-level proteinuria can be due to tubular injury, histopathological analysis of kidney tissue has revealed different patterns of glomerular injury in patients infected with SARS-CoV-2.

COVID-19–Associated Nephropathy

The predominate glomerular lesion described in the literature is collapsing glomerulopathy associated with COVID-19 infection, commonly referred to as COVID-associated nephropathy (COVAN).[28] Multiple case reports and small case series describe patients with collapsing focal segmental glomerulosclerosis (FSGS) lesions.[22,23,29-38] FSGS is a glomerular disorder defined as glomerular scarring in a focal (involving <50% of glomeruli) and segmental (affecting <50% of each glomerulus) pattern. One of the histological patterns of FSGS is a collapsing variant with features of glomerular-tuft collapse associated with hypertrophy and hyperplasia of the overlying visceral epithelial cells that can form pseudocrescents, as well as severe tubular injury, tubular microcysts, and severe foot process effacement.[39] Clinically, patients often present with nephrotic syndrome, which consists of significant proteinuria (≥3.5 g/day), hypoalbuminemia (<3.5 g/dL), hypercholesterolemia, and peripheral edema. The patients selected for biopsy that showed COVAN all had AKI and/or nephrotic-range proteinuria or nephrotic syndrome.

The vast majority of patients diagnosed with COVAN are of African ancestry,[40] with a few exceptions, including reports of COVAN in a Hispanic patient[22] and a patient of Asian heritage.[37] Patients of African ancestry are at risk for another viral-induced collapsing glomerulopathy, human immunodeficiency virus (HIV)-associated nephropathy, if they are homozygous for apolipoprotein L1 (APOL1) high-risk allele variants (G1 and G2).[41] In our review of the current literature, 100% (N = 28) of patients diagnosed with COVAN who underwent genetic analysis had high-risk APOL1 genotypes (G1/G1, G1/G2, or G2/G2).[a] This includes

_____

[a]References 18, 22, 23, 30, 31, 33, 38.

the case of a Hispanic patient with collapsing glomer-ulopathy.[22] The high-risk *APOL1* genotype can also predispose patients infected with COVID-19 to develop other podocytopathies such as minimal change disease.[23]

Reports of Other Glomerulonephritis

A variety of other glomerular lesions in patients infected with COVID-19 have been reported in the current lit-erature. There are reports of de novo or recurrent anti–glomerular basement membrane (anti-GBM) disease,[23,42-44] with an additional case of de novo anti-GBM disease diagnosed by positive serum testing for anti-GBM in a patient with pulmonary-renal syndrome without a confirmatory kidney biopsy.[45] There also have been cases of pauci-immune glomerulonephritis,[46] mem-branous nephropathy,[23] and Ig-A vasculitis.[47,48] It is unclear if these lesions are directly the result of SARS-CoV-2 infections or if the viral infection acts as a "second hit" in susceptible individuals provoking the different patterns of kidney injury. It has been hypoth-esized that infection or inflammation resulting in endo-thelial cell injury could unmask antigens, such as the noncollagenous domain of the alpha-3 chain of type IV collagen or phospholipase A2 receptor, resulting in an autoimmune response.[23,42] In one report of eight cases of anti-GBM over a 5-month period during the pan-demic, the five patients tested for SARS-CoV-2 infection by viral RNA testing were all negative. However, four of the eight patients had immunoglobulin M (IgM) and/or IgG antibodies to the spike protein suggestive of recent infection.[44] In a case of IgA vasculitis, the nephritic syndrome developed a total of 5 weeks after the patient's COVID-19 diagnosis.[47] These delayed pre-sentations suggest an inflammatory reaction secondary to SARS-CoV-2 that then triggers endothelial cell and subsequent glomerular injury.

Thrombotic Microangiopathy

Thrombotic microangiopathy (TMA) has been reported in kidney biopsies from COVID-19 patients as either the primary lesion or in addition to other histological find-ings.[21,22,33,49] In six of eight described cases, patients had laboratory findings concerning for TMA, including AKI, thrombocytopenia, and hemolytic anemia.[21,22] The mechanism of injury is not definitively the result of SARS-CoV-2, because patients often were exposed to other reported causes of TMA, including malignant hypertension, cocaine use, and medications (gemcit-abine, hydroxychloroquine, or calcineurin inhibitors).[21,22,50,51]

Findings in the literature that suggest COVID-19 infection results in complement dysregulation, which can lead to a TMA pattern of kidney injury.[22,49,52,53] Com-plement dysregulation results in formation of the membrane attack complex, resulting in endothelial cell damage. One case report indicated alternative comple-ment pathway activation resulting from low serum C3 levels and normal C4 levels,[22] whereas another case report detected a complement defect based on findings of low factor H complement antigen and elevated plasma CBb and SC5b-9 levels.[49] In a study of pediatric patients with SARS-CoV-2 infection, soluble C5b9 (sC5b9) was measured as a biomarker of complement dysregulation and TMA.[52] They demonstrated elevated levels of sC5b9 in patients with either mild or severe COVID-19 disease or multisystem inflammatory syn-drome in children (MIS-C) compared with healthy con-trols.[52] In addition, they found an association with elevated plasma sC5b9 levels in patients with AKI and with clinical criteria for TMA.[52] These findings support a complement-mediated mechanism of injury rather than TMA secondary to sepsis-induced coagulopathy.

Proposed Mechanisms

Whether there is direct viral infection of glomerular epithelial cells has been debated. There were early reports of detection of SARS-CoV-2 RNA by immuno-histochemistry and virion particles seen on electron microscopy of kidney biopsies and in autopsy studies.[18,19,35,54] However, subsequent case reports and case series using staining for SARS-CoV-2 RNA, spike protein, and nucleocapsid protein on immunohisto-chemistry in addition to electron microscopy have failed to consistently detect the presence of SARS-COV-2.[20-23,29,33] Despite the possible mechanism of cell entry by binding to ACE2 and transmembrane protease serine 2 receptors located on podocytes, there currently is no definitive evidence confirming any direct viral infection of the kidney.

Rather than acting directly on the kidney paren-chyma, the viral infection also could be acting as a second hit in individuals susceptible to glomerular injury. As alluded to earlier, there is a clearer under-standing of the pathological processes behind *APOL1* high-risk alleles and podocytopathies. Research studies have shown that interferon is a regulator of *APOL1* levels in both low- and high-risk human podocytes.[55] Upregulation of *APOL1* high-risk variants can result in disruption of autophagy and mitochondrial hemostasis, ultimately resulting in glomerular epithelial cell death.[55] Elevated interferon levels in COVID-19 patients have been inferred from the visualization of glomerular endo-thelial tubulorecticular inclusions by electron micros-copy.[23,56] This finding is not limited to patients with COVAN. One case series of 17 patients visualized tub-uloreticular inclusions in 6 of 10 cases that had glom-eruli available for electron microscopy, including cases of ATI, membranous glomerulopathy, and minimal change disease.[23] In patients without high-risk *APOL1* genotype, glomerular injury is also likely driven by endothelial cell dysfunction and cytokine storm induced by viral infection.[11,57]

Management of COVID-19 Acute Kidney Injury

As we have discussed, the pathogenesis of AKI in patients with COVID-19 is multifactorial. There is no specific evidence that COVID-19 should be managed differently from other causes of AKI. Therefore, in all patients at high risk for AKI, using the standard of care to prevent and manage multiorgan failure is recommended.[58,59]

Close monitoring of hemodynamics, serum markers of kidney function, individualized fluid management, and decreasing exposure to nephrotoxic drugs are important strategies to decrease risk for kidney injury.

Hypovolemia is common in the early COVID-19 infection course of hospitalized patients likely due to sepsis related to COVID-19 infection.[60] Using balanced crystalloids over normal saline as initial management to expand intravascular volume has been shown to decrease rates of persistent kidney dysfunction and need for RRT in critically ill patients and in sepsis.[61]

In patients who develop AKI, further considerations in AKI management include medical management of fluid and electrolyte strategies.[62] To avoid hypervolemia, consideration of fluid restriction to 10 mL/kg per day and use of high-dose diuretics. To decrease the risk for hyperkalemia, restriction of oral potassium intake, and using potassium binders can be started early in the AKI course. Metabolic acidosis can be managed with oral or intravenous bicarbonate solutions. In the event of AKI progression, close attention to drug dosing and altered pharmacokinetics is important to avoid drug toxicity.

In the event conservative management fails, indications for RRT are the same for patients with AKI and COVID-19 as in AKI events not related to COVID-19. These include oliguria with refractory hypervolemia, hyperkalemia, severe acidosis, or azotemia.

Medication Treatment

At the time of publication, there is no strong evidence that any medication used to treat COVID-19 decreases the likelihood of development of AKI or attenuates the severity, although data analysis remains ongoing, so this may change with time. However, it is important to discuss what treatments have been studied in patients with kidney failure of any type and if there are important dose modifications based on GFR.

Antivirals: Remdesivir

As we have previously discussed, there is some evidence that SARS-CoV-2 has direct viral tropism to tubular cells and podocytes by ACE2 receptors.[19] So treatment with antivirals could theoretically be a treatment to ameliorate COVID-19–induced AKI.

Remdesivir is a nucleotide analog that inhibits viral RNA-dependent RNA polymerase. The ACCT-1 trial showed that remdesivir decreased recovery time for hospitalized patients.[63] In that trial, the reported cases of decreased kidney function or AKI were slightly less in the remdesivir-treated group (85/532 [15.9%], 105/516 [20.3%]).[63]

Notably, most trials excluded patients with severe AKI or end-stage kidney disease (ESKD) based on GFR cutoffs (either 50 or 30 mL/min/1.73 m²). Additionally, remdesivir has limited water solubility, and the intravenous formulation requires a carrier of sulfobutylether-beta-cyclodextrin (SBECD). This carrier is also excreted by the kidneys and has been associated with nephrotoxicity.[64]

Some small trials have evaluated the safety of remdesivir in patients with GFR cutoffs below initial trials and do suggest that there is no overt toxicity in patients with reduced GFR or in patients already on dialysis.[65-67] As mentioned earlier, evidence that antivirals reduce kidney-related events is only limited or indirect.

Immunomodulatory Agents: Tocilizumab and Baricitinib

Severe SARS-CoV-2 infection is thought to be secondary to proinflammatory state with increased interleukin-1 (IL-1), IL-6, tumor necrosis factor, and other cytokines. Immunomodulatory agents can decrease cytokine production or block cytokine receptor activation, thereby decreasing the overall inflammatory response.[58]

Tocilizumab is a humanized IgG1 monoclonal antibody that is directed against the IL-6 receptor. IL-6 is thought to be an important cytokine in COVID-19–related immune dysregulation and development of severe COVID-19 and acute respiratory distress syndrome (ARDS).[68] Data are currently conflicting on the impact of tocilizumab in severe COVID-19 illness.[69,70] Kidney injury occurred at similar rates in the groups.[70] Because tocilizumab is a monoclonal antibody, dose adjustment is not needed for decreased GFR.

Baricitinib is an oral selective inhibitor of Janus kinase (JAK) 1 and 2 and inhibits intracellular cytokine signaling, thereby mitigating the immune response and presumed therapeutic target for the hyperinflammatory state of severe COVID-19.

A follow-up to the ACCT-1 trial investigated treatment with a combination of baricitinib and remdesivir over remdesivir alone for the treatment of hospitalized patients with COVID-19 pneumonia. Baricitinib plus remdesivir was superior to remdesivir alone in reducing recovery time and accelerating improvement, particularly in patients receiving high-flow oxygen or noninvasive mechanical ventilation. Safety analysis showed that kidney events occurred at a similar rate in both groups in this trial.[71]

Data are limited for baricitinib in patients with severe kidney impairment. Baricitinib is not recommended for patients who are on dialysis, have ESKD, or have AKI.

Corticosteroids

Low-dose dexamethasone was found to reduce mortality in hospitalized patients with severe or critical COVID-19 requiring supplemental oxygen or mechanical ventilation. A secondary outcome in this study was the new requirement for RRT. In this study, there were fewer patients receiving RRT at 28 days in the dexamethasone group than in the usual care group (relative risk [RR] 0.61; 95% confidence interval [CI], 0.48–0.76).[72]

Dexamethasone is primarily metabolized hepatically, and there are no dose adjustments required in patients with kidney failure receiving dialysis.

Niacinamide

Niacinamide is the base form of vitamin B_3 and has been suggested to increase nicotinamide adenine dinucleotide (NAD+) level safely. NAD+ shortage has been proposed as a mechanism for acute tubular necrosis; thus increasing NAD+ availability theoretically could help prevent cell damage and ATN.[73,74] In a small prospective study, niacinamide use was associated with decreased frequency of RRT needs and mortality among stage 2/3 AKI, but no differences were seen in outcomes among patients with stage 1 AKI.[75]

Monoclonal Antibodies

Bamlanivimab and etesevimab are neutralizing monoclonal antibodies that bind to spike proteins of the COVID-19 virus. The BLAZE trial showed reduction of SARS-CoV-2 viral load at day 11 among nonhospitalized patients with mild to moderate COVID-19 illness who were treated with bamlanivimab and etesevimab compared with placebo.[76,77] No dose adjustment is recommended in kidney failure. Notably, kidney failure (acute and chronic) was not an exclusion criterion for BLAZE trial participants. Currently, no data exist on whether monoclonal antibodies decrease the development of or attenuate the severity of AKI.

Renin-Angiotensin-Aldosterone System Inhibition

Normally in the body, when blood flow to the kidney is reduced, juxtaglomerular cells convert prorenin to renin. Renin then converts angiotensinogen to angiotensin-1. Angiotensin-1 is converted to angiotensin-2 by ACE. Angiotensin-2 then causes vasoconstriction resulting in increased blood pressure. The ACE2 receptor is a membrane-bound receptor that counteracts this effect by hydrolyzing angiotensin-2. ACE2, as discussed previously, is the entry point into cells by the SARS-CoV-2 virus. Acutely, angiotensin-2 decreases ACE2 receptor expression.

ACE inhibitors (ACEIs) block the conversion of angiotensin-1 to angiotensin-2, and angiotensin receptor blockers (ARBs) block the binding of angiotensin-2 to the angiotensin-1 receptor (AT1R). Experimental animal models have suggested that ACEIs and ARBs increase ACE2 expression in kidney and heart tissue.[78] It was hypothesized early in the course of the pandemic that ACEIs and ARBs may be either beneficial or harmful in the setting of COVID-19 illness.[79] The harm hypothesis comes from ACEIs and ARBs increasing ACE2 expression, leading to increased viral entry and injury. In the beneficial hypothesis, the decreasing of angiogenin-2 production with an ACEI or by blocking the AT1R with an ARB diminishes the inflammation and fibrosis caused by angiotensin-2.

At the time of publication, there are multiple ongoing randomized controlled trials (RCTs) investigating this area. Results have returned from the BRACE-CORONA trial, which randomized patients chronically on an ACEI or ARB hospitalized with mild to moderate COVID-19 to temporarily suspend or continue their medication.[80] There was no difference in mortality between the two groups. Adverse events, including AKI requiring hemodialysis, were similar between the two groups. Data from large observational studies also have not supported an increased risk in patients taking ACEIs or ARBs.[81,82] Thus the recommendations from many professional societies are to continue ACEIs and ARBs unless clinically contraindicated.

Systemic Anticoagulation

SARS-CoV-2 is associated with a prothrombotic state, and thrombi in the kidney microvasculature may contribute to the risk for AKI and/or AKI progression. No data have shown decreased risk for AKI with systemic anticoagulation at this time. Systemic anticoagulation strategies in AKI requiring RRT are important for filter patency, especially in continuous RRT.[58]

Renal Replacement Therapy

The timing of initiation of RRT can be a challenge among critically ill patients. A number of clinical trials and meta-analyses have evaluated initiation of RRT in the critically ill and have not shown a difference in mortality or kidney recovery in the absence of emergent indication.[83-85] There is no current evidence to suggest a different strategy (i.e., earlier initiation) is more effective in management of COVID-19–related AKI.

We recommend conservative management of AKI and the initiation of dialysis to manage the

Table 10.2 Summary of Pros and Cons of Dialysis Modalities in the COVID-19 Pandemic

Dialysis Modality	Pro	Con
CRRT	Easier to remove fluid in hemodynamically unstable patients.	The machines and nurses to run these machines may be in short supply.
PIRRT	Can use either iHD or CRRT machine. Machines can be used for multiple patients in a day. Hemodynamically unstable patients can better tolerate fluid removal with its prolonged nature.	Many hospitals may not have a protocol for this, so nurses may be unexperienced at running these treatments.
iHD	Machines are widely available. One machine can treat multiple patients in a day.	Fluid removal can be difficult in hemodynamically unstable patients.
PD	Do not need a water supply. Well tolerated in hemodynamically unstable patients. Thrombosis is not an issue.	Expertise not widely available and there is a risk for pericatheter leaks.

CRRT, Continuous renal replacement therapy; *iHD,* intermittent hemodialysis; *PD,* peritoneal dialysis. *PIRRT,* prolonged intermittent renal replacement therapy.

life-threatening complications of AKI, including hyperkalemia, acidemia, and/or fluid volume overload.

Modality of RRT can be more complicated in the setting of the COVID-19 pandemic because of the volumes of patients in need and lack of dialysis resources (dialysate, dialyzer filters, anticoagulation medications), machines, and appropriately trained staff.[62]

No study has evaluated outcomes of one modality over another in COVID-19, but there are practical concerns in the determination of modality. Selection should be based on patient needs, local expertise, and availability of staff and resources. The various modalities and their pros and cons are discussed in the following section and are summarized in Table 10.2.

Continuous Renal Replacement Therapy

Continuous renal replacement therapy (CRRT) can be delivered as continuous venovenous hemofiltration (convective clearance), continuous venovenous hemodialysis (diffusive clearance), or continuous venovenous hemodiafiltration (combination of both).

This modality is a rational option for patients with hemodynamic instability or marked fluid overload or when shifts in fluid balance are poorly tolerated. This modality is also the preferred modality for patients in

the intensive care unit (ICU) and at the timing of new initiation of RRT with adequate staffing and resources.

The recommended dose for CRRT is an effluent volume of 25 to 30 mL/kg per hour.[86] This dose could be decreased once metabolic or fluid status has been adequately achieved in the setting of ongoing concerns on the availability of resources (dialysate solutions/filters).

Prolonged Intermittent Renal Replacement Therapy (PIRRT)

Prolonged intermittent renal replacement therapy (PIRRT) is a hybrid therapy with longer treatment duration (8–12 hours) delivered daily or on alternative days.[87] PIRRT can be performed using either a CRRT machine with higher effluent rates (40–50 mL/kg per hour) or an intermittent hemodialysis (iHD) machine (also referred to as sustained low-efficiency dialysis [SLED]) with lower blood flows (300 mL/min) and dialysate flows (200 mL/min). It is another rational option for patients with hemodynamic instability, patients who have marked fluid overload, or when shifts in fluid balance are poorly tolerated.

Advantages to PIRRT include that it can be administered by trained ICU nurses (rather than hemodialysis nurses) and multiple patients can be treated in a single day.

Intermittent Hemodialysis

iHD is the preferred modality in a hemodynamically stable patient. Its advantages include being widely available, allowing treatment of multiple patients with the same machine in a given day. In addition, iHD uses higher blood flow rates that can reduce the risk for clotting.

KDIGO suggests iHD three times per week with delivered single-pool Kt/V urea of 1.3 per session.[86]

Some concerns with intermittent hemodialysis in critically ill patients include that it can lead to the exacerbation of hemodynamic instability. Additionally, the staffing requires a dedicated dialysis nurse with the addition of a bedside ICU nurse. Because of its intermittent schedule, it can be less effective in reaching daily fluid balance goals. Requiring more frequent iHD, especially in the ICU setting for solute removal or management of fluid removal should prompt consideration of switching to a continuous modality.

Peritoneal Dialysis

Acute peritoneal dialysis (PD) or urgent-start PD should be considered when acute surges in patient volume has led to shortages in resources or contraindications to anticoagulation exist.

Acute/urgent-start PD requires the placement of a PD catheter. In critically ill patients, a cuffed PD catheter is preferred.[88] Initial dialysate volumes should be low (1–1.5 L) to decrease the risk for pericatheter leaks. These low-dialysate volume exchanges can be performed with a rapid timeline (exchange time of 1–2 hours) to achieve higher solute clearance, and rapid fluid removal can be achieved by using higher dextrose solutions.

Advantages of acute PD include it being less likely to exacerbate hemodynamic instability, it does not require vascular access, and thrombosis is less likely to affect the PD circuit.

Challenges to acute PD include that currently acute PD protocols, policies, and expertise are not widely available. These generally are limited to centers with acute or urgent start practices. Additionally, using automated cycler machines may be limited because of availability and ICU nursing staff are often not trained in their use. Finally, prone positioning can compromise PD functionality and should be avoided in these circumstances.

Anticoagulation Strategies

Patients with COVID-19 are at high risk for thromboembolism.[89] In patients with AKI requiring initiation of CRRT, clotting events can lead to disruption of the treatment, decreased clearance, and increased use of resources (filters, tubing). Thus keeping the patency of the filter and dialysis circuit can be more challenging in the management of AKI with CRRT in critically ill COVID-19 patients. The CRRT circuit can be maintained without any anticoagulation, but early anticoagulation in these patients can improve the patency of the filter and decrease disruptions to the treatment. A single-center study of hospitalized patients with COVID-19 showed that there were fewer clotting events and filters maintained patency longer in patients who were receiving anticoagulation therapy (124/350, 35% anticoagulated vs. 79/152, 52%, no anticoagulation).[90]

Heparin and citrate anticoagulation can be used in CRRT as anticoagulation strategies to maintain patency. Heparin is commonly used throughout hospital settings and can be applied to the CRRT circuit either through a systemic approach or directly in the CRRT circuit at the prefilter site. Partial thromboplastin time (PTT) levels are generally used to monitor heparin levels, but severe COVID-19 has been associated with coagulation abnormalities, including thrombocytopenia and prolonged prothrombin time (PT)/PTT.[91] In these circumstances, PTT levels have been found to not be as reliable in COVID-19 and instead factor Xa levels can be used for monitoring of heparin in CRRT.[92]

Regional citrate anticoagulation is a local anticoagulation strategy. Citrate complexes calcium, preventing the coagulation cascades and platelet activation. Citrate is added within the dialysis circuit to deplete circuit calcium, and then calcium is added back after the circuit

to maintain physiological levels of calcium in the patient. This form of anticoagulation has been shown to be effective and improve mean treatment duration of CRRT in COVID-19 patients.[90,93] Not all centers have the same experience with citrate as with heparin, which can limit its use and availability, but it should be considered if center expertise allows, especially in patients with contraindications to other anticoagulation options.

Interruptions in CRRT because of clotting increase the risk for inadequate electrolyte, acid-base, and fluid balance control, so it is important to minimize interruptions and maximize kidney replacement therapies.

Unique Kidney Populations and COVID-19

The next part of this chapter transitions to discussion of two unique populations of kidney patients: ESKD and kidney transplant recipients. Both populations have high rates of comorbidities that are known to increase risk for mortality from COVID-19, including diabetes mellitus and hypertension. As will be discussed in the next section, both populations have been affected in distinct ways during the course of the pandemic and have seen high rates of mortality with COVID-19 illness.

End-Stage Kidney Disease and COVID-19

Patients with ESKD represent a portion of our population at significant risk for exposure to the SARS-CoV-2 virus. Patients on in-center hemodialysis must travel to dialysis units three times weekly (sometimes by public transportation), interact with staff and other patients, and sit for hours while receiving dialysis and may not be able to be appropriately socially distanced. Home dialysis patients are a little more protected, but they usually need to go to dialysis clinic visits at least monthly. Not surprisingly, hemodialysis centers have been found to be high-risk settings for transmission of the SARS-CoV-2 virus.[94,95] Patients on in-center hemodialysis in New York City had a prevalence of 14% of COVID-19 compared with only 2.6% in the general population.[96] COVID-19 has been found to occur much less frequently in home dialysis patients than in-center hemodialysis patients.[94]

Patients with ESKD appear to have a dichotomous presentation with COVID-19. Some patients are asymptomatic or only mildly symptomatic; however, some develop fatal multiorgan failure.[97] Mortality in retrospective analyses of ESKD patients has varied based on geographic location between 16% and 32%.[97-100] Risk factors for death from COVID-19 in the setting of ESKD include older age, higher levels of inflammatory markers, fever, longer time on HD, and need for mechanical ventilation.[97,99,101]

Transplant and COVID-19

Acute Kidney Injury in Kidney Transplant Recipients

The previously described glomerular pathological conditions, vascular complications, and tubular injury that can occur in patients infected with SARS-CoV-2 can also occur in kidney transplant recipients. There have been a small number of case reports of ATI,[22,23,33,102] cortical infarction,[23,103,104] FSGS not otherwise specified variant,[102] TMA,[105] and collapsing glomerulopathy in kidney transplant recipients.[30,106] Transplant patients have additional risk factors for some of these histological findings, such as calcineurin inhibitor toxicity, concurrent rejection, or recurrence of native disease. The lymphopenia and increased inflammatory cytokines seen in SARS-CoV-2 infection could possibly increase the risk for BK virus (BKV) reactivation.[107] There is a case report of a patient with increasing BKV PCR levels after COVID-19 infection despite a reduction in immunosuppressive medications.[108] This patient did have a history of BK viremia, so the resurgence may not reflect a direct effect of COVID-19, but one should consider screening for BK viremia in a kidney transplant recipient with AKI and/or proteinuria in the setting of SARS-CoV-2 infection.

Although a multicenter cohort of 104 patients did not have any reports of allograft rejection,[109] there have been a few reports of transplant patients who had evidence of T-cell–mediated and/or antibody-mediated allograft rejection at time of presentation with COVID-19 or in the weeks after COVID-19 diagnosis.[22,23] The development of allograft rejection in the setting of the virus could be secondary to reduction of immunosuppression or potentially stimulation of the immune system in response to viral infection.[110] The clinician should have an understanding that any kidney injury can occur in a transplanted kidney and consider the additional possibilities of graft rejection, opportunistic infections, and drug toxicity when evaluating AKI in a kidney transplant recipient.

Mortality of COVID-19 Infection in Kidney Transplant

Mortality rates reported in kidney transplant recipients in the current literature range from 13% to 50%, with the majority of data coming from small single-center studies.[111] Larger multicenter studies and international registries have reports of 19% to 32% mortality in kidney transplant recipients with COVID-19.[109,112-115] Some of the registry data were incomplete at time of publication because they included patients with active infection.[113,115] A prospective cohort study screened their transplant patient population for symptoms of COVID-19.[116] During the study period, 5% (66/1216) of the transplant recipients were diagnosed with COVID-19, which was greater than the incidence of 0.3% in the general population in France at that time. Ultimately, 91% (60/66) of transplant patients with COVID-19 required hospital admission, with 22% of the patients requiring ICU care. In this cohort, 24% of the patients infected with COVID-19 died.[116] It is important to note that these studies reflect a sicker patient population because they either excluded patients who were not hospitalized or predominately involved hospitalized patients.

Transplant patients could be at increased risk for complications from SARS-CoV-2 because of a higher rate of high-risk comorbidities. Current literature reports a high prevalence of hypertension (50%–100%), cardiovascular disease (8%–50%), obesity (29%–69%), and diabetes (15%–90%) in transplant patients who present with COVID-19.[111] In addition, the occurrence of AKI during COVID-19 infection is relatively high, with reports of 43% to 51% of kidney transplant recipients developing AKI[12,15,18] compared with a reported incidence of AKI in 14% to 35% of critically ill patiets.[57,109,112,115] Factors associated with higher mortality in kidney transplant recipients include older age,[b] decreased kidney function,[112,115] cardiovascular disease,[115] pneumonia,[113] ARDS,[109] and dyspnea on presentation.[115,119] There have been inconsistent results when trying to determine if transplant status is an independent risk factor for mortality.[118-121] In a matched-cohort study involving 273 kidney transplant recipients and 273 nontransplanted controls, the 30-day mortality in kidney transplant recipients was 17.9% versus 11.4% in the control group. The controls were matched for age, body mass index, and other comorbidities, but more transplant patients had hypertension (91.3% vs. 49.8%).[119] In this study and others, transplant status was not identified as an independent risk factor for mortality.[111,117,119] The observed mortality rate may be due to higher rates of comorbidities and a higher incidence of AKI, rather than transplant recipient status or use of immunosuppression.

Impact on Kidney Transplantation and Medication Management

No evidenced-based guidelines exist regarding management of immunosuppressive medication in kidney transplant recipients infected with SARS-CoV-2. A working group of the European Renal Association and European Dialysis and Transplant Association (ERA-EDTA) published a consensus statement regarding general guidance for immunosuppressive medication management in kidney transplant recipients who are more than 3 to

---

[b]References 109, 112, 113, 115, 117, 118.

6 months post their transplant.[122] For patients with mild symptoms, the consensus group recommended holding mycophenolate, azathioprine, or mammalian target of rapamycin (mTOR) inhibitors and continuing prednisone and calcineurin inhibitors if on triple therapy. If on steroid-free dual therapy, it is recommended to consider replacing mycophenolate or mTOR inhibitors with low-dose steroids. If the patient does not clinically improve, one can consider reducing the calcineurin inhibitor. In patients with more severe infection or high-risk patients with mild pneumonia, the group recommended also stopping calcineurin inhibitors and increasing the dose of steroids.[122] A retrospective single-center cohort study involving 38 kidney transplant recipients did not find any association with mortality and immunosuppressant management aside from increased prednisone equivalents in the patients who died, reflecting their more severe disease.[123] The general consensus is to tailor the medications on a patient-by-patient basis based on their risk factors and severity of illness.

An additional impact of the COVID-19 pandemic was a reduction in kidney transplants as centers suspended or reduced transplant surgeries because of the risk of high-dose immunosuppression and to help conserve essential medical supplies. This created a dilemma of balancing the risk of transplantation versus remaining on the waitlist. Studies have indicated similar overall rates of mortality in transplant recipients and waitlist candidates who tested positive for SARS-CoV-2.[124,125] This finding was attributed to higher rates of infection in waitlist candidates but a higher all-cause mortality rate in transplant recipients who tested positive for SARS-CoV-2.[124,126] In contrast, a single-center study in New York had a higher case fatality rate for waitlisted patients with COVID-19.[127] However, it is unclear if all waitlisted patients were "active" candidates, and the waitlist patient population in the study had higher rates of diabetes, cardiovascular disease, and smoking history compared with transplant recipients.[127] Similarly, a French registry indicated a higher daily incidence of deaths in waitlisted individuals compared with transplant recipients from March to June 2020 compared with the same time period in 2018 and 2019.[128] This difference was mainly seen in areas with low viral risk and could have been affected by the inclusion of "inactive" patients on the waitlist.[128] There has been conflicting evidence regarding the impact of COVID-19 infection on mortality within the first year of transplant.[124,125,127,128] Analysis of these results is limited because of the retrospective study design, small sample sizes, and/or insufficient clinical characteristics included in databases. As with studies of the general population during this time, the data are also limited mainly to patients being tested for the virus and thus not able to adequately capture outcomes of asymptomatic individuals. The future impact of the COVID-19 vaccine on these findings is also currently unknown.

Conclusion

COVID-19 illness increases the risk for AKI significantly, and the development of AKI in COVID-19 substantially increases the risk for death. The most common cause of AKI is ATI; however, glomerular lesions, particularly COVAN, have been seen. If a patient recovers from COVID-19 and survives the hospitalization, few require ongoing RRT at discharge; however, they appear to be at risk for more rapid loss of their GFR in the long term after COVID-19 infection. No large RCT of any therapeutics in the setting of COVID-19 has demonstrated significant reduction in the risk for AKI from COVID-19; however, the risk for AKI has seemed to decrease as the pandemic has progressed, suggesting possibly that improved clinical care overall may be decreasing the AKI risk. Treatment of COVID-19–associated AKI remains good supportive care with RRT as needed for the normal indications.

Patients with ESKD on chronic RRT and patients with kidney transplants represent a portion of our population at high risk for morbidity and mortality from COVID-19 illness. Patients with ESKD have frequent health care visits to dialysis centers, and dialysis centers have been shown to be high-risk centers of transmission of the SARS-CoV-2 virus. Kidney transplant patients are chronically immunosuppressed, and decisions on reduction in immunosuppressants in patients with COVID-19 must be made on a case-by-case basis.

More research is needed in the areas of long-term outcomes after COVID-19–associated AKI, improving mortality in patients with AKI or ESKD and in kidney transplant recipients, and in understanding the pathogenesis of AKI in COVID-19 and creating targeted treatments to prevent and/or decrease severity of AKI.

REFERENCES

1. Khwaja A. KDIGO clinical practice guidelines for acute kidney injury. *Nephron Clin Pract.* 2012;120(4):c179–c184. doi:10.1159/000339789.
2. Robbins-Juarez SY, Qian L, King KL, et al. Outcomes for patients with COVID-19 and acute kidney injury: a systematic review and meta-analysis. *Kidney Int Rep.* Aug. 2020;5(8):1149–1160. doi:10.1016/j.ekir.2020.06.013.
3. Chan L, Chaudhary K, Saha A, et al. AKI in hospitalized patients with COVID-19. *J Am Soc Nephrol.* 2021;32(1):151–160. doi:10.1681/ASN.2020050615.
4. Moledina DG, Simonov M, Yamamoto Y, et al. The association of COVID-19 with acute kidney injury independent of severity of illness: a multicenter cohort study. *Am J Kidney Dis.* 2021;77(4):490–499. e1. doi:10.1053/j.ajkd.2020.12.007.
5. Birkelo BC, Parr SK, Perkins AM, et al. Comparison of COVID-19 versus influenza on the incidence, features, and recovery from acute kidney injury in hospitalized United States Veterans. *Kidney Int.* 2021;100(4):894–905. doi:10.1016/j.kint.2021.05.029.

6. Zhou S, Xu J, Xue C, Yang B, Mao Z, Ong ACM. Coronavirus-associated kidney outcomes in COVID-19, SARS, and MERS: a meta-analysis and systematic review. *Ren Fail.*Nov 09 2020;43(1):1-15. doi:10.1080/0886022X.2020.1847724

7. Hirsch JS, Ng JH, Ross DW, et al. Acute kidney injury in patients hospitalized with COVID-19. *Kidney Int.* 2020;98(1):209–218. doi:10.1016/j.kint.2020.05.006.

8. Gupta S, Hayek SS, Wang W, et al. Factors associated with death in critically ill patients with coronavirus disease 2019 in the US. *JAMA Intern Med.* 2020;180(11):1436–1447. doi:10.1001/jamainternmed.2020.3596.

9. Tejpal A, Gianos E, Cerise J, et al. Sex-based differences in COVID-19 outcomes. *J Womens Health (Larchmt).* 2021;30(4):492–501. doi:10.1089/jwh.2020.8974.

10. Fisher M, Neugarten J, Bellin E, et al. AKI in hospitalized patients with and without COVID-19: a comparison study. *J Am Soc Nephrol.* 2020;31(9):2145–2157. doi:10.1681/ASN.2020040509.

11. Gupta A, Madhavan MV, Sehgal K, et al. Extrapulmonary manifestations of COVID-19. *Nat Med.* 2020;26(7):1017–1032. doi:10.1038/s41591-020-0968-3.

12. Chen YT, Shao SC, Lai EC, Hung MJ, Chen YC. Mortality rate of acute kidney injury in SARS, MERS, and COVID-19 infection: a systematic review and meta-analysis. *Crit Care.* 2020;24(1):439. doi:10.1186/s13054-020-03134-8.

13. Richards-Belle A, Orzechowska I, Gould DW, et al. COVID-19 in critical care: epidemiology of the first epidemic wave across England, Wales and Northern Ireland. *Intensive Care Med.* 2020;46(11):2035–2047. doi:10.1007/s00134-020-06267-0.

14. Bowe B, Cai M, Xie Y, Gibson AK, Maddukuri G, Al-Aly Z. Acute Kidney Injury in a National Cohort of Hospitalized US Veterans with COVID-19. *Clin J Am Soc Nephrol.* 2020;16(1):14–25. doi:10.2215/CJN.09610620.

15. Charytan DM, Parnia S, Khatri M, et al. Decreasing Incidence of Acute Kidney Injury in Patients with COVID-19 Critical Illness in New York City. *Kidney Int Rep.* 2021;6(4):916–927. doi:10.1016/j.ekir.2021.01.036.

16. Gupta S, Coca SG, Chan L, et al. AKI Treated with Renal Replacement Therapy in Critically Ill Patients with COVID-19. *J Am Soc Nephrol.* 2021;32(1):161–176. doi:10.1681/ASN.2020060897.

17. Nugent J, Aklilu A, Yamamoto Y, et al. Assessment of Acute Kidney Injury and Longitudinal Kidney Function After Hospital Discharge Among Patients With and Without COVID-19. *JAMA Netw Open.* 2021;4(3):e211095. doi:10.1001/jamanetworkopen.2021.1095.

18. Su H, Yang M, Wan C, et al. Renal histopathological analysis of 26 postmortem findings of patients with COVID-19 in China. *Kidney Int.* 2020;98(1):219–227. doi:10.1016/j.kint.2020.04.003.

19. Puelles VG, Lütgehetmann M, Lindenmeyer MT, et al. Multiorgan and Renal Tropism of SARS-CoV-2. *N Engl J Med.* 2020;383(6):590–592. doi:10.1056/NEJMc2011400.

20. Santoriello D, Khairallah P, Bomback AS, et al. Postmortem Kidney Pathology Findings in Patients with COVID-19. *J Am Soc Nephrol.* 2020;31(9):2158–2167. doi:10.1681/ASN.2020050744.

21. Sharma P, Uppal NN, Wanchoo R, et al. COVID-19-Associated Kidney Injury: A Case Series of Kidney Biopsy Findings. *J Am Soc Nephrol.* 2020;31(9):1948–1958. doi:10.1681/ASN.2020050699.

22. Akilesh S, Nast CC, Yamashita M, et al. Multicenter Clinico-pathologic Correlation of Kidney Biopsies Performed in COVID-19 Patients Presenting With Acute Kidney Injury or Proteinuria. *Am J Kidney Dis.* 2021;77(1):82–93. doi:10.1053/j.ajkd.2020.10.001 e1.

23. Kudose S, Batal I, Santoriello D, et al. Kidney Biopsy Findings in Patients with COVID-19. *J Am Soc Nephrol.* 2020;31(9):1959–1968. doi:10.1681/ASN.2020060802.

24. Huang C, Wang Y, Li X, et al. Clinical features of patients infected with 2019 novel coronavirus in Wuhan, China. *Lancet.* 2020;395(10223):497–506. doi:10.1016/S0140-6736(20)30183-5.

25. Zhu Z, Cai T, Fan L, et al. Clinical value of immune-inflammatory parameters to assess the severity of coronavirus disease 2019. *Int J Infect Dis.* 2020;95:332–339. doi:10.1016/j.ijid.2020.04.041.

26. Abdulkader RC, Ho YL, de Sousa Santos S, Caires R, Arantes MF, Andrade L. Characteristics of acute kidney injury in patients infected with the 2009 influenza A (H1N1) virus. *Clin J Am Soc Nephrol.* 2010;5(11):1916–1921. doi:10.2215/CJN.00840110.

27. Pei G, Zhang Z, Peng J, et al. Renal Involvement and Early Prognosis in Patients with COVID-19 Pneumonia. *J Am Soc Nephrol.* 2020;31(6):1157–1165. doi:10.1681/ASN.2020030276.

28. Velez JCQ, Caza T, Larsen CP. COVAN is the new HIVAN: the re-emergence of collapsing glomerulopathy with COVID-19. *Nat Rev Nephrol.* 2020;16(10):565–567. doi:10.1038/s41581-020-0332-3.

29. Wu H, Larsen CP, Hernandez-Arroyo CF, et al. AKI and Collapsing Glomerulopathy Associated with COVID-19 and. *J Am Soc Nephrol.* 2020;31(8):1688–1695. doi:10.1681/ASN.2020050558.

30. Shetty AA, Tawhari I, Safar-Boueri L, et al. COVID-19-Associated Glomerular Disease. *J Am Soc Nephrol.* 2021;32(1):33–40. doi:10.1681/ASN.2020060804.

31. Magoon S, Bichu P, Malhotra V, et al. COVID-19-Related Glomerulopathy: A Report of 2 Cases of Collapsing Focal Segmental Glomerulosclerosis. *Kidney Med.* 2020;2(4):488–492. doi:10.1016/j.xkme.2020.05.004.

32. Malik IO, Ladiwala N, Chinta S, Khan M, Patel K. Severe Acute Respiratory Syndrome Coronavirus 2 Induced Focal Segmental Glomerulosclerosis. *Cureus.* 2020;12(10):e10898. doi:10.7759/cureus.10898.

33. Ferlicot S, Jamme M, Gaillard F, et al. The spectrum of kidney biopsies in hospitalized patients with COVID-19, acute kidney injury, and/or proteinuria. *Nephrol Dial Transplant.* 2021. doi:10.1093/ndt/gfab042.

34. Kadosh BS, Pavone J, Wu M, Reyentovich A, Gidea C. Collapsing glomerulopathy associated with COVID-19 infection in a heart transplant recipient. *J Heart Lung Transplant.* 2020;39(8):855–857. doi:10.1016/j.healun.2020.05.013.

35. Kissling S, Rotman S, Gerber C, et al. Collapsing glomerulopathy in a COVID-19 patient. *Kidney Int.* 2020;98(1):228–231. doi:10.1016/j.kint.2020.04.006.

36. Izzedine H, Brocheriou I, Arzouk N, et al. COVID-19-associated collapsing glomerulopathy: a report of two cases and literature review. *Intern Med J.* 2020;50(12):1551–1558. doi:10.1111/imj.15041.

37. Gupta RK, Bhargava R, Shaukat AA, Albert E, Leggat J. Spectrum of podocytopathies in new-onset nephrotic syndrome

following COVID-19 disease: a report of 2 cases. *BMC Nephrol.* 2020;21(1):326. doi:10.1186/s12882-020-01970-y.

38. Sharma Y, Nasr SH, Larsen CP, Kemper A, Ormsby AH, Williamson SR. COVID-19-Associated Collapsing Focal Segmental Glomerulosclerosis: A Report of 2 Cases. *Kidney Med.* 2020;2(4):493–497. doi:10.1016/j.xkme.2020.05.005.

39. D'Agati VD, Kaskel FJ, Falk RJ. Focal segmental glomerulosclerosis. *N Engl J Med.* 2011;365(25):2398–2411. doi:10.1056/NEJMra1106556.

40. Sharma P, Ng JH, Bijol V, Jhaveri KD, Wanchoo R. Pathology of COVID-19-associated acute kidney injury. *Clin Kidney J.* 2021;14(Suppl 1):i30–i39. doi:10.1093/ckj/sfab003.

41. Kopp JB, Nelson GW, Sampath K, et al. APOL1 genetic variants in focal segmental glomerulosclerosis and HIV-associated nephropathy. *J Am Soc Nephrol.* 2011;22(11):2129–2137. doi:10.1681/ASN.2011040388.

42. Winkler A, Zitt E, Sprenger-Mähr H, Soleiman A, Cejna M, Lhotta K. SARS-CoV-2 infection and recurrence of anti-glomerular basement disease: a case report. *BMC Nephrol.* 2021;22(1):75. doi:10.1186/s12882-021-02275-4.

43. Koc NS, Yildirim T, Saglam A, Arici M, Erdem Y. A patient with COVID-19 and anti-glomerular basement membrane disease. *Nefrologia.* 2021;41(4):471–473. doi:10.1016/j.nefro.2020.08.003.

44. Prendecki M, Clarke C, Cairns T, et al. Anti-glomerular basement membrane disease during the COVID-19 pandemic. *Kidney Int.* 2020;98(3):780–781. doi:10.1016/j.kint.2020.06.009.

45. Nahhal S, Halawi A, Basma H, Jibai A, Ajami Z. Anti-Glomerular Basement Membrane Disease as a Potential Complication of COVID-19: A Case Report and Review of Literature. *Cureus.* 2020;12(12):e12089. doi:10.7759/cureus.12089.

46. Uppal NN, Kello N, Shah HH, et al. ANCA-Associated Vasculitis With Glomerulonephritis in COVID-19. *Kidney Int Rep.* 2020;5(11):2079–2083. doi:10.1016/j.ekir.2020.08.012.

47. Suso AS, Mon C, Oñate Alonso I, et al. IgA Vasculitis With Nephritis (Henoch-Schönlein Purpura) in a COVID-19 Patient. *Kidney Int Rep.* 2020;5(11):2074–2078. doi:10.1016/j.ekir.2020.08.016.

48. Li NL, Papini AB, Shao T, Girard L. Immunoglobulin-A Vasculitis With Renal Involvement in a Patient With COVID-19: A Case Report and Review of Acute Kidney Injury Related to SARS-CoV-2. *Can J Kidney Health Dis.* 2021;8:2054358121991684. doi:10.1177/2054358121991684.

49. Jhaveri KD, Meir LR, Flores Chang BS, et al. Thrombotic microangiopathy in a patient with COVID-19. *Kidney Int.* 2020;98(2):509–512. doi:10.1016/j.kint.2020.05.025.

50. Fromm LM. Suspected hydroxychloroquine-induced thrombotic thrombocytopaenic purpura. *Journal of Pharmacy Practice and Research.* 2018;48:72–75.

51. Al-Nouri ZL, Reese JA, Terrell DR, Vesely SK, George JN. Drug-induced thrombotic microangiopathy: a systematic review of published reports. *Blood.* 2015;125(4):616–618. doi:10.1182/blood-2014-11-611335.

52. Diorio C, McNerney KO, Lambert M, et al. Evidence of thrombotic microangiopathy in children with SARS-CoV-2 across the spectrum of clinical presentations. *Blood Adv.* 2020;4(23):6051–6063. doi:10.1182/bloodadvances.2020003471.

53. Merrill JT, Erkan D, Winakur J, James JA. Emerging evidence of a COVID-19 thrombotic syndrome has treatment implications. *Nat Rev Rheumatol.* 2020;16(10):581–589. doi:10.1038/s41584-020-0474-5.

54. Braun F, Lütgehetmann M, Pfefferle S, et al. SARS-CoV-2 renal tropism associates with acute kidney injury. *Lancet.* 2020;396(10251):597–598. doi:10.1016/S0140-6736(20)31759-1.

55. Beckerman P, Bi-Karchin J, Park AS, et al. Transgenic expression of human APOL1 risk variants in podocytes induces kidney disease in mice. *Nat Med.* 2017;23(4):429–438. doi:10.1038/nm.4287.

56. Gaillard F, Ismael S, Sannier A, et al. Tubuloreticular inclusions in COVID-19-related collapsing glomerulopathy. *Kidney Int.* 2020;98(1):241. doi:10.1016/j.kint.2020.04.022.

57. Perico L, Benigni A, Casiraghi F, Ng LFP, Renia L, Remuzzi G. Immunity, endothelial injury and complement-induced coagulopathy in COVID-19. *Nat Rev Nephrol.* 2021;17(1):46–64. doi:10.1038/s41581-020-00357-4.

58. Nadim MK, Forni LG, Mehta RL, et al. COVID-19-associated acute kidney injury: consensus report of the 25th Acute Disease Quality Initiative (ADQI) Workgroup. *Nat Rev Nephrol.* 2020;16(12):747–764. doi:10.1038/s41581-020-00356-5.

59. Ronco C, Reis T, Husain-Syed F. Management of acute kidney injury in patients with COVID-19. *Lancet Respir Med.* 2020;8(7):738–742. doi:10.1016/S2213-2600(20)30229-0.

60. Xia P, Wen Y, Duan Y, et al. Clinicopathological Features and Outcomes of Acute Kidney Injury in Critically Ill COVID-19 with Prolonged Disease Course: A Retrospective Cohort. *J Am Soc Nephrol.* 2020;31(9):2205–2221. doi:10.1681/ASN.2020040426.

61. Brown RM, Wang L, Coston TD, et al. Balanced Crystalloids versus Saline in Sepsis. A Secondary Analysis of the SMART Clinical Trial. *Am J Respir Crit Care Med.* 2019;200(12):1487–1495. doi:10.1164/rccm.201903-0557OC.

62. Burgner A, Ikizler TA, Dwyer JP. COVID-19 and the Inpatient Dialysis Unit: Managing Resources during Contingency Planning Pre-Crisis. *Clin J Am Soc Nephrol.* 2020;15(5):720–722. doi:10.2215/CJN.03750320.

63. Beigel JH, Tomashek KM, Dodd LE, et al. Remdesivir for the Treatment of Covid-19 - Final Report. *N Engl J Med.* 2020;383(19):1813–1826. doi:10.1056/NEJMoa2007764.

64. Adamsick ML, Gandhi RG, Bidell MR, et al. Remdesivir in Patients with Acute or Chronic Kidney Disease and COVID-19. *J Am Soc Nephrol.* 2020;31(7):1384–1386. doi:10.1681/ASN.2020050589.

65. Thakare S, Gandhi C, Modi T, et al. Safety of Remdesivir in Patients With Acute Kidney Injury or CKD. *Kidney Int Rep.* 2021;6(1):206–210. doi:10.1016/j.ekir.2020.10.005.

66. Estiverne C, Strohbehn IA, Mithani Z, et al. Remdesivir in Patients With Estimated GFR < 30 ml/min per 1.73 m. *Kidney Int Rep.* 2021;6(3):835–838. doi:10.1016/j.ekir.2020.11.025.

67. Aiswarya D, Arumugam V, Dineshkumar T, et al. Use of Remdesivir in Patients With COVID-19 on Hemodialysis: A Study of Safety and Tolerance. *Kidney Int Rep.* 2021;6(3):586–593. doi:10.1016/j.ekir.2020.12.003.

68. Aziz M, Fatima R, Assaly R. Elevated interleukin-6 and severe COVID-19: A meta-analysis. *J Med Virol.* 2020;92(11):2283–2285. doi:10.1002/jmv.25948.

69. Gordon AC, Mouncey PR, Al-Beidh F, et al. Interleukin-6 Receptor Antagonists in Critically Ill Patients with Covid-19. *N Engl J Med.* 2021;384(16):1491–1502. doi:10.1056/NEJMoa2100433.

70. Rosas IO, Bräu N, Waters M, et al. Tocilizumab in Hospitalized Patients with Severe Covid-19 Pneumonia. *N Engl J Med.* 2021;384(16):1503–1516. doi:10.1056/NEJMoa2028700.

71. Kalil AC, Patterson TF, Mehta AK, et al. Baricitinib plus Remdesivir for Hospitalized Adults with Covid-19. *N Engl J Med.* 2021;384(9):795–807. doi:10.1056/NEJMoa2031994.

72. Horby P, Lim WS, Emberson JR, et al. Dexamethasone in Hospitalized Patients with Covid-19. *N Engl J Med.* 2021;384(8):693–704. doi:10.1056/NEJMoa2021436.

73. Tran MT, Zsengeller ZK, Berg AH, et al. PGC1α drives NAD biosynthesis linking oxidative metabolism to renal protection. *Nature.* 2016;531(7595):528–532. doi:10.1038/nature17184.

74. Poyan Mehr A, Tran MT, Ralto KM, et al. De novo NAD. *Nat Med.* 2018;24(9):1351–1359. doi:10.1038/s41591-018-0138-z.

75. Raines NH, Ganatra S, Nissaisorakarn P, et al. Niacinamide May Be Associated with Improved Outcomes in COVID-19-Related Acute Kidney Injury: An Observational Study. *Kidney360.* 2021;2(1):33–41. doi:10.34067/kid.0006452020.

76. Gottlieb RL, Nirula A, Chen P, et al. Effect of Bamlanivimab as Monotherapy or in Combination With Etesevimab on Viral Load in Patients With Mild to Moderate COVID-19: A Randomized Clinical Trial. *JAMA.* 2021;325(7):632–644. doi:10.1001/jama.2021.0202.

77. Chen P, Nirula A, Heller B, et al. SARS-CoV-2 Neutralizing Antibody LY-CoV555 in Outpatients with Covid-19. *N Engl J Med.* 2021;384(3):229–237. doi:10.1056/NEJMoa2029849.

78. Ferrario CM, Jessup J, Chappell MC, et al. Effect of angiotensin-converting enzyme inhibition and angiotensin II receptor blockers on cardiac angiotensin-converting enzyme 2. *Circulation.* 2005;111(20):2605–2610. doi:10.1161/CIRCULATIONAHA.104.510461.

79. South AM, Tomlinson L, Edmonston D, Hiremath S, Sparks MA. Controversies of renin-angiotensin system inhibition during the COVID-19 pandemic. *Nat Rev Nephrol.* 2020;16(6):305–307. doi:10.1038/s41581-020-0279-4.

80. Lopes RD, Macedo AVS, de Barros E, Silva PGM, et al. Effect of Discontinuing vs Continuing Angiotensin-Converting Enzyme Inhibitors and Angiotensin II Receptor Blockers on Days Alive and Out of the Hospital in Patients Admitted With COVID-19: A Randomized Clinical Trial. *JAMA.* 2021;325(3):254–264. doi:10.1001/jama.2020.25864.

81. Mehta N, Kalra A, Nowacki AS, et al. Association of Use of Angiotensin-Converting Enzyme Inhibitors and Angiotensin II Receptor Blockers With Testing Positive for Coronavirus Disease 2019 (COVID-19). *JAMA Cardiol.* 2020;5(9):1020–1026. doi:10.1001/jamacardio.2020.1855.

82. de Abajo FJ, Rodríguez-Martín S, Lerma V, et al. Use of renin-angiotensin-aldosterone system inhibitors and risk of COVID-19 requiring admission to hospital: a case-population study. *Lancet.* 2020;395(10238):1705–1714. doi:10.1016/S0140-6736(20)31030-8.

83. Gaudry S, Hajage D, Schortgen F, et al. Initiation Strategies for Renal-Replacement Therapy in the Intensive Care Unit. *N Engl J Med.* 2016;375(2):122–133. doi:10.1056/NEJMoa1603017.

84. Barbar SD, Clere-Jehl R, Bourredjem A, et al. Timing of Renal-Replacement Therapy in Patients with Acute Kidney Injury and Sepsis. *N Engl J Med.* 2018;379(15):1431–1442. doi:10.1056/NEJMoa1803213.

85. Gaudry S, Hajage D, Benichou N, et al. Delayed versus early initiation of renal replacement therapy for severe acute kidney injury: a systematic review and individual patient data meta-analysis of randomised clinical trials. *Lancet.* 2020;395(10235):1506–1515. doi:10.1016/S0140-6736(20)30531-6.

86. Group KDIGO KAKIW. KDIGO Clinical Practice Guideline for Acute Kidney Injury. *Kidney Int.* 2012;Supplement(2):1–138.

87. Burgner A, Golper T. Walkaway PIRRT (as SLED) for Acute Kidney Injury. *Clin J Am Soc Nephrol.* 2020;16(1):138–140. doi:10.2215/CJN.07510520.

88. Srivatana V, Aggarwal V, Finkelstein FO, Naljayan M, Crabtree JH, Perl J. Peritoneal Dialysis for Acute Kidney Injury Treatment in the United States: Brought to You by the COVID-19 Pandemic. *Kidney360.* 2020;1(5):410–415. doi:10.34067/kid.0002152020.

89. Malas MB, Naazie IN, Elsayed N, Mathlouthi A, Marmor R, Clary B. Thromboembolism risk of COVID-19 is high and associated with a higher risk of mortality: A systematic review and meta-analysis. *EClinicalMedicine.* 2020;29:100639. doi:10.1016/j.eclinm.2020.100639.

90. Shankaranarayanan D, Muthukumar T, Barbar T, et al. Anticoagulation Strategies and Filter Life in COVID-19 Patients Receiving Continuous Renal Replacement Therapy: A Single-Center Experience. *Clin J Am Soc Nephrol.* 2020;16(1):124–126. doi:10.2215/CJN.08430520.

91. Bikdeli B, Madhavan MV, Jimenez D, et al. COVID-19 and Thrombotic or Thromboembolic Disease: Implications for Prevention, Antithrombotic Therapy, and Follow-Up: JACC State-of-the-Art Review. *J Am Coll Cardiol.* 2020;75(23):2950–2973. doi:10.1016/j.jacc.2020.04.031.

92. Endres P, Rosovsky R, Zhao S, et al. Filter clotting with continuous renal replacement therapy in COVID-19. *J Thromb Thrombolysis.* 2021;51(4):966–970. doi:10.1007/s11239-020-02301-6.

93. Arnold F, Westermann L, Rieg S, et al. Comparison of different anticoagulation strategies for renal replacement therapy in critically ill patients with COVID-19: a cohort study. *BMC Nephrol.* 2020;21(1):486. doi:10.1186/s12882-020-02150-8.

94. Corbett RW, Blakey S, Nitsch D, et al. Epidemiology of COVID-19 in an Urban Dialysis Center. *J Am Soc Nephrol.* 2020;31(8):1815–1823. doi:10.1681/ASN.2020040534.

95. Xiong F, Tang H, Liu L, et al. Clinical Characteristics of and Medical Interventions for COVID-19 in Hemodialysis Patients in Wuhan, China. *J Am Soc Nephrol.* 2020;31(7):1387–1397. doi:10.1681/ASN.2020030354.

96. Weiss S, Bhat P, Del Pilar Fernandez M, Bhat JG, Coritsidis GN. COVID-19 Infection in ESKD: Findings from a Prospective Disease Surveillance Program at Dialysis Facilities in New York City and Long Island. *J Am Soc Nephrol.* 2020;31(11):2517–2521. doi:10.1681/ASN.2020070932.

97. Alberici F, Delbarba E, Manenti C, et al. A report from the Brescia Renal COVID Task Force on the clinical characteristics and short-term outcome of hemodialysis patients with SARS-CoV-2 infection. *Kidney Int.* 2020;98(1):20–26. doi:10.1016/j.kint.2020.04.030.

98. Zhang J, Cao F, Wu SK, et al. Clinical characteristics of 31 hemodialysis patients with 2019 novel coronavirus: a retrospective study. *Ren Fail.* 2020;42(1):726–732. doi:10.1080/0886022X.2020.1796705.

99. Valeri AM, Robbins-Juarez SY, Stevens JS, et al. Presentation and Outcomes of Patients with ESKD and COVID-19. *J Am Soc Nephrol.* 2020;31(7):1409–1415. doi:10.1681/ASN.2020040470.

100. Ng JH, Hirsch JS, Wanchoo R, et al. Outcomes of patients with end-stage kidney disease hospitalized with COVID-19. *Kidney Int.* 12. 2020;98(6):1530–1539. doi:10.1016/j.kint.2020.07.030.

101. Hsu CM, Weiner DE, Aweh G, et al. COVID-19 Among US Dialysis Patients: Risk Factors and Outcomes From a National Dialysis Provider. *Am J Kidney Dis.* 2021;77(5):748–756.e1. doi:10.1053/j.ajkd.2021.01.003.

102. Oniszczuk J, Moktefi A, Mausoleo A, et al. De Novo Focal and Segmental Glomerulosclerosis After COVID-19 in a Patient With a Transplanted Kidney From a Donor With a High-risk APOL1 Variant. *Transplantation.* 2021;105(1):206–211. doi:10.1097/TP.0000000000003432.

103. Webb C, Davidson B, Jones ESW, et al. COVID-19-Associated Graft Loss From Renal Infarction in a Kidney Transplant Recipient. *Kidney Int Rep.* 2021;6(4):1166–1169. doi:10.1016/j.ekir.2021.01.009.

104. Xu JJ, Samaha D, Mondhe S, Massicotte-Azarniouch D, Knoll G, Ruzicka M. Renal infarct in a COVID-19-positive kidney-pancreas transplant recipient. *Am J Transplant.* 2020;20(11):3221–3224. doi:10.1111/ajt.16089.

105. Jespersen Nizamic T, Huang Y, Alnimri M, Cheng M, Chen LX, Jen KY. COVID-19 Manifesting as Renal Allograft Dysfunction, Acute Pancreatitis, and Thrombotic Microangiopathy: A Case Report. *Transplant Proc.* 2021;53(4):1211–1214. 0. doi:10.1016/j.transproceed.2020.10.048.

106. Lazareth H, Péré H, Binois Y, et al. COVID-19-Related Collapsing Glomerulopathy in a Kidney Transplant Recipient. *Am J Kidney Dis.* 2020;76(4):590–594. doi:10.1053/j.ajkd.2020.06.009.

107. Chen Y, Trofe J, Gordon J, et al. Interplay of cellular and humoral immune responses against BK virus in kidney transplant recipients with polyomavirus nephropathy. *J Virol.* 2006;80(7):3495–3505. doi:10.1128/JVI.80.7.3495-3505.2006.

108. Masset C, Ville S, Halary F, et al. Resurgence of BK virus following Covid-19 in kidney transplant recipients. *Transpl Infect Dis.* 2021;23(1):e13465. doi:10.1111/tid.13465.

109. Favà A, Cucchiari D, Montero N, et al. Clinical characteristics and risk factors for severe COVID-19 in hospitalized kidney transplant recipients: A multicentric cohort study. *Am J Transplant.* 2020;20(11):3030–3041. doi:10.1111/ajt.16246.

110. D'Orsogna L, van den Heuvel H, van Kooten C, Heidt S, Claas FHJ. Infectious pathogens may trigger specific allo-HLA reactivity via multiple mechanisms. *Immunogenetics.* 2017;69(8-9):631–641. doi:10.1007/s00251-017-0989-3.

111. Azzi Y, Bartash R, Scalea J, Loarte-Campos P, Akalin E. COVID-19 and Solid Organ Transplantation: A Review Article. *Transplantation.* 2021;105(1):37–55. doi:10.1097/TP.0000000000003523.

112. Cravedi P, Mothi SS, Azzi Y, et al. COVID-19 and kidney transplantation: Results from the TANGO International Transplant Consortium. *Am J Transplant.* 2020;20(11):3140–3148. doi:10.1111/ajt.16185.

113. Sánchez-Álvarez JE, Pérez Fontán M, Jiménez Martín C, et al. [SARS-CoV-2 infection in patients on renal replacement therapy. Report of the COVID-19 Registry of the Spanish Society of Nephrology (SEN)]. *Nefrologia.* 2020;40(3):272–278. doi:10.1016/j.nefro.2020.04.002.

114. Jager KJ, Kramer A, Chesnaye NC, et al. Results from the ERA-EDTA Registry indicate a high mortality due to COVID-19 in dialysis patients and kidney transplant recipients across Europe. *Kidney Int.* 2020;98(6):1540–1548. doi:10.1016/j.kint.2020.09.006.

115. Caillard S, Anglicheau D, Matignon M, et al. An initial report from the French SOT COVID Registry suggests high mortality due to COVID-19 in recipients of kidney transplants. *Kidney Int.* 2020;98(6):1549–1558. doi:10.1016/j.kint.2020.08.005.

116. Elias M, Pievani D, Randoux C, et al. COVID-19 Infection in Kidney Transplant Recipients: Disease Incidence and Clinical Outcomes. *J Am Soc Nephrol.* 2020;31(10):2413–2423. doi:10.1681/ASN.2020050639.

117. Azzi Y, Parides M, Alani O, et al. COVID-19 infection in kidney transplant recipients at the epicenter of pandemics. *Kidney Int.* 2020;98(6):1559–1567. doi:10.1016/j.kint.2020.10.004.

118. Chaudhry ZS, Williams JD, Vahia A, et al. Clinical characteristics and outcomes of COVID-19 in solid organ transplant recipients: A cohort study. *Am J Transplant.* 2020;20(11):3051–3060. doi:10.1111/ajt.16188.

119. Caillard S, Chavarot N, Francois H, et al. Is COVID-19 infection more severe in kidney transplant recipients?. *Am J Transplant.* 2021;21(3):1295–1303. doi:10.1111/ajt.16424.

120. Chavarot N, Gueguen J, Bonnet G, et al. COVID-19 severity in kidney transplant recipients is similar to nontransplant patients with similar comorbidities. *Am J Transplant.* 2021;21(3):1285–1294. doi:10.1111/ajt.16416.

121. Williamson EJ, Walker AJ, Bhaskaran K, et al. Factors associated with COVID-19-related death using OpenSAFELY. *Nature.* 2020;584(7821):430–436. doi:10.1038/s41586-020-2521-4 08.

122. Maggiore U, Abramowicz D, Crespo M, et al. How should I manage immunosuppression in a kidney transplant patient with COVID-19? An ERA-EDTA DESCARTES expert opinion. *Nephrol Dial Transplant.* 2020;35(6):899–904. doi:10.1093/ndt/gfaa130.

123. Santeusanio AD, Menon MC, Liu C, et al. Influence of patient characteristics and immunosuppressant management on mortality in kidney transplant recipients hospitalized with coronavirus disease 2019 (COVID-19). *Clin Transplant.* 2021;35(4):e14221. doi:10.1111/ctr.14221.

124. Clarke C, Lucisano G, Prendecki M, et al. Informing the risk of kidney transplantation versus remaining on the waitlist in the coronavirus disease 2019 era. *Kidney Int Rep.* 2021;6(1):46–55. doi:10.1016/j.ekir.2020.10.032.

125. Mamode N, Ahmed Z, Jones G, et al. Mortality rates in transplant recipients and transplantation candidates in a high-prevalence COVID-19 environment. *Transplantation.* 2021;105(1):212–215. doi:10.1097/TP.0000000000003533.

126. Ravanan R, Callaghan CJ, Mumford L, et al. SARS-CoV-2 infection and early mortality of waitlisted and solid organ transplant recipients in England: a national cohort study. *Am J Transplant.* 2020;20(11):3008–3018. doi:10.1111/ajt.16247.

127. Craig-Schapiro R, Salinas T, Lubetzky M, et al. COVID-19 outcomes in patients waitlisted for kidney transplantation and kidney transplant recipients. *Am J Transplant.* 2021;21(4):1576–1585. doi:10.1111/ajt.16351.

128. Thaunat O, Legeai C, Anglicheau D, et al. IMPact of the COVID-19 epidemic on the moRTAlity of kidney transplant recipients and candidates in a French Nationwide registry sTudy (IMPORTANT). *Kidney Int.* 2020;98(6):1568–1577. doi:10.1016/j.kint.2020.10.008.

CHAPTER

11 Ophthalmic Manifestations of COVID-19

Behin Barahimi, MD, Cullen P. Moran, MD, Alexander De Castro-Abeger, MD, and Sylvia Groth, MD

OUTLINE

Introduction and Historical Perspectives

In late December 2019, an ophthalmologist named Li Wenliang sent a message to a group of fellow physicians in Wuhan, China, warning them of an emerging respiratory illness that he thought bore resemblance to severe acute respiratory syndrome (SARS). Weeks later, after local authorities admonished him for "spreading rumors," Dr. Li contracted the virus from one of his glaucoma patients and passed away.[2]

Ophthalmological manifestations of members of the *Coronaviridae* family were documented long before SARS-CoV-2 surfaced in humans. In the mid-20th century, a murine coronavirus was demonstrated to infect central nervous system cells[3] and was later shown to cause a biphasic infection of the mouse retina characterized by early vasculitis and subsequent retinal degeneration.[4] Later, with the first outbreak of the SARS pandemic in 2003, it was demonstrated that SARS-CoV-1 could cause conjunctivitis in humans[5,6] and was detectable in tear samples.[7] In fact, the first diagnosis of a new SARS-CoV-1 strain was made in a 7-month-old child with conjunctivitis.[5] It was also hypothesized that transmission of SARS-CoV-1 could occur through the ocular surface, because contact with SARS patient secretions without eye protection was an independent risk factor for transmission of the virus.[8]

Since Dr. Li's death, ophthalmologists have remained on the front lines of the COVID-19 pandemic and will continue to play an important role in prevention and detection of SARS-CoV-2 in the months and years to come. The physical examination is a critical component of an ophthalmology visit, and the close proximity necessitated by the slit-lamp examination is well within the range of droplets expelled by conversation and normal breathing that may harbor the virus.[9,10] Therefore it is essential that all health care workers who care for patients with eye conditions be prepared to recognize the role that the ocular surface plays in transmission of the virus, the ophthalmic manifestations of COVID-19, and the therapeutic interventions.

Role of the Eye in Transmission and Prevention

The surface of the eye is an important route of transmission for many pathogens, and coronaviruses are no exception. Surface proteins angiotensin-converting enzyme-2 (ACE2) and transmembrane protease serine 2 must be present for SARS-CoV-2 to invade human cells, and both receptors have been shown to be consistently expressed on the cornea, pointing to a possible route of ocular infection.[11] ACE2 expression also has been demonstrated on the conjunctiva and in the aqueous humor.[12]

In addition to being a potential site of inoculation, the eye also may play a role in viral shedding. Studies of a feline coronavirus have demonstrated that the offspring of infected cats have detectable live coronavirus on the conjunctiva, suggesting that ocular secretions are potentially infectious.[13] Studies conducted in China early in the pandemic showed that a small number of patients had tear samples that were positive for SARS-CoV-2 antigens.[14,15] In a more recent study conducted in Italy, SARS-CoV-2 RNA was detected on the surface of the eye in 52 of 91 patients with COVID-19.[16]

Lending further credence to the idea that SARS-CoV-2 transmission may occur through the ocular surface, a study conducted in China found that patients who wore eyeglasses daily may be less likely to contract the virus.[17] This finding prompted many health care institutions to require eye protection for all employees who encounter patients during the pandemic. The decreased susceptibility to infection in eyeglass wearers suggests that the barrier provided by the glasses prevents contact of the ocular surface with droplets that may be expelled by patients as they cough, speak, or breathe. Alternatively, glasses could provide a deterrent to inadvertent touching of the eyes with hands that are contaminated with viral particles. Contact lens wearers are not afforded the same protection, but they also are not at any increased risk for infection, despite regularly touching their eyes to place and remove contact lenses.[18]

Ocular Manifestations

Epidemiology

Reports of the prevalence of ophthalmic manifestations of COVID-19 vary across studies. Most systematic reviews estimate the range is from 4% to 11%,[19,20] but some case series place the prevalence as high as 47%.[1] The most common ophthalmic manifestation is conjunctivitis. Ocular disease beyond conjunctivitis is rare and not widely reported in the literature. In one comprehensive review, only 8 of 43 studies reported additional ophthalmic manifestations, including keratitis, nodular scleritis, neuroophthalmological manifestations, and optic nerve findings.[20] Other case series and reports have identified signs and symptoms of COVID-19 in the orbit, eyelid, retina, microvasculature, and uvea (see Table 11.1). These reports are limited in their scope and must be approached with the understanding that more data are needed before it can be determined with certainty whether any given eye complaint is a result of a SARS-CoV-2 infection or if the patient was simply experiencing an unrelated eye condition when he or she contracted COVID-19.

The remainder of this section will discuss the current literature at the time of publication for reported manifestations of COVID-19 in the anterior segment of the eye, orbit, eyelid, retina, microvasculature, and uvea and neuroophthalmological manifestations and specific considerations for pediatric populations. The information here will undoubtedly change as the ophthalmology community learns more about the effects of SARS-CoV-2 on the eyes, and thus it will be updated accordingly in future editions.

Anterior Segment

The conjunctiva is a mucous membrane that covers the surface of the eye and the inner surface of the eyelids. Inflammation of the conjunctiva, called conjunctivitis, is the most common ocular manifestation of COVID-19, with an overall rate of 1.1% and representing an estimated 88% of ocular disease in COVID-19 patients.[19,21]

Table 11.1 Structures of the Eye and Orbit and Their Associated COVID-19 Manifestations

Structure	Pathology
Anterior segment	Conjunctivitis, episcleritis, keratitis, uveitis
Retina	Central retinal artery occlusion, central retinal vein occlusion, retinal nerve fiber layer edema, vitreous hemorrhage
Cranial nerves and optic pathway	Neuromyelitis optica spectrum disorder (NMOSD), Miller-Fisher syndrome, CN II–XII palsies, myasthenia gravis, encephalitis, opsoclonus-myoclonus, cavernous sinus thrombosis
Eyelids and orbit	Blepharitis, orbital cellulitis, orbital myositis

Reported signs and symptoms of COVID-19 conjunctivitis range from mild tearing and foreign body sensation to severe symptoms such as photophobia, mucous secretions, and eyelid swelling.[20] Other reported symptoms include eye pain, burning sensation, itching, conjunctival hyperemia, chemosis, and dry eye.[20,22] One systematic review reported findings of fibrin and inflammatory cell pseudomembranes on the tarsal conjunctiva, as well as tarsal petechiae, hemorrhages, and mucus filaments.[20] Systemic findings associated with conjunctivitis, in addition to the known respiratory and constitutional symptoms of COVID-19, include lymphadenopathy in the preauricular, submandibular, and cervical chains.

One meta-analysis found an association between conjunctivitis and a higher severity of COVID-19, with conjunctivitis being present in 3% of severely ill patients and 0.7% of patients with milder symptoms.[21] This finding indicates that providers should recognize conjunctivitis as a possible sign of more severe disease in COVID-19 patients and further underscores the importance of eye protection for health workers when caring for COVID-19 patients. More data are needed to evaluate the utility of such reports in the larger context of ocular manifestations of COVID-19.

Despite conjunctivitis being the most common ocular manifestation of COVID-19, the association between SARS-CoV-2 positivity on conjunctival swab and conjunctivitis remains ambiguous. In a study of 30 patients with COVID-19, only 1 patient had conjunctivitis and on polymerase chain reaction (PCR) evaluation was found to have SARS-CoV-2 RNA in the tear film.[14] In a separate study that included 10 COVID-19 patients with ocular symptoms, SARS-CoV-2 was not detected in tear samples of any patients.[22] Yet another study found a prevalence of ocular symptoms of 32%, with only 5% of the patients having SARS-CoV-2 nucleotides in conjunctival specimens.[23] From these studies it is clear that ocular symptoms can occur even in the absence of viral shedding in tears.

Keratitis and episcleritis, or inflammation of the cornea and the episcleral coat of the eye, also have been noted in case reports.[24–26] One case report notes pseudodendrites like those seen in herpetic keratitis that later evolved into dozens of subepithelial infiltrates with overlying epithelial defects across the cornea.[24]

Uvea

The uvea is the middle layer of the eye involving the choroid, ciliary body, iris, and the associated vasculature of these structures. Uveitis is inflammation of the uvea and nearby structures such as the sclera, vitreous, and retina. The uveitides are a collection of about 30 different diseases.[27] They are organized by location of primary inflammation (anterior, intermediate, posterior, and panuveitis) and whether they are infectious, associated with systemic autoinflammatory/autoimmune disease, or immune-mediated and limited to the eye without other signs of systemic inflammation.[28] Although there have been reports of SARS-CoV-2 on the ocular surface, studies have yet to demonstrate active virus intraocularly.[29,30] Therefore it is suspected that any uveitis associated with COVID-19 is more likely a result of systemic or autoimmune inflammation.

Two case reports demonstrate autoinflammatory-mediated uveitis in the context of COVID-19. In the first report, a 54-year-old woman presented to an ophthalmology clinic with 2 weeks of bilateral blurry vision after being managed as an inpatient for COVID-19 multisystem inflammatory syndrome. Her ophthalmic examination had evidence of anterior chamber inflammation, keratic precipitates, corneal edema with Descemet folds, and decreased vision. She was managed successfully with topical steroids and cycloplegics.[31] A second case report by Alonso et al.[32] describes a patient with anterior uveitis associated with ocular hypertension, which was also thought to be secondary to multisystem inflammatory syndrome.

Although the described cases presented after a known infection of COVID-19, there have been cases in which the manifesting sign of COVID-19 was uveitis. A 60-year-old woman presented to the emergency department with ocular pain, redness, and decreased vision in her left eye. On examination she had anterior chamber inflammation, vitreous inflammation, and optic nerve edema consistent with acute panuveitis. Initial infectious serological studies for syphilis, toxoplasmosis, and human immunodeficiency virus were negative. She was presumed to have Vogt-Koyanagi-Harada disease and was started on oral steroids. Ten days later she developed a cough and systemic symptoms and tested positive for COVID-19. She was treated systemically and did well, including improved visual acuity in the left eye. Even in this case, anterior chamber PCR was negative for the SARS-CoV-2 virus.[33]

Retina

In studies of coronavirus in animal models, the JMHV strain was demonstrated to affect cells that are found in the retina and posterior pole of mice,[13] specifically glial cells, astrocytes, oligodendrocytes, and microglia. Moreover, COVID-19 infection has been associated with microvascular disease and coagulation disorders.[34] With these neuronal and vascular manifestations of coronaviruses in mind, it is no surprise that retinal findings have been noted in some patients with COVID-19. In one cross-sectional study, patients with known COVID-19 (n = 54) demonstrated dilated veins (27.7%), tortuosity of vasculature (12.9%), retinal hemorrhages (9.25%), and cotton-wool spots (7.4%) on fundus photos. In addition, there was a significant increase in diameter of the retinal arteries and veins in the COVID-19 patients compared with those in controls, and the mean vein diameter was positively associated with COVID-19 in severe and nonsevere cases compared with unexposed controls. However, dilated veins are not always visible by clinical examination and require computer programming for accurate interpretation.[35]

Overall, the retinal manifestations of COVID-19, like the uveitic manifestations, mostly likely are sequelae of the infection rather than acute infection itself. The most common retinal findings in COVID-19 patients are microangiographic changes and consequences of microvascular compromise. These findings are likely related to both hypoxia and the cytokines associated with the inflammatory response to the virus. Gonzalez-Lopez et al.[36] reported a case of a 50-year-old patient in the late phase of acute COVID-19 infection receiving inpatient treatment for severe infection requiring antivirals, hydroxychloroquine, systemic steroids, and high-flow oxygen therapy.[36] On day 7 of his care, he noted an inferior "crescent-shaped" blind spot that had been increasing without pain or other symptoms. Although his vision was good and the anterior segment examination was normal, fundus examination revealed peripapillary cotton wool spots in both eyes without hemorrhages. Optical coherence tomography (OCT) demonstrated retinal nerve fiber layer edema in the area associated with his scotoma.

Other microvascular retinal findings in patients with COVID-19 include central retinal artery occlusion (CRAO) and central retinal vein occlusion (CRVO). CRAO is the ophthalmic equivalent of a stroke and is due to a lack of blood flow through the central retinal artery (see Figure 11.1). Usually, a CRAO manifests as monocular central vision loss and in one case report was the manifesting symptom of a patient with severe COVID-19 who required intensive care unit treatment with intubation.[37] Other case reports describe CRAOs that developed in patients who were recovering from severe COVID-19 infections.[38,39] CRVOs, on the other hand, are due to venous outflow stasis from the retina. The suspected

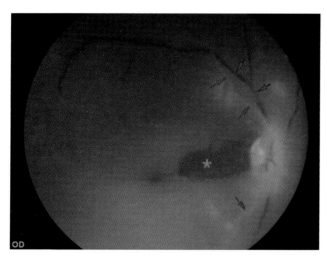

Fig. 11.1 FundusImage From the Right Eye of a COVID-19 Patient With Central Retinal Artery Occlusion (CRAO). The retinal arteries are not perfused *(red arrows)*, and there is retinal vein "boxcarring" *(blue arrows)*. There is cilioretinal artery sparing *(green asterisk)*, but it does not extend to the fovea. There is retinal whitening and a "cherry red" fovea, corresponding to diffuse nerve fiber layer edema. (From Murchison AP, Sweid A, Dharia R, et al. Monocular visual loss as the presenting symptom of COVID-19 infection. *Clin Neurol Neurosurg.* 2021;201:106440. doi:10.1016/j.clineuro.2020.106440.)

pathophysiology of CRVO in COVID-19 is related to endothelial cell damage and inflammation leading to stasis. CRVOs have been reported in a wide range of patients from a previously healthy 33-year-old[40] to a case of bilateral CRVOs in an obese patient with COVID-19.[41]

In addition, a case of paracentral acute middle maculopathy (PAMM), or irregularities seen in the middle layers on the retina on OCT, was diagnosed in a patient who developed a CRAO after a mild case of COVID-19. Two weeks after his COVID-19 diagnosis, this patient's vision declined severely, and on fundoscopic examination a CRAO was seen. Of note, the hypercoagulable workup was negative. He had an OCT demonstrating diffuse reflectance and thickening of the inner nuclear layer of the retina consistent with PAMM.[42]

Neuroophthalmology

Previous coronaviruses have demonstrated neurological complications in both animal and human models. A murine coronavirus has been shown to lead to demyelination,[43] and a coronavirus that affects nonhuman primates has been found in high concentrations in perivascular neural tissue.[44] Previous studies in humans discovered SARS in the cytoplasm of hypothalamic and cortical neurons,[45] and there is one report of a child who was clinically diagnosed with acute disseminated encephalomyelitis and the only detected microbe in the cerebrospinal fluid was a coronavirus.[46]

One of the most common symptoms of SARS-CoV-2 is loss of taste and smell, thought to be secondary to direct involvement of the virus with the olfactory nerve.[47] As the virus commonly affects the first cranial nerve (CN I), it should come as no surprise that the optic nerve can also be affected. Each optic nerve is a collection of approximately 1.5 million nerve fibers that coalesce from the retinal nerve fiber layer and travel to the brain. Diseases of the optic nerve associated with COVID-19 include direct neuronal inflammation, such as optic neuritis, as well as microvascular compromise to the nerve, such as ischemic optic neuropathy (ION). There have been two reported cases of anterior ION, a disease associated with microvascular compromise of the anterior optic nerve head.[48,49]

Neuromyelitis optica spectrum disorder (NMOSD) is an inflammatory condition of the nervous system that often involves the optic nerves and spinal cord with known causes (anti–aquaporin-4 and myelin oligodendrocyte glycoprotein–immunoglobulin G [MOG-IgG] antibodies, among others) and seronegative/idiopathic causes. As we are discovering, COVID-19 may be an inciting factor for NMOSD. In one report, a 15-year-old boy in the Netherlands presented with 7 days of worsening vision loss with associated flashing lights and headache a few weeks after being diagnosed with a mild nonspecific viral illness, which was presumed by the study authors to be COVID-19. He was found to have bilateral optic disc edema with decreased vision in both eyes. Magnetic resonance imaging (MRI) of the brain and orbits demonstrated longitudinal enhancement of bilateral optic nerves consistent with NMOSD, and follow-up serological testing confirmed MOG-IgG positivity.[50] In another study, an 11-year-old boy presented with redness and pain in both eyes after a febrile illness. Two weeks later, he developed sudden severe vision loss in the right eye and was found to have right optic nerve edema with an associated relative afferent pupillary defect. He was later found to be positive for both COVID-19 and MOG-IgG, and MRI findings were consistent with NMOSD.[51] The patients in both cases responded well to steroid therapy. In another case, a 39-year-old woman with previously diagnosed anti-MOG NMOSD was found to have a flare of her optic neuritis and confirmed COVID-19 positive on nasal swab.[52]

There have been multiple reports of CN palsies associated with COVID-19 infection, from both microvascular compromise and direct neuronal inflammation. MRI findings of enhancement and thickening of the nerves have been associated with direct inflammation or postinfectious nerve palsy. With respect to CN III palsies, they are most often reported as a postinfectious/inflammatory change associated with COVID-19 and/or associated with systemic inflammation in a Miller-Fisher syndrome subtype of Guillain-Barré syndrome.[53,54] There are also reports of CN III palsies resulting from microvascular compromise. In one case, a previously healthy 67-year-old man presented with double vision 1 month after being diagnosed with COVID-19 and was found to have a left CN III palsy (see

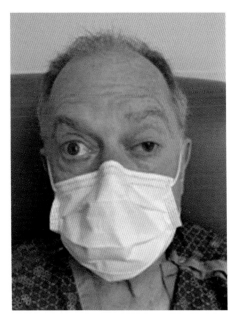

Fig. 11.2 COVID-19 Patient Presenting With a Cranial Nerve III Palsy. (Image used with permission from John Fitzpatrick.)

Figure 11.2). An MRI of the brain demonstrated scattered nonspecific changes of the affected oculomotor nerve, which indicates microvascular ischemic changes. He was found to have an elevated D-dimer and otherwise negative workup, including systemic causes of microvascular disease. It is postulated that COVID-19 led to microvascular compromise of the left CN III.[55] Similarly, there have been multiple case reports of CN IV and CN VI palsies in suspected microvascular and postinflammatory cranial neuropathy.[56,57] Finally, there have been cases of myasthenia gravis after infection with COVID-19, indicating an autoimmune mechanism. There are three reported cases of acetylcholine receptor antibody–positive myasthenia gravis with a wide array of manifesting symptoms, including ptosis and diplopia roughly 5 to 7 days after febrile illness from presumed COVID-19.[58]

As we move further posteriorly in the anatomy of the ophthalmic system, there have been case reports of eye movement abnormalities associated with COVID-19 encephalitis,[59,60] postinfectious brainstem syndrome,[61] and opsoclonus-myoclonus.[62]

Larger vascular compromise and hypercoagulable disorders such as cavernous sinus thrombosis (CST) and cerebral venous sinus thrombosis (CVST) are a growing concern after COVID-19. CST has been reported in the acute infectious period[63] and after recovery from the infection.[64] Some providers recommend excluding the diagnosis of CVST in COVID-19–positive patients presenting with focal neurological deficits, progressive headaches, and/or other signs of increased intracranial pressure as a result of its prevalence.

Eyelids and Orbit

SARS-CoV-2 infection has been shown to have ophthalmic manifestations that extend beyond the globe to involve the eyelids and orbit. In one cohort study out of Italy, 11 of 29 patients hospitalized for COVID-19 presented with signs of blepharitis, including crusting of the eyelashes, lid margin hyperemia and telangiectasias, and alterations in the meibomian orifices.[22] Other reports have noted that orbital infections can occur in the setting of COVID-19 secondary to nasal congestion and sinus obstruction.[65,66] Additionally, the immune response to SARS-CoV-2 has been linked in one study to the development of unilateral orbital myositis, or inflammation of the extraocular muscles.[67]

Pediatric Ophthalmic Manifestations

The systematic course of COVID-19 infection in children has been milder than in adults, as have the ocular manifestations.[20] However, there have been increasing reports of multisystem inflammatory syndrome, a syndrome similar to Kawasaki disease in which conjunctivitis is common.[68] Furthermore, some newborns with suspected COVID-19 were found to have hemorrhagic conjunctivitis with serous chemosis and fundus findings of cotton wool spots and vitreous hemorrhage.[69] As in adults, the relationship between ocular symptoms and SARS-CoV-2 positivity on conjunctival swab in pediatric patients is unclear; in one study, all pediatric patients with ocular manifestations of COVID-19 had negative PCR results of ocular samples, despite being positive for SARS-CoV-2 IgG by serology.[70]

Conclusion

Eye care providers play an important role in the detection and prevention of COVID-19. In the context of the COVID-19 pandemic, and considering the data presented in this chapter, providers should proceed with an increased index of suspicion for patients presenting with common ocular complaints such as conjunctivitis. As we learn more about the natural history of COVID-19, our understanding of ocular manifestations of the disease will continue to improve, as will our strategies for treating its still emerging ophthalmic sequelae.

REFERENCES

1. Gangaputra SS, Patel SN. Ocular symptoms among nonhospitalized patients who underwent COVID-19 testing. *Ophthalmology*. 2020;127(10):1425–1427. doi:10.1016/j.ophtha.2020.06.037.
2. Green A. Li wenliang (obituary). *The Lancet*. 2020;395(10225):682. doi:10.1016/S0140-6736(20)30382-2.
3. Bailey OT, Pappenheimer AM, Cheever FS, Daniels JB. A murine virus (JHM) causing disseminated encephalomyelitis with extensive destruction of myelin. *The Journal of Experimental*

Medicine. 1949;90(3):195–212. https://www.ncbi.nlm.nih.gov/pmc/articles/PMC2135909/.

4. Hooks JJ, Percopo C, Wang Y, Detrick B. Retina and retinal pigment epithelial cell autoantibodies are produced during murine coronavirus retinopathy. *The Journal of Immunology.* 1993;151(6):3381–3389. https://www-jimmunol-org.proxy.library.vanderbilt.edu/content/151/6/3381.

5. van der Hoek L, Pyrc K, Jebbink MF, et al. Identification of a new human coronavirus. *Nature Medicine.* 2004;10(4):368–373. doi:10.1038/nm1024.

6. Vabret A, Mourez T, Dina J, et al. Human coronavirus NL63, France. *Emerging Infectious Diseases.* 2005;11(8):1225–1229. doi:10.3201/eid1108.050110

7. Loon S-C, Teoh SCB, Oon LLE, et al. The severe acute respiratory syndrome coronavirus in tears. *The British Journal of Ophthalmology.* 2004;88(7):861–863. doi:10.1136/bjo.2003.035931.

8. Raboud J, Shigayeva A, McGeer A, et al. Risk factors for SARS transmission from patients requiring intubation: a multicentre investigation in Toronto, Canada. *PLoS ONE.* 2010;5(5):e10717. doi:10.1371/journal.pone.0010717.

9. Abkarian M, Mendez S, Xue N, Yang F, Stone HA. Speech can produce jet-like transport relevant to asymptomatic spreading of virus. *Proceedings of the National Academy of Sciences.* 2020;117(41):25237–25245. doi:10.1073/pnas.2012156117.

10. Wen JC. Bacterial dispersal associated with speech in the setting of intravitreous injections. *Archives of Ophthalmology.* 2011;129(12):1551. doi:10.1001/archophthalmol.2011.227.

11. Ma D, Chen C-B, Jhanji V, et al. Expression of SARS-CoV-2 receptor ACE2 and TMPRSS2 in human primary conjunctival and pterygium cell lines and in mouse cornea. *Eye.* 2020;34(7):1212–1219. doi:10.1038/s41433-020-0939-4.

12. Holappa M, Vapaatalo H, Vaajanen A. Many faces of renin-angiotensin system: focus on eye. *The Open Ophthalmology Journal.* 2017;11:122–142. doi:10.2174/1874364101711010122.

13. Seah I, Agrawal R. Can the coronavirus disease 2019 (COVID-19) affect the eyes? A review of coronaviruses and ocular implications in humans and animals. *Ocular Immunology and Inflammation.* 2020;28(3):391–395. doi:10.1080/09273948.2020.1738501.

14. Xia J, Tong J, Liu M, Shen Y, Guo D. Evaluation of coronavirus in tears and conjunctival secretions of patients with SARS-CoV-2 infection. *Journal of Medical Virology.* 2020;92(6):589–594. doi:10.1002/jmv.25725.

15. Li M, Yang Y, He T, et al. Detection of SARS-CoV-2 in the ocular surface in different phases of COVID-19 patients in Shanghai, China. *Annals of Translational Medicine.* 2021;9(2):100. doi:10.21037/atm-20-6026.

16. Azzolini C, Donati S, Premi E, et al. SARS-CoV-2 on Ocular Surfaces in a Cohort of Patients With COVID-19 From the Lombardy Region, Italy. *JAMA Ophthalmology.* 2021;139(9):956–963. doi:10.1001/jamaophthalmol.2020.5464.

17. Zeng W, Wang X, Li J, et al. Association of Daily Wear of Eyeglasses With Susceptibility to Coronavirus Disease 2019 Infection. *JAMA Ophthalmology.* 2020;138(11):1196. doi:10.1001/jamaophthalmol.2020.3906.

18. Jones L, Walsh K, Willcox M, Morgan P, Nichols J. The COVID-19 pandemic: Important considerations for contact lens practitioners. *Contact Lens & Anterior Eye.* 2020;43(3):196–203. doi:10.1016/j.clae.2020.03.012.

19. Nasiri N, Sharifi H, Bazrafshan A, Noori A, Karamouzian M, Sharifi A. Ocular Manifestations of COVID-19: A Systematic Review and Meta-analysis. *Journal of Ophthalmic & Vision Research.* 2021;16(1):103–112. doi:10.18502/jovr.v16i1.8256.

20. Badawi AE, Elsheikh SS, Addeen SZ, et al. An ophthalmic insight into novel coronavirus 2019 disease: A comprehensive review of the ocular manifestations and clinical hazards. *Journal of Current Ophthalmology.* 2020;32(4):315–328. doi:10.4103/JOCO.JOCO_255_20.

21. Loffredo L, Pacella F, Pacella E, Tiscione G, Oliva A, Violi F. Conjunctivitis and COVID-19: A meta-analysis. *Journal of Medical Virology.* 2020;92(9):1413–1414. doi:10.1002/jmv.25938.

22. Meduri A, Oliverio GW, Mancuso G, et al. Ocular surface manifestation of COVID-19 and tear film analysis. *Scientific Reports.* 2020;10(1):20178. doi:10.1038/s41598-020-77194-9.

23. Wu P, Duan F, Luo C, et al. Characteristics of Ocular Findings of Patients With Coronavirus Disease 2019 (COVID-19) in Hubei Province, China. *JAMA Ophthalmology.* 2020;138(5):575. doi:10.1001/jamaophthalmol.2020.1291.

24. Cheema M, Aghazadeh H, Nazarali S, et al. Keratoconjunctivitis as the initial medical presentation of the novel coronavirus disease 2019 (COVID-19). *Canadian Journal of Ophthalmology Journal Canadien D'Ophtalmologie.* 2020;55(4):e125–e129. doi:10.1016/j.jcjo.2020.03.003.

25. Bostanci Ceran B, Ozates S. Ocular manifestations of coronavirus disease 2019. *Graefe's Archive for Clinical and Experimental Ophthalmology.* 2020;258(9):1959–1963. doi:10.1007/s00417-020-04777-7.

26. Méndez Mangana C, Barraquer Kargacin A, Barraquer RI. Episcleritis as an ocular manifestation in a patient with COVID-19. *Acta Ophthalmologica.* 2020;98(8):e1056–e1057. doi:10.1111/aos.14484.

27. Jabs DA, Busingye J. Approach to the diagnosis of the uveitides. *American Journal of Ophthalmology.* 2013;156(2):228–236. doi:10.1016/j.ajo.2013.03.027.

28. Burkholder BM, Jabs DA. Uveitis for the non-ophthalmologist. *The BMJ.* 2021;372. doi:10.1136/bmj.m4979.

29. Lauermann P, Storch M, Weig M, et al. There is no intraocular affection on a SARS-CoV-2 - Infected ocular surface. *American Journal of Ophthalmology Case Reports.* 2020;20:100884. doi:10.1016/j.ajoc.2020.100884.

30. List W, Regitnig P, Kashofer K, et al. Occurrence of SARS-CoV-2 in the intraocular milieu. *Experimental Eye Research.* 2020;201:108273. doi:10.1016/j.exer.2020.108273.

31. Bettach E, Zadok D, Weill Y, Brosh K, Hanhart J. Bilateral anterior uveitis as a part of a multisystem inflammatory syndrome secondary to COVID-19 infection. *Journal of Medical Virology.* 2021;93(1):139–140. doi:10.1002/jmv.26229.

32. Alonso RS, Alonso F de OM, Fernandes BF, Ecard V de O, Ventura MP. COVID-19 Related Ocular Hypertension Secondary to Anterior Uveitis as Part of a Multi-systemic Inflammatory Syndrome. *Journal of Glaucoma.* 2021;30(5):e256–e258. doi:10.1097/IJG.0000000000001835.

33. Benito-Pascual B, Gegúndez JA, Díaz-Valle D, et al. Panuveitis and Optic Neuritis as a Possible Initial Presentation of the Novel Coronavirus Disease 2019 (COVID-19). *Ocular Immunology and Inflammation.* 2020;28(6):922–925. doi:10.1080/09273948.2020.1792512.

34. Helms J, Tacquard C, Severac F, et al. High risk of thrombosis in patients with severe SARS-CoV-2 infection: a multicenter

prospective cohort study. *Intensive Care Medicine.* 2020;46(6):1089–1098. doi:10.1007/s00134-020-06062-x.

35. Invernizzi A, Torre A, Parrulli S, et al. Retinal findings in patients with COVID-19: Results from the SERPICO-19 study. *EClinicalMedicine.* 2020;27:100550. doi:10.1016/j.eclinm.2020.100550.

36. Gonzalez Lopez JJ, Felix Espinar B, Ye-Zhu C. Symptomatic Retinal Microangiopathy in a Patient with Coronavirus Disease 2019 (COVID-19): Single Case Report. *Ocular Immunology and Inflammation.* 2021;29(4):642–644. doi:10.1080/09273948.2020.1852260.

37. Murchison AP, Sweid A, Dharia R, et al. Monocular visual loss as the presenting symptom of COVID-19 infection. *Clinical Neurology and Neurosurgery.* 2021;201:106440. doi:10.1016/j.clineuro.2020.106440.

38. Acharya S, Diamond M, Anwar S, Glaser A, Tyagi P. Unique case of central retinal artery occlusion secondary to COVID-19 disease. *IDCases.* 2020;21:e00867. doi:10.1016/j.idcr.2020.e00867.

39. Montesel A, Bucolo C, Mouvet V, Moret E, Eandi CM. Case Report: Central Retinal Artery Occlusion in a COVID-19 Patient. *Frontiers in Pharmacology.* 2020;11:588384. doi:10.3389/fphar.2020.588384.

40. Yahalomi T, Pikkel J, Arnon R, Pessach Y. Central retinal vein occlusion in a young healthy COVID-19 patient: A case report. *American Journal of Ophthalmology Case Reports.* 2020;20:100992. doi:10.1016/j.ajoc.2020.100992.

41. Gaba WH, Ahmed D, al Nuaimi RK, Dhanhani AA, Eatamadi H. Bilateral Central Retinal Vein Occlusion in a 40-Year-Old Man with Severe Coronavirus Disease 2019 (COVID-19) Pneumonia. *The American Journal of Case Reports.* 2020;21:e927691. doi:10.12659/AJCR.927691.

42. Turedi N, Onal Gunay B. Paracentral acute middle maculopathy in the setting of central retinal artery occlusion following COVID-19 diagnosis. *European Journal of Ophthalmology.* 2021:1120672121995347. doi:10.1177/1120672121995347.

43. Wege H, Schluesener H, Meyermann R, Barac-Latas V, Suchanek G, Lassmann H. Coronavirus infection and demyelination. Development of inflammatory lesions in Lewis rats. *Advances in Experimental Medicine and Biology.* 1998;440:437–444.

44. Cabirac GF, Soike KF, Zhang J-Y, et al. Entry of coronavirus into primate CNS following peripheral infection. *Microbial Pathogenesis.* 1994;16(5):349-357. doi:10.1006/mpat.1994.1035.

45. Gu J, Gong E, Zhang B, et al. Multiple organ infection and the pathogenesis of SARS. *The Journal of Experimental Medicine.* 2005;202(3):415–424. doi:10.1084/jem.20050828.

46. Yeh EA, Collins A, Cohen ME, Duffner PK, Faden H. Detection of coronavirus in the central nervous system of a child with acute disseminated encephalomyelitis. *Pediatrics.* 2004;113(1 Pt 1):e73–e76. doi:10.1542/peds.113.1.e73.

47. Martin Paez Y, Bennett JL, Subramanian PS, Pelak VS. Considerations for the Treatment of Inflammatory Neuro-Ophthalmologic Disorders During the COVID-19 Pandemic. *Journal of Neuro-Ophthalmology.* 2020;40(3):305–314. doi:10.1097/WNO.0000000000001016.

48. Rho J, Dryden SC, McGuffey CD, Fowler BT, Fleming J. A Case of Non-Arteritic Anterior Ischemic Optic Neuropathy with COVID-19. *Cureus.* 2020;12(12):e11950. doi:10.7759/cureus.11950.

49. Finsterer J, Scorza FA, Scorza CA, Fiorini AC. Vascular Damage May Mimic Retinitis and Optic Neuritis in COVID-19. *Current Eye Research.* 2021;46(12):1934–1935. doi:10.1080/02713683.2021.1896743.

50. de Ruijter NS, Kramer G, Gons RAR, Hengstman GJD. Neuromyelitis optica spectrum disorder after presumed coronavirus (COVID-19) infection: A case report. *Multiple Sclerosis and Related Disorders.* 2020;46:102474. doi:10.1016/j.msard.2020.102474.

51. Khan A, Panwala H, Ramadoss D, Khubchandani R. Myelin Oligodendrocyte Glycoprotein (MOG) Antibody Disease in a 11 Year Old with COVID-19 Infection. *Indian Journal of Pediatrics.* 2021;88(5):488–489. doi:10.1007/s12098-020-03656-7.

52. Woodhall M, Mitchell JW, Gibbons E, Healy S, Waters P, Case Huda S. Report: Myelin Oligodendrocyte Glycoprotein Antibody-Associated Relapse With COVID-19. *Frontiers in Neurology.* 2020;11:598531. doi:10.3389/fneur.2020.598531.

53. Dinkin M, Gao V, Kahan J, et al. COVID-19 presenting with ophthalmoparesis from cranial nerve palsy. *Neurology.* 2020;95(5):221–223. doi:10.1212/WNL.0000000000009700.

54. Gutiérrez-Ortiz C, Méndez-Guerrero A, Rodrigo-Rey S, et al. Miller Fisher syndrome and polyneuritis cranialis in COVID-19. *Neurology.* 2020;95(5):e601–e605. doi:10.1212/WNL.0000000000009619.

55. Fitzpatrick JC, Comstock J, Longmuir R, Donahue S, Fitzpatrick JM, Bond JBI. Cranial Nerve III Palsy in the Setting of COVID-19 Infection. *Journal of Neuro-Ophthalmology.* 2021;41(3):e286–e287.

56. Greer CE, Bhatt JM, Oliveira CA, Dinkin MJ. Isolated Cranial Nerve 6 Palsy in 6 Patients With COVID-19 Infection. *Journal of Neuro-Ophthalmology.* 2020;40(4):520–522. doi:10.1097/WNO.0000000000001146.

57. Falcone MM, Rong AJ, Salazar H, Redick DW, Falcone S, Cavuoto KM. Acute abducens nerve palsy in a patient with the novel coronavirus disease (COVID-19). *Journal of AAPOS.* 2020;24(4):216–217. doi:10.1016/j.jaapos.2020.06.001.

58. Restivo DA, Centonze D, Alesina A, Marchese-Ragona R. Myasthenia Gravis Associated With SARS-CoV-2 Infection. *Annals of Internal Medicine.* 2020;173(12):1027–1028. doi:10.7326/L20-0845.

59. Wong PF, Craik S, Newman P, et al. Lessons of the month 1: A case of rhombencephalitis as a rare complication of acute COVID-19 infection. *Clinical Medicine.* 2020;20(3):293–294. doi:10.7861/clinmed.2020-0182.

60. Llorente Ayuso L, Torres Rubio P, do Rosário RF, Giganto Arroyo ML, Sierra-Hidalgo F. Bickerstaff encephalitis after COVID-19. *Journal of Neurology.* 2020;268(6):2035–2037 1-3. doi:10.1007/s00415-020-10201-1.

61. Khoo A, McLoughlin B, Cheema S, et al. Postinfectious brainstem encephalitis associated with SARS-CoV-2. *Journal of Neurology, Neurosurgery, and Psychiatry.* 2020;91(9):1013–1014. doi:10.1136/jnnp-2020-323816.

62. Sanguinetti SY, Ramdhani RA. Opsoclonus-myoclonus-ataxia syndrome related to the novel coronavirus (COVID-19). *Journal of Neuro-Ophthalmology.* 2021;41(3):e288–e289. doi:10.1097/WNO.0000000000001129.

63. Khacha A, Bouchal S, Ettabyaoui A, et al. Cavernous sinus thrombosis in a COVID-19 patient: a case report. *Radiology Case Reports.* 2021;16(3):480–482. doi:10.1016/j.radcr.2020.12.013.

64. Aljanabi KSK, Almaqbali T, Alkilidar AAH. A COVID-19 patient with cavernous sinus thrombosis post dental extraction: a diagnostic dilemma. *Indian Journal of Otolaryngology and Head and Neck Surgery.* 2021;1–4. doi:10.1007/s12070-021-02460-9.

65. Turbin RE, Wawrzusin PJ, Sakla NM, et al. Unusual cause of acute sinusitis and orbital abscess in COVID-19 positive patient: case report. *Orbit (Amsterdam, Netherlands)*. 2020;39(4):305–310. doi:10.1080/01676830.2020.1768560.

66. Shires CB, Klug T, Dryden S, Ford J. Unusual cause of acute sinusitis and orbital abscess in COVID-19 positive patient: Case report. *International Journal of Surgery Case Reports*. 2021;79:164–168. doi:10.1016/j.ijscr.2021.01.043.

67. Mangan MS, Yildiz E. New onset of unilateral orbital myositis following mild COVID-19 infection. *Ocular Immunology and Inflammation*. 2021;29(4):670–699. doi:10.1080/09273948.2021.1887282.

68. Chiotos K, Bassiri H, Behrens EM, et al. Multisystem inflammatory syndrome in children during the coronavirus 2019 pandemic: A case series. *Journal of the Pediatric Infectious Diseases Society*. 2020;9(3):393–398. doi:10.1093/JPIDS/PIAA069.

69. Pérez-Chimal LG, Cuevas GG, Di-Luciano A, Chamartín P, Amadeo G, Martínez-Castellanos MA. Ophthalmic manifestations associated with SARS-CoV-2 in newborn infants: a preliminary report. *Journal of American Association for Pediatric Ophthalmology and Strabismus*. 2021;25(2):102–104. doi:10.1016/j.jaapos.2020.11.007.

70. Fernández Alcalde C, Granados Fernández M, Nieves Moreno M, Calvo Rey C, Falces Romero I, Noval Martín S. COVID-19 ocular findings in children: a case series. *World Journal of Pediatrics*. 2021;17(3):329–334. 1–6. doi:10.1007/s12519-021-00418-z.

CHAPTER

12 Psychiatric Manifestations of COVID-19

Karen E. Giles, MD, MS, Charles B. Nemeroff, MD, PhD, and William M. McDonald, MD

Introduction

Neuropsychiatric sequelae of viral infections have been described in the literature and are well known from studies of influenza pandemics[1,2], human immunodeficiency virus (HIV) infections,[3] and viral encephalitis.[4] Perhaps the most researched neuropsychiatric disorder after a viral infection was the development of encephalitis lethargica after the Spanish flu outbreak in the last century. Encephalitis lethargica had prominent parkinsonian symptoms, psychosis, and catatonia.

Prominent neuropsychiatric syndromes were described in two more current coronavirus pandemics: severe acute respiratory syndrome (SARS) in 2002 and Middle Eastern respiratory syndrome (MERS) in 2012. In the acute stage of SARS or MERS infections, confusion (suggesting delirium) occurred in 27.9% of patients, and depression, anxiety, and insomnia were relatively common.[5] In follow-up studies of patients who had contracted SARS or MERS that ranged from 6 weeks to 39 months after recovery from the acute infection, more than 15% of patients reported sleep disorders, recurrent traumatic memories, emotional lability, impaired concentration, fatigue, or impaired memory.[5] Survivors of critical illnesses had the most risk for psychiatric comorbidities at 1 year, with about one-third experiencing significant anxiety, depression, or posttraumatic symptoms.[5]

The severe acute respiratory syndrome coronavirus 2 (SARS-CoV-2) was first identified in Wuhan, China in late 2019, and it soon became clear that the virus can spread beyond the respiratory tract to other vital organs, including the central nervous system (CNS). Clinical evidence of CNS involvement was substantiated by the detection of coronaviruses in the cerebrospinal fluid of patients with neuropsychiatric sequelae[6-8]; early cases of dizziness, headache, delirium, cerebrovascular disease, encephalopathy, neuromuscular disorders, anosmia, and ageusia[9,10]; and psychiatric disorders,[11] including suicides among older adults.[5]

In terms of psychiatric disorders, the infection presents two potential risks. The risk for psychiatric sequelae is clearly increased by the psychosocial and economic stress associated with the COVID-19 pandemic.[12-15] In addition, the viral infection of the CNS, the hyperinflammatory state,[16] and medications used to treat the infection (e.g., exogenous corticosteroids) increased the risk for the development of acute psychiatric disorders.

The COVID-19 pandemic is associated with an increase in psychiatric symptoms, most notably anxiety, depression, and posttraumatic stress disorder (PTSD), and these symptoms are disabling.[5,8,17] Some patients who recovered from the acute phase of COVID-19 had continued neuropsychiatric symptoms. These patients were described in the literature as "long haulers," who over time develop a variety of neuropsychological symptoms, including poor concentration (or "brain fog"), fatigue, and multiple psychiatric symptoms such as depression, anxiety, PTSD, obsessive-compulsive symptoms, psychosis, and an increased risk for suicide (Fig. 12.1).[18] These patients also have symptoms that can masquerade as psychiatric symptoms (e.g., chronic fatigue, insomnia, concentration difficulties) and lead to significant disability.[19,20] This chapter will present the available data on both the acute and long-term incidence of psychiatric diagnoses related to SARS-CoV-2 infections.

Delirium

Coronaviruses target the angiotensin-converting enzyme-2 receptor (ACE2), which is found on glial cells

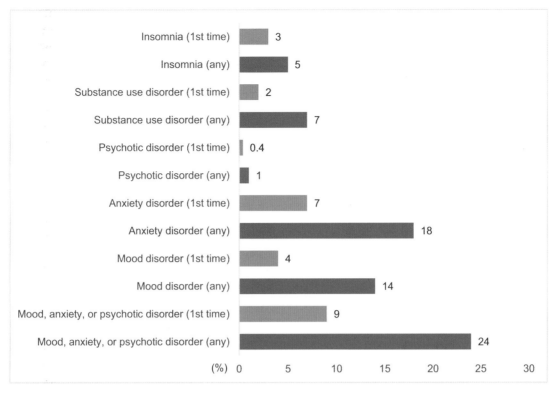

Fig. 12.1 Incidence (%) of Any and New (First Time) Psychiatric Sequelae in COVID-19 Survivors at 6 Months. (Data adapted from Taquet M, Geddes JR, Husain M, et al. 6-month neurological and psychiatric outcomes in 236 379 survivors of COVID-19: a retrospective cohort study using electronic health records. *Lancet Psychiat.* 2021;8[5]:416-427.)

in the brain. SARS-CoV-2 has been shown to enter the CNS though the olfactory epithelium or cribriform bone, by a breakdown of the blood–brain barrier during a viremic phase of the illness, or by peripheral nerve terminals.[21] Once the virus enters neuronal cells, viral RNA replicates and is released into the cerebrovascular circulation.

Delirium is an acute sign of brain dysfunction and has been reported in up to 50% of mechanically ventilated patients.[22] In some patients, particularly the elderly, delirium may be the initial or only presenting symptom of acute COVID-19.[23,24] Awareness of delirium as a common symptom of COVID-19 is even more essential in these patients for early diagnosis, treatment, and prevention of further spread of the virus.[23]

In a retrospective study in Italy, over a quarter of patients hospitalized for neurological conditions associated with COVID-19 experienced delirium.[25] This rate was over three times the incidence of delirium in patients hospitalized for other neurological conditions who had not contracted COVID-19 during the same time. A group in the United Kingdom (UK) reported that over 30% of patients hospitalized with COVID-19 experienced altered mental status and more than half (59%) met criteria for a psychiatric diagnosis, including psychosis and affective symptoms.[26] About half of the patients with altered mental status were under 60 years old.

Delirium is associated with higher mortality and long-term cognitive and functional decline.[27] COVID-19

patients are at particularly high risk for delirium given that they are often prescribed higher doses of sedating medication (e.g., benzodiazepines and propofol) than other mechanically ventilated patients and have a higher risk for delirium because of multiple medical complications (e.g., neuroinflammation, cerebrovascular accidents from hypercoagulability, multisystem organ failure, and social isolation).[28] Agitated delirium tends to be the more prominent type of delirium in patients with COVID-19 and has been reported in nearly 70% of patients hospitalized with severe COVID-19 symptoms.[29] This type of delirium is more overt and easily identifiable than hypoactive delirium, and therefore it is likely that patients with hypoactive delirium are underreported.

COVID-19 patients are also at a higher risk for hypoxic brain injury from an immune-mediated reaction described as a cytokine storm.[21] A cytokine storm is the result of the inflammatory response to the infection and can result in vascular leakage and end organ damage. Delirium also can be the primary manifesting syndrome in COVID-19 patients even before the respiratory symptoms are apparent.

Importantly, delirium during hospitalization in COVID-19 patients is linked to an increased risk for death during hospitalization[30] and an increased need for support on discharge from the hospital.[31] Physical functioning after discharge was notably impaired in patients who were diagnosed with delirium during their hospitalization.[27] A COVID-19 post–intensive care syndrome has been identified that includes cognitive impairment, depression, anxiety, and physical signs such as weakness.[32]

In a multicenter cohort study conducted in 69 adult intensive care units (ICUs) with 2000 patients across 14 countries (half the patients were in Spain) admitted with COVID-19, investigators identified variables associated with delirium and coma.[28] In this study, 55% of patients were delirious for an average duration of 3 days. Significant factors associated with delirium included older age, higher Simplified Acute Physiology Score (assessing the risk for death in ICU patients), male sex, smoking or alcohol abuse at baseline, use of vasopressors on day 1, and invasive mechanical ventilation on day 1 (all $P < .01$). In this study, the investigators identified two modifiable risk factors associated with a decreased incidence of delirium: lower benzodiazepine use and more frequent family visitations in the ICU (either in person or virtually). The investigators outlined interventions to lower the incidence of delirium, including decreasing sedatives, increasing mobility, breathing trials off ventilation, and encouraging families to visit. Other strategies could include circadian rhythm regulation using medications such as melatonin.[33]

The US Food and Drug Administration has not approved any medications to treat delirium. The primary interventions recommended are behavioral, including family involvement. Off-label medication treatments used to manage COVID-19–related delirium include alpha-2 agonists, low-potency antipsychotics, valproic acid, and trazodone.[33]

Impact of Preexisting Psychiatric Disorders on COVID-19 Outcomes

The impact of a preexisting mental health disorder on the emergence of psychiatric symptoms during or after SARS-CoV-2 infection is well documented. Patients with severe mental illness are at particularly high risk for contracting COVID-19 and transmitting the virus. These patients may not adhere to protocols to decrease transmission (e.g., mask wearing), have less access to medical clinics for vaccinations and medical care, and are more at risk for an exacerbation of their underlying psychiatric symptoms.[34]

Two large-scale meta-analyses found associations between COVID-19 mortality and preexisting psychiatric conditions. A recent meta-analysis of studies from seven countries and over 19,000 patients with COVID-19 found an increased risk for mortality (odds ratio [OR], 1.75) in patients with a mental health condition.[35] Patients with more severe psychiatric conditions, such as schizophrenia and bipolar affective disorder, were over two times at risk for mortality from COVID-19

compared to patients without a mental health diagnosis.

A meta-analysis compiling data from 21 studies with 90 million COVID-19 patients detected a higher likelihood of hospitalization and death if a preexisting affective disorder was present (OR, 1.31 and 1.51, respectively). There was no association between mood disorders and risk for infection of SARS-CoV-2.[36] The data from these two meta-analyses make clear that patients with preexisting psychiatric disorders are at high risk for hospitalization and death when infected with SARS-CoV-2. The risk for significant short- and long-term psychiatric symptoms in an individual patient with a premorbid psychiatric diagnosis who contracts SARS-CoV-2 is clearly increased,[37] and these patients should be monitored carefully.

Anxiety, Depression, Mania, and Suicide Risk

Psychopathology is relatively common in patients recovering from COVID-19, with more than half showing significant symptoms of at least one psychiatric disorder 1 month after infection (i.e., PTSD, depression, anxiety, or obsessive-compulsive symptoms).[17] Multiple other studies also found high rates of depression and anxiety after SARS-CoV-2 infection.[38-43] The reasons for patients developing anxiety and depressive symptoms during and after COVID-19 disease are multifactorial. A previous psychiatric diagnosis,[17,39,44] female sex,[17,39,43,44] younger age,[38,43] lower socioeconomic status,[41,42,44] and unemployment[39,43] are all linked to higher rates of psychological distress after COVID-19. Interestingly, the prevalence of depression and anxiety was similar in health care workers with COVID-19 compared with the general public in one meta-analysis[44] and other reviews,[41] although nurses had a high burden of mood symptoms.[44,45]

The medications used to treat COVID-19 include several with known adverse drug reactions, including mania or hypomania. High-dose steroids are heavily used in hospitalized patients with severe COVID-19, particularly those requiring supplemental oxygen, and case reports suggest that some patients developed mania with grandiosity, hyper-religiosity, elevated energy, and insomnia severe enough to warrant psychiatric hospitalization and treatment with psychotropic medication, including mood stabilizers and antipsychotics.[46,47] Furthermore, quinolone antibiotics, which have been initiated to treat secondary infections in patients with COVID-19 are also known to provoke hypomania and euphoria in some patients.[47] At the time of writing, no reports of new-onset mania have been reported in patients with COVID-19 who did not receive medications known to elicit manic symptoms.

Suicide risk is also increased in patients with COVID-19 infections,[34,37,48–50] although the data are still preliminary.[51] The precipitants for a potential increase in suicide rates secondary to the pandemic are multifactorial and related to social isolation, socioeconomic stresses such as high rates of unemployment, and the risk for psychiatric symptoms in persons with preexisting psychiatric disorders.[51,52] Insomnia is also associated with COVID-19 and can significantly increase the risk for suicide; it should be evaluated and addressed in this patient population.[53]

There are protective factors to prevent the development of depression and anxiety after COVID-19, including sufficient medical resources to manage the illness, current information, confidence in the reports on the status of the pandemic,[38,44] being married, connection to family, and exercise.[43] Social isolation is a factor that can potentially be addressed to decrease the risk for depression and anxiety.[44,54] The dyad of fear and isolation is a clear precipitant to the development of anxiety, depression, and potentially suicide in this patient population.[34]

There are limited medication trials for anxiety and depression related to COVID-19, but there would be no reason to think that the psychotropic medications used to manage major depression, PTSD, and anxiety disorders would not be effective in this population. In fact, serotonin reuptake inhibitors have been shown to be protective in developing COVID-19 symptoms.[55]

Posttraumatic Stress Disorder and Trauma-Related Symptoms

PTSD in COVID-19 survivors has been diagnosed as early as 7 weeks after discharge from the hospital. At 3 months, 10% of patients who had been hospitalized for COVID-19 met the criteria for PTSD.[56] By 4 months after discharge, 17% of patients who had been hospitalized for COVID-19 had symptoms of PTSD.[57] One study comparing patients who required hospitalization to those who did not followed patients between 1 and 6 months after COVID-19 diagnosis and found no significant difference in the prevalence of PTSD between these groups.[58]

Longer-term symptoms also have been reported in a cross-sectional survey of 284 patients who were followed an average of 50 days after their COVID-19 diagnosis.[37] In this survey, significant PTSD symptoms (assessed by the self-report questionnaire the Impact of Event Scale–Revised) were the most common psychiatric condition and moderate to severe PTSD was associated with an increase in suicidal thoughts. Risk factors for PTSD symptoms also included female sex, a history of traumatic events, how concerned the patient was that COVID-19 was a serious threat, and feeling stigmatized by contracting the virus.

Young adults (18–30 years old) reported particularly high rates of PTSD symptoms, with 31.8% of patients in the sample scoring 45 or greater on the PTSD Checklist-Civilian Version (>33 is considered clinically significant symptoms on this scale).[59] In this cross-sectional online study of PTSD symptoms, the respondents also had high levels of depression and anxiety and psychiatric symptoms were associated with loneliness, COVID-19 concerns, and low distress tolerance. Social support after contracting the virus, particularly from the patient's family, was shown to be protective.

Psychosis and Catatonia

The risk for psychosis has been documented in previous flu epidemics.[5] Corticosteroids have been a significant contributor to psychosis and mania in previous viral pandemics.[5]

Rare cases of brief psychotic disorder in the setting of acute COVID-19 infection are documented in a single-site retrospective study in Spain.[60] Ten patients without previous episodes of psychosis, severe mental health history, or substance use history who had contracted COVID-19 were evaluated for new-onset psychosis. Within this study, delusions (particularly those of persecution, prejudice, and referential beliefs) were present in all of the psychotic patients. The majority (60%) of patients with psychosis had difficulties with orientation and attention, and many reported auditory (40%) or visual hallucinations (10%). The majority (80%) of patients did not develop psychosis for several weeks after physical symptoms of COVID-19 and had resolution of psychosis with low doses of antipsychotics within 2 weeks. Disorientation and inattention resolved faster than delusions. In this study, iatrogenic factors could not be ruled out, because most patients had received corticosteroids and hydroxychloroquine, which have been associated with psychosis. There has been a case of brief psychotic disorder in a patient with COVID-19 who had not been exposed to any medications known to precipitate psychosis.[61]

A surveillance study of over 150 patients with COVID-19 in the United Kingdom revealed that 43% of patients who developed neuropsychiatric symptoms with acute SARS-CoV-2 infection had new-onset psychosis, which was a considerably higher incidence compared with the development of mood disorders in this patient population.[26]

Catatonia has been observed in patients with acute COVID-19.[62,63] Catatonia is a psychomotor condition that in itself may be life threatening. It can manifest from a medical condition such as COVID-19 but also may be a symptom of an underlying psychiatric state. Patients classically may be mute and rigid, stop eating and drinking, and have autonomic instability. In a review of 10 cases of catatonia in patients with COVID-19, all patients exhibited akinetic mutism.[62] Patients with catatonia associated with COVID-19 have reportedly responded to benzodiazepine treatment, the standard of care.[63]

Psychiatric Symptoms Directly Linked to Viral Infection

Not surprisingly, the pandemic in and of itself has created a "second wave" of psychiatric morbidity in all populations as a result of the stress of social isolation, persistent feelings of uncertainty or loss of control, sense of powerlessness, and secondary traumatization. Therefore it can be difficult to decipher how much of the psychiatric sequelae in patients with COVID-19 is related to the stress of the pandemic compared with direct effects from the virus. Several studies have provided evidence that suggests the viral infection plays a significant role in the relatively high incidence of psychiatric symptoms.

Hospitalized patients with COVID-19 have been compared with age- and sex-matched patients hospitalized during the pandemic for other respiratory illnesses. Patients with COVID-19 had significantly higher rates of mood, anxiety, or psychotic disorders compared with controls.[64]

Higher levels of the inflammatory marker C-reactive protein were detected in COVID-19 survivors who developed severe depression compared with normal controls, suggesting that the inflammatory response from the virus may be inducing neuropsychiatric symptoms.[65] In this study, duration of hospitalization did not have an impact on risk for depression, suggesting that the hospital experience and possibly severity of COVID-19 (if duration is a proxy for disease severity) may not be contributing to development of depression.

Conclusion

Significant psychiatric comorbidities are relatively common in patients with COVID-19 and can lead to significant disability, which can persist for months to years in vulnerable populations. There are no established somatic treatments, although using selective serotonin reuptake inhibitors and evidenced-based psychotherapies such as cognitive-behavioral therapy and prolonged exposure therapy are reasonable approaches. However, data to support their efficacy in COVID-19 are limited.

There are also public health approaches that have been shown to be effective in limiting the psychiatric comorbidities of COVID-19. Decreasing social isolation (e.g., providing Meals on Wheels, telepsychiatry groups, visits by family members), increasing knowledge about the pandemic in regular and reliable public service announcements, and decreasing stigma associated with contracting the virus should all be addressed by broader public health measures. Disseminating reliable information on the pandemic with the proliferation of social media has been challenging and should be addressed. The public should be confident in the information they are receiving and referred to the Centers for Disease Control and Prevention and other public health agencies that are current and reliable. This may be difficult but should be immediately addressed.

Stigmatization for contracting the virus will be particularly difficult to address in patients who declined to get vaccinated and contracted the disease. This may be a problem not only for the general public but also health care workers and is reminiscent of the issues surrounding other "self-induced" illnesses such as cirrhosis in an alcoholic patient or lung cancer in a chronic smoker. Perhaps public service announcements or other information outlining why people declined the vaccination would be helpful in personalizing an individual's decision.

There are also specific patient groups that should be targeted as at high risk for developing psychiatric symptoms, including those patients with previous psychiatric diagnoses or presently in psychiatric treatment. Female sex was a significant risk factor for psychiatric symptoms and could lead to some targeted strategies such as asking gynecologists to screen COVID-19–positive patients carefully for psychiatric symptoms.

Clearly, physicians managing patients with acute COVID-19 should be alert to the potential for the emergence of psychiatric symptoms both in the acute phase and over time. These patients are at significant risk for disabling psychiatric syndromes. Decreasing the psychiatric comorbidities should include public health measures (e.g., decreasing social isolation, increasing accurate information on the pandemic) and monitoring patients for symptoms, particularly those in high-risk populations (e.g., premorbid psychiatric conditions, low socioeconomic status). Treatment with antidepressant medications and psychotherapy should be considered in symptomatic patients.

REFERENCES
1. Menninger KA. Influenza and schizophrenia. An analysis of post-influenzal "dementia precox," as of 1918, and five years later further studies of the psychiatric aspects of influenza. 1926. *Am J Psychiatry*. 1994;151(Suppl. 6): 182–187.
2. Kępińska AP, Iyegbe CO, Vernon AC, Yolken R, Murray RM, Pollak TA. Schizophrenia and influenza at the centenary of the 1918-1919 Spanish influenza pandemic: mechanisms of psychosis risk. *Front Psychiatry*. 2020;11:72.
3. Dubé B, Benton T, Cruess DG, Evans DL. Neuropsychiatric manifestations of HIV infection and AIDS. *J Psychiatry Neurosci*. 2005;30(4):237–246.
4. Arciniegas DB, Anderson CA. Viral encephalitis: neuropsychiatric and neurobehavioral aspects. *Curr Psychiatry Rep*. 2004;6(5):372–379.

5. Rogers JP, Chesney E, Oliver D, Pollak TA, McGuire P, Fusar-Poli P, Zandi MS, Lewis G, David AS. Psychiatric and neuropsychiatric presentations associated with severe coronavirus infections: a systematic review and meta-analysis with comparison to the COVID-19 pandemic. *Lancet Psychiatry*. 2020;7(7):611–627.

6. Alexopoulos H, Magira E, Bitzogli K, Kafasi N, Vlachoyiannopoulos P, Tzioufas A, Kotanidou A, Dalakas MC. Anti-SARS-CoV-2 antibodies in the CSF, blood-brain barrier dysfunction, and neurological outcome: Studies in 8 stuporous and comatose patients. *Neurol Neuroimmunol Neuroinflamm*. 2020;7(6):e893.

7. Espíndola OM, Brandão CO, Gomes YCP, Siqueira M, Soares CN, Lima M, Leite A, Torezani G, Araujo AQC, Silva MTT. Cerebrospinal fluid findings in neurological diseases associated with COVID-19 and insights into mechanisms of disease development. *Int J Infect Dis*. 2021;102:155–162.

8. Liu JM, Tan BH, Wu S, Gui Y, Suo JL, Li YC. Evidence of central nervous system infection and neuroinvasive routes, as well as neurological involvement, in the lethality of SARS-CoV-2 infection. *J Med Virol*. 2021;93(3): 1304–1313.

9. Mao L, Jin H, Wang M, Hu Y, Chen S, He Q, Chang J, Hong C, Zhou Y, Wang D, Miao X, Li Y, Hu B. Neurologic manifestations of hospitalized patients with coronavirus disease 2019 in Wuhan, China. *JAMA Neurol*. 2020;77(6):683–690.

10. de Sousa Moreira JL, Barbosa SMB, Vieira JG, Chaves NCB, Felix EBG, Feitosa PWG, da Cruz IS, da Silva CGL, Neto MLR. The psychiatric and neuropsychiatric repercussions associated with severe infections of COVID-19 and other coronaviruses. *Prog Neuropsychopharmacol Biol Psychiatry*. 2021;106:110159.

11. Hossain MM, Tasnim S, Sultana A, Faizah F, Mazumder H, Zou L, McKyer ELJ, Ahmed HU, Ma P. Epidemiology of mental health problems in COVID-19: a review. *F1000Res*. 2020;9:636.

12. Brooks SK, Webster RK, Smith LE, Woodland L, Wessely S, Greenberg N, Rubin GJ. The psychological impact of quarantine and how to reduce it: rapid review of the evidence. *Lancet*. 2020;395(10227):912–920.

13. Davide P, Andrea P, Martina O, Andrea E, Davide D, Mario A. The impact of the COVID-19 pandemic on patients with OCD: Effects of contamination symptoms and remission state before the quarantine in a preliminary naturalistic study. *Psychiatry Res*. 2020;291:113213.

14. Greenberg N, Docherty M, Gnanapragasam S, Wessely S. Managing mental health challenges faced by healthcare workers during covid-19 pandemic. *Bmj*. 2020;368:m1211.

15. Troyer EA, Kohn JN, Hong S. Are we facing a crashing wave of neuropsychiatric sequelae of COVID-19? Neuropsychiatric symptoms and potential immunologic mechanisms. *Brain Behav Immun*. 2020;87:34–39.

16. Johansson A, Mohamed MS, Moulin TC, Schiöth HB. Neurological manifestations of COVID-19: A comprehensive literature review and discussion of mechanisms. *J Neuroimmunol*. 2021;358:577658.

17. Mazza MG, De Lorenzo R, Conte C, Poletti S, Vai B, Bollettini I, Melloni EMT, Furlan R, Ciceri F, Rovere-Querini P, Benedetti F. Anxiety and depression in COVID-19 survivors: Role of inflammatory and clinical predictors. *Brain Behav Immun*. 2020;89:594–600.

18. Sher L. Post-COVID syndrome and suicide risk. *Qjm*. 2021;114(2):95–98.

19. Carfi A, Bernabei R, Landi F. Persistent Symptoms in Patients After Acute COVID-19. *Jama*. 2020;324(6):603–605.

20. Townsend L, Dyer AH, Jones K, Dunne J, Mooney A, Gaffney F, O'Connor L, Leavy D, O'Brien K, Dowds J, Sugrue JA, Hopkins D, Martin-Loeches I, Ni Cheallaigh C, Nadarajan P, McLaughlin AM, Bourke NM, Bergin C, O'Farrelly C, Bannan C, Conlon N. Persistent fatigue following SARS-CoV-2 infection is common and independent of severity of initial infection. *PLoS One*. 2020;15(11):e0240784.

21. Ahmad I, Rathore FA. Neurological manifestations and complications of COVID-19: A literature review. *J Clin Neurosci*. 2020;77:8–12.

22. Girard TD, Exline MC, Carson SS, Hough CL, Rock P, Gong MN, Douglas IS, Malhotra A, Owens RL, Feinstein DJ, Khan B, Pisani MA, Hyzy RC, Schmidt GA, Schweickert WD, Hite RD, Bowton DL, Masica AL, Thompson JL, Chandrasekhar R, Pun BT, Strength C, Boehm LM, Jackson JC, Pandharipande PP, Brummel NE, Hughes CG, Patel MB, Stollings JL, Bernard GR, Dittus RS, Ely EW. Haloperidol and Ziprasidone for Treatment of Delirium in Critical Illness. *N Engl J Med*. 2018;379(26):2506–2516.

23. Ward CF, Figiel GS, McDonald WM. Altered Mental Status as a Novel Initial Clinical Presentation for COVID-19 Infection in the Elderly. *Am J Geriatr Psychiatry*. 2020;28(8):808–811.

24. Butt I, Sawlani V, Geberhiwot T. Prolonged confusional state as first manifestation of COVID-19. *Ann Clin Transl Neurol*. 2020;7(8):1450–1452.

25. Benussi A, Pilotto A, Premi E, Libri I, Giunta M, Agosti C, Alberici A, Baldelli E, Benini M, Bonacina S, Brambilla L, Caratozzolo S, Cortinovis M, Costa A, Cotti Piccinelli S, Cottini E, Cristillo V, Delrio I, Filosto M, Gamba M, Gazzina S, Gilberti N, Gipponi S, Imarisio A, Invernizzi P, Leggio U, Leonardi M, Liberini P, Locatelli M, Masciocchi S, Poli L, Rao R, Risi B, Rozzini L, Scalvini A, Schiano di Cola F, Spezi R, Vergani V, Volonghi I, Zoppi N, Borroni B, Magoni M, Pezzini A, Padovani A. Clinical characteristics and outcomes of inpatients with neurologic disease and COVID-19 in Brescia, Lombardy, Italy. *Neurology*. 2020;95(7):e910–e920.

26. Varatharaj A, Thomas N, Ellul MA, Davies NWS, Pollak TA, Tenorio EL, Sultan M, Easton A, Breen G, Zandi M, Coles JP, Manji H, Al-Shahi Salman R, Menon DK, Nicholson TR, Benjamin LA, Carson A, Smith C, Turner MR, Solomon T, Kneen R, Pett SL, Galea I, Thomas RH, Michael BD, Allen C, Archibald N, Arkell J, Arthur-Farraj P, Baker M, Ball H, Bradley-Barker V, Brown Z, Bruno S, Carey L, Carswell C, Chakrabarti A, Choulerton J, Daher M, Davies R, Di Marco Barros R, Dima S, Dunley R, Dutta D, Ellis R, Everitt A, Fady J, Fearon P, Fisniku L, Gbinigie I, Gemski A, Gillies E, Gkrania-Klotsas E, Grigg J, Hamdalla H, Hubbett J, Hunter N, Huys A-C, Ihmoda I, Ispoglou S, Jha A, Joussi R, Kalladka D, Khalifeh H, Kooij S, Kumar G, Kyaw S, Li L, Littleton E, Macleod M, Macleod MJ, Madigan B, Mahadasa V, Manoharan M, Marigold R, Marks I, Matthews P, McCormick M, McInnes C, Metastasio A, Milburn-McNulty P, Mitchell C, Mitchell D, Morgans C, Morris H, Morrow J, Mubarak Mohamed A, Mulvenna P, Murphy L, Namushi R, Newman E, Phillips W, Pinto A, Price DA, Proschel H, Quinn T, Ramsey D, Roffe C, Ross Russell A, Samarasekera

N, Sawcer S, Sayed W, Sekaran L, Serra-Mestres J, Snowdon V, Strike G, Sun J, Tang C, Vrana M, Wade R, Wharton C, Wiblin L, Boubriak I, Herman K, Plant G. Neurological and neuropsychiatric complications of COVID-19 in 153 patients: a UK-wide surveillance study. *The Lancet Psychiatry*. 2020;7(10):875–882.

27. McLoughlin BC, Miles A, Webb TE, Knopp P, Eyres C, Fabbri A, Humphries F, Davis D. Functional and cognitive outcomes after COVID-19 delirium. *Eur Geriatr Med*. 2020;11(5):857–862.

28. Pun BT, Badenes R, Heras La Calle G, Orun OM, Chen W, Raman R, Simpson BK, Wilson-Linville S, Hinojal Olmedillo B, Vallejo de la Cueva A, van der Jagt M, Navarro Casado R, Leal Sanz P, Orhun G, Ferrer Gómez C, Núñez Vázquez K, Piñeiro Otero P, Taccone FS, Gallego Curto E, Caricato A, Woien H, Lacave G, O'Neal Jr HR, Peterson SJ, Brummel NE, Girard TD, Ely EW, Pandharipande PP. Prevalence and risk factors for delirium in critically ill patients with COVID-19 (COVID-D): a multicentre cohort study. *Lancet Respir Med*. 2021;9(3):239–250.

29. Helms J, Kremer S, Merdji H, Clere-Jehl R, Schenck M, Kummerlen C, Collange O, Boulay C, Fafi-Kremer S, Ohana M, Anheim M, Meziani F. Neurologic Features in Severe SARS-CoV-2 Infection. *N Engl J Med*. 2020;382(23):2268–2270.

30. Garcez FB, Aliberti MJR, Poco PCE, Hiratsuka M, Takahashi SF, Coelho VA, Salotto DB, Moreira MLV, Jacob-Filho W, Avelino-Silva TJ. Delirium and Adverse Outcomes in Hospitalized Patients with COVID-19. *J Am Geriatr Soc*. 2020;68(11):2440–2446.

31. Welch C. Age and frailty are independently associated with increased COVID-19 mortality and increased care needs in survivors: results of an international multi-centre study. *Age Ageing*. 2021;50(3):617–630.

32. Kotfis K, Roberson SWilliams, Wilson J, Pun B, Ely EW, Jeżowska I, Jezierska M, Dabrowski W. COVID-19: What do we need to know about ICU delirium during the SARS-CoV-2 pandemic?. *Anaesthesiol Intensive Ther*. 2020;52(2):132–138.

33. Baller EB, Hogan CS, Fusunyan MA, Ivkovic A, Luccarelli JW, Madva E, Nisavic M, Praschan N, Quijije NV, Beach SR, Smith FA. Neurocovid: Pharmacological Recommendations for Delirium Associated With COVID-19. *Psychosomatics*. 2020;61(6):585–596.

34. Yao H, Chen JH, Xu YF. Patients with mental health disorders in the COVID-19 epidemic. *Lancet Psychiatry*. 2020;7(4):e21.

35. Fond G, Nemani K, Etchecopar-Etchart D, Loundou A, Goff DC, Lee SW, Lancon C, Auquier P, Baumstarck K, Llorca P-M, Yon DK, Boyer L. Association Between Mental Health Disorders and Mortality Among Patients With COVID-19 in 7 Countries: A Systematic Review and Meta-analysis. *JAMA Psychiatry*. 2021.

36. Ceban F, Nogo D, Carvalho IP, Lee Y, Nasri F, Xiong J, Lui LMW, Subramaniapillai M, Gill H, Liu RN, Joseph P, Teopiz KM, Cao B, Mansur RB, Lin K, Rosenblat JD, Ho RC, McIntyre RS. Association Between Mood Disorders and Risk of COVID-19 Infection, Hospitalization, and Death: A Systematic Review and Meta-analysis. *JAMA Psychiatry*. 2021.

37. Poyraz B, Poyraz CA, Olgun Y, Gürel Ö, Alkan S, Özdemir YE, Balkan İ, Karaali R. Psychiatric morbidity and protracted symptoms after COVID-19. *Psychiatry Res*. 2021;295:113604.

38. Bäuerle A, Teufel M, Musche V, Weismüller B, Kohler H, Hetkamp M, Dörrie N, Schweda A, Skoda EM. Increased generalized anxiety, depression and distress during the COVID-19 pandemic: a cross-sectional study in Germany. *J Public Health (Oxf)*. 2020;42(4):672–678.

39. Xiong J, Lipsitz O, Nasri F, Lui LMW, Gill H, Phan L, Chen-Li D, Iacobucci M, Ho R, Majeed A, McIntyre RS. Impact of COVID-19 pandemic on mental health in the general population: A systematic review. *J Affect Disord*. 2020;277:55–64.

40. Deng J, Zhou F, Hou W, Silver Z, Wong CY, Chang O, Huang E, Zuo QK. The prevalence of depression, anxiety, and sleep disturbances in COVID-19 patients: a meta-analysis. *Ann N Y Acad Sci*. 2021;1486(1):90–111.

41. Rehman U, Shahnawaz MG, Khan NH, Kharshiing KD, Khursheed M, Gupta K, Kashyap D, Uniyal R. Depression, Anxiety and Stress Among Indians in Times of Covid-19 Lockdown. *Community Ment Health J*. 2021;57(1):42–48.

42. Rudenstine S, McNeal K, Schulder T, Ettman CK, Hernandez M, Gvozdieva K, Galea S. Depression and Anxiety During the COVID-19 Pandemic in an Urban, Low-Income Public University Sample. *J Trauma Stress*. 2021;34(1):12–22.

43. Shah SMA, Mohammad D, Qureshi MFH, Abbas MZ, Aleem S. Prevalence, Psychological Responses and Associated Correlates of Depression, Anxiety and Stress in a Global Population, During the Coronavirus Disease (COVID-19) Pandemic. *Community Ment Health J*. 2021;57(1):101–110.

44. Luo M, Guo L, Yu M, Jiang W, Wang H. The psychological and mental impact of coronavirus disease 2019 (COVID-19) on medical staff and general public - A systematic review and meta-analysis. *Psychiatry Res*. 2020;291:113190.

45. Lai J, Ma S, Wang Y, Cai Z, Hu J, Wei N, Wu J, Du H, Chen T, Li R, Tan H, Kang L, Yao L, Huang M, Wang H, Wang G, Liu Z, Hu S. Factors Associated With Mental Health Outcomes Among Health Care Workers Exposed to Coronavirus Disease 2019. *JAMA Netw Open*. 2020;3(3):e203976.

46. Correa-Palacio AF, Hernandez-Huerta D, Gómez-Arnau J, Loeck C, Caballero I. Affective psychosis after COVID-19 infection in a previously healthy patient: a case report. *Psychiatry Res*. 2020;290:113115.

47. Lu S, Wei N, Jiang J, Wu L, Sheng J, Zhou J, Fang Q, Chen Y, Zheng S, Chen F, Liang T, Hu S. First report of manic-like symptoms in a COVID-19 patient with no previous history of a psychiatric disorder. *J Affect Disord*. 2020;277:337–340.

48. Devitt P. Can we expect an increased suicide rate due to Covid-19?. *Ir J Psychol Med*. 2020;37(4):264–268.

49. Mamun MA, Ullah I. COVID-19 suicides in Pakistan, dying off not COVID-19 fear but poverty? - The forthcoming economic challenges for a developing country. *Brain Behav Immun*. 2020;87:163–166.

50. Thakur V, Jain A. COVID 2019-suicides: A global psychological pandemic. *Brain Behav Immun*. 2020;88:952–953.

51. Niederkrotenthaler T, Gunnell D, Arensman E, Pirkis J, Appleby L, Hawton K, John A, Kapur N, Khan M, O'Connor RC, Platt S. Suicide Research, Prevention, and COVID-19. *Crisis*. 2020;41(5):321–330.

52. Gunnell D, Appleby L, Arensman E, Hawton K, John A, Kapur N, Khan M, O'Connor RC, Pirkis J. Suicide risk and prevention during the COVID-19 pandemic. *Lancet Psychiatry*. 2020;7(6):468–471.

53. Sher L. COVID-19, anxiety, sleep disturbances and suicide. *Sleep Med*. 2020;70:124.

54. Armitage R, Nellums LB. COVID-19 and the consequences of isolating the elderly. *Lancet Public Health.* 2020;5(5):e256.

55. Lenze EJ, Mattar C, Zorumski CF, Stevens A, Schweiger J, Nicol GE, Miller JP, Yang L, Yingling M, Avidan MS, Reiersen AM. Fluvoxamine vs Placebo and Clinical Deterioration in Outpatients With Symptomatic COVID-19: A Randomized Clinical Trial. *Jama.* 2020;324(22):2292–2300.

56. Tarsitani L, Vassalini P, Koukopoulos A, Borrazzo C, Alessi F, Di Nicolantonio C, Serra R, Alessandri F, Ceccarelli G, Mastroianni CM, d'Ettorre G. Post-traumatic Stress Disorder Among COVID-19 Survivors at 3-Month Follow-up After Hospital Discharge. *J Gen Intern Med.* 2021;36(6):1702–1707.

57. Bellan M, Soddu D, Balbo PE, Baricich A, Zeppegno P, Avanzi GC, Baldon G, Bartolomei G, Battaglia M, Battistini S, Binda V, Borg M, Cantaluppi V, Castello LM, Clivati E, Cisari C, Costanzo M, Croce A, Cuneo D, De Benedittis C, De Vecchi S, Feggi A, Gai M, Gambaro E, Gattoni E, Gramaglia C, Grisafi L, Guerriero C, Hayden E, Jona A, Invernizzi M, Lorenzini L, Loreti L, Martelli M, Marzullo P, Matino E, Panero A, Parachini E, Patrucco F, Patti G, Pirovano A, Prosperini P, Quaglino R, Rigamonti C, Sainaghi PP, Vecchi C, Zecca E, Pirisi M. Respiratory and Psychophysical Sequelae Among Patients With COVID-19 Four Months After Hospital Discharge. *JAMA Netw Open.* 2021;4(1):e2036142.

58. Einvik G, Dammen T, Ghanima W, Heir T, Stavem K. Prevalence and Risk Factors for Post-Traumatic Stress in Hospitalized and Non-Hospitalized COVID-19 Patients. *Int J Environ Res Public Health.* 2021;18(4):2079.

59. Liu CH, Zhang E, Wong GTF, Hyun S, Hahm HC. Factors associated with depression, anxiety, and PTSD symptomatology during the COVID-19 pandemic: Clinical implications for U.S. young adult mental health. *Psychiatry Res.* 2020;290:113172.

60. Parra A, Juanes A, Losada CP, Álvarez-Sesmero S, Santana VD, Martí I, Urricelqui J, Rentero D. Psychotic symptoms in COVID-19 patients. A retrospective descriptive study. *Psychiatry Res.* 2020;291:113254.

61. Smith CM, Komisar JR, Mourad A, Kincaid BR. COVID-19-associated brief psychotic disorder. *BMJ Case Rep.* 2020;13(8).

62. Scheiner NS, Smith AK, Wohlleber M, Malone C, Schwartz AC. COVID-19 and catatonia: a case series and systematic review of existing literature. *Journal of the Academy of Consultation-Liaison Psychiatry.* 2021.

63. Caan MP, Lim CT, Howard M. A case of catatonia in a man with COVID-19 Case of Catatonia in a Man With COVID-19. *Psychosomatics.* 2020;61(5):556–560.

64. Taquet M, Geddes JR, Husain M, Luciano S, Harrison PJ. 6-month neurological and psychiatric outcomes in 236 379 survivors of COVID-19: a retrospective cohort study using electronic health records. *The Lancet Psychiatry.* 2021;8(5):416–427.

65. Guo Q, Zheng Y, Shi J, Wang J, Li G, Li C, Fromson JA, Xu Y, Liu X, Xu H, Zhang T, Lu Y, Chen X, Hu H, Tang Y, Yang S, Zhou H, Wang X, Chen H, Wang Z, Yang Z. Immediate psychological distress in quarantined patients with COVID-19 and its association with peripheral inflammation: a mixed-method study. *Brain Behav Immun.* 2020;88:17–27.

Fetus, Newborn, Infants, Children

Impact of Maternal SARS-CoV-2 Infection on the Fetus and Newborn

Amelie Pham, MD, David M. Brooks, MD, Susan M. Lopata, MD,
Jennifer L. Thompson, MD, and Jörn-Hendrik Weitkamp, MD

History of Perinatal Coronavirus Infections

Before the worldwide pandemic, data on coronavirus infection in pregnancy were limited despite two previous large epidemics. A 2020 systematic review and meta-analysis found only 12 cases of Middle East respiratory syndrome coronavirus (MERS-CoV) and 33 cases of severe acute respiratory syndrome coronavirus-2 (SARS-CoV-2) infections in pregnancy, all of which were from case reports, case series, or small retrospective cohort studies.[1] However, evidence showed that the case fatality rate appeared higher in pregnant women with more disease severity than in nonpregnant individuals. A case-control study compared 10 pregnant to 40 nonpregnant women affected by severe acute respiratory syndrome (SARS) in Hong Kong and showed a 60% rate of intensive care unit (ICU) admission in pregnancy compared with 17.5% in nonpregnant patients. Case fatality rate was also increased in pregnant patients at 40% compared with no deaths in nonpregnant individuals.[2] A total of 11 cases of MERS in pregnancy were found in one literature review that reported a 64% ICU admission rate and a 27% case fatality rate.[3] A more recent review quoted the overall maternal mortality rate at 18% and 25%, for the SARS-CoV-1 and MERS-CoV epidemics, respectively.[4]

Pregnancy Outcomes During Previous Coronavirus Epidemics

Pregnancy outcomes from prior coronavirus epidemics can provide some insight into disease severity in pregnancy during the current SARS-CoV-2 pandemic (Table 13.1). A systematic review and meta-analysis

evaluated different clinical features of pregnant patients infected with one of the coronaviruses known to cause severe disease in humans. Fever, cough, and fatigue were the most common clinical features, with prevalence ranging from 50% to 78% in MERS-CoV and 80% to 97% in SARS-CoV-1, and the pooled prevalence of all clinical symptoms was 26% (95% CI, 15.2–40.1).[1] Pneumonia was the most common diagnosis in pregnant patients with a prevalence of 71.4% in MERS-CoV and 88.9% in SARS-CoV-1. Lymphocytopenia and elevated C-reactive protein (CRP) were the most common laboratory findings. MERS-CoV was the predominant causative agent of severe cases among infected pregnant women, with a prevalence of 77%, followed by SARS-CoV-1 (48%). None of the studies reported documented transmission of MERS-CoV or SARS-CoV-1 from the mother to the fetus.

Impacts of SARS-CoV-2 Infection on the Pregnant Mother

Epidemiology of Maternal SARS-CoV-2 Infection

As the SARS-CoV-2 pandemic continues to evolve, more data become available on the impact on pregnant patients. As of June 14, 2021, the Centers for Disease Control and Prevention (CDC) has reported 97,293 cases in pregnancy and 106 maternal deaths related to SARS-CoV-2 infection in the United States alone.[5] In June 2020, the CDC released surveillance data evaluating SARS-CoV-2-related outcomes in pregnancy. Among 326,335 women aged 15 to 44 years with positive test results for SARS-CoV-2, pregnant women (which encompassed only 28% of all women of reproductive age)

Table 13.1 Summary of Perinatal Outcomes During the SARS-CoV-1 and MERS-CoV Epidemics

Perinatal Effects	SARS-CoV-1 (n = 33)	MERS-CoV (n = 12)
First-trimester miscarriage	38.1% miscarriage[1]	No data on miscarriage[1]
Second-/third-trimester loss	One fetus in a twin gestation[3]	Two fetuses (at 20 wk and at 34 wk)[3]
Prematurity	12% <34 wk preterm birth 21.7% <37 wk preterm birth 12.5% preterm premature rupture of membrane[1]	33.3% <34 wk preterm birth[1]
Fetal growth and placental effects	12.5% fetal growth restriction No cases of preeclampsia[1]	Single placental abruption at 37 wk[3] 5.7% preeclampsia[1]
Delivery and postnatal outcomes	38.5% >37 wk birth 50% cesarean delivery 22.2% "normal" vaginal delivery 33% fetal distress 10% perinatal deaths None of the studies reported Apgar score <7 at 5 min, neonatal asphyxia, or NICU admission[1]	80% >37 wk birth 66.7% cesarean delivery 16.7% "normal" vaginal delivery 33.3% perinatal deaths No report of fetal distress, Apgar score <7 at 5 min, neonatal asphyxia, or NICU admission[1]
Maternal outcomes	54.5% maternal ICU admission 12.5% maternal death[1]	33.3% maternal ICU admission 40% maternal death[1]
Neonatal outcomes	No report of maternal vertical transmission[3] RDS and bowel perforation in neonate at 26 wk[143] RDS, necrotizing enterocolitis, and patent ductus arteriosus in neonate at 28 wk[143]	No report of maternal vertical transmission[3] 1 neonatal death at 24 wk (birth weight 240 g because of extreme prematurity)[143] 2 stillbirths[143]

ICU, Intensive care unit; NICU, neonatal ICU; RDS, respiratory distress syndrome.

were more likely to be hospitalized, admitted to an ICU, and receive mechanical ventilation. However, the overall absolute increase in rates of ICU admission and mechanical ventilation were low among pregnant and nonpregnant women (1.5% vs. 0.9% for ICU admission, respectively, and 0.5% vs. 0.3% for mechanical ventilation, respectively). Moreover, SARS-CoV-2–related death rates were similar in the pregnant and nonpregnant populations.[6]

Since the onset of the first reported case in 2019, over 6200 new studies have been published on maternal and child health and nutrition related to SARS-CoV-2 per the repository compiled by the Johns Hopkins Center for Humanitarian Health. This rapid and overwhelming increase in available evidence results from studies with varying degrees of bias and quality.[7] Early reports found that SARS-CoV-2 during pregnancy was likely to be associated with severe maternal morbidity similar to prior coronavirus epidemics.[8] However, the SARS-CoV-2 virus has surprised scientists in that it behaves like no other respiratory infection, involving multiple extrapulmonary organs.[9] More recent data suggest that the mortality rate of pregnant patients due to SARS-CoV-2 is lower than with SARS-CoV-1 and MERS-CoV,[10] but still higher than in the nonpregnant population.[11] Finally, similar to the nonpregnant population, disparities in social determinants of health among Hispanic and Black pregnant patients exist and act as barriers to health and well-being, which has led to disproportionate SARS CoV-2 infection rates and deaths in these populations.[12]

Today, the data continue to evolve. Initial studies available early in the pandemic focused mostly on infections occurring in the last trimester of pregnancy near delivery. In addition, early testing availability was variable, which affected the reported number of cases and outcomes related to them. In comparison, more recent studies include infections occurring in all trimesters, as well as in the periconception and postpartum periods.[13] As with other congenital infections, as data and cases become more readily available, the clinical findings and recommendations in pregnancy will continue to evolve.

Maternal SARS-CoV-2 Infection

Physiological Changes in Pregnancy

Physiological changes that occur in pregnancy may help explain the effects seen on morbidity and mortality in pregnancies affected by SARS-CoV-2 infection (see Table 13.1). Those most significantly affected are the respiratory and immunological systems, and hypercoagulability increases in pregnancy.

Respiratory System

Lung physiology is altered in pregnancy secondary to hormonal patterns. Progesterone leads to decreased plasma partial pressure of carbon dioxide, higher tidal volumes, and lower functional residual capacity (FRC) (by 9.5%–25%).[14] Reduced FRC subsequently causes functional ventilation-perfusion mismatch and ineffective airway clearance, potentially contributing to the enhanced severity of lower respiratory tract infections.[9]

Expiratory reserve volume decreases during the second half of pregnancy (8%–40% at term), as a result of reduction in residual volume by 7% to 22%. Inspiratory capacity increases and maintains a stable total lung capacity.[14] Because the respiratory rate remains unchanged in pregnancy, minute ventilation increases significantly (by up to 48%) during the first trimester and plateaus in the second and third trimesters.[14] The increase in minute ventilation results in a physiological respiratory alkalosis. Finally, the increased metabolic demand of pregnancy increases oxygen consumption by 20%.

These respiratory changes ensure appropriate oxygenation of the fetus, potentially at the expense of the mother, whose ability to compensate is reduced during respiratory illness. For example, during the 2009 H1N1 influenza epidemic, pregnant mothers were at a significantly higher risk for respiratory complications and hospitalization.[15] SARS-CoV-2 disease affects the lower respiratory tract and can lead to rapid bilateral lung involvement.[16] This may predispose pregnant patients to an increased risk for hypoxic respiratory failure. If pregnancy is further complicated by other comorbidities, such as obesity, expiratory reserve volume, functional residual capacity, and lung compliance are more compromised, triggering increased disease severity.[17]

The Immune System

The immunological changes that occur during pregnancy allow a genetically and immunologically foreign fetus to survive.[18] This requires significant maternal immunomodulation, with a delicate balance between innate and humoral immunity. The consequence of this immunosuppression has been postulated to increase maternal susceptibility to various pathogens, including viruses.[4]

Peripheral blood mononuclear cells (PBMCs) are the primary immune cells of the immune system. They include T, B, and natural killer (NK) cells, as well as circulating monocytes. Recognition of pathogens by these cells produces a cascade of immune molecules, including cytokines and chemokines. There is strong evidence demonstrating a shift in cytokine profile of successful pregnancies, such that there is a reduction in T helper type 1 (Th1) cytokines (interferon-gamma [IFN-g] and interleukin-2 [IL-2]) with a simultaneous increase in Th2 cytokines (IL-4 and IL-10), compared with nonpregnant patients. On the other hand, there is an increased ratio of Th1 to Th2 cytokine production in failed pregnancies.[19]

Additionally, research has demonstrated that the balance between Th17 and T regulator (Treg) cells also plays a role in pregnancy. Th17 cells produce predominately inflammatory cytokines such as IL-17A. In contrast, Treg cells produce mainly antiinflammatory cytokines, such as IL-4 and transforming growth factor-beta (TGF-β), and inhibit autoimmune responses.[20]

In pregnancy, the ratio of Treg/Th17 is shifted such that a higher level of Treg cells help support the mother's immune tolerance to the fetus.[21]

The severity of SARS-CoV-2 disease can be reflected in the cytokine profile. Studies of nonpregnant patients found activation of both Th1 and Th2-biased immune cells.[4] Patients requiring ICU-level care were found to have higher plasma levels of IL-2, IL-7, IL-10, granulocyte colony-stimulating factor, and tumor necrosis factor-α.[22] Additionally, the ratio of Treg/Th17 cells shifted in favor of Th17 cells (proinflammatory) in patients with more severe SARS-CoV-2 infections.[4] The immunological changes that occur in pregnancy were initially thought to impair adaptive immune response and increase release of proinflammatory cytokines, leading to systemic inflammation and potentially severe organ damage. However, more recent data are now supporting the theory that the physiological shift toward a Th2- and Treg-predominant environment in pregnancy may in fact result in a less severe form of COVID-19, by preventing the excessive inflammatory response usually observed in SARS-CoV-2 patients with severe disease.[23,24] However, characterization of the immune response in pregnant patients with COVID-19 has yet to be fully elucidated.

Hypercoagulable State and Endothelial Dysfunction

Pregnancy is a physiologically hypercoagulable state.[25] Most notably there is a significant change in coagulation, with increased factor VII, VIII, and X; von Willebrand factor activity; and marked increases in fibrinogen and D-dimer (increases to 50% above baseline normal range of 0.3–1.7 mg/L[26] by the third trimester).[27] Thrombin generation markers (prothrombin F1 and 2 as well as thrombin-antithrombin complexes) are also increased. Protein S and activated protein C levels decrease during pregnancy.[28] Fibrinolytic activity is reduced with plasminogen activator inhibitor type 1 (PAI-1) levels increased by five-fold and increases in placentally derived PAI-2, particularly during the third trimester.[29] Pregnancy is associated with a four- to six-fold increased risk of venous thromboembolism (VTE), and this risk is further increased in the postpartum period.[25]

Disruption of the endothelium is thought to occur during SARS-CoV-2 infection, and concern has been raised for possible exacerbation of an enhanced thrombotic state in pregnancy. Endothelial disruption occurs either directly through signaling effects or indirectly through increased proinflammatory mediator production and subsequent deregulation of the coagulation cascade.[30] Pericytes with high expression of angiotensin-converting enzyme-2 (ACE2) are the target cells of SARS-CoV-2, found in most organs such as heart, lung, kidney, vessels, brain, and others, including the placenta,[9] and result in endothelial cell and microvascular dysfunction. Severe SARS-CoV-2 appears to resemble complement-mediated thrombotic microangiopathies. Autopsy studies revealed generalized thrombotic microangiopathy and endothelial dysfunction together with pulmonary embolus and deep venous thrombosis in SARS-CoV-2 infected patients.[30] Some suggested that inactivation and downregulation of ACE2 occurs by formation of viral-ACE2 complex after SARS-CoV-2 placental infection. This then causes lowering of plasma angiotensin levels, which in return potentiates vasoconstriction and procoagulopathic state, leading to early-onset, severe preeclampsia.[9] The extent of the clinical impacts of endothelial dysfunction during SARS-CoV-2 infection in pregnancy remains to be fully evaluated.

Clinical Findings of Maternal SARS-CoV-2 Infection

Clinical presentation of SARS-CoV-2 varies in pregnancy. A systematic review of 571 pregnancies reported an asymptomatic rate of 15% in pregnant women with SARS-CoV-2–positive tests.[17] The clinical findings are similar to those of nonpregnant women. Fever, cough, and dyspnea are the most common symptoms.[17,31] Others included myalgia, malaise, sore throat, diarrhea, and shortness of breath.[32] Overall, presence of any SARS-CoV-2 symptoms is thought to be associated with increased maternal morbidity and mortality. Specifically, severe pregnancy and neonatal complication rates were highest in pregnant patients if fever and shortness of breath were present for 1 to 4 days, reflecting systemic disease.[11]

There are no major differences between pregnant and nonpregnant women with SARS-CoV-2 in terms of laboratory findings, with elevated CRP being the most common finding (99%). Lymphopenia is another common biomarker.[10] In nonpregnant individuals, significantly elevated D-dimer level (up to 12- to 17-fold the upper normal range in pregnancy) is considered a poor prognostic indicator of SARS-CoV-2 disease.[27,33] One study found higher D-dimer levels in those requiring ICU admission versus those who did not (median D-dimer 2.4 mg/L vs. 0.5 mg/L $P = .0042$).[22] Another study observed higher D-dimer levels in nonsurvivors compared with survivors of SARS-CoV-2 disease (2.12 mg/L vs. 0.6 mg/L, $P \leq .001$).[34] Given the expected rise in D-dimer level during pregnancy, it remains unclear whether D-dimer elevation would indicate a similarly poor prognosis in pregnancy. The International Society of Thrombosis and Hemostasis (ISTH) suggests that those with a significant D-dimer elevation may warrant hospitalization regardless of symptoms.[35] Prothrombin time (PT), activated partial thromboplastin time (aPTT), fibrinogen, and platelets are also considered valuable markers in pregnancy. There have been reports of increased hematological complications in pregnant women with COVID-19 compared with those without infection, although the evidence is still limited.[26]

The majority of pregnant patients with pulmonary findings on chest imaging had ground-glass opacities (81.6%), bilateral lung involvement (79.2%), or a consolidation (17.6%), similar to nonpregnant patients.[4]

Maternal and Obstetric Outcomes in SARS-CoV-2 Infection

Although the body of evidence on maternal outcomes in pregnancies affected by SARS-CoV-2 infection continues to expand at a rapid pace, several comprehensive studies have been published. A large study conducted by the Maternal-Fetal Medicine Unit (MFMU) Network including 1219 patients from 33 hospitals in 14 states reported that mothers with severe or critical SARS-CoV-2 disease and their neonates are at increased risk for a number of perinatal complications, including cesarean birth, hypertensive disorders of pregnancy, preterm birth, VTE, neonatal ICU (NICU) admission, and lower birth weight, compared with asymptomatic mothers.[36] However, data remain incomplete and, at times, inconsistent with many studies because of a large degree of heterogeneity regarding methods and included populations.

Maternal Morbidity and Mortality

SARS-CoV-2 infection in pregnancy is consistently associated with substantial increases in severe maternal morbidity and mortality.[11] The MFMU Network study found the rate of severe to critical SARS-CoV-2 disease to be 12% in pregnant patients. Maternal ICU admission occurred in 4.8%, and maternal death occurred in 0.3% of this population.[36] Another large systematic review reported a maternal mortality rate of 0.02%, ICU admission rate of 4%, mechanical ventilation rate of 3%, and extracorporeal membrane oxygenation (ECMO) rate of 0.2% among pregnant women.[37] Conversely, Karimi et al.[38] conducted a systematic review that investigated 117 published reports involving 11,758 pregnant women from high- and middle-income countries and found a mortality rate for COVID-19 of 1.30% and a rate of severe pneumonia of up to 14%.[38] A 2021 multinational cohort study including 18 countries found a similar risk for maternal mortality of 1.6%.[11] Mortality was reported to be 22 times higher in pregnant women with COVID-19 compared with nonpregnant women. These rates exceed reported rates from studies conducted in the United States likely because of disparities of maternity services between lower- and higher-income countries.[39] However, one factor that all studies agree on is the high prevalence of comorbidities in pregnant women with increased rates of severe morbidity and mortality associated with COVID-19.[37] Karimi et al.[38] reported a comorbidity rate of 20% in deceased pregnant individuals. Advanced maternal age was most prevalent; other comorbidities included diabetes, obesity, asthma, and cardiovascular disease, including essential hypertension, gestational hypertension, preeclampsia, and hemolysis, elevated liver enzymes, and low platelets (HELLP) syndrome.[38]

Mode of Delivery

Although the safest mode of delivery in patients with SARS-CoV-2 infection is not clear, overall an increased rate of cesarean delivery (CD) in women with COVID-19 has been reported. The MFMU Network study reported a cesarean birth rate of 36.9%. This rate was even higher (59.6%) in expecting mothers with severe or critical COVID-19.[36] One summary of 39 systematic reviews reported a CD rate between 52.3% and 95.8%.[40] Rates of CD, in which the primary indication was COVID-19, varied between 7.7% and 60.4%.[40] In particular, one review found that maternal SARS-CoV-2 infection was the primary indication for 49.6% (59/119) of preterm CD and 65.7% (159/242) of term CD.[41] Vaginal delivery rates ranged between 4.2% and 44.7%.[40]

Hypertensive Disorder of Pregnancy

An increase in hypertensive disorders of pregnancy has been reported in pregnant patients diagnosed with SARS-CoV-2 infection. The overall risk of a hypertensive disorder in pregnancies affected by COVID-19 was 23.4%, with 40.4% in women with severe to critical disease.[36] A multinational cohort study reported by Villar et al.[11] found a rate of pregnancy- induced hypertension of 8.2% in those with SARS-CoV-2 disease compared with 5.6% in unaffected pregnancies. Furthermore, 8.4% of pregnancies complicated by COVID-19 had a diagnosis of preeclampsia, eclampsia, or HELLP syndrome, compared with 4.4% of those without.[11]

Risk for Preterm Birth, Preterm Labor, and Premature Rupture of Membranes

Infection with SARS-CoV-2 during pregnancy has a demonstrated increased risk for preterm birth. In a large network study conducted in the United States, overall risk for preterm birth before 37 weeks was reported as 16.9% in pregnancies complicated by COVID-19.[36] In this study, the rate of preterm birth was 41.8% in patients with severe to critical COVID-19 compared with 11.9% in asymptomatic women. Villar et al.[11] reported a 22.5% rate of preterm birth before 37 weeks in patients with COVID-19 compared with 13.6% in unaffected pregnancies. Overall, reported rates of preterm deliveries vary between 14.3% and 63.8% for pregnancies complicated by COVID-19.[40] Two large studies found spontaneous preterm birth rates of 5%[42] and 6.4%,[37] and another review reported a medically indicated preterm birth rate of 21.4%.[42] Another study described a medically indicated preterm birth rate of 18.8% in pregnant women with COVID-19 compared with 8.9% in normal pregnancies.[11] Reported rates of preterm labor range between 22.7% and 32.2%.[40] Premature rupture of membranes (PROM) also ranges

between 2.5% and 26.5%.[7] Data for preterm PROM are even more limited, with a reported range of 6.4% to 16.1%.[40]

Miscarriage and Pregnancy Loss

Currently available data on rates of miscarriage and pregnancy loss are limited and inconsistent. Overall reported miscarriage rates associated with SARS-CoV-2 infection reported by moderate- to high-quality studies are low at less than 2.5%.[40] However, one review including 637 participants reported miscarriage rates of 16.1% and 3.6% for first- and second trimester infections, respectively.[41] Although miscarriage may occur in the setting of COVID-19, determining causality has been challenging. Metz et al.[36] found 3 fetal deaths before 20 weeks gestation among 141 pregnancies complicated by critical to severe COVID-19 compared with 6 among 499 patients with mild to moderate disease, and 4 among 579 women with asymptomatic SARS-CoV-2 infection.[36] Few studies have reported rates of pregnancy termination; however, one study reported a rate of 0.1% in a cohort of patients with first- and second-trimester infections. Indications for termination were related to the patient's anxiety for potential SARS-CoV-2–associated adverse pregnancy outcomes.[41]

Fetal Outcomes

Data on fetal outcomes continue to evolve. Rates of fetal distress in pregnancies complicated by SARS-CoV-2 infection vary between 7.8% and 61.1%,[40] with the largest sample reporting a rate of 8.5%.[37] Within a multinational cohort study conducted by Villar et al.,[11] fetal distress was reported in 12.3% of pregnancies complicated by SARS-CoV-2 infection compared with 8.4% in those without. Reported rates of stillbirth are low, with the two largest collected series of deliveries reporting a rate of 0.6% and 0.9%.[37,42] Additionally, Metz et al.[36] found the rates of fetal death reported in pregnant patients with severe or critical COVID-19 after 20 weeks gestation were 1 in 141 (0.07%) compared with 4 in 499 (0.008%) with mild to moderate disease and 5 in 579 (0.009%) among asymptomatic pregnancies.

Overall, pregnancies complicated by underlying comorbidities in addition to SARS-COV-2 infection are at higher risk for adverse outcomes compared with pregnancies complicated by SARS-COV-2 infection alone.[43] However, data remain incomplete and inconsistent, with many studies containing a large degree of heterogeneity regarding methods and included populations. Data available early in the pandemic focused mostly on infections in the last trimester and near delivery. In addition, testing availability was not universal, which affected the reported number of cases and related outcomes. Moreover, not all studies stratify data by classification of disease severity (mild, severe, critical) but rather between asymptomatic and symptomatic women.

Manifestations of SARS-CoV-2 in the Placenta and Other Organs

Vertical Transmission: Why Are We Concerned?

Teratogenicity and fetal morbidity are known to be associated with many viral infections, such as Zika virus and so-called TORCH infections (toxoplasmosis, other [parvovirus B19, syphilis, varicella zoster virus (VZV)], etc.), rubella, cytomegalovirus (CMV), and herpes simplex virus (HSV). The transmission rates for these pathogens range from as low as 0.2% to 0.4% for CMV and VZV, to as high as 17% to 33% for parvovirus B19. The transplacental passage of infectious pathogens tends to occur with increasing frequency as gestational age increases, whereas detrimental effects on the fetus increase at earlier gestational age.[44]

The teratogenic risk associated with SARS-CoV-2 infection in pregnancy remains unknown. At the beginning of the pandemic, there was a concern that SARS-CoV-2 infection in pregnancy may have detrimental effects similar to those of other TORCH infections; however, that has not been the case. Vertical transmission rates have been reported as high as 7.9%,[17] but most studies have found a much lower rate, around 3.2%.[44] However, these data remain limited by the indirect measures of possible vertical transmission used by most studies. Fetal infection can be conclusively determined only by the direct demonstration of the presence of the SARS-CoV-2 virus in fetal tissues, which often are not available for study.[44]

In addition to direct in-utero fetal infection, indirect fetal effects are also a concern with maternal SARS-CoV-2 infection. One systematic review found several cohort studies and case reports describing an association between maternal SARS-CoV-2 infection and placental evidence of maternal vascular malperfusion, particularly with maternal vessel injury and intervillous thrombi. One may speculate that SARS-CoV-2 may result in the activation of endothelial damage pathways predisposing to the development of hypertensive disorders of pregnancy, which in itself is associated with poor maternal and neonatal outcomes (i.e., prematurity, growth restriction, low birth weight) in the short and long term. This is one of the many issues that remain open for study.[44]

Data From Neonatal RT-PCR Tests on Nasopharyngeal Swab, Amniotic Fluid, Placenta, Urine, Cord Blood, and Anal or Rectal Swabs

Nasopharyngeal Sampling

Both the American Academy of Pediatrics (AAP) and the CDC recommend nasopharyngeal reverse transcription polymerase chain reaction (RT-PCR) testing of all neonates born to mothers with suspected or confirmed SARS-CoV-2 infection during pregnancy.[45,46] Case reports, single-center cohort studies, retrospective reviews, and systematic reviews have published data on nasopharyngeal RT-PCR testing of neonates born to mothers with COVID-19 during pregnancy. The overwhelming majority of neonates in these studies had negative nasopharyngeal RT-PCR testing.[47–56] Mirbeyk et al.[57] published a systematic review including 37 studies containing 365 pregnant women with SARS-CoV-2 infection and 302 of their neonates. Of the 302 neonates, 219 underwent nasopharyngeal RT-PCR testing with only 11 in 219 (5%) testing positive. Similarly, Villar et al.[11] conducted a multinational cohort study on mothers with SARS-CoV-2 infection in pregnancy and their neonates. Nasopharyngeal testing was performed on 416 neonates born to SARS-CoV-2–infected mothers. Of the 416 neonates, 54 (12.9%) had positive test results within the first 48 hours after birth.[11] Studies reporting positive nasopharyngeal RT-PCR results in neonates were variable in timing of specimen collection from shortly after birth to up to 1 week of life.[51,52,58–62] Currently, there are no recommendations for routine RT-PCR testing of amniotic fluid, placenta, cord blood, urine, and/or anal or rectal samples for SARS-CoV-2 in exposed neonates. Most of the data collected from these sites comes from case reports or small cohort studies.

Amniotic Fluid

The majority of RT-PCR testing performed on amniotic fluid produced negative results.[a] A single case report documented positive RT-PCR testing of amniotic fluid in a mother with severe COVID-19.[68] Neonatal cord blood and nasopharyngeal RT-PCR testing obtained at 2 hours after birth were negative. However, amniotic fluid and repeat nasopharyngeal testing obtained at 24 hours after birth were positive.

Placental Tissue

Testing of placental tissue is uncommon and has yielded predominantly negative results.[46,50,51,54,64–67] A placental analysis from eight cohort or case series studies yielded a pooled positive RT-PCR rate of 7.7% (2/26) of all tested placentas of SARS-CoV-2–infected mothers.[44] However, evidence of placental viral infection does not guarantee intrauterine vertical transmission to the fetus.[69] Transplacental infection not only requires detection of viral RNA in the placenta but also in amniotic fluid before the onset of labor; cord or neonatal blood, body fluid, or respiratory samples; or demonstration of viral particles by electron microscopy, immunohistochemistry studies, or in situ hybridization in fetal/neonatal tissues.[53]

One case report demonstrated positive placenta RT-PCR testing in a mother and neonate with positive

---

[a]References 48, 50, 52, 54, 56, 63–67.

nasopharyngeal RT-PCR swabs.[58] Histological examination of placental tissue showed multiple areas of infiltration with inflammatory cells and early infarction. One study reported histopathological findings in 16 placentas from mothers with SARS-CoV-2 infection during pregnancy. Despite lack of significant differences in acute or chronic inflammatory pathological processes compared with controls, placentas of SARS-CoV-2–infected mothers did have higher rates of decidual arteriopathy and other maternal vascular malperfusion features that have been associated with adverse outcomes.[70] Two additional case reports found SARS-CoV-2 localization and damage predominantly to the syncytiotrophoblast cells at the maternofetal interface.[71,72] In contrast, a single-center review compared 101 placentas from mothers with SARS-CoV-2 infection during pregnancy to 121 controls and found no significant difference in chorioamnionitis, fetal vascular malperfusion, or maternal vascular malperfusion between the two groups.[59]

Cord Blood and Urine

Testing umbilical cord blood of neonates born to mothers with SARS-CoV-2 infection during pregnancy has largely produced negative results.[b] Although rarely performed, two studies including 20 neonates reported negative urine RT-PCR results in all neonates.[63,64]

Anal and Rectal Swabs

Anal and rectal RT-PCR swabs performed on neonates also produced predominantly negative results.[c] In a cohort study of 33 neonates born to mothers with SARS-CoV-2 infection, only 3 had positive anal swab samples, which were obtained on postpartum days 2 and 4.[61]

Conflicting Data on Antibody Testing in Neonates

In adults, SARS-CoV-2 immunoglobulin M (IgM) and IgG antibody testing is a useful tool for detecting recent or past infection. IgM antibodies are produced early in the immune response and are the first immunoglobulin class synthesized by infants. IgG antibodies are produced later and remain present after IgM levels fall. Unlike IgG, IgM antibodies do not cross the placenta. In neonates, although the presence of SARS-CoV-2 IgG antibodies likely represents transplacental transfer of maternal immunoglobulins, IgM presence shortly after birth may provide support for intrauterine vertical transmission. Currently, antibody testing is not recommended to evaluate for acute infection in neonates and children.[45]

Studies evaluating antibody testing shortly after birth on neonates born to mothers with confirmed

SARS-CoV-2 infection during pregnancy have produced conflicting results. Three studies from Wuhan, China evaluated 36 neonates born to SARS-CoV-2–positive mothers with RT-PCR and antibody testing shortly after birth. Of the 36 neonates, 26 and 9 had IgG and IgM levels above the normal reference range, respectively. However, all neonates were asymptomatic and none had positive RT-PCR swabs of the throat or anus.[75-77] In a separate study, cord blood samples of 37 neonates born to SARS-CoV-2–positive mothers were evaluated for IgG and IgM antibodies. Of the 37 neonates tested, 23 had elevated cord blood IgG and 1 had elevated IgM levels. In the neonate with IgM antibodies, nasopharyngeal RT-PCR testing was negative and placental pathology was indicative of feto-maternal hemorrhage, which suggested leakage of IgM antibodies into the fetal circulation rather than intrauterine vertical transmission.[77]

It is plausible that the presence of IgM antibodies in infants from these studies was the result of leakage from maternal to fetal circulation, which is supported by the absence of symptoms or positive RT-PCR results in these infants. Conversely, the presence of IgM antibodies in these infants may provide evidence for intrauterine vertical transmission. At this time, both hypotheses remain plausible, but more research is needed.

Transplacental passage of IgG antibodies from mother to neonate may confer passive immunity to the neonate in utero and after birth. Kubiak et al.[78] evaluated IgG antibody levels in mothers with SARS-CoV-2 infection during pregnancy and in their neonates after birth. A strong, direct relationship was found between maternal IgG level and maternal oxygen requirement and neonate IgG levels, suggesting that maternal disease severity is associated with higher IgG levels in neonates at birth.[78] A study by Mo et al.[76] examined the duration of elevated IgG levels in neonates born to mothers with SARS-CoV-2 infection. In that study, neonatal IgG levels remained elevated for up to 180 days after birth, and maternal infection in the second trimester was associated with a longer duration of IgG elevation compared with the third trimester. What remains unknown, however, is the IgG level needed to provide immunity to neonates after birth.

Treatment and Interventions in Pregnancy

Treatment and interventions vary between the outpatient and inpatient setting. The management of hospitalized pregnant women with SARS-CoV-2 infection is not substantially different from that of nonpregnant patients.[79] However, pregnancy status may confer a lower threshold for admission.[80] Inpatient monitoring may be necessary for pregnant patients with moderate to severe signs and symptoms of SARS-CoV-2 infection, oxygen saturation less than 95%, presence of comorbid

[b]References 48, 50, 52, 54–56, 64, 65, 67.
[c]References 50, 58, 63, 64, 66, 67, 73, 74.

conditions (uncontrolled hypertension, inadequately controlled gestational or pregestational diabetes, chronic renal disease, chronic cardiopulmonary disease, or immunosuppressive states), or fevers greater than 39°C despite acetaminophen.

Once admitted, management requires a multispecialty team-based approach that may include consultation with obstetrics, maternal-fetal medicine, infectious disease, pulmonary and critical care, neonatology, and pediatric specialists. Fetal and uterine contraction monitoring should be performed when appropriate, based on gestational age, and delivery planning should be individualized. In most cases, the timing of delivery should be dictated by obstetric indications rather than maternal diagnosis of SARS-CoV-2 infection. Most importantly, potentially effective treatment for SARS-CoV-2 infection should not be withheld from pregnant women because of theoretical concerns related to the safety of therapeutic agents in pregnancy.[6]

Diagnostic chest radiographs and chest computed tomography (CT) scans may be required. Although radiation exposure during pregnancy should be minimized, radiography, CT, or nuclear medicine imaging techniques in addition to ultrasonography or magnetic resonance imaging (MRI) should not be withheld from pregnant patients, if medically indicated.[81] If these techniques are necessary, in addition to ultrasonography or MRI, they should not be withheld from pregnant patients.

A large number of medical therapeutic options have been investigated for the treatment of SARS-CoV-2 infection, but data remain limited in pregnancy. Proposed therapies have included antiviral drugs, corticosteroids, monoclonal antibodies, and convalescent plasma. None of these therapies have absolute contraindications in pregnancy; however, pregnant patients have been excluded from almost all clinical trials. The RECOVERY trial is an ongoing randomized clinical trial (RCT) investigating use of multiple therapies to prevent death in patients with SARS-CoV-2. This trial was the first to include pregnant women.[79]

Corticosteroids

Corticosteroids are well-known immunomodulators that can reduce inflammatory response.[82] The RECOVERY trial demonstrated that dexamethasone for up to 10 days resulted in lower 28-day mortality among people requiring invasive mechanical ventilation and a small but statistically significant decrease in mortality risk among those requiring supplemental oxygen but not intubation for SARS-CoV-2. However, this benefit was not seen in patients not requiring respiratory support.[83] Use of dexamethasone in pregnancy has been associated with risk for cleft palate and impaired fetal growth when used in the first trimester.[84,85] Neonatal concerns

regarding its use later in pregnancy include maternal hyperglycemia leading to neonatal hypoglycemia and the potential for the development of maternal adrenal insufficiency.[86] However, given the significant benefit of reduction in mortality among patients with SARS-CoV-2, this treatment should not be withheld from pregnant COVID-19 patients. The maternal benefits outweigh the risks of neonatal harm.[87] If glucocorticoids are indicated for fetal lung maturity, dexamethasone can be dosed at 6 mg intramuscularly (IM) every 12 hours for 48 hours (four doses) followed by up to a total of 10 days of 6 mg dexamethasone orally (PO) or intravenously (IV) daily to provide transplacental fetal benefit. If glucocorticoids are not indicated for fetal lung maturity, 6 mg dexamethasone (PO/IV) daily for up to 10 days has been recommended for nonpregnant patients.[88]

Remdesivir

Remdesivir is a broad-spectrum antiviral drug that effectively inhibits replication of SARS-CoV-2 in vitro.[89] To date, data are mixed about its clinical use in patients with SARS-CoV-2 infection and data on use in pregnancy are limited. A single small case series of six pregnant women exposed to remdesivir while being treated for Ebola did not find any adverse pregnancy outcomes.[90] It should be noted that remdesivir was given outside of the first trimester in all case reports. A case series of 86 women (67 were pregnant, 19 immediately postpartum) given remdesivir on a compassionate use basis for severe SARS-CoV-2 infection found a high rate of clinical recovery, but rates of preterm delivery were high (likely related to severe SARS-CoV-2).[91] Nevertheless, these data are difficult to quantify in the absence of a control arm. Remdesivir can be given in pregnancy if the benefits outweigh the potential risks and could be offered to pregnant patients meeting criteria for compassionate use.[88]

Immune Modulators

Monoclonal antibodies inhibit a single cytokine and thus have the benefit of molecular precision. These agents provide a focused inhibition of a single pathway, avoiding the broad side effect profile of corticosteroids. On the other hand, monoclonal antibodies are also exceedingly expensive and often have limited availability. Tocilizumab is an IL-6 monoclonal antibody that can cause immune suppression by inhibiting IL-6, a proinflammatory cytokine associated with the SARS-CoV-2–related cytokine storm.[92] It is commonly used for treatment of rheumatoid arthritis. It has been offered for SARS-CoV-2 treatment as part of the RECOVERY trial. Small trials in nonpregnant adult patients showed that tocilizumab reduced the chance of progression to the composite outcome of mechanical ventilation or death in hospitalized patients with SARS-CoV-2 pneumonia who were not receiving mechanical ventilation.[93]

Janus kinase (JAK) inhibitors, such as baricitinib, are a different type of immunomodulator with the ability to inhibit the intracellular signaling pathway of multiple cytokines known to be elevated in severe COVID-19, including IL-2, IL-6, IL-10, IFN-g, and granulocyte-macrophage colony-stimulating factor (GM-CSF). It also acts against SARS-CoV-2 through the impairment of AP2-associated protein kinase 1 (AAK-1), which regulates endocytosis in alveolar type II cells, and prevents SARS-CoV-2 cellular entry and infectivity. Finally, it improves lymphocyte counts in infected patients.[94] In three case series, baricitinib treatment was associated with both an improvement in oxygenation and a reduction in select inflammatory markers. A recent clinical trial (ACTT-2 Trial) showed that combination treatment with baricitinib and remdesivir was safe and superior to remdesivir alone for the treatment of hospitalized patients with COVID-19 complicated by pneumonia.[95]

Based on experimental animal studies, use of immunomodulators is not expected to increase the risk for congenital malformations, but data are scarce in pregnancy. Because these agents are potentially effective against SARS-CoV-2 infection, use should be considered on an individual basis and not be withheld from pregnant women because of theoretical concerns related to safety of the fetus.

Convalescent Plasma

In previous epidemics, patients with SARS, MERS, H1N1 influenza, and Ebola infections have been treated using plasma collected from recovered patients.[96,97] One explanation for the efficacy of convalescent plasma therapy is that antibodies from convalescent plasma might suppress viremia.[97] Two RCTs of nonpregnant patients with severe or life-threatening COVID-19 failed to show a difference in clinical status or overall mortality between patients treated with convalescent plasma compared with placebo or standard treatment.[96,98] Despite these findings, several cases have reported using convalescent plasma in the management of pregnancies complicated by SARS-CoV-2 infection with rapid deterioration.[99,100] At this time, pharmacological use of convalescent plasma is considered investigational and efficacy remains unclear.[88]

Unique Considerations in Pregnancy

Antithrombotic Prophylaxis

As mentioned earlier, pregnancy is a hypercoagulable state that poses an increased risk for venous thrombotic events. Hemostatic and thromboembolic complications have been reported in 0.98% and 0.28% of pregnant women with SARS-CoV-2 infection, respectively.[26] Additional studies demonstrated that hematological complications are more commonly observed in pregnant

women with SARS-CoV-2 infection (1.26%) than in pregnant women without (0.45%).[26] There is no consensus on antepartum and postpartum anticoagulation guidelines at this time; however, various recommendations have been made.

The Royal College of Obstetricians and Gynaecologists (RCOG) current guidelines (as of February 2021) recommend that all pregnant women and women who are within 6 weeks postpartum, admitted with confirmed or suspected SARS-CoV-2 infection, be offered prophylactic low-molecular-weight heparin (LMWH) during admission and continued for at least 10 days after discharge. One study demonstrated that hematological complications are more commonly observed in pregnant women with SARS-CoV-2 infection (1.26%) than in pregnant women without (0.45%).[26,101]

The Canadian ISTH (Subcommittee for Women's Health Issues in Thrombosis and Hemostasis) has also suggested weight-adjusted VTE prophylaxis with LMWH in all pregnant and postpartum women admitted to hospital with SARS-CoV-2 infection in the absence of active bleeding and with a platelet count above 30×10^9/L, provided urgent delivery is not anticipated or timing is beyond 24 hours postpartum. They also recommended careful and individualized VTE risk assessment for outpatient anticoagulation after discharge from the hospital, varying between a 10- to 14-day course of LMWH to 2 to 6 weeks for postpartum women. For women at low risk for VTE, hydration, appropriate nutrition, mobilization, and control of pyrexia were encouraged. Use of antiembolic stockings at home may be beneficial but the authors acknowledge that these recommendations are based on limited evidence.[25]

Cardiomyopathy

Although SARS-CoV-2 presents predominantly with pulmonary manifestations, there are reports of cardiovascular complications such as cardiomyopathy, viral myocarditis, myocardial infarction, and arrhythmias.[102] Data are limited to case reports; however, a 33% incidence of cardiomyopathy has been reported.[103,104] It is unknown whether the rate of developing SARS-CoV-2–associated cardiomyopathy is exacerbated in the pregnant population or similar to the rate in nonpregnant patients. One theory involves a higher level of inflammatory markers, such as IL-6, as a common pathophysiology for pregnancy-associated cardiomyopathy and SARS-CoV-2–related cardiomyopathy.[102] Zeng et al.[105] reviewed inflammatory markers in over 3900 SARS-CoV-2 patients and found that survivors had lower levels of IL-6 than nonsurvivors.

Further studies are needed to investigate whether pregnancy affects the chance of developing SARS-CoV-2–related cardiomyopathy compared with that of the general population.[102] Moreover, cardiomyopathy should be considered in the differential of pregnant patients with worsening clinical status in cases of severe COVID-19 and an echocardiographic evaluation should be considered given the assumed higher risk for cardiovascular complications after SARS-CoV-2 infection.[4]

Mechanical Ventilation

Mechanical ventilation includes both noninvasive and invasive modalities. Both modalities are used in patients with worsening severe respiratory distress syndrome related to SARS-CoV-2.[4] Among obstetric patients, the most common diagnosis of a severe respiratory illness requiring mechanical ventilation is acute respiratory distress syndrome (ARDS) caused by infection or preeclampsia. ARDS is a main finding in patients with critical SARS-CoV-2 pneumonia; however, to date there are still only a few reported cases of mechanical ventilation as a result of SARS-CoV-2 infection in pregnancy. A systematic review of 295 pregnant women found a rate of 1.8% for invasive mechanical ventilation and of 12.4% for noninvasive ventilation.[4]

Extracorporeal Membrane Oxygenation

ECMO can provide respiratory support (venovenous [VV]-ECMO) or both respiratory and circulatory support (venoarterial [VA]-ECMO).[106] Acute respiratory distress in the obstetric population because of viral pneumonia requiring ECMO during the midtrimester of pregnancy is rare. Until 2016, only 45 cases of ECMO in pregnancy had been reported in the literature worldwide, and most cases occurred during the H1N1 pandemic.[107]

ECMO in the setting of pregnancy presents unique challenges. Major hemorrhage is the most common complication, with bleeding occurring in various sites: intracranial, uterine, lung, upper gastrointestinal (GI), and the cannulation site. If major bleeding is present, immediate delivery is necessary. Cannula dislodgement, thrombosis, hemolysis, and infections are additional concerns of ECMO in pregnancy.[107]

Reported survival rates for pregnant patients on ECMO have been significantly higher than the overall survival for nonpregnant adults requiring ECMO for pulmonary (59%) or cardiac (43%) causes, with maternal survival rates ranging from 70% to 80% and fetal survival rates from 65% to 72%.[108] However, the data are inadequate about the safety of ECMO in pregnancy.[107] In a 10-year study of ECMO in 54 pregnant women with cardiopulmonary failure, only 60% of mothers and fetuses survived.[109] Another systematic review showed that ECMO in the peripartum period has been successfully used with a maternal survival rate of 75.4%.[108] Survival varied depending on the indication for ECMO. Nevertheless, ECMO has the potential to increase the survival rates of both mother and fetus and should be considered as salvage therapy for peripartum women with reversible forms of cardiorespiratory failure.[109] Multidisciplinary care is necessary for optimal management of the mother and fetus in patients affected by severe respiratory failure related to SARS-CoV-2 refractory to conventional therapies.[4]

Vaccine in Pregnancy

Several vaccines are now available for use worldwide. Although pregnant individuals were excluded from initial phase III vaccine trials, professional organizations continue to support vaccines not being withheld from pregnant and lactating persons.[88] Regarding vaccine safety in pregnancy, developmental and reproductive toxicity studies have not found adverse outcomes related to fetal development, pregnancy, delivery, or postpartum complication.[110] Early data from the CDC SARS-CoV-2 vaccine symptom monitoring system, V-safe, demonstrated no difference in side effects between pregnant and nonpregnant individuals who received the mRNA SARS-CoV-2 vaccines.[111] Furthermore, no differences in adverse pregnancy outcomes, including miscarriage, small for gestational age, preterm birth, or neonatal death were found in 827 completed pregnancies compared with historical rates before the SARS-CoV-2 pandemic.[111]

Antibody response is similar in those vaccinated during pregnancy compared with nonpregnant individuals. A study evaluating 131 pregnant individuals found similar levels of vaccine-induced antibody titers from mRNA SARS-CoV-2 vaccines compared with those in nonpregnant individuals. Moreover, pregnant individuals who received the vaccine in pregnancy had higher antibody titers than those observed from natural SARS-CoV-2 infection in pregnancy.[112]

Vaccination during pregnancy may provide fetal protection through passive immunity. Multiple studies have demonstrated the presence of vaccine-produced antibodies in cord blood and breast milk.[112–114] Increased rates of vaccine-associated IgG antibodies were found in cord blood samples of patients who received both doses of SARS-CoV-2 mRNA vaccine (Pfizer/BioNTech or Moderna) before delivery.[113,114] Additionally, cord blood antibodies were present in samples obtained more than 3 weeks after vaccine administration.[113,114] In summary, SARS-CoV-2 vaccines have the ability to reduce the risk for severe maternal morbidity and mortality and provide protection to neonates through passive immunity.

Breastfeeding

The SARS-CoV-2 pandemic has raised concerns regarding the possibility and effects of mother-infant transmission of SARS-CoV-2 through breastfeeding and close infant contact.[115] Breastfeeding has many benefits for both mothers and neonates. One case report described detection of SARS-CoV-2 RNA in milk samples from a mother for 4 consecutive days, coinciding with mild maternal symptoms and a SARS-CoV-2–positive diagnostic test of the newborn.[116] A case series of 15 mothers with SARS-CoV-2 infection found detectable RNA in breastmilk samples of 4 mothers (26.7%).[117] The throat swab samples from these mothers' infants were also found to be positive for SARS-CoV-2 RNA. Three of the four mothers were breastfeeding. Although it is not known whether SARS-CoV-2 can be transmitted through breastmilk, or if any potentially transmitted viral components are infectious, suspected or confirmed maternal SARS-CoV-2 infection is not considered a contraindication to infant feeding with breastmilk. Moreover, the benefits of breastfeeding may outweigh the risks of SARS-CoV-2 infection in infants.

Individuals with suspected or confirmed SARS-CoV-2 can still transmit the virus through respiratory droplets while in close contact with the infant, including while breastfeeding. Nevertheless, evidence supports the safety of direct breastfeeding in SARS-CoV-2–positive mothers who practice infection prevention measures.[118,119] Therefore obstetrician-gynecologists and other maternal care practitioners should counsel women with suspected or confirmed SARS-CoV-2 who intend to feed their infants with breastmilk on how to minimize the risk for transmission, including breastmilk expression with a manual or electric breast pump and precautions to avoid spreading the virus (hand hygiene and wearing a mask or cloth face covering, if possible, while breastfeeding).[120]

Impact of SARS-CoV-2 Infections on the Fetus and Newborn

Prevention of Neonatal SARS-CoV-2 Infection

At the beginning of the pandemic, the lack of understanding of peripartum transmission risk to the neonate led to varying management of SARS-CoV-2–exposed neonates among hospitals regarding rooming-in versus separation of the mother-infant dyad and allowance of direct breastfeeding. Not surprisingly, breastfeeding rates were lower in separated neonates. Despite this heterogeneity in care, none of the 70 exposed neonates in a US study tested positive for SARS-CoV-2.[53] Fortunately, time has afforded the medical community the ability to understand peripartum transmission risk and develop evidence-based best practices to aid in prevention of neonatal infection. Close contact with a SARS-CoV-2–positive mother or caretaker is likely the primary route of infection in neonates rather than vertical transmission.[45,121] Interestingly, maternal SARS-CoV-2 viral load does not appear to be associated with neonatal positivity or severity of illness.[122]

After delivery, neonates with suspected or confirmed perinatal exposure do not necessarily require NICU admission unless the neonate needs intensive care for other reasons or a facility lacks the means to care for a neonate requiring isolation.[45] Previously, there were concerns about the safety of rooming-in. An observational multicenter cohort study followed perinatally exposed neonates who roomed-in. These neonates could participate in skin-to-skin care and breastfeed. Mothers wore surgical masks when near their neonates and practiced infection prevention hygiene. All neonates were kept in a closed isolette when not being held. Results support the notion that perinatal transmission of SARS-CoV-2 is unlikely to occur if infection prevention measures are undertaken. None of the neonates tested positive on serial screening.[118] Similarly, a multicenter study in Italy examining rooming-in found this practice to be safe.[119]

Society recommendations have evolved throughout the pandemic. At present, the World Health Organization (WHO), CDC, and AAP support rooming-in with proper infection prevention measures and direct breastfeeding.[45,46,123] The AAP and CDC suggest that placing the neonate in an isolette incubator in the mother's room may facilitate distancing and provide protection from aerosolized viral particles.[45,46] The WHO and AAP endorse skin-to-skin care.[46,123] The AAP also supports delayed cord clamping when indicated.[46] The CDC advises against neonates wearing masks or plastic face shields.[45] SARS-CoV-2–positive mothers can discontinue isolation and precautions when it has been at least 10 days since the onset of symptoms, she has been afebrile for at least 24 hours, and her symptoms have improved.[45]

Neonatal SARS-CoV-2 Infection

Neonatal SARS-CoV-2 infections have been recognized in the literature. The number of cases in neonates is low compared with that in adults.[124] Theories to explain the low infection rates include research demonstrating that SARS-CoV-2 enters cells by ACE2 receptors located in the respiratory tract epithelium and lung parenchyma, which is immature in young children, thus decreasing viral invasion ability. There also may be a decreased intracellular response induced by ACE2 in children.[124] Neonates appear to have protection from SARS-CoV-2 as a result of the presence of fetal hemoglobin, which comprises alpha and gamma chains but not beta chains. SARS-CoV-2 virus attacks the heme on the beta chain in adult hemoglobin leading to hypoxia.[124,125] The passage of maternal IgG antibodies across the placenta against SARS-CoV-2 also likely provides protection.[105] One interesting study described developmental regulation and lower expression levels of SARS-CoV-2 spike protein primer transmembrane protease serine 2 (TMPRSS2) in lung tissues of infants and children, possibly adding to their increased protection from severe respiratory illness associated with SARS-CoV-2 infection.[126]

Neonatal infection from perinatal SARS-CoV-2 exposure varies across studies and ranges from 2% to 10.7%.[46,122,127,128] In a retrospective observational study performed in India, SARS-CoV-2 testing was performed in neonates with suspected infection (including neonates with both SARS-CoV-2–positive and SARS-CoV-2–negative mothers); 10.6% (21/198) of neonates were positive. Two of the positive neonates were born to mothers with negative testing.[129] In another retrospective study in India evaluating outborn neonates admitted to the NICU, 4.25% (18/423) were positive. Just 50% of SARS-CoV-2–positive neonates in this study had positive mothers or caretakers.[130] At present, there has not yet been a confirmed case of neonatal mortality as a result of SARS-CoV-2 infection during birth hospitalization.[46] Neonatal fatalities associated with COVID-19 are very rare in general.[36,40]

Symptoms

Largely, SARS-CoV-2 infection is less severe in children compared with adults. A decreased systemic inflammatory response in children with SARS-CoV-2 may contribute to less severe manifestations.[125] However, when illness severity is compared in children, neonates appear to have more severe infections.[131,132] Acquired immunity from other viruses may provide some protection in older children. Neonates have not yet had the time to develop this cross immunity.[125] In addition, airways are still small and underdeveloped in neonates, possibly placing them at higher risk for respiratory compromise. Gotzinger et al.[133] found that age younger than 1 month was a significant risk factor for requiring intensive care.

Neonates with SARS-CoV-2 infection are often asymptomatic.[122,127] In a meta-analysis of 176 published cases of neonatal SARS-CoV-2, 55% of infected neonates had clinical manifestations.[134] The most common reported symptoms were respiratory distress, fever, neurological sequelae, and GI symptoms.[135] Respiratory symptoms included tachypnea, retractions, and rhinitis. Neurological manifestations comprised abnormalities in tone, irritability, and apnea. GI features were primarily feeding-related difficulties, diarrhea, and emesis. Other noted symptoms included conjunctivitis and rashes.[134] Severe lung disease requiring mechanical ventilation has been reported.[136] It may be difficult to ascertain whether these clinical signs were due to prematurity-related pathological conditions or SARS-CoV-2 in this population. Because SARS-CoV-2–positive neonates were more likely being born prematurely, required respiratory support may be more a complication of prematurity rather than SARS-CoV-2 infection.[122]

Multisystem inflammatory syndrome in children (MIS-C) is a rare and potentially life-threatening condition involving fever, multisystem dysfunction (≥ 2 organs), inflammation, and current or recent SARS-CoV-2 infection with no alternative diagnosis.[137] Cases appear to be postinfectious rather than related to acute infection.[138] The CDC reports only 3% of MIS-C cases are in those younger than 1 year of age.[139] Despite its rarity, there are documented cases of MIS-C in the neonatal population. Kappanayil et al.[140] reported MIS-C in

a neonate born to a mother with SARS-CoV-2 infection at 31 weeks gestation. The mother was negative for SARS-CoV-2 at delivery. The infant became symptomatic with cardiogenic shock and multiorgan dysfunction on day 22 of life. MIS-C was diagnosed given the temporal association with prenatal SARS-CoV-2, evidence of IgG antibodies to SARS-CoV-2, and lack of other plausible explanations.[140]

Laboratory and Radiographic Findings

Neonatal SARS-CoV-2 infection can exhibit relatively nonspecific laboratory abnormalities such as leukopenia and lymphopenia, elevated transaminases and elevated nonspecific inflammatory markers, including procalcitonin and CRP.[134,135] In a meta-analysis, 64% of infected neonates had abnormal lung imaging on ultrasound or chest x-ray with an interstitial alveolar pattern or a CT scan with ground-glass opacities.[134]

Testing

All neonates born to mothers with either suspected or confirmed SARS-CoV-2 infection should undergo testing irrespective of symptomatology.[45,46] The ideal time to test exposed neonates is unknown. Contamination from maternal fluids containing SARS-CoV-2 can cause false positives in those tested early. Additionally, early testing may lead to false-negative results because RNA may not yet be at detectable levels.[45] The CDC and AAP recommend testing at 24 hours of age.[45,46] Repeat testing at 48 hours of age is suggested.[46] The CDC recommends repeat testing at 48 hours in those testing negative at 24 hours of life or if results are still pending.[45] If hospital discharge is planned before 48 hours of life, a single test can be performed close to discharge from 24 to 48 hours of life.[45,46] If the initial test is positive, the AAP recommends considering follow-up testing at 48- to 72-hour intervals for neonates admitted to the NICU until the neonate has had two negative tests indicating mucosal viral clearance.[46] Testing should be performed using RT-PCR for SARS-CoV-2 RNA. Serological testing is not recommended.[45]

Management

All neonates with suspected or confirmed perinatal exposure to SARS-CoV-2 infection should be bathed directly after birth to help remove possible virus on the skin.[46] Currently, there are no established guidelines for the treatment of neonates with confirmed SARS-CoV-2 infection. Treatment remains largely supportive. Various medications have been used in the treatment of neonatal SARS-CoV-2 infection, including hydroxychloroquine, azithromycin, and remdesivir.[131,136,141] Data from large trials on therapies is lacking at this time, and further studies are needed to evaluate the safety and efficacy of such medications in the neonatal population. Similarly, treatment of MIS-C is aimed at reducing inflammation and supporting organ function, including mechanical ventilation, inotropic support, antibiotics to treat secondary infections, intravenous immunoglobulin, and steroids as noted in case reports of neonatal MIS-C.[138,140] In asymptomatic neonates with SARS-CoV-2 infection diagnosed after birth, outpatient follow-up through 14 days of life is recommended.[46]

Neonatal Outcomes

In addition to pregnancy outcomes associated with SARS-CoV-2 infection, knowledge of neonatal outcomes is essential to develop the best plan of care for these patients. According to data acquired from 15 reviews, low birth weight ranged from 5.3% to 47.4%.[40] The data on Apgar score in neonates is highly heterogenous. Two reviews reported six neonates with scores less than 7 at 1 and 5 minutes. These infants were all born preterm because of fetal distress in mothers with critical SARS-CoV-2 disease.[41,142] The meta-analysis by Allotey et al.,[37] which included the largest number of neonates for this outcome, calculated 2.2% (11/500) of neonates with "abnormal" Apgar scores at 5 minutes. The need for admission to the neonatal ICU varied between 10% and 76.9%.[40] Neonatal mortality rates have been reported at 0.3%, although no deaths have been directly associated with a neonatal SARS-CoV-2 infection.[40] Metz et al.[36] found 2 neonatal deaths in 141 pregnancies with critical to severe COVID-19 compared with 1 in 499 pregnant mothers with mild to moderate disease and 2 in 579 pregnant individuals with asymptomatic disease.

Currently, there is a lack of data on the long-term outcomes of neonatal SARS-CoV-2 infection. It remains to be seen what chronic effects SARS-CoV-2 has on the developing fetus and newborn. Additional research is needed to elucidate the ramifications of neonatal SARS-CoV-2 infection.

Conclusion

SARS-CoV-2–related maternal morbidity and mortality are higher in pregnant compared with nonpregnant individuals. However, the management of SARS-CoV-2 infection in pregnancy remains similar to that in non-pregnant patients. Most importantly, potentially effective treatment for SARS-CoV-2 infection should not be withheld from pregnant women because of theoretical concerns related to safety concerns for the fetus.[6] As data continue to evolve at a rapid pace, key questions remain regarding maternal care considerations during SARS-CoV-2 infection. Despite a higher complication rate in pregnant patients, data on neonatal infectivity rate, development, and outcomes remain reassuring. In general, professional society recommendations support the use of mRNA and adenovirus vaccines approved by the US Food and Drug Administration in pregnancy and the postpartum period, and breastfeeding or using human milk, as medically indicated, from mothers with SARS-CoV-2 infection. Although the risk for vertical transmission is thought to be low, currently there is a lack of data on the long-term outcomes of neonatal SARS-CoV-2 infection.

REFERENCES

1. Diriba K, Awulachew E, Getu E. The effect of coronavirus infection (SARS-CoV-2, MERS-CoV, and SARS-CoV) during pregnancy and the possibility of vertical maternal-fetal transmission: a systematic review and meta-analysis. *Eur J Med Res*. 2020;25(1):39. doi:10.1186/s40001-020-00439-w.
2. Lam CM, Wong SF, Leung TN, et al. A case-controlled study comparing clinical course and outcomes of pregnant and non-pregnant women with severe acute respiratory syndrome. *BJOG*. 2004;111(8):771–774. doi:10.1111/j.1471-0528.2004.00199.x.
3. Mullins E, Evans D, Viner RM, O'Brien P, Morris E. Coronavirus in pregnancy and delivery: rapid review. *Ultrasound obstetrics & gynecology*. 2020;55(5):586–592. doi:10.1002/uog.22014.
4. Thompson JL, Nguyen LM, Noble KN, Aronoff DM. COVID-19-related disease severity in pregnancy. *Am J Reprod Immunol*. 2020;84(5):e13339. doi:10.1111/aji.13339.
5. Tracker CCD. Data on COVID-19 during Pregnancy: Severity of Maternal Illness. 2021. Accessed May 13 2021, https://covid.cdc.gov/covid-data-tracker/?CDC_AA_refVal=https%3A%2F%2Fwww.cdc.gov%2Fcoronavirus%2F2019-ncov%2Fcases-updates%2Fspecial-populations%2Fpregnancy-data-on-covid-19.html#pregnant-population
6. Australian Government Department of Health. Guidelines NC-T. Special Considerations in Pregnancy 2020. *Pregnancy care guidelines 2019 edition*; Pregnancy care guidelines 2019 edition. https://www.health.gov.au/sites/default/files/pregnancy-care-guidelines_0.pdf.
7. Vergara-Merino L, Meza N, Couve-Pérez C, et al. Maternal and perinatal outcomes related to COVID-19 and pregnancy: an overview of systematic reviews. *Acta Obstet Gynecol Scand*. 2021;100(7):1200–1218. doi:10.1111/aogs.14118.
8. Zaigham M, Andersson O. Maternal and perinatal outcomes with COVID-19: A systematic review of 108 pregnancies. *Acta Obstet Gynecol Scand*. 2020;99(7):823–829. doi:10.1111/aogs.13867.
9. Wong YP, Khong TY, Tan GC. The effects of COVID-19 on placenta and pregnancy: what do we know so far? *Diagnostics (Basel)*. 2021;11(1):94. doi:10.3390/diagnostics11010094.
10. Makvandi S, Mahdavian M, Kazemi-Nia G, et al. The 2019 novel coronavirus disease in pregnancy: a systematic review. *Adv Exp Med Biol*. 2021;1321:299–307. doi:10.1007/978-3-030-59261-5_27.
11. Villar J, Ariff S, Gunier RB, et al. Maternal and neonatal morbidity and mortality among pregnant women with and without COVID-19 infection: the INTERCOVID multinational cohort study. *JAMA Pediatr*. 2021;175(8):817–826. doi:10.1001/jamapediatrics.2021.1050.
12. Riley LE, Beigi R, Jamieson DJ, et al. Vaccinating pregnant and lactating patients against COVID-19. *ACOG*. Dec 2020. www.paobgyn.org/news/9428373.
13. Boyton RJ, Altmann DM. Risk of SARS-CoV-2 reinfection after natural infection. *Lancet*. 2021;397(10280):1161–1163. doi:10.1016/S0140-6736(21)00662-0.

14. LoMauro A, Aliverti A. Respiratory physiology of pregnancy: Physiology masterclass. *Breathe (Sheff)*. 2015;11(4):297–301. doi:10.1183/20734735.008615.

15. Chamseddine RS, Wahbeh F, Chervenak F, Salomon LJ, Ahmed B, Rafii A. Pregnancy and neonatal outcomes in SARS-CoV-2 Infection: a systematic review. *J Pregnancy*. 2020;2020:4592450. doi:10.1155/2020/4592450.

16. Shi H, Han X, Jiang N, et al. Radiological findings from 81 patients with COVID-19 pneumonia in Wuhan, China: a descriptive study. *Lancet Infect Dis*. 2020;20(4):425–434. doi:10.1016/s1473-3099(20)30086-4.

17. Karimi L, Vahedian-Azimi A, Makvandi S, Sahebkar A. A systematic review of 571 pregnancies affected by COVID-19. *Adv Exp Med Biol*. 2021;1321:287–298. doi:10.1007/978-3-030-59261-5_26.

18. Poole JA, Claman HN. Immunology of pregnancy. Implications for the mother. *Clin Rev Allergy Immunol*. 2004;26(3):161–170. doi:10.1385/CRIAI:26:3:161.

19. Sherer ML, Posillico CK, Schwarz JM. The psychoneuroimmunology of pregnancy. *Front Neuroendocrinol*. 2018;51:25–35. doi:10.1016/j.yfrne.2017.10.006.

20. Lee GR. The balance of Th17 versus treg cells in autoimmunity. *Int J Mol Sci*. 2018;19(3):730. doi:10.3390/ijms19030730.

21. Figueiredo AS, Schumacher A. The T helper type 17/regulatory T cell paradigm in pregnancy. *Immunology*. 2016;148(1):13–21. doi:10.1111/imm.12595.

22. Huang C, Wang Y, Li X, et al. Clinical features of patients infected with 2019 novel coronavirus in Wuhan, China. *Lancet*. 2020;395(10223):497–506. doi:10.1016/S0140-6736(20)30183-5.

23. Sarapultsev A, Sarapultsev P. Immunological environment shifts during pregnancy may affect the risk of developing severe complications in COVID-19 patients. *Am J Reprod Immunol*. 2020;84(3):e13285. doi:10.1111/aji.13285.

24. Chen L, Jiang H, Zhao Y. Pregnancy with COVID-19: Management considerations for care of severe and critically ill cases. *Am J Reprod Immunol*. 2020;84(5):e13299. doi:10.1111/aji.13299.

25. Kadir RA, Kobayashi T, Iba T, et al. COVID-19 coagulopathy in pregnancy: Critical review, preliminary recommendations, and ISTH registry-Communication from the ISTH SSC for Women's Health. *J Thromb Haemost*. 2020;18(11):3086–3098. doi:10.1111/jth.15072.

26. Servante J, Swallow G, Thornton JG, et al. Haemostatic and thrombo-embolic complications in pregnant women with COVID-19: a systematic review and critical analysis. *BMC Pregnancy Childbirth*. 2021;21(1):108. doi:10.1186/s12884-021-03568-0.

27. Vlachodimitropoulou Koumoutsea E, Vivanti AJ, Shehata N, et al. COVID-19 and acute coagulopathy in pregnancy. *J Thromb Haemost*. 2020;18(7):1648–1652. doi:10.1111/jth.14856.

28. Szecsi PB, Jorgensen M, Klajnbard A, Andersen MR, Colov NP, Stender S. Haemostatic reference intervals in pregnancy. *Thromb Haemost*. 2010;103(4):718–727. doi:10.1160/TH09-10-0704.

29. McLean KC, Bernstein IM, Brummel-Ziedins KE. Tissue factor-dependent thrombin generation across pregnancy. *Am J Obstet Gynecol*. 2012;207(2):135 e1-6. doi:10.1016/j.ajog.2012.05.027.

30. Gavriilaki E, Anyfanti P, Gavriilaki M, Lazaridis A, Douma S, Gkaliagkousi E. Endothelial Dysfunction in COVID-19: Lessons Learned from Coronaviruses. *Curr Hypertens Rep*. 2020;22(9):63. doi:10.1007/s11906-020-01078-6.

31. Rodríguez-Morales AJ, Cardona-Ospina JA, Gutiérrez-Ocampo E, et al. Clinical, laboratory and imaging features of COVID-19: A systematic review and meta-analysis. *Travel Med Infect Dis*. 2020;34:101623. doi:10.1016/j.tmaid.2020.101623.

32. Yang H, Wang C, Poon LC. Novel coronavirus infection and pregnancy. *Ultrasound in obstetrics & gynecology*. 2020;55(4):435–437. doi:10.1002/uog.22006.

33. Savla SR, Prabhavalkar KS, Bhatt LK. Cytokine storm associated coagulation complications in COVID-19 patients: Pathogenesis and Management. *Expert Rev Anti Infect Ther*. 19 2021:1–17. doi:10.1080/14787210.2021.1915129.

34. Tang N, Li D, Wang X, Sun Z. Abnormal coagulation parameters are associated with poor prognosis in patients with novel coronavirus pneumonia. *J Thromb Haemost*. 2020;18(4):844–847. doi:10.1111/jth.14768.

35. Thachil J, Tang N, Gando S, et al. ISTH interim guidance on recognition and management of coagulopathy in COVID-19. *J Thromb Haemost*. 2020;18(5):1023–1026. doi:10.1111/jth.14810.

36. Metz TD, Clifton RG, Hughes BL, et al. Disease Severity and Perinatal Outcomes of Pregnant Patients With Coronavirus Disease 2019 (COVID-19). *Obstet Gynecol*. 2021;137(4):571–580. doi:10.1097/AOG.0000000000004339.

37. Allotey J, Stallings E, Bonet M, et al. Clinical manifestations, risk factors, and maternal and perinatal outcomes of coronavirus disease 2019 in pregnancy: living systematic review and meta-analysis. *BMJ*. 2020;370:m3320. doi:10.1136/bmj.m3320.

38. Karimi L, Makvandi S, Vahedian-Azimi A, Sathyapalan T, Sahebkar A. Effect of COVID-19 on Mortality of Pregnant and Postpartum Women: A Systematic Review and Meta-Analysis. *J Pregnancy*. 2021;2021:8870129. doi:10.1155/2021/8870129.

39. Menezes MO, Takemoto MLS, Nakamura-Pereira M, et al. Risk factors for adverse outcomes among pregnant and postpartum women with acute respiratory distress syndrome due to COVID-19 in Brazil. *Int J Gynaecol Obstet*. 2020;151(3):415–423. doi:10.1002/ijgo.13407.

40. Papapanou M, Papaioannou M, Petta A, et al. Maternal and Neonatal Characteristics and Outcomes of COVID-19 in Pregnancy: An Overview of Systematic Reviews. *Int J Environ Res Public Health*. 2021;18(2). doi:10.3390/ijerph18020596.

41. Turan O, Hakim A, Dashraath P, Jeslyn WJL, Wright A, Abdul-Kadir R. Clinical characteristics, prognostic factors, and maternal and neonatal outcomes of SARS-CoV-2 infection among hospitalized pregnant women: A systematic review. *Int J Gynaecol Obstet*. 2020;151(1):7–16. doi:10.1002/ijgo.13329.

42. Khalil A, Kalafat E, Benlioglu C, et al. SARS-CoV-2 infection in pregnancy: A systematic review and meta-analysis of clinical features and pregnancy outcomes. *EClinicalMedicine*. 2020;25:100446. doi:10.1016/j.eclinm.2020.100446.

43. D'Antonio F, Sen C, Mascio DD, et al. Maternal and perinatal outcomes in high compared to low risk pregnancies complicated by severe acute respiratory syndrome coronavirus 2 infection (phase 2): the World Association of Perinatal Medicine working group on coronavirus disease 2019. *Am J Obstet Gynecol MFM*. 2021;3(4):100329. doi:10.1016/j.ajogmf.2021.100329.

44. Kotlyar AM, Grechukhina O, Chen A, et al. Vertical transmission of coronavirus disease 2019: a systematic review and meta-analysis. *Am J Obstet Gynecol*. 2021;224(1):35–53 e3. doi:10.1016/j.ajog.2020.07.049.

45. Centers for Disease Control and Prevention. Evaluation and Management Considerations for Neonates At Risk for COVID-19. 12/8/2020. https://stacks.cdc.gov/view/cdc/88194.

46. American Academy of Pediatrics. FAQs: Management of Infants Born to Mothers with Suspected or Confirmed COVID-19. 02/11/2021 https://aap.org/en/pages/2019-novel-coronavirus-covid-19-infections/clinical-guidance/.

47. Zhu H, Wang L, Fang C, et al. Clinical analysis of 10 neonates born to mothers with 2019-nCoV pneumonia. *Transl Pediatr*. 2020;9(1):51–60. doi:10.21037/tp.2020.02.06.

48. Chen H, Guo J, Wang C, et al. Clinical characteristics and intrauterine vertical transmission potential of COVID-19 infection in nine pregnant women: a retrospective review of medical records. *Lancet*. 2020;395(10226):809–815. doi:10.1016/S0140-6736(20)30360-3.

49. Liu W, Cheng H, Wang J, et al. Clinical Analysis of Neonates Born to Mothers with or without COVID-19: A Retrospective Analysis of 48 Cases from Two Neonatal Intensive Care Units in Hubei Province. *Am J Perinatol*. 2020;37(13):1317–1323. doi:10.1055/s-0040-1716505.

50. Peng Z, Wang J, Mo Y, et al. Unlikely SARS-CoV-2 vertical transmission from mother to child: A case report. *J Infect Public Health*. 2020;13(5):818–820. doi:10.1016/j.jiph.2020.04.004.

51. Chen S, Huang B, Luo DJ, et al. Pregnancy with new coronavirus infection: clinical characteristics and placental pathological analysis of three cases. *Zhonghua Bing Li Xue Za Zhi*. 2020;49(5):418–423. doi:10.3760/cma.j.cn112151-20200225-00138.

52. Zamaniyan M, Ebadi A, Aghajanpoor S, Rahmani Z, Haghshenas M, Azizi S. Preterm delivery, maternal death, and vertical transmission in a pregnant woman with COVID-19 infection. *Prenat Diagn*. 2020;40(13):1759–1761. doi:10.1002/pd.5713.

53. Congdon JL, Kair LR, Flaherman VJ, et al. Management and Early Outcomes of Neonates Born to Women with SARS-CoV-2 in 16 U.S. Hospitals. *Am J Perinatol*. 2021;38(6):622–631. doi:10.1055/s-0041-1726036.

54. Fan C, Lei D, Fang C, et al. Perinatal Transmission of 2019 Coronavirus Disease-Associated Severe Acute Respiratory Syndrome Coronavirus 2: Should We Worry? *Clin Infect Dis*. 2021;72(5):862–864. doi:10.1093/cid/ciaa226.

55. Kalafat E, Yaprak E, Cinar G, et al. Lung ultrasound and computed tomographic findings in pregnant woman with COVID-19. *Ultrasound in obstetrics & gynecology*. 2020;55(6):835–837. doi:10.1002/uog.22034.

56. Yang P, Wang X, Liu P, et al. Clinical characteristics and risk assessment of newborns born to mothers with COVID-19. *J Clin Virol*. 2020;127:104356. doi:10.1016/j.jcv.2020.104356.

57. Mirbeyk M, Saghazadeh A, Rezaei N. A systematic review of pregnant women with COVID-19 and their neonates. *Arch Gynecol Obstet*. 2021;304(1):5–38. doi:10.1007/s00404-021-06049-z.

58. Kirtsman M, Diambomba Y, Poutanen SM, et al. Probable congenital SARS-CoV-2 infection in a neonate born to a woman with active SARS-CoV-2 infection. *CMAJ*. 2020;192(24):E647–E650. doi:10.1503/cmaj.200821.

59. Zhang P, Heyman T, Greechan M, et al. Maternal, neonatal and placental characteristics of SARS-CoV-2 positive mothers. *J Matern Fetal Neonatal Med*. 2021:1–9. doi:10.1080/14767058.2021.1892637.

60. Yu N, Li W, Kang Q, et al. Clinical features and obstetric and neonatal outcomes of pregnant patients with COVID-19 in Wuhan, China: a retrospective, single-centre, descriptive study. *Lancet Infect Dis*. 2020;20(5):559–564. doi:10.1016/S1473-3099(20)30176-6.

61. Zeng L, Xia S, Yuan W, et al. Neonatal Early-Onset Infection With SARS-CoV-2 in 33 Neonates Born to Mothers With COVID-19 in Wuhan, China. *JAMA Pediatr*. 2020;174(7):722–725. doi:10.1001/jamapediatrics.2020.0878.

62. Breslin N, Baptiste C, Gyamfi-Bannerman C, et al. Coronavirus disease 2019 infection among asymptomatic and symptomatic pregnant women: two weeks of confirmed presentations to an affiliated pair of New York City hospitals. *Am J Obstet Gynecol MFM*. 2020;2(2):100118. doi:10.1016/j.ajogmf.2020.100118.

63. Liu W, Wang J, Li W, Zhou Z, Liu S, Rong Z. Clinical characteristics of 19 neonates born to mothers with COVID-19. *Front Med*. 2020;14(2):193–198. doi:10.1007/s11684-020-0772-y.

64. Li Y, Zhao R, Zheng S, et al. Lack of Vertical Transmission of Severe Acute Respiratory Syndrome Coronavirus 2, China. *Emerg Infect Dis*. 2020;26(6):1335-1336. doi:10.3201/eid2606.200287

65. Wang X, Zhou Z, Zhang J, Zhu F, Tang Y, Shen X. A Case of 2019 Novel Coronavirus in a Pregnant Woman With Preterm Delivery. *Clin Infect Dis*. 2020;71(15):844–846. doi:10.1093/cid/ciaa200.

66. Xiong X, Wei H, Zhang Z, et al. Vaginal delivery report of a healthy neonate born to a convalescent mother with COVID-19. *J Med Virol*. 2020;92(9):1657–1659. doi:10.1002/jmv.25857.

67. Liao X, Yang H, Kong J, Yang H. Chest CT Findings in a Pregnant Patient with 2019 Novel Coronavirus Disease. *Balkan Med J*. 2020;37(4):226–228. doi:10.4274/balkanmedj.galenos.2020.2020.3.89.

68. Farhadi R, Mehrpisheh S, Ghaffari V, Haghshenas M, Ebadi A. Clinical course, radiological findings and late outcome in preterm infant with suspected vertical transmission born to a mother with severe COVID-19 pneumonia: a case report. *J Med Case Rep*. 2021;15(1):213. doi:10.1186/s13256-021-02835-0.

69. Robbins JR, Bakardjiev AI. Pathogens and the placental fortress. *Curr Opin Microbiol*. 2012;15(1):36–43. doi:10.1016/j.mib.2011.11.006.

70. Shanes ED, Mithal LB, Otero S, Azad HA, Miller ES, Goldstein JA. Placental pathology in COVID-19. *medRxiv*. 2020;154(1):23–32. doi:10.1101/2020.05.08.20093229.

71. Schoenmakers S, Snijder P, Verdijk RM, et al. Severe Acute Respiratory Syndrome Coronavirus 2 Placental Infection and Inflammation Leading to Fetal Distress and Neonatal Multi-Organ Failure in an Asymptomatic Woman. *J Pediatric Infect Dis Soc*. 2020;10(5):556–561. doi:10.1093/jpids/piaa153.

72. Hosier H, Farhadian SF, Morotti RA, et al. SARS-CoV-2 infection of the placenta. *J Clin Invest*. 2020;130(9):4947–4953. doi:10.1172/JCI139569.

73. Khan S, Jun L, Nawsherwan, et al. Association of COVID-19 with pregnancy outcomes in health-care workers and

general women. *Clin Microbiol Infect.* 2020;26(6):788–790. doi:10.1016/j.cmi.2020.03.034.

74. Khan S, Peng L, Siddique R, et al. Impact of COVID-19 infection on pregnancy outcomes and the risk of maternal-to-neonatal intrapartum transmission of COVID-19 during natural birth. *Infect Control Hosp Epidemiol.* 2020;41(6):748–750. doi:10.1017/ice.2020.84.

75. Gao J, Li W, Hu X, et al. Disappearance of SARS-CoV-2 Antibodies in Infants Born to Women with COVID-19, Wuhan, China. *Emerg Infect Dis.* 2020;26(10):2491–2494. doi:10.3201/eid2610.202328.

76. Mo H, Wang M, Wang M, Han Y, Zhang Y, Hu K. Detectable antibodies against SARS-CoV-2 in newborns from mothers infected with COVID-19 at different gestational ages. *Pediatr Neonatol.* 2021;62(3):321–323. doi:10.1016/j.pedneo.2021.03.011.

77. Edlow AG, Li JZ, Collier AY, et al. Assessment of Maternal and Neonatal SARS-CoV-2 Viral Load, Transplacental Antibody Transfer, and Placental Pathology in Pregnancies During the COVID-19 Pandemic. *JAMA Netw Open.* 2020;3(12):e2030455. doi:10.1001/jamanetworkopen.2020.30455.

78. Kubiak JM, Murphy EA, Yee J, et al. Severe acute respiratory syndrome coronavirus 2 serology levels in pregnant women and their neonates. *Am J Obstet Gynecol.* 2021;225(1):73. e1–73.e7. doi:10.1016/j.ajog.2021.01.016.

79. Gupta A, Madhavan MV, Sehgal K, et al. Extrapulmonary manifestations of COVID-19. *Nat Med.* 2020;26(7):1017–1032. doi:10.1038/s41591-020-0968-3.

80. Ellington S, Tong VT, Woodworth K, Galang RR, et al. Characteristics of Women of Reproductive Age with Laboratory-Confirmed SARS-CoV-2 Infection by Pregnancy Status — United States, January 22–June 7, 2020. *CDC Morbidity and Mortality Weekly Report (MMWR).* 2020;69(25):769–775.

81. American College of Obstetricians and Gynecologists. Guidelines for Diagnostic Imaging During Pregnancy and Lactation. pdf. *ACOG committee opinion.* Number 723 2018;132(3):786.

82. McFee RB. COVID-19: Therapeutics and interventions currently under consideration. *Dis Mon.* 2020;66(9):101058. doi:10.1016/j.disamonth.2020.101058.

83. Group RC, Horby P, Lim WS, et al. Dexamethasone in Hospitalized Patients with Covid-19. *N Engl J Med.* 2021;384(8):693–704. doi:10.1056/NEJMoa2021436.

84. Skuladottir H, Wilcox AJ, Ma C, et al. Corticosteroid use and risk of orofacial clefts. *Birth Defects Res A Clin Mol Teratol.* 2014;100(6):499–506. doi:10.1002/bdra.23248.

85. Reinisch JM, Simon NG, Karow WG, Gandelman R. Prenatal exposure to prednisone in humans and animals retards intrauterine growth. *Science.* 1978;202(4366):436–438. doi:10.1126/science.705336.

86. American College of Obstetricians and Gynecologists. Antenatal Corticosteroid Therapy for Fetal Maturation. *Committee Opinion.* 2020; Number 713. http://www.acog.org/clinical/clinical-guidance/committee-opinion/articles/2017/08/antenatal-corticosteroid-therapy-for-fetal-maturation.

87. Jacobson J, Antony K, Beninati M, Alward W, Hoppe KK. Use of dexamethasone, remdesivir, convalescent plasma and prone positioning in the treatment of severe COVID-19 infection in pregnancy: A case report. *Case Rep Womens Health.* 2021;29:e00273. doi:10.1016/j.crwh.2020.e00273.

88. Society for Maternal-Fetal Medicine. Provider Considerations for Engaging in COVID-19 Vaccine Counseling With Pregnant and Lactating Patients. SMFM. 2021. https://s3.amazonaws.com/cdn.smfm.org/media/2858/Provider_Considerations_for_Engaging in COVID_Vaccination Considerations_4-1-21_(final).pdf?mc_cid=9d123dc-38b&mc_eid=1b22292cbf

89. Singh AK, Singh A, Singh R, Misra A. Remdesivir in COVID-19: A critical review of pharmacology, pre-clinical and clinical studies. *Diabetes Metab Syndr.* 2020;14(4):641–648. doi:10.1016/j.dsx.2020.05.018.

90. Mulangu S, Dodd LE, Davey Jr RT, et al. A Randomized, Controlled Trial of Ebola Virus Disease Therapeutics. *N Engl J Med.* 2019;381(24):2293–2303. doi:10.1056/NEJMoa1910993.

91. Burwick RM, Yawetz S, Stephenson KE, et al. Compassionate Use of Remdesivir in Pregnant Women with Severe Covid-19. *Clin Infect Dis.* 2020;73(11):e3996–e4004. doi:10.1093/cid/ciaa1466.

92. Group RC. <Tocilizumab in patients admitted to hospital with COVID-19 (RECOVERY)- a randomised, controlled, open-label, platform trial.pdf>. *The Lancet.* 2021; 397(10285):1637–1645. doi:10.1016/S0140-6736(21) 00676-0.

93. Salama C, Han J, Yau L, et al. Tocilizumab in Patients Hospitalized with Covid-19 Pneumonia. *N Engl J Med.* 2021;384(1):20–30. doi:10.1056/NEJMoa2030340.

94. Weisberg E, Parent A, Yang PL, et al. Repurposing of Kinase Inhibitors for Treatment of COVID-19. *Pharm Res.* 2020;37(9):167. doi:10.1007/s11095-020-02851-7.

95. Kalil AC, Patterson TF, Mehta AK, et al. Baricitinib plus Remdesivir for Hospitalized Adults with Covid-19. *N Engl J Med.* 2021;384(9):795–807. doi:10.1056/NEJMoa2031994.

96. Li L, Zhang W, Hu Y, et al. Effect of Convalescent Plasma Therapy on Time to Clinical Improvement in Patients With Severe and Life-threatening COVID-19: A Randomized Clinical Trial. *JAMA.* Aug 4 2020;324(5):460–470. doi:10.1001/jama.2020.10044.

97. Chen L, Xiong J, Bao L, Shi Y. Convalescent plasma as a potential therapy for COVID-19. *Lancet Infect Dis.* 2020; 20(4):398–400. doi:10.1016/S1473-3099(20)30141-9.

98. Simonovich VA, Burgos Pratx LD, Scibona P, et al. A Randomized Trial of Convalescent Plasma in Covid-19 Severe Pneumonia. *N Engl J Med.* 2021;384(7):619–629. doi:10.1056/NEJMoa2031304.

99. Grisolia G, Franchini M, Glingani C, et al. Convalescent plasma for coronavirus disease 2019 in pregnancy: a case report and review. *Am J Obstet Gynecol MFM.* 2020;2(3):100174. doi:10.1016/j.ajogmf.2020.100174.

100. Magallanes-Garza GI, Valdez-Alatorre C, Dávila-González D, et al. Rapid improvement of a critically ill obstetric patient with SARS-CoV-2 infection after administration of convalescent plasma. *Int J Gynaecol Obstet.* 2021;152(3):439–441. doi:10.1002/ijgo.13467.

101. Royal College of Obstetricians and Gynaecologists. Coronavirus (COVID-19) Infection in Pregnancy. 2021; https://www.rcog.org.uk/coronavirus-pregnancy.

102. Nejadrahim R, Khademolhosseini S, Kavandi H, Hajizadeh R. Severe acute respiratory syndrome coronavirus-2- or pregnancy-related cardiomyopathy, a differential to be considered in the current pandemic: a case report. *J Med Case Rep.* 2021;15(1):143. doi:10.1186/s13256-021-02751-3.

103. Guo T, Fan Y, Chen M, et al. Cardiovascular Implications of Fatal Outcomes of Patients With Coronavirus Disease 2019 (COVID-19). *JAMA Cardiol.* 2020;5(7):811–818. doi:10.1001/jamacardio.2020.1017.

104. Juusela A, Nazir M, Gimovsky M. Two cases of coronavirus 2019-related cardiomyopathy in pregnancy. *Am J Obstet Gynecol MFM.* 2020;2(2):100113. doi:10.1016/j.ajogmf.2020.100113.

105. Zeng H, Xu C, Fan J, et al. Antibodies in Infants Born to Mothers With COVID-19 Pneumonia. *JAMA.* 2020;323(18):1848–1849. doi:10.1001/jama.2020.4861.

106. Pacheco LD, Saade GR, Hankins GDV. Extracorporeal membrane oxygenation (ECMO) during pregnancy and postpartum. *Semin Perinatol.* 2018;42(1):21–25. doi:10.1053/j.semperi.2017.11.005.

107. Tambawala ZY, Hakim ZT, Hamza LK, Al Rayes M. Successful management of severe acute respiratory distress syndrome due to COVID-19 with extracorporeal membrane oxygenation during mid-trimester of pregnancy. *BMJ Case Rep.* 2021;14(2). doi:10.1136/bcr-2020-240823.

108. Naoum EE, Chalupka A, Haft J, et al. Extracorporeal Life Support in Pregnancy: A Systematic Review. *J Am Heart Assoc.* 2020;9(13):e016072. doi:10.1161/JAHA.119.016072.

109. Webster CM, Smith KA, Manuck TA. Extracorporeal membrane oxygenation in pregnant and postpartum women: a ten-year case series. *Am J Obstet Gynecol MFM.* 2020;2(2):100108. doi:10.1016/j.ajogmf.2020.100108.

110. Riley LE, Jamieson DJ, Hughes BL, Swamy G, et al. Vaccinating Pregnant and Lactating Patients Against COVID-19 _ ACOG.pdf >. Updated April 28, 2021. https://www.acog.org/clinical/clinical-guidance/practice-advisory/articles/2020/12/vaccinating-pregnant-and-lactating-patients-against-covid-19

111. Shimabukuro TT, Kim SY, Myers TR, et al. Preliminary Findings of mRNA Covid-19 Vaccine Safety in Pregnant Persons. *N Engl J Med.* 2021;384(24):2273–2282. doi:10.1056/NEJMoa2104983.

112. Gray KJ, Bordt EA, Atyeo C, et al. COVID-19 vaccine response in pregnant and lactating women: a cohort study. *Am J Obstet Gynecol.* 2021;225(3):303.e1–303.e17. doi:10.1016/j.ajog.2021.03.023.

113. Prabhu M, Murphy EA, Sukhu AC, et al. Antibody Response to Coronavirus Disease 2019 (COVID-19) Messenger RNA Vaccination in Pregnant Women and Transplacental Passage Into Cord Blood. *Obstet Gynecol.* 2021;138(2):278–280. doi:10.1097/AOG.0000000000004438.

114. Mithal LB, Otero S, Shanes ED, Goldstein JA, Miller ES. Cord blood antibodies following maternal coronavirus disease 2019 vaccination during pregnancy. *Am J Obstet Gynecol.* 2021;225(2):192–194. doi:10.1016/j.ajog.2021.03.035.

115. Rollins N, Minckas N, Jehan F, et al. A public health approach for deciding policy on infant feeding and mother-infant contact in the context of COVID-19. *Lancet Glob Health.* 2021;9(4):e552–e557. doi:10.1016/S2214-109X(20)30538-6.

116. Gross R, Conzelmann C, Muller JA, et al. Detection of SARS-CoV-2 in human breastmilk. *Lancet.* 2020;395(10239):1757–1758. doi:10.1016/S0140-6736(20)31181-8.

117. Kilic T, Kilic S, Berber NK, Gunduz A, Ersoy Y. Investigation of SARS-CoV-2 RNA in milk produced by women with COVID-19 and follow-up of their infants: A preliminary study. *Int J Clin Pract.* 2021:e14175. doi:10.1111/ijcp.14175.

118. Salvatore CM, Han JY, Acker KP, et al. Neonatal management and outcomes during the COVID-19 pandemic: an observation cohort study. *Lancet Child Adolesc Health.* 2020;4(10):721–727. doi:10.1016/S2352-4642(20)30235-2.

119. Ronchi A, Pietrasanta C, Zavattoni M, et al. Evaluation of Rooming-in Practice for Neonates Born to Mothers With Severe Acute Respiratory Syndrome Coronavirus 2 Infection in Italy. *JAMA Pediatr.* 2021;175(3):260–266. doi:10.1001/jamapediatrics.2020.5086.

120. American College of Obstetricians and Gyaenocologists. 756 ACO. Optimizing Support for Breastfeeding as Part of Obstetric Practice.pdf. *ACOG.* 2018;132(4):1086–1088.

121. Altendahl M, Afshar Y, de St Maurice A, Fajardo V, Chu A. Perinatal Maternal-Fetal/Neonatal Transmission of COVID-19: A Guide to Safe Maternal and Neonatal Care in the Era of COVID-19 and Physical Distancing. *Neoreviews.* 2020;21(12):e783–e794. doi:10.1542/neo.21-12-e783.

122. Anand P, Yadav A, Debata P, Bachani S, Gupta N, Gera R. Clinical profile, viral load, management and outcome of neonates born to COVID 19 positive mothers: a tertiary care centre experience from India. *Eur J Pediatr.* 2021;180(2):547–559. doi:10.1007/s00431-020-03800-7.

123. World Health Organization. Coronavirus disease (COVID-19): Pregnancy and childbirth. 9/2/2020. https://www.who.int/news-room/questions-and-answers/item/coronavirus-disease-covid-19-pregnancy-and-childbirth.

124. Rawat M, Chandrasekharan P, Hicar MD, Lakshminrusimha S. COVID-19 in Newborns and Infants-Low Risk of Severe Disease: Silver Lining or Dark Cloud? *Am J Perinatol.* 2020;37(8):845–849. doi:10.1055/s-0040-1710512.

125. Sotoudeh E, Sotoudeh H. A hypothesis about the role of fetal hemoglobin in COVID-19. *Med Hypotheses.* 2020;144:109994. doi:10.1016/j.mehy.2020.109994.

126. Schuler BA, Habermann AC, Plosa EJ, et al. Age-determined expression of priming protease TMPRSS2 and localization of SARS-CoV-2 in lung epithelium. *J Clin Invest.* 2021;131(1):e140766. doi:10.1172/JCI140766.

127. Bachani S, Arora R, Dabral A, et al. Clinical Profile, Viral Load, Maternal-Fetal Outcomes of Pregnancy With COVID-19: 4-Week Retrospective, Tertiary Care Single-Centre Descriptive Study. *J Obstet Gynaecol Can.* 2021;43(4):474–482. doi:10.1016/j.jogc.2020.09.021.

128. Woodworth KR, Olsen EO, Neelam V, et al. Birth and Infant Outcomes Following Laboratory-Confirmed SARS-CoV-2 Infection in Pregnancy - SET-NET, 16 Jurisdictions, March 29-October 14, 2020. *MMWR Morb Mortal Wkly Rep.* 2020;69(44):1635–1640. doi:10.15585/mmwr.mm6944e2.

129. Nanavati R, Mascarenhas D, Goyal M, Haribalakrishna A, Nataraj G. A single-center observational study on clinical features and outcomes of 21 SARS-CoV-2-infected neonates from India. *Eur J Pediatr.* 2021;180(6):1895–1906. doi:10.1007/s00431-021-03967-7.

130. Shah B, Dande V, Rao S, Prabhu S, Bodhanwala M. Outcome of Covid-19 Positive Newborns Presenting to a Tertiary Care Hospital. *Indian Pediatr.* 2021;58(2):177–179.

131. Coronado Munoz A, Nawaratne U, McMann D, Ellsworth M, Meliones J, Boukas K. Late-Onset Neonatal Sepsis in a Patient with Covid-19. *N Engl J Med.* 2020;382(19):e49. doi:10.1056/NEJMc2010614.

132. Liguoro I, Pilotto C, Bonanni M, et al. Correction to: SARS-COV-2 infection in children and newborns: a systematic

review. *Eur J Pediatr.* 2021;180(7):2343. doi:10.1007/s00431-021-03961-z.

133. Gotzinger F, Santiago-Garcia B, Noguera-Julian A, et al. COVID-19 in children and adolescents in Europe: a multinational, multicentre cohort study. *Lancet Child Adolesc Health.* 2020;4(9):653–661. doi:10.1016/S2352-4642(20)30177-2.

134. Raschetti R, Vivanti AJ, Vauloup-Fellous C, Loi B, Benachi A, De Luca D. Synthesis and systematic review of reported neonatal SARS-CoV-2 infections. *Nat Commun.* 2020;11(1):5164. doi:10.1038/s41467-020-18982-9.

135. Karabay M, Çinar N, Karakaya Suzan O, Yalnizoğlu Çaka S, Karabay O. Clinical characteristics of confirmed COVID-19 in newborns: a systematic review. *J Matern Fetal Neonatal Med.* 2020:1–12. doi:10.1080/14767058.2020.1849124.

136. Sagheb S, Lamsehchi A, Jafary M, Atef-Yekta R, Sadeghi K. Two seriously ill neonates born to mothers with COVID-19 pneumonia: a case report. *Italian Journal of Pediatrics.* 2020;46(1):137. doi:10.1186/s13052-020-00897-2.

137. Centers for Disease Control and Prevention. Multisystem Inflammatory Syndrome in Children (MIS-C) Associated with Coronavirus Disease 2019 (COVID-19). May 14, 2020. https://pubmed.ncbi.nlm.nih.gov/33180746/.

138. Nakra NA, Blumberg DA, Herrera-Guerra A, Lakshminrusimha S. Multi-system inflammatory syndrome in children (MIS-C) following SARS-CoV-2 infection: review of clinical presentation, hypothetical pathogenesis, and proposed management. *Children (Basel).* 2020;7(7):69. doi:10.3390/children7070069.

139. Centers for Disease Control and Prevention. Health Department-Reported Cases of Multisystem Inflammatory Syndrome in Children (MIS-C) in the United States. May 3, 2021. https://pubmed.ncbi.nlm.nih.gov/33295957/.

140. Kappanayil M, Balan S, Alawani S, et al. Multisystem inflammatory syndrome in a neonate, temporally associated with prenatal exposure to SARS-CoV-2: a case report. *Lancet Child Adolesc Health.* 2021;5(4):304–308. doi:10.1016/S2352-4642(21)00055-9.

141. Wardell H, Campbell JI, VanderPluym C, Dixit A. Severe acute respiratory syndrome coronavirus 2 infection in febrile neonates. *J Pediatric Infect Dis Soc.* 2020;9(5):630–635. doi:10.1093/jpids/piaa084.

142. Pettirosso E, Giles M, Cole S, Rees M. COVID-19 and pregnancy: a review of clinical characteristics, obstetric outcomes and vertical transmission. *Aust N Z J Obstet Gynaecol.* 2020;60(5):640–659. doi:10.1111/ajo.13204.

143. Shek CC, Ng PC, Fung GP, et al. Infants born to mothers with severe acute respiratory syndrome. *Pediatrics.* 2003;112(4):e254. doi:10.1542/peds.112.4.e254.

COVID-19 in Children and Adolescents

Ritu Banerjee, MD, PhD

Coronavirus Infections in Children and Adolescents

Coronaviruses are enveloped single-stranded RNA viruses comprising four genera: alpha, beta, gamma, and delta. They infect humans and animals and were first described in the 1960s as causative agents of mild upper respiratory tract infections. Four human coronaviruses caused up to 35% of upper respiratory tract infections in humans: 2229E, NL63 (both alpha coronaviruses), and HKU1 and OC43 (beta coronaviruses).[1] OC43 was thought to cause the most disease and was prevalent in children younger than 5 years.[2] In rare instances, severe infections have been described in immunosuppressed children with NL63.[3] These endemic human coronaviruses are often identified in coinfections with other respiratory viruses, making it difficult to determine their true role in disease.[4,5]

In evaluations of children with respiratory symptoms and respiratory virus testing, approximately 2% to 10% had human coronavirus.[2,4–6] Human coronavirus was also detected in 10% of asymptomatic control children.[5] Additionally, 33% to 68% had coinfections of human coronavirus and another virus, most commonly rhinovirus or respiratory syncytial virus (RSV).[2,4,5] Human coronavirus infections were present throughout the year but peaked in the winter months in North America and Europe.[4,5] Clinical manifestations of human coronavirus were indistinguishable from those of other respiratory viruses.[4,7] In rare cases, human coronavirus could cause lower respiratory tract infection in children with underlying medical conditions.[2]

Over the past 20 years, three new beta coronaviruses emerged and caused severe, sometimes fatal illness in humans: severe acute respiratory syndrome coronavirus-1 (SARS-CoV-1), Middle Eastern respiratory syndrome coronavirus (MERS-CoV), and, more recently, SARS-CoV-2. SARS-CoV-1 was described in 2003 in Southeast Asia and is thought to have originated from bats. It caused over 8000 cases and more than 700 deaths and had a mortality rate of 10% in adults but caused no deaths in the 135 pediatric cases reported.[8] No further cases of SARS-CoV-1 have been reported since 2004. MERS-CoV is thought to have been transmitted from bats to camels to humans and was identified in 2012 in Saudi Arabia. It infected more than 2400 people and caused severe respiratory illness and a mortality rate of 36%. However, in children most cases of MERS-CoV infection were asymptomatic.[9] MERS-CoV continues to occur sporadically, primarily in the Middle East.

In both SARS-CoV-1 and MERS-CoV outbreaks, children had less severe manifestations than adults and infected children were commonly identified during contact investigations of adult patients.[8,10–12] The clinical manifestations of children infected with SARS-CoV-1 or MERS-CoV were nonspecific and ranged from asymptomatic to mild, nonspecific respiratory symptoms such as fever, cough, and rhinorrhea. Some infected children developed opacities on their chest radiographs and laboratory abnormalities, including lymphopenia, thrombocytopenia, and elevated transaminases.[8,12]

Epidemiology of SARS-CoV-2 Infection in Children and Adolescents

SARS-CoV-2 was first recognized as the cause of the COVID-19 pandemic by the World Health Organization (WHO) in March 2020, at which time 118,000 cases had occurred in 114 countries and nearly 4300 people had died.[13] By September 27, 2021, approximately 18 months later, there had been more than 231 million confirmed cases of COVID-19 and more than 4 million deaths globally.[14] Our understanding of SARS-CoV-2 transmission dynamics, infectiousness, clinical manifestations, and outcomes continues to evolve during the pandemic.

Throughout the pandemic there has been great geographic variation in the burden of COVID-19. At the time of this writing, the highest number of COVID-19 cases has been reported by the United States, at more than 42 million cases, followed by India with more than 33 million cases and Brazil with 21 million cases.[14] These three countries also report the greatest number of COVID-19–associated deaths. In contrast, by September 2021 all of Europe reported 69 million cases, Southeast Asia reported 42 million cases, and Africa reported 6 million cases. All of these numbers are underestimates because of imperfect reporting systems and limited capacity for SARS-CoV-2 testing in many parts of the world. Additionally, the true burden of infection in children is likely to be much higher, because many places preferentially tested for SARS-CoV-2 among symptomatic, hospitalized patients early in the pandemic, and these patients tended to be adult patients.

Hospitalization and mortality rates for SARS-CoV-2 have been consistently lower among children than adults. Despite variability in testing and reporting of SARS-CoV-2 infections and deaths, reports from most parts of the world show that pediatric cases account for 1% to 2% of infections documented.[15–18] As of September 16, 2021, the United States reported over 5.5 million pediatric SARS-CoV-2 infections, representing 15% of all cases, 1% to 4% of total hospitalizations and less than 1% of all COVID-19 deaths.[17] Children 5 to 11 years had lower hospitalization rates compared with younger and older children (Fig. 14.1).[19] Among 121 people younger than 21 years of age who died from SARS-CoV-2 in the United States between February and July 2020, 10% were infants younger than 1 year and 70% were between the ages of 10 and 20 years.[20]

Although hospital admissions for COVID-19 among children and adolescents are rare, it is important to consider that COVID-19 has caused more pediatric hospitalizations than influenza. Among US adolescents, COVID-19–associated hospitalizations between October 2020 and April 2021 were almost three times higher than influenza-associated hospitalizations from three previous influenza seasons (Fig. 14.2).[19] In children, as in adults, SARS-CoV-2 infection and hospitalization rates and mortality vary by race and ethnicity. Hispanic, Black, or American Indian/Alaskan Native persons composed 75% of a US cohort of persons younger than 21 years who died from COVID.[20,21]

In the summer of 2021, the B.1.617.2 (delta) variant of SARS-CoV-2 emerged and spread in the United States.

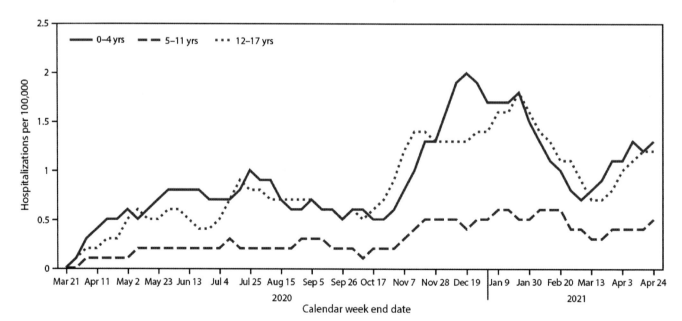

Fig. 14.1 Three-week moving average COVID-19–associated hospitalization rates among children and adolescents in the United States, aged younger than 18 years by age group. (Data from COVID-NET, March 2020-April 2021. From Havers FP, Whitaker M, Self JL, et al. Hospitalization of adolescents aged 12-17 years with laboratory-confirmed COVID-19-COVID-NET, U.S. states, March 1, 2020-April 24, 2021. *MMWR Morb Mortal Wkly Rep.* 2021;70:851-857.)

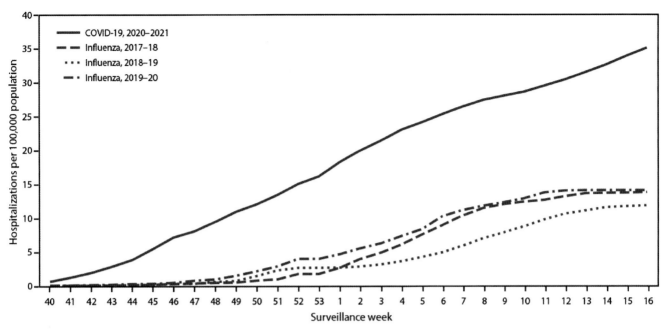

Fig. 14.2 COVID-19–associated hospitalizations versus influenza-associated hospitalizations among adolescents aged 12 to 17 years. (Data from COVID-Net and FluSurve-NET, 14 U.S. states 2017-2021. From Havers FP, Whitaker M, Self JL, et al. Hospitalization of adolescents aged 12-17 years with laboratory-confirmed COVID-19-COVID-NET, 14 states, March 1, 2020-April 24, 2021. *MMWR Morb Mortal Wkly Rep.* 2021;70:851-857.)

This fourth surge of SARS-CoV-2 coincided with off-season circulation of RSV and return to in-person school for children after summer vacation, resulting in high numbers of pediatric SARS-CoV-2 infections and hospitalizations in the United States.[17,22] The delta variant appears to be more transmissible than SARS-CoV-2 variants that circulated earlier in the pandemic.[23] Although the delta variant has caused increased numbers of pediatric COVID infections, thus far it does not seem to cause more severe disease than earlier variants. Hospitalization rates and outcomes of children infected with delta variant have not been different from those seen with earlier variants.[22,24]

Susceptibility of Children to SARS-CoV-2 Infection

SARS-CoV-2 is transmitted person to person by respiratory droplets generated during coughing, sneezing, and speaking and from contact with fomites.[25] Unlike for SARS-CoV-1, asymptomatic and presymptomatic individuals infected with SARS-CoV-2 can transmit the virus, which has led to challenges controlling viral spread during the pandemic. Transmissibility of SARS-CoV-2 appears to be greatest 2 days before until 3 days after symptom onset.[26]

The significantly higher burden of COVID-19 infection and severe disease in adults suggests that children may be less susceptible to SARS-CoV-2 infection than adults. This hypothesis has biological plausibility because children have been found to have fewer copies

of angiotensin-converting enzyme-2 (ACE2), the receptor for SARS-CoV-2, in their nasal epithelium.[27] ACE2 gene expression increases with age, potentially protecting the youngest children, who tend to be the least symptomatic from COVID-19, from acquiring infection.[27] Another explanation is that unlike adults, children have frequent and recent exposure to endemic human coronaviruses, and thus may have some cross-protective antibodies against SARS-CoV-2, preventing the hyperinflammation associated with severe COVID-19.

It is unclear what role children have played in the spread of SARS-CoV-2. Unlike other respiratory viruses such as influenza, which is commonly spread by children to others in the community, SARS-CoV-2 transmission was initially thought to be driven by adult infections, which were so much more prevalent than pediatric infections. However, SARS-CoV-2 viral loads in respiratory secretions and stool have been high in children. Some reports suggest prolonged periods of viral shedding among children, although it is controversial whether children routinely have higher viral loads than adults. A comparison of reverse transcription polymerase chain reaction (RT-PCR) cycle threshold values from respiratory specimens of children in California between April and August 2020 found that cycle threshold values were lower (and therefore viral loads were higher) in children younger than 5 years and in symptomatic versus asymptomatic children.[28] Similarly, in a retrospective evaluation of nine US institutions performing pediatric SARS-CoV-2 testing between March and July 2020, viral loads were

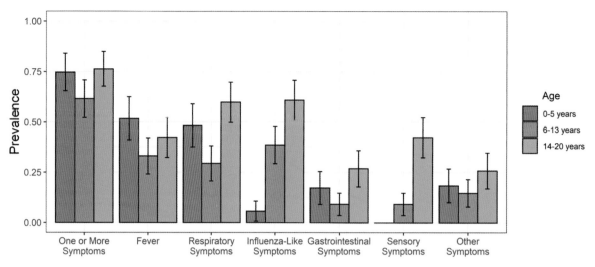

Fig. 14.3 Prevalence of symptoms among 293 SARS-CoV-2–infected children by age group. Symptom complexes were broken down into respiratory symptoms (cough, difficulty breathing, congestion, rhinorrhea), influenza-like symptoms (headache, myalgias, pharyngitis), gastrointestinal symptoms (abdominal pain, diarrhea, vomiting), and sensory symptoms (anosmia or dysgeusia). (From Hurst JH, Heston SM, Chambers HN, et al. SARS-CoV-2 infections among children in the biospecimens from respiratory virus-exposed kids (BRAVE Kids) study. *Clin Infect Dis.* 2021;7[9]:e2875-e2882.)

10-fold lower in specimens from asymptomatic compared with symptomatic children.[29] In a single-center study of 145 specimens, conducted in Chicago, viral loads from respiratory specimens were highest in children younger than 5 years of age and viral loads were similar between children older than 5 years and adults.[30] However, other studies reported that viral loads in respiratory specimens did not differ by age.[31] The discrepancies between these studies may be due to differences in testing practices (e.g., preferential testing of symptomatic vs. asymptomatic individuals), differences in timing of testing, inconsistencies in classifying symptoms, and differences in the assays used.

Although early reports did not suggest that children contributed significantly to SARS-CoV-2 spread, larger studies conducted later in the pandemic suggest children can efficiently transmit SARS-CoV-2, including within households. A systematic review and meta-analysis of 87 studies representing over 1 million households across 30 countries reported a household secondary attack rate of SARS-CoV-2 of 18.9%.[32] In a large cohort study conducted in Ontario, Canada of 6280 households with pediatric index SARS-CoV-2 cases, 27% of households experienced secondary transmission. Furthermore, within these households, children younger than 3 years had the highest odds of transmitting SARS-CoV-2 to household contacts compared with older children.[33] This may be because young children have higher viral loads in their nasopharynx, are less commonly symptomatic, and have more frequent physical contact with household members compared with older children.

Clinical Manifestations of SARS-CoV-2 Infection in Infants and Children

As observed with the other human coronaviruses, the clinical presentation of SARS-CoV-2 is milder in young children than in adolescents and adults. It is estimated that approximately 15% to 35% of infected children can be asymptomatic.[34] When children do exhibit symptoms, they range from mild fever, with or without respiratory symptoms (cough, rhinorrhea, congestion, sore throat), gastrointestinal symptoms (nausea, vomiting, diarrhea), and other systemic symptoms (headache, myalgias, fatigue), to acute respiratory distress syndrome and respiratory failure and death.[35] An early report comparing 291 children to over 10,000 adults suggested that children experience fever, cough, or shortness of breath less commonly than do adults.[15] In general, it is difficult to distinguish SARS-CoV-2 infection from other viral illnesses based on symptoms alone. SARS-CoV-2 infection also has been associated with extrarespiratory symptoms, including neurological manifestations such as loss of taste and/or smell; cerebrovascular accidents and seizures; Guillain-Barré syndrome; cutaneous findings, including chilblain-like (pernio) lesion, erythema multiforme, and urticaria[36]; conjunctivitis[37]; myocarditis[38,39]; and liver and renal dysfunction.[40,41] In addition, thrombotic complications are commonly seen in COVID-19 patients with critical illness.[42] The constellation of symptoms appears to vary by age of the child, with adolescents having more respiratory, influenza-like, and sensory symptoms than younger children (Fig. 14.3).[31,43]

Children with asymptomatic or mild COVID-19 may have mild lymphopenia and thrombocytopenia.[44] Those with moderate to severe symptoms are more likely to have laboratory abnormalities, including lymphopenia, thrombocytopenia, coagulopathy, and elevated inflammatory markers such as C-reactive protein and procalcitonin. A wide spectrum of abnormalities can be seen on chest radiographs among children with COVID-19 pneumonia, including unilateral or bilateral infiltrates, often with peripheral and lower lung zone predominance, peribronchial thickening or opacities, ground-glass opacities, and consolidations.[45] To date, bacterial superinfection has been seen in only a small proportion of hospitalized adults with COVID-19.[46,47] This is likely also true in hospitalized children, although pediatric data are still emerging.

Duration of symptoms is generally short, with symptom resolution occurring in 45% by 5 days and in 94% by 1 month in an assessment of 1000 infected children.[43] Postacute sequelae of SARS-CoV-2 infection (PASC), commonly referred to as long-COVID, has been reported in many adults after SARS-CoV-2 infection but appears to be rare among children.[48] Among 366 adults in California who had a positive SARS-CoV-2 infection between April and December 2020, 128 (35%) endorsed ongoing symptoms 2 months later.[48] In contrast, in a large prospective cohort study of SARS-CoV-2–infected children in the United Kingdom in which parents reported data about their symptomatic children using a mobile application, median illness duration in positive children was 6 days and only 25 of 1379 (1.8%) experienced symptoms for at least 56 days.[49] However, emerging data suggest that PASC may be more common in children than previously reported and warrants further study.[50]

Risk Factors for Hospitalization and Severe COVID-19 in Children

Risk factors for severe COVID-19 disease and hospitalization in children and adolescents are incompletely understood. Early descriptions of severe disease in children were single-center studies with small sample sizes and identified older age, comorbid conditions, and elevated CRP as risk factors for severe COVID-19.[18,51-55] As the pandemic has continued and more children have become infected or hospitalized, larger studies have similarly demonstrated that underlying medical conditions are associated with hospitalization for COVID-19 in children. However, it is unclear whether the increased hospitalization rate among children with comorbidities is due to lower threshold for admission or more severe COVID-19 disease.

Numerous studies have identified specific comorbid conditions as risk factors for severe COVID or hospitalization in children. In a cross-sectional study across 46 pediatric intensive care units (ICUs) conducted in North America between March and April 2020, 40 of 48 (83%) children admitted to ICUs had preexisting medical conditions (Table 14.1).[56] Likewise, in a retrospective case series of 112 persons younger than 21 years reported to the Centers for Disease Control and Prevention (CDC) with suspected SARS-CoV-2–associated deaths, 86% had at least one underlying condition, most commonly obesity, asthma, or developmental disorders.[57] In a retrospective single-center cohort study of the first 1000 SARS-CoV-2–infected children in a health system in the US Southeast, comorbid conditions, Black race, Hispanic ethnicity, and dyspnea and vomiting at presentation were associated with pediatric hospitalization.[43] An analysis using a large US health care claims database included over 43,000 children younger than 18 years with emergency department (ED) or inpatient encounters for COVID-19 and demonstrated that the risk for hospitalization was greatest in children with complex chronic diseases, specifically type 1 diabetes, obesity, and congenital cardiac or circulatory diseases, with adjusted risk ratios of 4.6, 3.07, and 2.12, respectively.[58] Hospitalization was also associated with infants younger than 1 year with history of prematurity. Although this was a very large study, it relied on diagnostic codes and had no adjudication of the primary reason for admission and thus may have misclassified and overestimated COVID-19 hospitalizations.

Additionally, an analysis using the Coronavirus Diseases 2019 Associated Hospitalization Surveillance Network (COVID-NET) found that among children, hospitalization rates were lowest in children aged 5 to 11 years and higher in the 0 to 4 and 12 to 17 age groups.[19,24] Among 376 adolescents hospitalized between January and March 2021, obesity (defined as body mass index [BMI] $\geq$ 95th percentile for age and sex); chronic lung disease; neurological disorders; chronic metabolic disease, including diabetes; immunocompromised condition; blood disorder, including

Table 14.1 Risk Factors for COVID-Associated Hospitalization or Severe Disease in Children and Adolescents

Comorbid conditions
Obesity
Type 1 diabetes mellitus
Chronic respiratory diseases
Medical technology dependence (e.g., tracheostomy)
Congenital cardiac or circulatory diseases
Neurological/neuromuscular disorders
Immunocompromising condition
Sickle cell anemia
Black race or Hispanic ethnicity
Dyspnea, hypoxia, or vomiting at presentation

sickle cell anemia; and cardiovascular disease were more commonly seen in those hospitalized for COVID-19 than among those hospitalized for other reasons.[19] In a multicenter evaluation of hospitalized children with COVID from eight sites in three states in the Northeastern United States, obesity and hypoxia on admission were predictive of severe respiratory disease.[59] Antoon et al.[21] conducted a retrospective cohort study of pediatric patients with a primary diagnosis of COVID-19 and discharged from the ED or inpatient units of 45 free-standing US hospitals. They observed that 20% of encounters resulted in hospital admission and that factors associated with ICU admission among hospitalized patients were obesity, older age, and preexisting conditions, including cardiovascular disease, obesity, type 2 diabetes mellitus, and pulmonary, neurological, or neuromuscular conditions.[21] Importantly, in several studies, Black and Hispanic or other non-White race were associated with higher hospitalization rates and disease severity in children, demonstrating that health disparities have affected children as well as adults during this pandemic.[21,43,51,60]

Multisystem Inflammatory Syndrome in Children

A rare but serious consequence of SARS-CoV-2 infection first identified in children in the United Kingdom and Italy in April 2020 is multisystem inflammatory syndrome in children (MIS-C).[44,61-63] A similar syndrome has been identified in adults, called MIS-A.[64] MIS-C typically manifests 2 to 6 weeks after a COVID-19 infection or exposure. Therefore MIS-C hospitalizations typically peak weeks after COVID-19 surges.[65] Notably, about two-thirds of MIS-C cases in the United States have occurred in Hispanic or Black children. By the end of August 2021, in the United States there had been 4661 cases of MIS-C reported and 41 MIS-C–associated deaths.[66]

MIS-C appears to be a delayed immunological response to SARS-CoV-2 infection and has features resembling Kawasaki disease and toxic shock syndrome, with evidence of inflammation in multiple organ systems. It is unclear why MIS-C disproportionately occurs in children and young adults compared to older patients. In May 2020, the CDC created a case definition of MIS-C and made it a reportable disease.[67] The case definition consists of a patient younger than 21 years with fever, laboratory evidence of inflammation, and evidence of clinically severe illness requiring hospitalization, with multisystem organ involvement (cardiovascular, dermatological, gastrointestinal, hematological, neurological, renal, or respiratory) who has tested positive for SARS-CoV-2 or had exposure to COVID-19. Clinical manifestations and laboratory abnormalities associated with MISC vary by age (Fig. 14.4).[68] More than 95% of children with MIS-C have a positive SARS-CoV-2 PCR or antibody test at time of diagnosis.

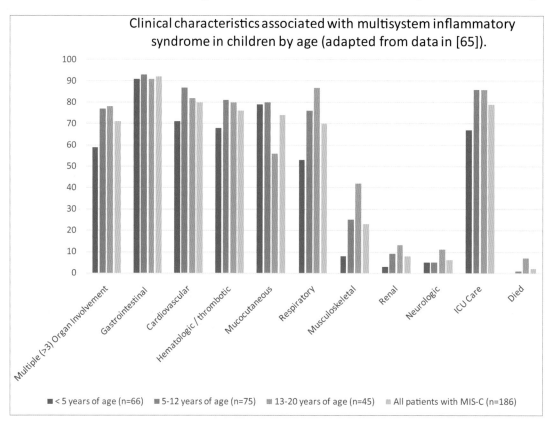

Fig. 14.4 Prevalence of Laboratory Abnormalities Associated With Multisystem Inflammatory Syndrome in Children, by Age. (From Feldstein LR, Rose EB, Horwitz SM, et al. Multisystem inflammatory syndrome in U.S. Children and Adolescents. *N Engl J Med.* 2020;383[4]:334-346.)

In a large cross-sectional cohort study including 1733 patients with MIS-C, the most common symptoms in addition to fever were abdominal pain (65%), vomiting (64%), and rash (56%), diarrhea (53%), and conjunctivitis (54%).[68] Respiratory symptoms were less common. Half of patients had hypotension, slightly over a third developed shock, 58% were admitted to intensive care, and 1.4% died. Cardiac dysfunction was reported in 31% and was more common in adolescents and young adults than in younger children.

Recently the CDC identified three classes of MIS-C patients with differing illness manifestations.[69] Class 1 patients had a median age of 9 years, the highest number of involved organs, and did not have manifestations that overlapped with acute COVID-19 or Kawasaki disease. Class 2 patients had a median age of 10 years and had respiratory system involvement that overlapped with manifestations of acute COVID-19. Class 3 patients were younger, with a median age of 6 years and had the highest prevalence of rash and mucocutaneous lesions and coronary artery dilation or aneurysm that overlapped with complete Kawasaki disease.[69] Treatment with intravenous immunoglobulin (IVIG), steroids, or other immunomodulatory agents, such as the IL-1 receptor anatagonist anakinra, have shown favorable outcomes. In a follow-up study of 68 patients with MIS-C in the United Kingdom, nearly 90% of children had normal echocardiograms at 1 year after hospitalization, with no significant short- or long-term sequelae.[70]

Neonatal SARS-CoV-2 Infection

Neonatal SARS-CoV-2 infections are rare, but when they do occur, they are generally acquired postnatally from infected adult caregivers and associated with good outcomes.[71-73] Early in the pandemic, pregnant women with SARS-CoV-2 infection underwent cesarean section, were separated from their infants, and were advised not to breastfeed because of concerns for perinatally acquired infection. Since then, many studies have demonstrated that severe SARS-CoV-2 infection acquired in the neonatal period is unlikely when caregivers adhere to appropriate masking and hand hygiene. A population-based active surveillance study in the United Kingdom found that neonatal inpatient admission for SARS-CoV-2 infection occurred in only 5.6 per 10,000 livebirths. Additionally, SARS-CoV-2–infected neonates are generally asymptomatic or have relatively mild symptoms.[74] Accordingly, guidance from the WHO and many countries is to avoid separation of mother and baby.[75,76] For additional details, see Chapter 13.

SARS-CoV-2 Infections in Immunocompromised Children

The impact of SARS-CoV-2 infection on immunocompromised children is variable and depends on the extent of immunosuppression.[77] Some studies report mild symptoms with SARS-CoV-2, and the United Kingdom's National Institute of Health and Care Excellence (NICE) has stated that COVID-19 disease is not worse in immunocompromised children compared with immunocompetent children.[78-81] However, other studies report poor outcomes after SARS-COV-2 infection in immunocompromised children. Severe COVID-19 has been reported in children receiving intensive chemotherapy for leukemia and CAR T-cell therapy and in patients with hypogammaglobulinemia and lymphopenia.[82-85] Mortality after SARS-CoV-2 infection in hematopoietic stem cell transplant recipients is lower for pediatric than adult patients.[86] A study using the Global Registry of COVID-19 in Childhood Cancer, a global cohort of children with cancer or prior hematopoietic stem cell transplant who had laboratory-confirmed SARS-CoV-2 infection between April 2020 and February 2021 followed 1319 patients for 30 days. Investigators found that almost 20% of subjects had severe or critical infection, over half had modifications to cancer treatment, and 3.8% died from COVID-19 infection. Lymphopenia, neutropenia, and residence in a low- or middle-income country were associated with severe or critical illness.[77] It is known that patients receiving active chemotherapy or recent hematopoietic stem cell transplantation can shed viable SARS-CoV-2 for prolonged periods and for at least 2 months after infection in one case series.[87]

Pediatric patients with cancer in remission or solid organ transplant recipients have greater risk for severe COVID-19 than the general pediatric population but overall have done well after SARS-CoV-2 infection, likely because they have sufficiently functional immune responses targeting the virus.[88] In a case series of 25 pediatric kidney and liver transplant recipients in Israel who developed SARS-CoV-2 infection, 84% developed mild disease and 96% developed detectable antibodies at a median of 7 weeks after acute infection.[89] In a retrospective cohort study of 26 pediatric solid organ transplant recipients with a positive SARS-CoV-2 test between April and July 2020 at five US transplant centers, almost all had mild disease and few required hospitalization.[90] Among 24 pediatric kidney transplant recipients, over two-thirds were managed as outpatients, 8 were hospitalized, and, among these, 2 required ICU-level care. None had respiratory failure or allograft loss or died.[91] Pediatric patients receiving other immunosuppressive agents for treatment of rheumatological or inflammatory conditions do not appear to have increased risk for severe COVID.[92]

Treatment of Acute COVID-19 in Children

The safety and efficacy of treatments for acute COVID-19 have been evaluated almost exclusively in adult patients. Very few of these treatment trials included or reported data from pediatric participants. Expert panels have developed treatment guidelines for COVID-19 that, in the absence of pediatric-specific data, have been applied to the care of children with SARS-CoV-2 infection.[93–95] These therapies are summarized in Table 14.2. Benefits of most therapies are greatest if given early in the course of COVID-19 disease. Because there is a substantial inflammatory component to COVID-19 pathological processes, immunomodulatory therapies have been used to treat severe disease in hospitalized adults and children. Use of these therapies in children are reviewed in this guidance document.[96] To date, tolerability and safety of these therapies has been relatively unproblematic in the pediatric population, but future studies of SARS-CoV-2 therapeutics should include children.[97]

Two medications have US Food and Drug Administration (FDA) Emergency Use Authorization (EUA) for treatment of SARS-CoV-2 in children. The FDA EUA for remdesivir applies to patients weighing over 3.5 kg and applies to the lyophilized powder formulation only.[98] SARS-CoV-2–neutralizing monoclonal antibodies have been approved in the United States under an EUA for treatment of children who are 12 years or older and weigh 40 kg or more, have mild to moderate SARS-CoV-2 not requiring hospitalization and not requiring new or increased amounts of supplemental oxygen, are within 10 days of symptom onset, and have one or more comorbidities.[99] There are limited data to aid risk stratification of children at high risk for progression to severe COVID-19. Consensus guidelines developed by pediatric infectious disease experts suggest not to provide monoclonal antibodies routinely in all pediatric patients because a majority of children have mild disease and are not hospitalized with COVID-19.[100] The expert panel as well as the American Academy of Pediatrics suggests prioritizing monoclonal antibody therapy for adolescents with obesity, medical complexity with technology dependence, and severe immunocompromise, which are conditions that predispose to severe COVID-19 among adolescents.[100,101] The combination monoclonal antibodies casirivimab and imdevimab also have an EUA to be given as postexposure prophylaxis to children 12 years of age and older and weighing 40 kg or more who are not hospitalized, are not fully vaccinated, or are fully vaccinated but not expected to have an adequate immune response because of immunosuppression, after exposure to a SARS-CoV-2–infected household contact within the prior 96 hours.[102] Notably, although over 1500 participants were included in the postexposure prophylaxis trial, only 67 subjects were adolescents.[103]

Treatment guidelines from national societies have recommended against the use of several therapies that were used early in the pandemic but have since been shown to be ineffective or potentially harmful.[93,94,101] These include hydroxychloroquine, azithromycin, nitazoxanide, lopinavir/ritonavir, and other HIV protease inhibitors. In addition, these groups cite insufficient evidence to recommend for or against the antiparasitic drug ivermectin.[104]

Prevention of SARS-CoV-2 Infection

Vaccination is the most effective strategy for ending the SARS-CoV-2 pandemic. At the present time three vaccines against SARS-CoV-2 are approved for use in adults in the United States[105] and are highly effective at reducing severe disease and hospitalization. Initially in children, only the Pfizer-BioNTech mRNA vaccine was approved by the FDA under an EUA for persons 12 years and older.[106] As of writing, clinical trials to assess the safety, efficacy, and optimal dose of the mRNA vaccines in younger children are underway. Breakthrough infections can occur among fully vaccinated individuals, especially during the surge of the delta variant, but they remain rare. COVID-19–associated hospitalizations are significantly lower among vaccinated compared to unvaccinated children and adolescents and are lower in US states with higher COVID-vaccination rates than in states with lower vaccination rates.[22] Despite evidence for safety and efficacy of COVID-19 mRNA vaccinations, only 32% of all 12- to 17-year-old children in the United States had been fully vaccinated by July 2021, although vaccination coverage varies widely by state.[107,108] This has been the lowest vaccine uptake among all vaccine-eligible age groups in the United States and is due in part to vaccine hesitancy or anti-vaccination sentiments among parents and caregivers.[108] The CDC recommended an additional dose of mRNA COVID-19 vaccine at least 28 days after a second dose among people, including adolescents, with moderate to severe immune compromise.

Additional nonpharmaceutical mitigation measures, such as consistent masking, have reduced transmission of SARS-CoV-2, especially in indoor spaces, for example, schools.[109] In two counties in the United States, schools with no masking requirement for students and staff were 3.5 times more likely to have a school-associated COVID-19 outbreak than schools that implemented masking requirements.[110] Social distancing, limiting large gatherings, prompt case identification and isolation, and contact tracing and appropriate quarantine of exposed individuals are also effective public health measures that can reduce SARS-CoV-2 transmission.

COVID-19 Impact on Well-Being of Children

The COVID-19 pandemic has had negative impacts on the physical and mental health of children and their social, emotional, and academic development. Millions of children throughout the world transitioned from in-person school to virtual instruction in 2020, and many continued with remote learning throughout the entire school year. This has caused significant academic and social disruptions and widened the learning gap between children from high- and low-income households that

Table 14.2 Treatment Options for Acute COVID-19 in Children and Adolescents

Drug	Mechanism of Action	Possible Toxicities/Harms	Notes
Remdesivir	Inhibits viral RNA transcription	Do not use if GFR <30 mL/min.	Recommended for hospitalized patients with hypoxemia and need for supplemental oxygen but not invasive ventilation FDA EUA for patients >3.5 kg
Corticosteroid	Immunomodulation to address ARDS and systemic inflammation	Hyperglycemia, agitation/confusion, adrenal suppression, risk for bacterial and fungal infection.	Recommended for hospitalized patients with hypoxemia for 10 days or until discharge
Baricitinib	Janus kinase (JAK) 1 and 2 inhibitor. Has antiinflammatory and antiviral activity		Recommended for hospitalized patients with severe COVID and evidence of inflammation but not on invasive mechanical ventilation. Should not be given in conjunction with IL-6 inhibitors. Can be given in conjunction with remdesivir in patients who have contraindications to receipt of corticosteroid.
Tocilizumab	Monoclonal antibody blocking IL-6 receptor to reduce hyperinflammation	No AEs noted in the trials of COVID-19 patients. Bowel perforations have been reported in case reports.	Current shortage of this medication in the United States
SARS-CoV-2–neutralizing monoclonal antibodies	Directed at SARS-CoV-2 spike protein; passive immunity has potential to rapidly reduce viral load	Local injection site reactions, infusion-related reactions including fever, chills, shortness of breath, dizziness, abdominal pain, nausea, vomiting and flushing, and pruritus. Serious hypersensitivity reactions, including anaphylaxis, may also occur.	FDA EUA* for treatment of children ≥12 years and ≥40 kg, with mild to moderate SARS-CoV-2 not requiring hospitalization and not requiring new or increased amounts of supplemental oxygen, who are within 10 days of symptom onset, and have one or more comorbidities. FDA EUA for postexposure prophylaxis for children ≥12 years and ≥40 kg who are not fully vaccinated or are fully vaccinated but not expected to mount an adequate immune response because of immunosuppression, after exposure to a SARS-CoV-2–infected household contact. This is to be given optimally within 96 hours and maximally within 7 days after the SARS-CoV-2 exposure.

*Bamlanivimab, bamlanivimab/etesevimab, casirivimab/imdevimab, and sotrovimab are no longer authorized for use because they are ineffective against currently circulating variants of SARS-CoV-2. Bebtolovimab is approved for use.

AE, Adverse events; *EUA*, Emergency Use Authorization; *FDA*, Food and Drug Administration; *GFR*, glomerular filtration rate; *IL-6*, interleukin-6.

Data from Infectious Diseases Society of America. IDSA Guidelines on the Treatment and Management of Patients with COVID-19 2021. https://www.idsociety.org/practice-guideline/covid-19-guideline-treatment-and-management/.

may lack reliable internet connections, computers, or housing. The severe economic consequences of the pandemic, including parental job loss, have disproportionately affected low-income families and likely will exacerbate levels of child poverty, which, in turn, may have lasting impacts on childhood health and learning.[111] In a survey of nearly 1300 parents of children aged 5 to 12 years conducted in the United States, parents of children receiving virtual instruction were more likely to report loss of work and emotional distress than parents of children with in-person instruction.[112] Additionally, parents of children receiving virtual instruction reported that their children spent less time outside, engaged with friends, or doing physical activity, which can adversely affect children's physical and mental health. Virtual instruction for children was more common among Black,

Hispanic, and multiracial parents compared with White parents, so the negative impacts of remote learning may have disproportionately affected racial and ethnic communities and is an area of active investigation.[112]

The reduced physical activity, social isolation, stress, and disruptions in income, food, and other determinants of health that have occurred during the pandemic have had alarming psychosocial impacts on children. Anxiety, depression, eating disorders, and suicide attempts have all increased among youth during the pandemic.[112,113] There also has been an alarming increase in obesity among US children. In a recent evaluation by the CDC, among over 432,000 persons aged 2 to 19 years, the BMI doubled during the pandemic compared with a prepandemic period.[114] The scale of COVID-10 mortality has resulted in many children worldwide experiencing the death of one or more parents or caregivers. The number of children experiencing parental loss is estimated to be 17% to 20% higher now compared with prepandemic periods.[115] As of February 2021, it is estimated that 37,000 to 43,000 US children aged 0 to 17 years have lost at least one parent to COVID-19, and this number will grow as the pandemic continues. Black children appear to be disproportionately affected by parental loss.[115] Globally, between March 2020 and April 2021 over 1 million children are estimated to have experienced the death of a primary caregiver.[116]

Lockdowns, "stay at home" orders, and anxiety during the pandemic have resulted in decreased well-child visits, and, as a result, many children are behind on their routine childhood vaccinations. For all routine childhood vaccinations (diphtheria, tetanus, pertussis, measles, mumps, rubella, and human papillomavirus) significantly fewer doses were administered to US children between March and September 2020 than during comparable periods in 2018 and 2019 across 10 US jurisdictions.[108,117] This raises concern that outbreaks of vaccine-preventable infectious diseases may occur in undervaccinated populations. Preventive health care visits were especially disrupted among racial and ethnic minority groups.

Widespread use of masks, social distancing, and school closures resulted in significant reductions in seasonal respiratory viral illnesses, including RSV and influenza and other conditions thought to be triggered by viral infections, including Kawasaki disease.[118] This reduction in respiratory illness as well as national lockdowns have contributed to dramatic declines in health care encounters and antibiotic prescriptions for outpatient pediatric visits.[119–121] Unfortunately, this has led to delayed diagnoses of other conditions such as malignancy.[122] With relaxing of mitigation measures and resumption of in-person school and social gatherings, RSV rates have increased.[123] Notably, in both Australia and North America, in the 2021 to 2022 season, there has been a delayed surge in RSV so that this virus is circulating during the spring and summer months rather than the typical fall and winter months. The impact of masking and distancing on influenza virus dynamics during the 2021 to 2022 season is currently unknown.

Conclusion

Our understanding of the impact of the COVID-19 pandemic on children and adolescents continues to evolve with the ongoing pandemic. Although COVID-associated infections, hospitalizations, and deaths are lower in children than adults, it has become clear that severe COVID does occur in children, especially in those with comorbid conditions. Experience over the past 18 months has improved the diagnosis and management of the postinfectious complication of MIS-C, although the pathogenesis and risk factors for MIS-C remain unclear. Additionally, it has become clear that children and adolescents are capable of transmitting SARS-CoV-2

and contributing to its spread within households and communities, illustrating the importance of developing and distributing safe and effective vaccines and anti-SARS-CoV-2 therapies for children and adolescents as part of the global pandemic response. Equally importantly, the COVID-19 pandemic has had significant negative impacts on the mental health of children and their social, emotional, and academic development. The long-term effects of the COVID-19 pandemic on the physical and mental health of children remain unknown and will only be understood decades from now.

REFERENCES

1. Coronaviruses, including SARS-CoV-2, and MERS-CoV. *Red Book: Report of the Committee on Infectious Diseases*. Itasca, IL: American Academy of Pediatrics; 2021:280–285.
2. Lee J, Storch GA. Characterization of human coronavirus OC43 and human coronavirus NL63 infections among hospitalized children <5 years of age. *Pediatr Infect Dis J*. 2014;33(8):814–820.
3. Chiu SS, Chan KH, Chu KW, Kwan SW, Guan Y, Poon LLM, et al. Human coronavirus NL63 infection and other coronavirus infections in children hospitalized with acute respiratory disease in Hong Kong, China. *Clin Infect Dis*. 2005;40:1721–1729.
4. Calvo C, Alcolea S, Casas I, Pozo F, Iglesias M, Gonzalez-Esguevillas M, et al. A 14-year prospective study of human coronavirus infections in hospitalized children: comparison with other respiratory viruses. *Pediatr Infect Dis J*. 2020;39(8):653–657.
5. Heimdal I, Moe N, Krokstad S, Christensen A, Skanke LH, Nordbo SA, et al. Human coronavirus in hospitalized children with respiratory tract infections: a 9-year population-based study from Norway. *J Infect Dis*. 2019;219(8):1198–1206.
6. Chiu WK, Cheung PC, Ng KL, Ip PL, Sugunan VK, Luk DC, et al. Severe acute respiratory syndrome in children: experience in a regional hospital in Hong Kong. *Pediatr Crit Care Med*. 2003;4(3):279–283.
7. Talbot HK, Crowe Jr JE, Edwards KM, Griffin MR, Zhu Y, Weinberg GA, et al. Coronavirus infection and hospitalizations for acute respiratory illness in young children. *J Med Virol*. 2009;81(5):853–856.
8. Rajapakse N, Dixit D. Human and novel coronavirus infections in children: a review. *Paediatr Int Child Health*. 2021;41(1):36–55.
9. Memish ZA, Al-Tawfiq JA, Assiri A, AlRabiah FA, Al Hajjar S, Albarrak A, et al. Middle East respiratory syndrome coronavirus disease in children. *Pediatr Infect Dis J*. 2014;33(9):904–906.
10. Ng PC, Leung CW, Chiu WK, Wong SF. Hon EK. SARS in newborns and children. *Biol Neonate*. 2004;85(4):293–298.
11. Hon KLE, Leung CW, Cheng WTF, Chan PKS, Chu WCW, Kwan YW, et al. Clinical presentations and outcome of severe acute respiratory syndrome in children. *The Lancet*. 2003;361(9370):1701–1703.
12. Bitnun A, Allen U, Heurter H, King SM, Opavsky MA, Ford-Jones E.L., et al. Children hospitalized with severe acute respiratory syndrome-related illness in Toronto. *Pediatrics*. 2003;112:e261–e268.
13. World Health Organization. Coronavirus disease 2019 (COVID-19) Situation Report - 51. 2020.

14. Coronavirus disease (COVID-19) pandemic [Available from: https://covid19.who.int/?adgroupsurvey = {adgroupsurvey}&gclid = EAIaIQobChMIsLbth6GJ8gIVlcSGCh3PnQJ-SEAAYASABEgLdr_D_BwE.

15. Coronavirus Disease 2019 in children - United States, February 12-April 2, 2020. MMWR Morbidity and Mortality Weekly Report. 2020;69:422-426.

16. Tagarro A, Epalza C, Santos M, Sanz-Santaeufemia FJ, Otheo E, Moraleda C, et al. Screening and severity of coronavirus diseases 2019 (COVID-19) in Madrid, Spain. *JAMA Pediatr.* 2020;175:316–317.

17. Children and COVID-19: State Data Report. Itasca, IL: American Academy of Pediatrics and Children's Hospital Association. September 16, 2021.

18. Wang Y, Zhu F, Wang C, Wu J, Liu J, Chen X, et al. Children Hospitalized With Severe COVID-19 in Wuhan. *Pediatr Infect Dis J.* 2020;39(7):e91–e94.

19. Havers FP, Whitaker M, Self JL, Chai SJ, Kirley PD, Alden N, et al. Hospitalization of adolescents aged 12-17 years with laboratory-confirmed COVID-19- COVID-NET, 14 states, March 1, 2020-April 24, 2021. *Mmwr-Morbid Mortal W.* 2021;70:851–857.

20. Bixler D, Miller AD, Mattison CP, Taylor B, Komatsu K, Pompa X, et al. SARS-CoV-2-associated deaths among persons aged <21 years - United States, February 12-July 31, 2020. *Mmwr-Morbid Mortal W.* 2020;69:1324–1329.

21. Antoon JW, Grijalva CG, Thurm C, Richardson T, Spaulding AB, Teufel Ii RJ, et al. Factors Associated With COVID-19 Disease Severity in US Children and Adolescents. *Journal of Hospital Medicine. 2021.* 2021;16(10):603–610.

22. Siegel DA, Reses HE, Cool AJ, Shapiro CN, Hsu J, Boehmer TK, et al. Trends in COVID-19 cases, emergency department visits, and hospital admissions among children and adolescents aged 0-17 years- United States, August 2020-August 2021. *MMWR Morbidity and Mortality Weekly Report.* 2021;70:1–6.

23. Lam-Hine T, McCurdy SA, Santora L, Duncan L, Corbett-Detig R, Kapusinsky B, et al. Outbreak associated with SARS-CoV-2 B. 1.617.2 (Delta) variant in an elementary school - Marin County, California, May-June 2021. *MMWR Morbidity and Mortality Weekly Report.* 2021;70:1214–1219.

24. Delahoy MJ, Ujamaa D, Whitaker M, O'Halloran A, Anglin O, Burns E, et al. Hospitalizations associated with COVID-19 among children and adolescents, COVID-NET, 14 states, March 1, 2020-August 14, 2021. *Mmwr-Morbid Mortal W.* 2021;70:1–7.

25. Centers for Disease Control and Prevention. Scientific Brief: SARS-CoV-2 Transmission 2021 [Available from: https://www.cdc.gov/coronavirus/2019-ncov/science/science-briefs/sars-cov-2-transmission.html.

26. Ge Y, Martinez L, Sun S, Chen Z, Zhang F, Li F, et al. COVID-19 Transmission Dynamics Among Close Contacts of Index Patients With COVID-19: A Population-Based Cohort Study in Zhejiang Province, China. *JAMA Intern Med.* 2021;181(10):1343–1350.

27. Bunyavanich S, Do A, Vicencio A. Nasal gene expression of angiotensin-converting enzyme 2 in children and adults. *JAMA.* 2020;323:2427–2428.

28. Strutner J, Ramchandar N, Dubey S, Gamboa M, Vanderpool MK, Mueller T, et al. Comparison of RT-PCR Cycle Threshold Values from Respiratory Specimens in Symptomatic and Asymptomatic Children with SARS-CoV-2 Infection. *Clin Infect Dis.* 2021;73(10):1790–1794.

29. Kociolek LK, Muller WJ, Yee R, Dien Bard J, Brown CA, Revell PA, et al. Comparison of Upper Respiratory Viral Load Distributions in Asymptomatic and Symptomatic Children Diagnosed with SARS-CoV-2 Infection in Pediatric Hospital Testing Programs. *J Clin Microbiol.* 2020;59(1) e02593-20.

30. Heald-Sargent T, Muller WJ, Zheng X, Rippe J, Patel AB, Kociolek LK. Age related differences in nasopharyngeal severe acute respiratory syndrome coronavirus 2 (SARS-CoV-2) levels in patients with mild to moderate coronavirus disease 2019 (COVID-19). *JAMA Pediatr.* 2020;174:902–903.

31. Hurst JH, Heston SM, Chambers HN, Cunningham HM, Price MJ, Suarez L, et al. SARS-CoV-2 Infections Among Children in the Biospecimens from Respiratory Virus-Exposed Kids (BRAVE Kids) Study. *Clin Infect Dis.* 2021;73(9):e2875–e2882.

32. Madewell ZJ, Yang Y, Longini Jr IM, Halloran ME, Dean NE. Household Transmission of SARS-CoV-2: A Systematic Review and Meta-analysis. *JAMA Netw Open.* 2020;3(12):e2031756.

33. Paul LA, Daneman N, Schwartz KL, Science M, Brown KA, Whelan M, et al. Association of Age and Pediatric Household Transmission of SARS-CoV-2 Infection. *JAMA Pediatr.* 2021;175(11):1151–1158.

34. Cui X, Zhao Z, Zhang T, Guo W, Guo W, Zheng J, et al. A systematic review and meta-analysis of children with coronavirus disease 2019 (COVID-19). *J Med Virol.* 2021;93(2):1057–1069.

35. Parcha V, Booker KS, Kalra R, Kuranz S, Berra L, Arora G, et al. A retrospective cohort study of 12,306 pediatric COVID-19 patients in the United States. *Sci Rep.* 2021;11(1):10231.

36. Andina D, Belloni-Fortina A, Bodemer C, Bonifazi E, Chiriac A, Colmenero I, et al. Skin manifestations of COVID-19 in children: Part 1. *Clin Exp Dermatol.* 2021;46(3):444–450.

37. Danthuluri V, Grant MB. Update and Recommendations for Ocular Manifestations of COVID-19 in Adults and Children: A Narrative Review. *Ophthalmol Ther.* 2020;9(4):853–875.

38. Boehmer TK, Kompaniyets L, Lavery AM, Hsu J, Ko JY, Yusuf H, et al. Association between COVID-19 and myocarditis using hospital-based administrative data - United States March 2020-January 2021. *Mmwr-Morbid Mortal W.* 2021;70:1228–1232.

39. Singer ME, Taub IB, Kaelber DC. Risk of Myocarditis from COVID-19 Infection in People Under Age 20: A Population-Based Analysis. *medRxiv.* 2021.

40. Lai C-C, Ko W-C, Lee P-I, Jean S-S, Hsueh P-R. Extra-respiratory manifestations of COVID-19. *International Journal of Antimicrobial Agents.* 2020;56(2):106024.

41. Williams PCM, Howard-Jones AR, Hsu P, Palasanthiran P, Gray PE, McMullan BJ, et al. SARS-CoV-2 in children: spectrum of disease, transmission and immunopathological underpinnings. *Pathology.* 2020;52(7):801–808.

42. Al-Samkari H, Leaf RSK, Dzik WH, Carlson JCT, Fogerty AE, Waheed A, et al. COVID-19 and coagulation: bleeding and thrombotic manifestations of SARS-CoV-2 infection. *Blood Adv.* 2020;136:489–500.

43. Howard LM, Garguilo K, Gillon J, LeBlanc K, Seegmiller AC, Schmitz JE, et al. The first 1000 symptomatic pediatric SARS-CoV-2 infections in an integrated health care system: a prospective cohort study. *BMC Pediatr.* 2021;21(1):403.

44. Ben-Shimol S, Livni G, Megged O, Greenberg D, Danino D, Youngster I, et al. COVID-19 in a Subset of Hospitalized Children in Israel. *J Pediatric Infect Dis Soc.* 2021;10(7):757–765.

45. Foust AM, Phillips GS, Chu WC, Daltro P, Das KM, Garcia-Pena P, et al. International Expert Consensus Statement on Chest Imaging in Pediatric COVID-19 Patient Management. Imaging Findings, Imaging Study Reporting, and Imaging Study Recommendations. *Radiol Cardiothorac Imaging.* 2020;2(2):e200214.

46. Garcia-Vidal C, Sanjuan G, Moreno-Garcia E, Puerta-Alcalde P, Garcia-Pouton N, Chumbita M, et al. Incidence of co-infections and superinfections in hospitalized patients with COVID-19: a retrospective cohort study. *Clin Microbiol Infect.* 2021;27(1):83–88.

47. Goncalves Mendes Neto A, Lo KB, Wattoo A, Salacup G, Pelayo J, DeJoy 3rd R, et al. Bacterial infections and patterns of antibiotic use in patients with COVID-19. *J Med Virol.* 2021;93(3):1489–1495.

48. Yomogida K, Zhu S, Rubino F, Figueroa W, Balanji N, Holman E. Post-acute sequelae of SARS-CoV-2 infection among adults aged >18 years - Long Beach, California, April 1-December 10, 2020. *MMWR Morbidity and Mortality Weekly Report.* 2021;70:1274–1277.

49. Molteni E, Sudre CH, Canas LS, Bhopal SS, Hughes RC, Antonelli M, et al. Illness duration and symptom profile in symptomatic UK school-aged children tested for SARS-CoV-2. *The Lancet Child & Adolescent Health.* 2021;5(10):708–718.

50. Ludvigsson JF. Case report and systematic review suggest that children may experience similar long-term effects to adults after clinical COVID-19. *Acta Paediatr.* 2021;110(3):914–921.

51. Graff K, Smith C, Silveira L, Jung S, Curran-Hays S, Jarjour J, et al. Risk Factors for Severe COVID-19 in Children. *Pediatr Infect Dis J.* 2021;40(4):e137–e145.

52. DeBiasi RL, Song X, Delaney M, Bell M, Smith K, Pershad J, et al. Severe Coronavirus Disease-2019 in Children and Young Adults in the Washington, DC, Metropolitan Region. *J Pediatr.* 2020;223:199–203 e1.

53. Chao JY, Derespina KR, Herold BC, Goldman DL, Aldrich M, Weingarten J, et al. Clinical Characteristics and Outcomes of Hospitalized and Critically Ill Children and Adolescents with Coronavirus Disease 2019 at a Tertiary Care Medical Center in New York City. *J Pediatr.* 2020;223:14–19 e2.

54. Zachariah P, Johnson CL, Halabi KC, Ahn D, Sen AI, Fischer A, et al. Epidemiology, Clinical Features, and Disease Severity in Patients With Coronavirus Disease 2019 (COVID-19) in a Children's Hospital in New York City, New York. *JAMA Pediatr.* 2020;174(10):e202430.

55. Otto WR, Geoghegan S, Posch LC, Bell LM, Coffin SE, Sammons JS, et al. The Epidemiology of SARS-CoV-2 in a Pediatric Healthcare Network in the United States. *J Pediatric Infect Dis Soc.* 2020;9(5):523–529.

56. Shekerdemian LS, Mahmood NR, Wolfe KK, Riggs BJ, Ross CE, McKiernan CA, et al. Characteristics and Outcomes of Children With Coronavirus Disease 2019 (COVID-19) Infection Admitted to US and Canadian Pediatric Intensive Care Units. *JAMA Pediatr.* 2020;174(9):868–873.

57. McCormick DW, Richardson LC, Young PR, Viens LJ, Gould CV, Kimball A, et al. Deaths in Children and Adolescents Associated With COVID-19 and MIS-C in the United States. *Pediatrics.* 2021;148(5):e2021052273.

58. Kompaniyets L, Agathis NT, Nelson JM, Preston LE, Ko JY, Belay B, et al. Underlying Medical Conditions Associated With Severe COVID-19 Illness Among Children. *JAMA Netw Open.* 2021;4(6):e2111182.

59. Fernandes DM, Oliveira CR, Guerguis S, Eisenberg R, Choi J, Kim M, et al. Severe Acute Respiratory Syndrome Coronavirus 2 Clinical Syndromes and Predictors of Disease Severity in Hospitalized Children and Youth. *J Pediatr.* 2021;230:23–31 e10.

60. Bailey LC, Razzaghi H, Burrows EK, Bunnell HT, Camacho PEF, Christakis DA, et al. Assessment of 135794 Pediatric Patients Tested for Severe Acute Respiratory Syndrome Coronavirus 2 Across the United States. *JAMA Pediatr.* 2021;175(2):176–184.

61. Riphagen S, Gomez X, Gonzalez-Martinez C, Wilkinson N, Theocharis P. Hyperinflammatory shock in children during COVID-19 pandemic. *Lancet.* 2020;395(10237):1607–1608.

62. Grazioli S, Tavaglione F, Torriani G, Wagner N, Rohr M, L'Huillier AG, et al. Immunological Assessment of Pediatric Multisystem Inflammatory Syndrome Related to Coronavirus Disease 2019. *J Pediatric Infect Dis Soc.* 2021;10(6):706–713.

63. Cattaneo C, Drean M, Subiros M, Combe P, Abasse S, Chamouine A, et al. Multisystem Inflammatory Syndrome Associated With Severe Acute Respiratory Syndrome Coronavirus 2 in Children: A Case Series From Mayotte Island. *J Pediatric Infect Dis Soc.* 2021;10(6):738–741.

64. Morris S, B. Schwartz NG, Patel P, Abbo L, Beauchamps L, Balan S, et al. Case Series of Multisystem Inflammatory Syndrome in Adults Associated withSARS-CoV-2 Infection — United Kingdom and United States, March–August 2020. *MMWR Morbidity and Mortality Weekly Report.* 2020;69:1450–1456.

65. Feldstein LR, Rose EB, Horwitz SM, Collins JP, Newhams MM, Son MBF, et al. Multisystem Inflammatory Syndrome in U.S. Children and Adolescents. *N Engl J Med.* 2020;383(4):334–346.

66. Centers for Disease Control and Prevention. COVID Data Tracker 2021 [Available from: https://covid.cdc.gov/covid-data-tracker/#mis-national-surveillance.

67. Centers for Disease Control and Prevention. Information for Healthcare Providers about Multisystem Inflammatory Syndrome in Children (MIS-C) 2021 [Available from: https://www.cdc.gov/mis/mis-c/hcp/index.html?CDC_AA_refVal=https%3A%2F%2Fwww.cdc.gov%2Fmis%2Fhcp%2Findex.html.

68. Belay ED, Abrams J, Oster ME, Giovanni J, Pierce T, Meng L, et al. Trends in Geographic and Temporal Distribution of US Children With Multisystem Inflammatory Syndrome During the COVID-19 Pandemic. *JAMA Pediatr.* 2021;175(8):837–845.

69. Godfred-Cato S, Bryant B, Leung J, Oster ME, Conklin L, Abrams J, et al. COVID-19-associated multisystem inflammatory syndrome in children - United States, March-July 2020. *MMWR-Morbid Mortal W.* 2020;69:1074–1080.

70. Davies P, du Pre P, Lillie J, Kanthimathinathan HK. One-Year Outcomes of Critical Care Patients Post-COVID-19 Multisystem Inflammatory Syndrome in Children. *JAMA Pediatr.* 2021;175(12):1281–1283.

71. Shalish W, Lakshminrusimha S, Manzoni P, Keszler M, Sant'Anna GM. COVID-19 and Neonatal Respiratory Care:

Current Evidence and Practical Approach. *Am J Perinatol.* 2020;37(8):780–791.

72. Chen H, Guo J, Wang C, Luo F, Yu X, Zhang W, et al. Clinical characteristics and intrauterine vertical transmission potential of COVID-19 infection in nine pregnant women: a retrospective review of medical records. *The Lancet.* 2020;395(10226):809–815.

73. World Health Organization. *Definition and categorization of the timing of mother-to-child transmission of SARS-CoV-2.* Geneva: WHO; 2020.

74. Gale C, Quigley MA, Placzek A, Knight M, Ladhani S, Draper ES, et al. Characteristics and outcomes of neonatal SARS-CoV-2 infection in the UK: a prospective national cohort study using active surveillance. *The Lancet Child & Adolescent Health.* 2021;5(2):113–121.

75. Yeo KT, Oei JL, De Luca D, Schmolzer GM, Guaran R, Palasanthiran P, et al. Review of guidelines and recommendations from 17 countries highlights the challenges that clinicians face caring for neonates born to mothers with COVID-19. *Acta Paediatr.* 2020;109(11):2192–2207.

76. American Academy of Pediatrics FAQs: Management of infants born to mothers with suspected or confirmed COVID-19: AAP; 2021 [Available from: https://www.aap.org/en/pages/2019-novel-coronavirus-covid-19-infections/clinical-guidance/faqs-management-of-infants-born-to-covid-19-mothers/.

77. Mukkada S, Bhakta N, Chantada GL, Chen Y, Vedaraju Y, Faughnan L, et al. Global characteristics and outcomes of SARS-CoV-2 infection in children and adolescents with cancer (GRCCC): a cohort study. *The Lancet Oncology.* 2021;22(10):1416–1426.

78. Wise J. Covid-19 is no worse in immunocompromised children, says NICE. *BMJ.* 2020;369 m1802.

79. Rossoff J, Patel AB, Muscat E, Kociolek LK, Muller WJ. Benign course of SARS-CoV-2 infection in a series of pediatric oncology patients. *Pediatr Blood Cancer.* 2020;67(9):e28504.

80. Kamdar KY, Kim TO, Doherty EE, Pfeiffer TM, Qasim SL, Suell MN, et al. COVID-19 outcomes in a large pediatric hematology-oncology center in Houston, Texas. *Pediatr Hematol Oncol.* 2021:1–14.

81. Faura A, Rives S, Lassaletta A, Sebastian E, Madero L, Huerta J, et al. Initial report on Spanish pediatric oncologic, hematologic, and post stem cell transplantation patients during SARS-CoV-2 pandemic. *Pediatr Blood Cancer.* 2020;67(9):e28557.

82. Patel PA, Lapp SA, Grubbs G, Edara VV, Rostad CA, Stokes CL, et al. Immune responses and therapeutic challenges in paediatric patients with new-onset acute myeloid leukaemia and concomitant COVID-19. *Br J Haematol.* 2021;194(3):549–553.

83. Phillips L, Pavisic J, Kaur D, Dorrello NV, Broglie L, Hijiya N. Successful management of SARS-CoV-2 acute respiratory distress syndrome and newly diagnosed acute lymphoblastic leukemia. *Blood Adv.* 2020;4(18):4358–4361.

84. Andre N, Rouger-Gaudichon J, Brethon B, Phulpin A, Thebault E, Pertuisel S, et al. COVID-19 in pediatric oncology from French pediatric oncology and hematology centers: High risk of severe forms?. *Pediatr Blood Cancer.* 2020;67(7):e28392.

85. Hensley MK, Bain WG, Jacobs J, Nambulli S, Parikh U, Cillo A, et al. Intractable Coronavirus Disease 2019 (COVID-19) and Prolonged Severe Acute Respiratory Syndrome Coronavirus 2 (SARS-CoV-2) Replication in a Chimeric Antigen Receptor-Modified T-Cell Therapy Recipient: A Case Study. *Clin Infect Dis.* 2021;73(3):e815–e821.

86. Vicent MG, Martinez AP, Trabazo Del Castillo M, Molina B, Sisini L, Moron-Cazalilla G, et al. COVID-19 in pediatric hematopoietic stem cell transplantation: The experience of Spanish Group of Transplant (GETMON/GETH). *Pediatr Blood Cancer.* 2020;67(9):e28514.

87. Aydillo T, Gonzales-Reiche AS, Aslam S, van de Guchte A, Khan Z, Obla A, et al. Shedding of viable SARS-CoV-2 after immunosuppressive therapy for cancer. *N Engl J Med.* 2020;383:2586–2588.

88. Nazon C, Velay A, Radosavljevic M, Fafi-Kremer S, Paillard C. Coronavirus disease 2019 3 months after hematopoietic stem cell transplant: A pediatric case report. *Pediatr Blood Cancer.* 2020;67(9):e28545.

89. Talgam-Horshi E, Mozer-Glassberg Y, Waisbourd-Zinman O, Ashkenazi-Hoffnung L, Haskin O, Levi S, et al. Clinical Outcomes and Antibody Response in Covid-19-Positive Pediatric Solid Organ Transplant Recipients. *Pediatr Infect Dis J.* 2021;40(12):e514–e516.

90. Goss MB, Galvan NTN, Ruan W, Munoz FM, Brewer ED, O'Mahony CA, et al. The pediatric solid organ transplant experience with COVID-19: An initial multi-center, multi-organ case series. *Pediatr Transplant.* 2021;25(3):e13868.

91. Varnell Jr C, Harshman LA, Smith L, Liu C, Chen S, Al-Akash S, et al. COVID-19 in pediatric kidney transplantation: The Improving Renal Outcomes Collaborative. *Am J Transplant.* 2021;21(8):2740–2748.

92. Nicastro E, Verdoni L, Bettini LR, Zuin G, Balduzzi A, Montini G, et al. COVID-19 in Immunosuppressed Children. *Front Pediatr.* 2021;9:629240.

93. Infectious Diseases Society of America. IDSA Guidelines on the Treatment and Management of Patients with COVID-19 2021 [Available from: https://www.idsociety.org/practice-guideline/covid-19-guideline-treatment-and-management/.

94. National Institutes of Health. COVID-19 Treatment Guidelines 2021 [Available from: https://www.covid19treatmentguidelines.nih.gov/about-the-guidelines/whats-new/.

95. Chiotos K, Hayes M, Kimberlin DW, Jones SB, James SH, Pinninti SG, et al. Multicenter interim guidance on use of antivirals for children with coronavirus disease 2019/severe acute respiratory syndrome coronavirus 2. J Pediatric Infect Dis Soc.10:34-48.

96. Dulek DE, Fuhlbrigge RC, Tribble AC, Connelly JA, Loi MM, El Chebib H, et al. Multidisciplinary guidance regarding the use of immunomodulatory therapies for acute COVID-19 in pediatric patients. *Journal Ped Infect Dis Soc.* 2020;9(6):716–737.

97. Mak G, Dassner AM, Hammer BM, Hanisch BR. Safety and Tolerability of Monoclonal Antibody Therapies for Treatment of COVID-19 in Pediatric Patients. *Pediatr Infect Dis J.* 2021;40(12):e507–e509.

98. US Food and Drug Administration. Fact Sheet for Health Care Providers Emergency Use Authorization of Veklury (remdesivir) for Hospitalized Pediatric Patients 2020 [Available from: https://www.fda.gov/media/137566/download#:~:text=The%20U.S.%20Food%20and%20Drug,40%20kg%20or%20hospitalized%20pediatric.

99. US Food and Drug Administration. Fact Sheet for Health Care Providers Emergency Use Authorization (EUA) for Bamlanivimab and Etesevimab [Available from: https://www.fda.gov/media/145802/download.

100. Zachariah P. Updated Guidance on Use of Monoclonal Antibody Therapy for Treatment of COVID-19 in Children and Adolescents. *J Pediatric Infect Dis Soc.* 2021 in press.

101. American Academy of Pediatrics. Interim Clinical Guidance: Outpatient COVID-19 Management Strategies in Children and Adolescents 2021 [Available from: https://www.aap.org/en/pages/2019-novel-coronavirus-covid-19-infections/clinical-guidance/outpatient-covid-19-management-strategies-in-children-and-adolescents/.

102. US Food and Drug Administration. Fact Sheet for Health Care Providers Emergency Use Authorization of REGEN-COVTM (casirivimab and imdevimab) 2021 [Available from: https://www.fda.gov/media/145611/download.

103. O'Brien MP, Forleo-Neto E, Musser BJ, Isa F, Chan KC, Sarkar N, et al. Subcutaneous REGEN-COV Antibody Combination to Prevent Covid-19. *N Engl J Med.* 2021;385(13):1184–1195.

104. Lopez-Medina E, Lopez P, Hurtado IC, Davalos DM, Ramirez O, Martinez E, et al. Effect of Ivermectin on Time to Resolution of Symptoms Among Adults With Mild COVID-19: A Randomized Clinical Trial. *JAMA.* 2021;325(14):1426–1435.

105. Self WH, Tenforde MW, Rhoads JP, Gaglani M, Ginde AA, Douin DJ, et al. Comparative Effectiveness of Moderna, Pfizer-BioNTech, and Janssen (Johnson & Johnson) Vaccines in Preventing COVID-19 Hospitalizations Among Adults Without Immunocompromising Conditions — United States, March–August 2021. *MMWR Morbidity and Mortality Weekly Report.* 2021;70:1–7.

106. BioNTech P. COVID-19 Vaccine Fact Sheet for Healthcare Providers Administering Vaccine. Available from: https://labeling.pfizer.com/ShowLabeling.aspx?id=14471.

107. Centers for Disease Control and Prevention. COVID-19 Vaccinations in the United States 2021. Available from: https://covid.cdc.gov/covid-data-tracker/#vaccinations_vacc-total-admin-rate-total.

108. Murthy BP, Zell E, Saelee R, Murthy N, Meng L, Meador S, et al. COVID-19 vaccination coverage among adolescents aged 12-17 years - United States, December 14, 2020-July 31, 2021. *MMWR Morbidity and Mortality Weekly Report.* 2021;70:1206–1213.

109. Budzyn SE, Panaggio MJ, Parks SE, Papazian M, Magid J, Barrios LC. Pediatric COVID-19 Cases in Counties With and Without School Mask Requirements — United States, July 1–September 4, 2021. *MMWR Morbidity and Mortality Weekly Report.* 2021;70:1–3.

110. Jehn M, McCullough JM, Dale AP, Gue M, Eller B, Cullen T, et al. Association between K-12 school masks policies and school-associated COVID-19 outbreaks – Maricopa and Pima counties, Arizona, July-August 2021. *MMWR Morbidity and Mortality Weekly Report.* 2021;70:1–3.

111. Van Lancker W, Parolin Z. COVID-19, school closures, and child poverty: a social crisis in the making. *The Lancet Public Health.* 2020;5(5):e243–e244.

112. Verlenden JV, Pampati S, Rasberry CN, Liddon N, Hertz M, Kilmer G, et al. Association of children's mode of school instruction with child and parent experiences and well-being during the COVID-19 pandemic - COVID Experiences Survey, United States, October 8-November 13, 2020. *MMWR Morbidity and Mortality Weekly Report.* 2021;70:369–376.

113. Hawrilenko M, Kroshus E, Tandon P, Christakis D. The Association Between School Closures and Child Mental Health During COVID-19. *JAMA Netw Open.* 2021;4(9):e2124092.

114. Lange SJ, Kompaniyets L, Freedman DS, Kraus EM, Porter R, Blanck HM, et al. Longitudinal trends in body mass index before and during the COVID-19 pandemic among persons aged 2-19 years - United States, 2018-2020. *MMWR Morbidity and Mortality Weekly Report.* 2021;70:1278–1283.

115. Kidman R, Margolis R, Smith-Greenaway E, Verdery AM. Estimates and Projections of COVID-19 and Parental Death in the US. *JAMA Pediatr.* 2021;175(7):745–746.

116. Hillis SD, Unwin HJT, Chen Y, Cluver L, Sherr L, Goldman PS, et al. Global minimum estimates of children affected by COVID-19-associated orphanhood and deaths of caregivers: a modelling study. *The Lancet.* 2021;398(10298):391–402.

117. Santoli J.M., Lindley M.C., DeSilva M.B., Kharbanda E.O., Daley M.F., Galloway L., et al. Effects of the COVID-19 pandemic on routine pediatric vaccine ordering and administration—United States, 2020. MMWR-Morbid Mortal W. 69:591–593.

118. Shulman S, Geevarghese B, Kim KY, Rowley A. The impact of social distancing for COVID-19 upon diagnosis of Kawasaki disease. *J Pediatric Infect Dis Soc.* 2021;10(6):742–744.

119. Antoon JW, Williams DJ, Thurm C, Bendel-Stenzel M, Spaulding AB, Teufel 2nd RJ, et al. The COVID-19 pandemic and changes in healthcare utilization for pediatric respiratory and nonrespiratory illnesses in the United States. *J Hosp Med.* 2021;16(5):294–297.

120. Katz SE, Spencer H, Zhang M, Banerjee R. Impact of the COVID-19 pandemic on infectious diagnoses and antibiotic use in pediatric ambulatory practices. *J Pediatric Infect Dis Society.* 2020;10:62–64.

121. Hatoun J, Correa ET, Donahue SMA, Vernacchio L. Social distancing for COVID-19 and diagnoses of other infectious diseases in children. *Pediatrics.* 2020;146(4):e2020006460.

122. Lazzerini M, Barbi E, Apicella A, Marchetti F, Cardinale F, Trobia G. Delayed access or provision of care in Italy resulting from fear of COVID-19. *The Lancet Child & Adolescent Health.* 2020;4(5):e10–e11.

123. American Academy of Pediatrics. Interim Guidance for Use of Palivizumab Prophylaxis to Prevent Hospitalization From Severe Respiratory Syncytial Virus Infection During the Current Atypical Interseasonal RSV Spread 2021 [Available from: https://www.aap.org/en/pages/2019-novel-coronavirus-covid-19-infections/clinical-guidance/interim-guidance-for-use-of-palivizumab-prophylaxis-to-prevent-hospitalization/.

Special Topics: Emergency Medicine, Therapeutics, Novel Targets, Vaccines

CHAPTER

15 COVID-19: Emergency Medicine Perspectives

John C. Ray, MD, MBA, Matthew Chinn, MD, FAEMS, Jamie Aranda, MD, FAAEM, FACEP, Nancy Jacobson, MD, Ally Esch, DO, and Krishna Ramakrishnamenon Prasad, MD

Introduction

The challenges posed by the COVID-19 pandemic have affected all of humanity, as well as the full range of medical specialties, yet one of the single most affected specialties has been emergency medicine. Emergency medicine specialists have been at the forefront for decades confronting all human crises related to physical and mental health and are trained in a variety of life-, limb- and vision-saving interventions. However, the COVID-19 pandemic added additional burden to already strained emergency medicine departments. The pandemic adversely affected the care of non–COVID-19 patients, just as it affected the patients seeking service from other fields of medical specialties, including definitive and often elective treatments and procedures in oncology, cardiology, and orthopedics, to name a few.

COVID-19 can affect multiple organ systems and often manifests with confusing clinical scenarios and diverse ramifications.

The following sections of this chapter attempt to capture the various manifestations of COVID-19 infection as emergency situations for the patients; the challenges in arriving at a proper diagnosis; appropriate workup, including laboratory and imaging studies; and the rather uncharted territory of interventions and management protocols, including supportive care, medications, and invasive procedures. As more experience is gained in dealing with this pandemic, many aspects of clinical management will evolve and change, for the better, just as in the past 2 years.

Clinical Manifestations

The clinical manifestation of COVID-19 is highly variable and includes a wide range of reported symptoms, making early clinical differentiation of this disease process challenging within the emergency department (ED). In one review that included over 40,000 patients, at least 26 different clinical manifestations were reported.[1] Symptomatic manifestations can also range in severity from mild to critical. Additionally, time to recovery is also highly variable, with some individuals experiencing only a few days of symptoms and others having persistent symptoms and long-term sequalae. Of those individuals who develop symptoms, approximately 97.6% will do so within 11.5 days of the infection.[2–4]

The most common symptom of all patients diagnosed with COVID-19 is fever. After fever, in the general population, the following symptoms were most common: cough, dyspnea, fatigue, malaise, myalgias, nausea and/or vomiting or diarrhea, headache, and anosmia or ageusia. Less frequent symptoms reported include sore throat, chest pain, and abdominal pain.[1,5]

History

Patient-provided history is a crucial piece for any potential or confirmed COVID-19 patient. Initial history questions regarding travel, sick contacts, or known COVID-19–positive exposure can be collected during the triage process and can help guide appropriate clinical care, diagnostics, and subsequent isolation needs. Next, signs and symptoms provided by the patient, such as fevers, cough, shortness of breath, body aches, nausea and/or vomiting, and loss of taste or smell, will help further guide diagnostic workup and testing. A detailed investigation into immunocompromised status and additional comorbidities is also needed to help stratify risk as well as guide potential treatment modalities. Finally, general demographics questions such as occupation, age, race, surrounding population statistics, travel history, and socioeconomic status can all be helpful at this stage in an ED evaluation. In the advent of widespread vaccine availability, ascertaining a patient's previous positive or negative testing status along with their current vaccine status can additionally provide key details for the clinician.

Physical Examination

Physical examination findings are very diverse and can be nonspecific, and similar to those of other viral illnesses and common infections such as influenza, pneumonia, bronchitis, or gastroenteritis. Special attention to vital signs is an important first step of any ED evaluation as abnormalities in any of the vital signs can be seen with COVID-19. The most common, however, is fever ($>38°C$).

Pulmonary

COVID-19 predominately affects the respiratory system, making dyspnea (53%–80%) and cough (60%–86%) the most common symptoms and contributors to clinical presentation.[6,7] Special consideration to respiratory rate and pulse oximetry is critical in the ED because these play a critical role in disposition and potential inpatient and outpatient treatment strategies. Despite predominately affecting the respiratory system, auscultatory findings can be either normal or abnormal. Coarse breath sounds are the most common finding identified during auscultation. Fine and coarse crackles were the next most common. Hypoxia with or without associated symptoms was frequently reported. When hypoxia was observed without additional clinical manifestations, it was often referred to as "silent hypoxemia," which came to be an initial hallmark of SARS-CoV-2–infected individuals.[6–8]

Ear, Nose, and Throat

Ear, nose, and throat (ENT) symptoms and clinical findings are less common. A unique and distinctive feature of COVID-19 was sensory alterations to smell and/or taste. Although a loss of taste and smell has a wide variation in prevalence, ranging from 4.23% to 98.33%, it is a clear pointer to COVID-19 when elicited during a history or examination. Other ENT symptoms that have been documented are more nonspecific, making them less useful in isolation. These include sneezing, rhinitis, sore throat, rhinorrhea, and nasal congestion. Objective ENT physical examination findings are more uncommon with tonsillar swelling, throat congestion, and lymphadenopathy seen in less than 2% of patients.[9]

Neurological

Several neurological manifestations have been associated with COVID-19 infection. Reported symptoms include myalgias, headaches, and dizziness. Encephalopathy also can occur and is more frequent in the elderly. Cerebrovascular occlusions have been documented and attributed as a complication to COVID-19 manifesting with associated neurological deficits.[6,10,11]

Gastrointestinal

The most common gastrointestinal (GI) symptoms include anorexia, diarrhea, and nausea and/or vomiting. Abdominal pain and vomiting are recorded in approximately 5% of patients.[6] In one study, patients with GI symptoms had a longer time from onset to admission, which was thought to be related to delayed diagnosis given nonspecific symptoms. These nonspecific symptoms made diagnosis more challenging because 7% of the COVID-19 patients with GI symptoms had no other respiratory or ENT complaints.[6,12]

Diagnostic Workup and Investigation

The diagnostic evaluation of suspected patients with COVID-19 in the ED is discussed in the following section. These diagnostic tools serve as adjuncts to the clinical evaluation and treatment of life-threatening situations by the ED provider. A sample diagnostic and treatment pathway is shown in Fig. 15.1.

Laboratory Evaluation

COVID-19 Testing

COVID-19 testing should be performed in the emergency department (ED) to assist in the diagnosis of severe acute respiratory syndrome coronavirus-2 (SARS-CoV-2). While Although testing continues to evolve, there are two basic types of testing: viral testing (nucleic acid amplification tests ([NAATs]) and antigen tests)

Sample Emergency Department COVID-19 Pathway:

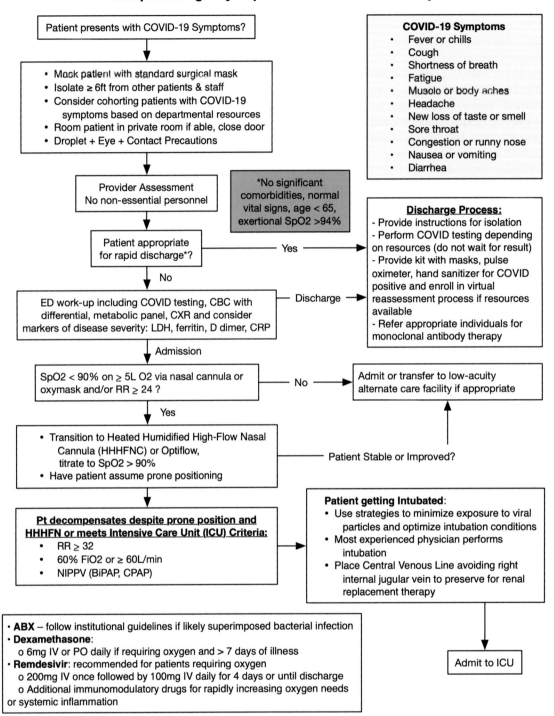

Fig. 15.1 Sample Diagnostic and Treatment Algorithm Used at a Large Academic Emergency Department With Adequate Staff and Space for Cohorting Suspected COVID-19 Patients. It uses recommendations from the Centers for Disease Control and Prevention and National Institutes of Health regarding management of patients and treatment guidelines. Discharge criteria and specific patient vital-sign parameters may need to be adjusted to account for potential mass-casualty scenarios, outpatient resources, and the unique culture and environment of the health care institution when applying the algorithm. *ABX,* antibiotics; *BiPAP,* bilevel positive airway pressure; *CPAP,* continuous positive airway pressure; *ICU,* intensive care unit; *NIPPV,* noninvasive positive pressure ventilation; *RR,* respiratory rate. (Data from Interim Clinical Guidance for Management of Patients with Confirmed Coronavirus Disease [COVID-19]. Centers for Disease Control and Prevention. https://www.cdc.gov/coronavirus/2019-ncov/hcp/clinical-guidance-management-patients.html; and National Institutes of Health. COVID-19 Treatment Guidelines Panel. Coronavirus Disease 2019 [COVID-19] Treatment Guidelines. https://www.covid19treatmentguidelines.nih.gov/.)

and antibody tests (serological tests). Antibody testing is mostly limited to identifying past infections and is less beneficial for ED testing of suspected patients; current literature suggests that they should not be used as a definitive test in a point-of-care hospital setting. Included in NAATs is the reverse transcriptase polymerase chain reaction (RT-PCR) test. RT-PCR and other NAATs are generally considered the preferred testing method for the ED as long as the hospital's laboratory has the appropriate equipment; laboratory-based NAATs are generally considered the most sensitive form of testing. Sensitivity and specificity are affected by several factors that include the analytical testing instrument used and the quality of acquisition of the sample. Nasopharyngeal samples are considered superior to throat samples.[13,14] Turnaround times (TATs) affect the utility of the test for the ED provider as because they can range from minutes to days. Ideally, an ED must perform rapid NAAT testing to confirm a diagnosis of COVID-19. Depending on capacity, an ED may choose to prioritize cohorts of patients into more rapid testing depending on disposition, severity, or other factors.

Supplemental Testing

A complete blood count is a commonly ordered study on many patients. A study with both outpatient- and inpatient-confirmed COVID-19 cases found a median white blood cell (WBC) count of 4700 mm^3, and another retrospective study of hospitalized patients found the median to be 7000 mm^3. A lymphopenia has been seen associated with COVID-19 in up to 83% of cases.[15] The basic metabolic panel, another commonly ordered test, does not seem to show any pathognomonic findings. Other laboratory tests that are often ordered, some to determine severity of disease, include D-dimer, C-reactive protein (CRP), lactate dehydrogenase (LDH), and procalcitonin. D-Dimer has been found to be elevated (≥ 0.5 mg/L) in 46.4% of all patients and 59.6% of those with severe disease. CRP of 10 mg/L or greater has been seen in 60.7% of patients, with a higher percentage of those with elevation with severe disease to 81.5%. LDH is found to be elevated in 41% of patients with a threshold of 250 U/L. Procalcitonin is often not found to be elevated; only 5.5% of all patients and 13.7% with severe disease had procalcitonin levels 0.5 ng/mL or greater. Testing for other respiratory infections, such as influenza, also may be performed concurrently based on prevalence of other infections at the time.[16–17]

Imaging

Chest x-ray is a common test ordered on patients with respiratory complaints and abnormalities, which are commonly noted in patients with COVID-19. A majority (59.1%) of patients who had a chest x-ray examination demonstrated an abnormality; among patients with increased disease severity, a higher proportion (76.7%) showed evidence of radiographical abnormalities. The most frequently found abnormalities in descending order of prevalence are bilateral patchy shadowing, local patchy shadowing, ground-glass opacity, and interstitial abnormalities. As expected, these findings increase with disease severity. Chest computed tomography (CT) is another imaging modality used to better evaluate lung pathological conditions in COVID-19 patients. Given the increased sensitivity of this imaging modality, a higher percentage of patients (86.2%) had a noted abnormality. In severely ill patients, this increased to almost 95%. Similar abnormalities to the chest radiographs were noted on chest CT. It should be noted, however, that one study found that 56% of patients who presented within 2 days of diagnosis had normal a CT image.[18] Pulmonary embolus is a known sequela of COVID-19 infection, and CT pulmonary angiograms should be considered in patients for whom there is a high clinical suspicion or who have not shown improvement along the expected recovery pattern.

Consultation

Consultation practices should follow the locally determined pathways for engagement with critical care services, infectious disease, and other specialists. Extracorporeal membrane oxygenation (ECMO) may be considered in the severely ill patient, and the appropriate teams should be considered based on the specific hospital's guidelines. Telemedicine consultation with specialists or other providers may be used in the appropriate circumstances to limit in-person contact and provide additional recommendations.[19–21]

Management

Treatment of SARS-CoV-2 (COVID-19) in the ED ranges from symptomatic and supportive care to identifying and treating associated end-organ dysfunction and invasive life-sustaining care for severe and critically ill patients. A sample diagnostic and treatment algorithm is shown in Fig. 15.1. Several medications are currently under investigation and may be appropriate for select patients (see medications section). The National Institutes of Health (NIH) has published information on caring for patients with COVID-19, and detailed information can be found at online at the NIH Coronavirus Disease 2019 (COVID-19) Treatment Guidelines.[22,23]

Symptomatic Support

Patients meeting criteria for mild to moderate disease without oxygen requirement or progressive dyspnea can be managed at home. Treatment consists of supportive care, education on preventing the spread of COVID-19 to others, and guidance on when to seek input from a health care provider or in-person evaluation. Patients with dyspnea may find prone positioning helpful while sleeping or resting. Supportive care includes antipyretics, analgesics, antitussives, and antiemetics. Rest and hydration should be emphasized, as well as signs and symptoms of dehydration that would prompt a need for return visit to the ED. Regarding antipyretics, there is current controversy over the use of nonsteroidal antiinflammatory drugs (NSAIDs), including ibuprofen; therefore it is reasonable to suggest acetaminophen as first-line therapy and using NSAIDs sparingly or for breakthrough fever and pain. Patients who are currently taking NSAIDs for comorbid conditions may continue using as directed. Opioids for pain are usually not indicated and may cause respiratory depression.

Home Oxygen

Depending on hospital capacity and the availability of alternative care facilities, some patients with mild to moderate dyspnea and limited supplemental oxygen requirement may be discharged from the ED with supplemental oxygen with planned virtual reassessment within 24 to 48 hours.

Medications

Since the emergence of the COVID-19 pandemic, recommendations for or against various treatment options have changed dynamically along with our understanding of this novel virus. As such, the recommendations found in this chapter are up to date as of its publication.

Antivirals

Remdesivir is currently the only medication approved by the FDA for the treatment of COVID-19. It is approved for mild to moderate COVID-19 in high-risk nonhospitalized patients and in hospitalized patients (aged > 12 years and weighing > 40 kg). The FDA does not recommend using remdesivir in patients with an eGFR of < 30 mL/min due to lack of data. It may be initiated in the ED as a 200-mg oral loading dose. The outpatient regimen is a 3-day course initiated within 7 days of symptom onset (200 mg IV on Day 1, followed by 100mg IV once daily on Days 2 and 3). Patients should be observed for >1 hour after infusion.

Ritonavir-boosted nirmatrelvir (Paxlovid) and molnupiravir have both received Emergency Use Authorizations from the FDA for the treatment of mild to moderate COVID-19 in patients aged >12 years and weighing > 40 kg who are within 5 days of symptom onset and at high risk of progressing to severe disease. The NIH COVID-19 Treatment Guidelines Panel recommends using nirmatrelvir 300mg with ritonavir 100mg (Paxlovid) orally twice daily for 5 days in nonhospitalized patients with mild to moderate COVID-19. Emergency physicians should carefully review the patient's medications to evaluate potential drug-drug interactions. Resources include the Liverpool COVID-19 Drug Interactions website, the EUA fact sheet for the ritonavir-boosted nirmatrelvir or pharmacist consultation. Molnupiravir should only be used if ritonavir-boosted nirmatrelvir or remdesivir cannot be used. The NIH COVID-19 Treatment Guidelines Panel recommends using molnupiravir 800mg orally (PO) twice daily for 5 days only when alternative therapies cannot be used. Treatment should be started as soon as possible and within 5 days of symptom onset.

Anti–SARS-CoV-2 Monoclonal Antibodies

Anti-Sars-CoV-2 monoclonal antibodies (mAbs) can be considered for the treatment of COVID-19 under Emergency Use Authorization by the FDA for nonhospitalizaed patients with mild to moderate COVID-19 who are at high risk for severe disease. Patients at risk for clinical decompensation who may benefit from monoclonal antibody treatment include those with a body mass index greater than 35, chronic kidney disease, diabetes mellitus, immunosuppressive disease or treatment, sickle cell anemia, age older than 65 years or older than 55 years with coronary artery disease, hypertension, or chronic lung diseases, including chronic obstructive pulmonary disease (COPD). Of note, SARS-CoV-2 variants may have reduced susceptibility to monoclonal antibodies because of mutations in the spike protein, and this may have an impact on effectiveness of treatment. Vaccination should be deferred for at least 90 days after treatment with anti–SARS-CoV-2 monoclonal antibodies. High-risk patients may receive monoclonal antibody therapy in the ED or be referred to an infusion clinic to initiate treatment. The NIH COVID-19 Treatment Guidelines Panel recommends bebtelovimab 175 mg IV in patients aged > 12 years as an alternative only when ritonavir-boosted nirmatrelvir (Paxlovid) and remdesivir are not available. Therapy should be initiated as soon as possible within 7 days of symptom onset and in a setting where the patient can be monitored and treated for severe hypersensitivity (including anaphylaxis) for one hour after injection. Treatment with bamlanivimab plus etesevimab or casirivimab plus imdevimab have been paused because the Omicron variant of concern and its subvariants are not susceptible to these agents

Antibiotics

There is insufficient evidence to recommend for or against empiric broad-spectrum antimicrobial therapy in the treatment of COVID pneumonia. However, if clinical suspicion suggests superimposed bacterial pneumonia (such as the presence of a lobar infiltrate on chest X-ray, leukocytosis, elevated serum lactate, microbiologic laboratory results or shock), clinicians should then follow routine Infectious Diseases Society of America (IDSA) guidelines for appropriate treatment of bacterial pneumonia.

Anticoagulation

Inpatients should be prophylactically anticoagulated with unfractionated or low-molecular-weight heparin if no contraindication exists. Patients with COVID-19 and a diagnosis of thromboembolism should receive the treatment dose of anticoagulation per usual guidelines. Patients being discharged from the ED or hospital with COVID-19 (and no thromboembolism) do not require anticoagulation unless they are at high-risk for thromboembolic disease, in which case, the decision to initiate anticoagulation therapy should be made on a case-by-case basis.

Steroids

There is no indication for steroid treatment in patients with COVID-19 being discharged from the ED who do not require supplemental oxygen. Additionally, the NIH recommends against the use of dexamethasone or other corticosteroids in hospitalized patients who do not require supplemental oxygen.[23] Patients requiring supplemental oxygen, high-flow nasal cannula (HFNC), noninvasive ventilation, invasive mechanical ventilation, or ECMO should be treated with dexamethasone 6 mg orally (PO) or intravenously (IV) daily.[24] If dexamethasone is unavailable, an alternative corticosteroid such as prednisone 40 mg, methylprednisolone 32 mg, or hydrocortisone 160 mg may be substituted. For patients being treated for septic shock and not already receiving a corticosteroid for treatment of COVID-19, the NIH recommends adding a steroid. Patients with COVID-19 being treated for asthma or COPD exacerbations who do not meet criteria for dexamethasone treatment for COVID-19 alone may be treated with an appropriate corticosteroid per the usual protocol.

Respiratory Support

Patient presentations to the ED with COVID-19 range from mild disease to overt respiratory failure. Mortality for intubated patients with COVID-19 is high, around 50%.[25] Many patients have been shown to tolerate hypoxia[25,26]; therefore it is reasonable to titrate from nasal cannula to nonrebreather, HFNC, and then noninvasive positive pressure ventilation (NIPPV) before progressing to intubation. In patients with acute hypoxemic respiratory failure, HFNC is recommended over NIPPV.[23] Symptomatic improvement and decreased work of breathing may be helpful indicators of respiratory status in the presence of permissive hypoxia.

Proning
Nebulizers and Metered-Dose Inhalers

Mild to moderate asthma and COPD exacerbations during the COVID pandemic can be managed with metered-dose inhalers (MDIs) and usual therapy, including steroids and magnesium. If a patient presents with acute respiratory failure or severe asthma or COPD exacerbation, nebulized bronchodilators can be given using inline administration by NIPPV or invasive mechanical ventilation with a viral filter. This should take place in a negative-pressure room, and staff must wear personal protective equipment (PPE) appropriate for aerosol-generating procedures. Finally, subcutaneous terbutaline or epinephrine may be viable alternatives to nebulized bronchodilators if negative-pressure rooms are unavailable.[30,32]

Coronavirus Disease–Associated Acute Respiratory Distress Syndrome and Intubation

There is some evidence that patients with COVID-19 who manifest acute respiratory syndrome represent a different pathophysiology than previously described patients with ARDS not related to COVID-19. Some have recommended referring to this unique entity as coronavirus disease–associated acute respiratory distress syndrome (CARDS).[32] A subset of these patients may

Table 15.1 Practical and Evidence-Based Strategies to Minimize Exposure to Viral Particles, Limit Traffic In and Out of Patient Rooms, and Optimize Intubation Conditions to Ensure First-Pass Success

Perform aerosol-generating procedures in a negative-pressure room (airborne infection isolation room)	Use video-laryngoscopy if available
The most-skilled provider with extensive airway management experience performs the intubation	Limit presence to only necessary personnel and equipment (totes or kits of intravenous or intubation supplies can be brought into the room)
Proper personal protective equipment is worn by all staff (N-95 with overlying mask, eye protection, bouffant/head covering, gown, booties, at least two pairs of gloves)	Designate a person to monitor and assist with doffing and designate a doffing area if available
Avoid bag-mask ventilation (connect endotracheal tube immediately to closed-loop system/ventilator after intubation)	Use a viral filter in ventilation circuits
Place additional lines (nasogastric or orogastric tube, central venous line) immediately after intubation to limit traffic in and out of room	Limit patient movement by obtaining portable x-ray films and avoid repeat imaging (perform chest x-ray after all lines have been placed)

retain normal lung compliance and thus can tolerate larger tidal volumes. Research is evolving in this area, and it is recommended that readers refer to the most up-to-date guidance from the Centers for Disease Control and Prevention (CDC) and the NIH.

Emergency physicians should proceed with intubation after a goals-of-care discussion with the patient and family giving careful consideration of age and comorbidities because of the high mortality associated with CARDS. If intubation becomes necessary, a provider with extensive airway management experience should perform the intubation. Strategies that can be implemented to optimize success and limit viral exposure are shown in Table 15.1.

Invasive Procedures and Hemodynamic Support

Central Line Placement

Maintain a low threshold for central venous line placement in intubated and critical patients with COVID-19 admitted through the ED. This is because of the risk for further decompensation and likely need for prone positioning that could pose challenges to obtaining central access. Placing a central line can take place around the same time as intubation to limit traffic in and out of the room and preserve resources (chest x-ray, PPE). Finally, in choosing a location for central venous line placement and considering the potential need for continuous renal replacement therapy, it behooves the ED provider to preserve the right internal jugular vein for a hemodialysis catheter. Femoral sites can be inconvenient in the prone patient. A left subclavian site could be considered; however, the risk for pneumothorax may be unacceptable in this patient population. Therefore the preferred location for central line placement is the left internal jugular vein if no contraindication exists.

Hemodynamic Support

Balanced crystalloid is the recommended resuscitation fluid for patients with COVID-19. Norepinephrine is the preferred first-line vasopressor, followed by the addition of vasopressin or epinephrine for additional support. Dobutamine may be used in the setting of cardiac dysfunction. Finally, corticosteroids are recommended for patients in shock who are not already receiving them as treatment for COVID-19.[23]

Extracorporeal Membrane Oxygenation

Although the NIH expert panel cites "insufficient data to recommend either for or against the use of ECMO in patients with COVID-19 and refractory hypoxemia,"[21] the emergency physician must keep this in mind as a potentially life-saving measure and advocate for its use in the appropriate patient. A recent report from the University Hospital Vienna demonstrated a good chance of survival with 75% of patients treated with ECMO between January 2020 and April 2021 surviving the study period of 28-days.[33] This represents an area of opportunity for further study and treatment of COVID-19 patients.

In conclusion, the treatment of COVID-19 in the ED requires a wide skillset, including symptomatic and supportive care for mild to moderate cases and thoughtful resuscitation and skilled performance of invasive procedures in the critically ill COVID-19 patient. Research in the treatment of COVID-19, including specialized therapies and unique respiratory physiology, continues to evolve. The CDC and NIH provide extensive online resources that are available to the emergency physician in real time.

Disposition

Throughout the COVID-19 pandemic, risk stratification and triage of patients with known or suspected COVID have posed significant challenges. Although rapid risk stratification is necessary for appropriate resource usage and patient safety, most evidence regarding risk for disease severity comes from expert recommendations, case studies, and predictive tools not yet validated for use in SARS-CoV-2 infection.[34,35] To mitigate uncertainty and facilitate the integration of new and emerging guidelines into clinical practice, many hospitals and health systems have developed pathways with agreed upon criteria for disposition and management of patients with known or suspected COVID-19.[36]

Nonetheless, disease severity spans a wide range: whereas some patients have no symptoms, others require ICU admission and even mechanical ventilation.[34] In one 2020 study at a large academic medical center ED in New York State, researchers found that of the 4404 persons under investigation for the SARS-CoV-2 virus presenting to the ED, 68% were discharged home, 29% were admitted to the medical floor, and 3% were admitted to the ICU. Of patients discharged from the ED, 6.2% had a repeat ED visit within the study period, 2.5% had repeat ED visits with medical floor admission, and less than 0.001% had repeat ED visits with admission directly to the ICU. Meanwhile, of patients admitted to the medical floor, 13% required transfer to the ICU.[37]

There are not any fixed criteria for hospital admission of patients with known or suspected SARS-CoV-2. Rather, disposition decisions must be made on a case-by-case basis.[38] Factors impacting disposition determination should include clinical factors, baseline medical and social needs, facility resource availability, potential adjunct to home care, patient, or caregiver ability to recognize and return for worsening symptoms.

Admission

Intensive Care Unit Admission

Patients with severe disease or requiring mechanical ventilation require disposition to a critical care setting. Clinical predictors of ICU admission include hypoxemia, opacities on imaging, male sex, insulin-dependent diabetes, and preexisting comorbidity.[34,37,39] Laboratory abnormalities that predict ICU admission include elevated anion gap, CRP, glucose, and LDH, as well as decreased albumin, calcium, and sodium. Additionally, male sex, hypoxemia, and increased respiratory rate predict requirement for mechanical ventilation, whereas history of COPD, age, and hypoxemia are predictors of mortality.[37]

Medical Floor Admission

Patients with moderate to severe symptoms, hypoxemia requiring oxygen supplementation, or high-risk features for clinical deterioration may require hospital admission for continued evaluation, monitoring, and management.[40] Risks for clinical deterioration or severe disease include age, hypertension, heart disease, obesity, chronic respiratory disease, transplant status, and chronic kidney disease.[34,39,41,42] Of all risk factors, age is the strongest, with case fatality rates highest in patients over 85 years.[41,42] Younger patients often have mild disease, but those with comorbid conditions such as asthma, insulin-dependent diabetes, malignancy, and obesity are at risk for severe disease.[39]

Alternative Care Site Admission

Since the onset of the COVID-19 pandemic, increased need for medical care paired with finite hospital resources has prompted jurisdictions to establish alternative care sites. Alternative care sites are set in nontraditional settings such as mobile field hospitals and can provide varying levels of care: nonacute care (ambulatory) for mild symptoms with other barriers to discharge home, hospital care (medical-surgical) for patients with hypoxia and nursing assistance, or acute care (ICU) for patients who require significant ventilatory support.[43] Local jurisdictions should have agreements in place with local health care facilities regarding patient transfers.[41] Appropriate disposition to alternative care facilities depends on the patient presentation, risk for clinical deterioration, level of care needed, and the capabilities of the local acute care facility.

Discharge

Discharge Home

Patients with mild symptoms and minimal risk factors for severe disease may be appropriate for discharge home.[39] In one study, of patients discharged from the ED with known or suspected SARS-CoV-2 infection, 6.2% had a repeat ED visit within the study period, but only 2.5% had repeat ED visit with admission to the medical floor, and less than 0.001% had repeat ED visits with admission directly to the ICU.[4] Nonetheless, factors beyond the clinical presentation of the patient must be considered when disposition planning home from the ED. In addition to clinical stability, patients must be able to adhere to home care isolation, recognize worsening symptoms, and return to the ED if needed.[38,41,42] For example, if a homeless person is diagnosed with COVID in the ED and discharged back to a communal shelter, that patient cannot reasonably self-isolate and may require temporary shelter or an alternative care facility.[40]

Adjuncts to Discharge Home

When hospital resources are exceeded, the discharge of adult patients with moderate symptoms or risk for potential clinical decline have been be discharged home with adjuncts to home care.[38] To augment traditional home care and monitor for stability, some health systems have established discharge protocols in which patients diagnosed with COVID are dispensed a pulse oximeter at discharge and telehealth visits are conducted following discharge.[44] The use of telehealth for patient reevaluation after ED discharge allows the patient to maintain self-isolation, decreases the incidence of infected patients visiting the health care setting, institutes effective remote assessment abilities, and enables ongoing follow-up for a large number of patients.[39] These adjuncts to home care are particularly useful for patients with mild disease but having risk factors for severe illness, because they need monitoring for development of severe symptoms.

Patient Education

Patient and caregiver education is vital to safe discharge home. Strict return precautions for worsening symptoms are of critical importance when discharging patients with known or suspected SARS-CoV-2 infection given potential for clinical deterioration in the second week after symptom onset.[39] Additionally, symptomatic patients should receive instructions on self-isolation practices at home. New and accumulating data support ending isolation precautions using a symptom-based strategy.[41,42] Educating patients on both the content and to access updated CDC guidelines for self-quarantine after diagnosis with SARS-CoV-2 is imperative.

COVID-19–Specific Follow-Up

Many patients diagnosed with the COVID-19 experience not only acute symptoms but also persistent physiological and psychological complications.[44,45] Although patients requiring ICU admission are most at risk for long-term effects of SARS-CoV-2 infection, even patients who do not require hospitalization may experience lingering symptoms.[45] To deliver high-quality care and streamline services, some hospitals and health care systems have developed integrated multidisciplinary outpatient services to support COVID-19 survivors with outpatient follow-up.[44,45] One such clinic is the Johns Hopkins Post-Acute COVID-19 Team (JH PACT) clinic, which includes specialists in pulmonology, physical medicine and rehabilitation, psychiatry, neurology, cardiology, infectious disease, nephrology, dermatology, hematology, hepatology, and otolaryngology.[45] Another such service at Beaumont Hospital comprises respiratory medicine, intensive care medicine, infectious diseases specialists, and psychiatry and psychology specialists.[44] These services were tasked with seeking large numbers of patients during the COVID-19 pandemic surge and have employed a hybrid virtual and in-person approach.[44,45] An integrated, multidisciplinary approach to follow-up for COVID-19 survivors has been shown to improve subjective outcomes and quality of life.[44]

Primary Care and Community Mental Health Follow-Up

When discharging patients with COVID-19 from the ED, availability of primary care follow-up should be considered.[41,42] Most discharging patients will be appropriate for primary care and community follow-up, and some COVID-19 survivor clinics enroll patients based on primary care consultation.[44,45]

Disposition of Special Populations

Patients Belonging to Minority Racial or Ethnic Groups

As a result of systemic social and health care inequities, various racial and ethnic minority groups are disproportionately affected by COVID-19. Studies have shown that racial and ethnic minority groups have increased mortality from SARS-CoV-2 infection, event at young ages. This has been attributed to health disparities resulting in young age and barriers to maintenance care for people belonging to minority groups.[42]

Pediatric Patients

Children and young people are often asymptomatic or only mildly symptomatic when infected with SARS-CoV-2. Nonetheless, some pediatric patients develop severe illness.[37–42] Like adults, pediatric patients with obesity, diabetes, lung disease, or immunosuppression are at increased risk for severe disease.[38–41] Additionally, children with genetic, metabolic, and neurological conditions; congenital heart disease; or sickle cell anemia are at risk for severe illness.[42] Discharge decisions

should be made on a case-by-case basis and should involve parents and specialists for comorbid conditions if specific questions or concerns arise.

Pregnant Patients

Most pregnant patients are young, otherwise healthy women, and overall risk for severe illness is relatively low. However, pregnancy causes an increased risk for severe illness from COVID-19. Additionally, infection with SARS-CoV-2 correlates with increased risk for preterm birth before 37 weeks in addition to other poor pregnancy outcomes. This should be considered during disposition planning. Patients and their obstetricians should be involved in disposition planning.[42]

Patients With Disabilities

Patients with medical or developmental disabilities are not inherently more at risk for severe COVID-19 disease than others. However, patients with disabilities may live in communal settings such as care facilities or group homes, may have difficulty understanding or adhering to instructions regarding safety measures, and may struggle to communicate new or worsening symptoms.[44] Despite no increased physiological risk for severe disease, these factors may contribute to worse outcomes for this patient population and affect disposition decision making.

Homeless Patients

Homelessness may portend worsened disease outcomes given that adults experiencing homelessness often suffer from underlying medical and mental health comorbidities.[42] Additionally, homelessness may be a barrier to recommended self-isolation and safety measures. This should be considered when disposition decisions are made for patients experiencing homelessness, and alternative shelter and alternative care facility disposition should be provided on a case-by-case basis.[38,42,43]

Special Considerations

The COVID-19 pandemic created many unique challenges for EDs around the world. This section will discuss several unique challenges within the ED setting.

Emergency Medical Services

Emergency medical services (EMS) is a vital piece of any ED and health care system and community. Their services play a key role in the access of emergency medical care both to and from EDs. Strong partnership and frequent communication between ED leadership and a local EMS agency is paramount during a pandemic. From a receiving ED's perspective, several challenges can be encountered.

Prearrival communication between EMS and the receiving ED that a COVID-19 patient under investigation is arriving is a critical alert step to ensure proper PPE precautions; immediate rooming procedures can also be undertaken to avoid unnecessary exposure of other patients and hospital staff.[46] Depending on an EMS service's resources and level of training, treatment with bilevel positive airway pressure (BPAP), continuous positive airway pressure (CPAP), high-flow oxygen, and nebulized breathing treatments may be used during transport; however, these treatment modalities, known as aerosol generating procedures, can create a potentially hazardous exposure environment as EMS agencies enter an ED.[46] Using a prearrival staging/screening area within an EMS arrival bay was found to be effective in certain circumstances, allowing time and preparation to place particle filtration devices such as high-efficiency particulate air (HEPA) filters before entering the ED halls. Additionally, prearrival staging areas can allow for a brief pause to ensure proper PPE and barrier equipment was being used by both the patient and the EMS crews.

By the nature of their position within a patient's care spectrum, EMS providers often were treating and transporting patients before any formal COVID-19 testing or status confirmation. This has implications in terms of EMS patients under investigation for exposure, subsequent need for isolation and screening, and ultimately EMS workforce ramifications. ED screening of EMS personnel on arrival to an ED can be considered depending on the individual practices and local oversight of the EMS group.[46]

A final consideration for EDs surrounding EMS transports was the need for rapid modification of prehospital care-based policies and protocols. Changes to protocols such as out of hospital cardiac arrest algorithms, use of NIVPP devices, or use of nebulized medications may need to be considered; thus frequent communication between EMS medical directors and the respective EDs should be undertaken.

Overall, a strong partnership between EMS leadership and ED leadership is needed to allow a health system to create a prearrival notification structure, a postexposure notification system, and rapid protocol adjustment process.

Personal Protective Equipment

One of the most important challenges that EDs faced during the COVID-19 pandemic was the education, training, and availability of proper PPE within the ED setting. With the uncertainty that surrounded a novel virus and its mode of transmission, there were many iterations to the best practice PPE advisories for both the patients and health care providers. Staying up to date, educating and communicating on the recommendations made by the CDC or equivalent government regulatory agency is imperative to adhering to best practices, allaying patient and health care provider fears

and creating a unified singular understanding of recommendations. It should be noted that many of the recommended PPE devices—powered air-purifying respirator (PAPR), controlled air-purifying respirator (CAPR), N-95 respirators, and elastomeric masks— require training and fitting before approved use. Fig. 15.2 depicts an example of an easy-to-follow guideline for proper PPE based on type of patient and exposure.

Supply chain constraints surrounding PPE created one of biggest challenges for emergency medicine health care personnel during the COVID-19 pandemic. During times of constraint several PPE conservation strategies emerged. Decontamination protocols and evidence-based guidelines for ultraviolet and vaporized hydrogen peroxide currently exist for repeated use of N-95 masks. Increased use of PAPR/CAPRs or reusable elastomeric masks, if available, allowed for conservation of N-95 masks. Organized local supply chain monitoring within the ED allowed for rapid up-stream awareness of any forthcoming concerns and subsequent need for supply chain pivoting.

Space Constraints and Modifications

ED overcrowding is a critical problem and is only exacerbated during a pandemic. Facility adjustment will be inevitable for all ED settings to help promote a safe caring environment during the COVID-19 pandemic for both patients presenting with COVID-19 concerns and those with other emergencies.[47,48] All patients presenting to the ED setting should be screened upon arrival to an ED for signs and symptoms of COVID-19. Although this will not capture asymptomatic or presymptomatic patients, screening remains an important piece of exposure mitigation so that proper cohorting and precautions can take place in an ED setting. Signage and visual alerts are an important engineering strategy to help promote routine source control measures such as social distancing, mask adherence, and hand hygiene. Social distancing along with PPE are the cornerstones of preventing spread of COVID-19.[48,49]

Social distancing within the ED setting is an onerous but crucial task for each ED to consider. Although all EDs will have unique constraints and unique solutions, there are several general areas for all EDs to pay close attention to: waiting room, vertical care or chair care internal waiting rooms, hallway patients, cohorting units, and physician/nursing stations.[48]

The waiting room of an ED often can be one of the most crowded and undistanced places within the health care setting. Although asking patients to maintain a 6-foot distance while waiting for a room is a key step, reengineered waiting room spaces are often necessary to create a safe environment for patients. Spacing of furniture and even possibly removing excess furniture may be necessary to promote social distancing. Physical

Standards
- PPE guidelines must be followed regardless of vaccination status.
- Hand hygiene, washing and/or sanitizing, should be performed before and after using PPE.
- Follow PPE conservation guidelines in the PPE playbook.
- If a patient is positive for SARS-CoV-2 and has an additional condition that warrants isolation precautions (i.e., MDRO, C. diff), the more restrictive PPE guidelines should be followed.
- Fluidshield masks should only be worn if anticipating splash or contamination with blood or body fluids.

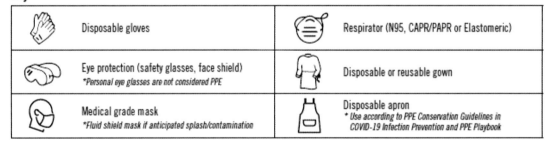

No patient contact or patient care. If you work within 6 feet of coworkers in nonclinical areas (i.e., office setting)	N/A	
If your role requires you to work within 6 feet of patients, the public or coworkers in clinical areas	All patient cares and interactions with patients or visitors	
Asymptomatic patients: • SARS-CoV-2 test pending	All asymptomatic patients that are pending a SARS-CoV-2 screening test should follow standard precautions	
Aerosol Generating Procedures (AGP)	Low-risk	
	Medium- and High-risk	
Direct patient care areas implementing droplet/contact precautions: • COVID-19 suspect, • SARS-CoV-2(+), • Inpatients who refuse testing • Clinic patients who are symptomatic and refuse testing	Inpatient	
	Ambulatory	

NOTE: See PPE playbook conservation guidelines section and isolation signage.

Infection Prevention and Control 1/08/2021

Key

	Disposable gloves		Respirator (N95, CAPR/PAPR or Elastomeric)
	Eye protection (safety glasses, face shield) *Personal eye glasses are not considered PPE*		Disposable or reusable gown
	Medical grade mask *Fluid shield mask if anticipated splash/contamination*		Disposable apron * Use according to PPE Conservation Guidelines in COVID-19 Infection Prevention and PPE Playbook

Fig. 15.2 Example Graphic for Proper Personal Protective Equipment *(PPE)* **Precautions Based on Clinical Setting and Exposure.** This is a sample PPE guideline chart internally created and drafted by the infection prevention department at a large academic hospital. It uses recommendations from the Centers for Disease Control and Prevention and National Institutes of Health regarding needed PPE for various clinical scenarios, treatments, and interventions. A detailed graphic key is provided with the chart to help health care providers quickly recognize the recommended PPE for each scenario. *CAPR,* Controlled air-purifying respirator; *C. diff, Clostridioidesdifficile; MDRO,* multidrug-resistant organism; *N/A,* not available; *PAPR,* powered air-purifying respirator; *PPE,* personal protective equipment.

barriers, signs, covers, drapes, or floor tape can be used to denote and demark appropriate distancing among patients. Remote triage facilities or, if the climate allows, outdoor assessment and triage stations could be considered. Overflow and waiting room surge spaces should be considered to accommodate times of peak volumes. Temporary isolation tents or ancillary building structures for either triage or low-acuity treatment area are options to help adhere to patient distancing as much as possible.[48]

Beyond the waiting room, EDs that use a vertical flow process or an internal waiting room will need to reconsider these care spaces where appropriate as 6 feet separation between patients may not be feasible, especially given that many lower acuity patients with milder respiratory complaints can be seen in this setting.[48]

Although unavoidable in many ED settings, secondary to space and volume constraints, the use of hallway spaces to care for patients would be considered less ideal especially for patients exhibiting concerning or infectious symptoms of COVID-19. Protocols restricting use of these hallway spaces for only specific presenting complaints could be a mitigating strategy when hallways beds are needed secondary to capacity constraints. Creation of specific cohorted units and triage spaces for patients presenting with respiratory complaints also can be considered to help reduce the spread of COVID-19.[48]

Consideration of the work environment for ED staff, nurses, and physicians should not be overlooked. Optimizing staff distancing can be challenging given close-quartered environments, workstations, and break rooms. When distancing is not feasible, strict adherence to PPE guidelines becomes an important priority.[49]

Finally, partnership with hospital engineering should be undertaken to improve indoor air quality and exchange. Optimization around the hospital's air-handling system may be needed to ensure maximized exchanged rates, filtration, and direction.[49,50]

Telehealth

A novel strategy that blossomed during the pandemic was the incorporation of telehealth modalities as an exposure reduction strategy. Telehealth services allowed for ongoing triage and care to select patient populations in the ED without increased exposure to patients, health care workers, or patient families and without the additional burden of space constraints. Use of real-time telephone or live audiovisual devices to interact and screen patients can be achieved safely and easily with smartphones, tablets, or computers.[7,19-21]

COVID-19 Vaccination in the Emergency Department

With more widespread availability of COVID-19 vaccines, additional opportunities for administration have become available for EDs around the world. Vaccine administration within the ED setting has some historical roots with administration of Tdap (tetanus toxoid, reduced diphtheria toxoid, and acellular pertussis) and influenza vaccines. However, mass distribution of investigational or EUA vaccines was not undertaken before the pandemic in ED settings. As it relates to the ED, administration of a two-dose vaccine series, rigorous extreme temperature control, and thawing requirements for mRNA COVID-19 vaccines makes operationalizing the distribution in the ED setting challenging. However, the single-dose vaccines that have less rigorous temperature and storing requirements have now made ED distribution more feasible. Specific attention to patient screening, patient education, storage, and information technology needs should be undertaken when developing a durable ED vaccination process.[51]

Conclusion

The preceding sections in this chapter address the current comprehensive approach to COVID-19–related emergencies. Further advancements in tackling the pandemic (diagnostics, vaccines, antiviral therapies, immunomodulator therapies etc.) will certainly dictate future changes in the clinical approach.

As the world knows, the COVID-19 pandemic has become a juxtaposition of triumphs and tragedies. The curses affecting health care are manifold. The outpatient specialties in health care had to adapt in various ways by incorporating phone visits and video visits and postponing essential and often lifesaving interventions and procedures. Emergency medicine was struck particularly hard, where the providers were faced with a range of unexpected clinical manifestations and incomplete guidelines for interventions and management, while having to use PPEs, robbing the opportunity of "face to face" interactions with the patients.

The striumphs must be considered as well. Technology companies came up with useful alternatives, including video conferencing platforms such as Zoom, WebEx, and Teams, etc., lowering costs for companies, organizations, and individuals and reducing environment-degrading emissions even as the transportation industry suffered. These innovations helped many medical specialties, and although not perfectly amenable to integration within traditional emergency medicine care, the telemedicine framework did begin to show various areas of opportunity within this specialty.

Medical science and research accelerated faster than usual to face up to the challenges posed by the COVID-19 pandemic. Biotech innovations including mRNA technology for fast-paced vaccine development, monoclonal antibodies, and antivirals have helped in providing supportive care supplementing proning, ventilator support, and ECMO.

We know that this is not the final statement about the COVID-19 pandemic and much will change as the scientific community continues to learn, adapt, and attack this virus. The United States has vacillated at various points toward some degree of normalcy as a result of the immunization, diagnostic and treament programs. However, multiple waves, surges, and various mutants also have been detected and loom on the forefront of this battle. We hope that the initial lessons learned from this pandemic will help prepare us better for similar or worse future outbreaks.

REFERENCES

1. da Rosa Mesquita R, Francelino Silva Junior LC, Santos Santana FM, et al. Clinical manifestations of COVID-19 in the general population: systematic review. *Wien Klin Wochenschr.* 2021;133(7-8):377–382. doi:10.1007/s00508-020-01760-4.
2. Wiersinga WJ, Rhodes A, Cheng AC, Peacock SJ, Prescott HC. Pathophysiology, transmission, diagnosis, and treatment of coronavirus disease 2019 (COVID-19): a review. *JAMA.* 2020;324(8):782–793. doi:10.1001/jama.2020.12839.

3. Nie X, Fan L, Mu G, et al. Epidemiological characteristics and incubation period of 7015 confirmed cases with coronavirus disease 2019 outside Hubei Province in China. *J Infect Dis*. 2020;222(1):26–33. doi:10.1093/infdis/jiaa211 Jun 16PMID: 32339231; PMCID: PMC7197553.

4. Lauer SA, Grantz KH, Bi Q, et al. The incubation period of coronavirus disease 2019 (COVID-19) from publicly reported confirmed cases: estimation and application. *Ann Intern Med*. 2020;172(9):577–582. doi:10.7326/M20-0504 May 5PMID: 32150748; PMCID: PMC7081172.

5. Richardson S, Hirsch JS, Narasimhan M, et al. Presenting characteristics, comorbidities, and outcomes among 5700 patients hospitalized with COVID-19 in the New York City area. *JAMA*. 2020;323(20):2052–2059. doi:10.1001/jama.2020.6775.

6. Johnson KD, Harris C, Cain JK, et al. Pulmonary and extra-pulmonary clinical manifestations of COVID-19. *Front Med (Lausanne)*. 2020;7:526. doi:10.3389/fmed.2020.00526.

7. Wang B, Liu Y, Wang Y, et al. Characteristics of pulmonary auscultation in patients with 2019 novel coronavirus in China. *Respiration*. 2020;99(9):755–763. doi:10.1159/000509610 PMID: 33147584.

8. Tobin MJ, Laghi F, Jubran A. Why COVID-19 silent hypoxemia is baffling to physicians. *Am J Respir Crit Care Med*. 2020;202(3):356–360. doi:10.1164/rccm.202006-2157CP.

9. Ibekwe TS, Fasunla AJ, Orimadegun AE. Systematic review and meta-analysis of smell and taste disorders in COVID-19. *OTO Open*. 2020;4(3):2473974X20957975. doi:10.1177/2473974X20957975.

10. Liotta EM, Batra A, Clark JR, et al. Frequent neurologic manifestations and encephalopathy-associated morbidity in Covid-19 patients. *Ann Clin Transl Neurol*. 2020;7(11):2221–2230. doi:10.1002/acn3.51210 PMID: 33016619; PMCID: PMC7664279.

11. Oxley TJ, Mocco J, Majidi S, et al. Large-vessel stroke as a presenting feature of COVID-19 in the young. *N Engl J Med*. 2020;382(20):e60. doi:10.1056/NEJMc2009787 PMID: 32343504; PMCID: PMC7207073.

12. Agarwal A, Chen A, Ravindran N, To C, Thuluvath PJ. Gastrointestinal and liver manifestations of COVID-19. *J Clin Exp Hepatol*. 2020;10(3):263–265. doi:10.1016/j.jceh.2020.03.001.

13. Centers for Disease Control and Prevention, "COVID-19 and Your Health." 11 Feb. 2020, https://www.cdc.gov/coronavirus/2019-ncov/symptoms-testing/testing.html.

14. Tang Yi-Wei, et al. Laboratory diagnosis of COVID-19: current issues and challenges. *Journal of Clinical Microbiology*. 2020;58(6). doi:10.1128/jcm.00512-20.

15. Guan W-J, Ni Z-Y, Hu Y, et al. Clinical characteristics of coronavirus disease 2019 in China. *New England Journal of Medicine*. 2020;382(18):1708–1720. doi:10.1056/nejmoa2002032.

16. Centers for Disease Control and Prevention, "Healthcare Workers." 11 Feb. 2020, http://www.cdc.gov/coronavirus/2019-ncov/hcp/clinical-guidance-management-patients.html.

17. Paranjpe I, Russak AJ, De Freitas JK, et al. Retrospective cohort study of clinical characteristics of 2199 hospitalised patients with COVID-19 in New York City. *BMJ Open*. 2020;10(11):e040736. doi:10.1136/bmjopen-2020-040736.

18. Bernheim A, Mei X, Huang M, et al. Chest CT findings in coronavirus disease-19 (COVID-19): relationship to duration of infection. *Radiology*. 2020;295(3):200463. doi:10.1148/radiol.2020200463.

19. Centers for Disease Control and Prevention. Using Telehealth to Expand Access to Essential Health Services during the COVID-19 Pandemic. https://www.cdc.gov/coronavirus/2019-ncov/hcp/telehealth.html. Accessed May 26, 2021

20. Russi CS, Heaton HA, Demaerschalk BM. Emergency medicine telehealth for COVID-19: minimize front-line provider exposure and conserve personal protective equipment. *Mayo Clin Proc*. 2020;95(10):2065–2068. doi:10.1016/j.mayocp.2020.07.025.

21. Hollander JE, Carr BG. Virtually Perfect? Telemedicine for Covid-19. *N Engl J Med*. 2020;382(18):1679–1681. doi:10.1056/NEJMp2003539 Apr 30PMID: 32160451.

22. Healthcare Workers: Information on COVID-19. Centers for Disease Control and Prevention. Available online: https://www.cdc.gov/coronavirus/2019-nCoV/hcp/index.html

23. Coronavirus Disease 2019 (COVID-19) Treatment Guidelines. National Institutes of Health. https://www.covid19treatmentguidelines.nih.gov

24. Horby P, Lim WS, Emberson JR, et al RECOVERY Collaborative Group. Dexamethasone in hospitalized patients with COVID-19. *N Engl J Med*. 2021;384(8):693–704. doi:10.1056/NEJMoa2021436 Feb 25PMID: 32678530; PMCID: PMC7383595.

25. Lim ZJ, Subramaniam A, Ponnapa Reddy M, et al. Case fatality rates for patients with COVID-19 requiring invasive mechanical ventilation: a meta-analysis. *Am J Respir Crit Care Med*. 2021;203(1):54–66. doi:10.1164/rccm.202006-2405OC Jan 1PMID: 33119402; PMCID: PMC7781141.

26. Voshaar T, Stais P, Köhler D, Dellweg D. Conservative management of COVID-19 associated hypoxaemia. *ERJ Open Res*. 2021;7(1):00026–02021. doi:10.1183/23120541.00026-2021 PMID: 33738306; PMCID: PMC7848791.

27. Guérin C, Reignier J, Richard JC, et al. Prone positioning in severe acute respiratory distress syndrome. *N Engl J Med*. 2013;368(23):2159–2168. doi:10.1056/NEJMoa1214103 Jun 6PMID: 23688302.

28. Elharrar X, Trigui Y, Dols AM, et al. Use of prone positioning in nonintubated patients with COVID-19 and hypoxemic acute respiratory failure. *JAMA*. 2020;323(22):2336–2338. doi:10.1001/jama.2020.8255 PMID: 32412581; PMCID: PMC7229532.

29. Sartini C, Tresoldi M, Scarpellini P, et al. Respiratory parameters in patients with COVID-19 after using noninvasive ventilation in the prone position outside the intensive care unit. *JAMA*. 2020;323(22):2338–2340. doi:10.1001/jama.2020.7861 PMID: 32412606; PMCID: PMC7229533.

30. Cazzola M, Ora J, Bianco A, Rogliani P, Matera MG. Guidance on nebulization during the current COVID-19 pandemic. *Respir Med*. 2021;176:106236. doi:10.1016/j.rmed.2020.106236 PMID: 33248363; PMCID: PMC7676318.

31. **KaneBG.Alternative treatments for acute asthma during COVID. COVID-19 Field Guide,ACEP.org.** https://www.acep.org/corona/covid-19-field-guide/treatment/alternative-treatments/#:~:text=Based%20on%20available%20evidence%2C%20injected,noted%20here%20is%20the%20deltoid.

32. Marini JJ. Dealing with the CARDS of COVID-19. *Crit Care Med*. 2020;48(8):1239–1241. doi:10.1097/CCM.0000000000004427 PMID: 32697499.

33. Covid-19: Good Chance of Survival Despite Severe Disease: Analyses Highlight Success of ECMO Treatment in Vienna. Cath Lab Digest. 2021 Apr. Access date: 05.21.2021. https://www.cathlabdigest.com/content/covid-19-good-chance-survival-despite-severe-disease-analyses-highlight-success-ecmo-treatment-vienna

34. Hao B, Sotudian S, Wang T, Xu T, Hu Y, Gaitanidis A, Breen K, Velmahos GC, Paschalidis IC. Early prediction of level-of-care requirements in patients with COVID-19. Elife. 2020 Oct 12;9:e60519. doi: 10.7554/eLife.60519. PMID: 33044170; PMCID: PMC7595731.

35. O'Brien H, Tracey MJ, Ottewill C, et al. An integrated multidisciplinary model of COVID-19 recovery care. *Ir J Med Sci*. 2021;190(2):461–468. doi:10.1007/s11845-020-02354-9 MayPMID: 32894436; PMCID: PMC7475726.

36. Patel H, Virapongse A, Baduashvili A, Devitt J, Barr R, Bookman K. Implementing a COVID-19 discharge pathway to improve patient safety. *Am J Med Qual*. 2021;36(2):84–89. doi:10.1097/01.JMQ.0000735436.50361.79 PMID: 33830095; PMCID: PMC8030876.

37. Singer AJ, Morley EJ, Meyers K, et al. Cohort of four thousand four hundred four persons under investigation for COVID-19 in a New York hospital and predictors of ICU care and ventilation. *Ann Emerg Med*. 2020;76(4):394–404. doi:10.1016/j.annemergmed.2020.05.011 OctPMID: 32563601; PMCID: PMC7211647.

38. Coronavirus Disease 2019 (COVID-19) Treatment Guidelines. National Institutes of Health. Access date: 05/21/2021. https://www.covid19treatmentguidelines.nih.gov

39. Stawicki SP, Jeanmonod R, Miller AC, et al. The 2019-2020 Novel Coronavirus (Severe Acute Respiratory Syndrome Coronavirus 2) Pandemic: A Joint American College of Academic International Medicine-World Academic Council of Emergency Medicine Multidisciplinary COVID-19 Working Group Consensus Paper. *J Glob Infect Dis*. 2020;12(2):47–93. doi:10.4103/jgid.jgid_86_20 PMID: 32773996; PMCID: PMC7384689.

40. Chavez S, Long B, Koyfman A, Liang SY. Coronavirus disease (COVID-19): a primer for emergency physicians. *Am J Emerg Med*. 2020. doi:10.1016/j.ajem.2020.03.036 Mar 24S0735-6757(20)30178-9PMID: 32265065; PMCID: PMC7102516.

41. Healthcare Workers: Information on COVID-19. Centers for Disease Control and Prevention. Access date: 05/21/2021. https://www.cdc.gov/coronavirus/2019-nCoV/hcp/index.html

42. Centers for Disease Control and Prevention. People at increased risk and other people who need to take extra precautions. Access date 5/27/2021. https://www.cdc.gov/coronavirus/2019-ncov/need-extra-precautions/index.html

43. Centers for Disease Control and Prevention. Considerations for alternate care sites. Access date 5/27/2021. https://www.cdc.gov/coronavirus/2019-ncov/need-extra-precautions/index.html

44. Brigham E, O'Toole J, Kim SY, et al. The Johns Hopkins Post-Acute COVID-19 Team (PACT): a multidisciplinary, collaborative, ambulatory framework supporting COVID-19 survivors. *Am J Med*. 2021;134(4):462–467.e1. doi:10.1016/j.amjmed.2020.12.009 PMID: 33444589; PMCID: PMC7801819.

45. O'Brien H, Tracey MJ, Ottewill C, et al. An integrated multidisciplinary model of COVID-19 recovery care. *Ir J Med Sci*. 2021;190(2):461–468. doi:10.1007/s11845-020-02354-9 MayPMID: 32894436; PMCID: PMC7475726.

46. Centers for Disease Control and Prevention. First Responders. https://www.cdc.gov/coronavirus/2019-ncov/hcp/guidance-for-ems.html. Accessed May 26, 2021.

47. Boyle AA, Henderson K. COVID-19: resetting ED care. *Emerg Med J*. 2020;37(8):458–459. doi:10.1136/emermed-2020-210282 AugPMID: 32665424; PMCID: PMC7418608.

48. Kirby JJ, Iloma C, Khong A, Magee M, Alanis N, Willis J, d'Etienne P, Smith JP. ACEP COVID-19 Field Guild: Facility Changes. https://www.acep.org/corona/covid-19-field-guide/work-safety/facility-changes/. Accessed May 26, 2021.

49. Centers for Disease Control and Prevention. Standard Operating Procedure (SOP) for Triage of Suspected COVID-19 Patients in non-US Healthcare Settings: Early Identification and Prevention of Transmission during Triage. https://www.cdc.gov/coronavirus/2019-ncov/hcp/non-us-settings/sop-triage-prevent-transmission.html. Accessed May 26, 2021.

50. Mousavi ES, Kananizadeh N, Martinello RA, Sherman JD. COVID-19 outbreak and hospital air quality: a systematic review of evidence on air filtration and recirculation. *Environ Sci Technol*. 2021;55(7):4134–4147. doi:10.1021/acs.est.0c03247.

51. Waxman MJ, Moschella P, Duber HC, et al. Emergency department-based COVID-19 vaccination: where do we stand?. *Acad Emerg Med*. 2021;28(6):707–709. doi:10.1111/acem.14261 PMID: 33825244.

CHAPTER

16 Therapeutics for COVID-19

Sriram Krishnaswami, PhD, Amparo de la Peña, PhD, Sarah Kim, and Sujatha S. Menon, M Pharm, MS Pharm, PhD

OUTLINE

Evolution of Therapeutic Approaches

The deadly novel coronavirus severe acute respiratory syndrome coronavirus 2 (SARS-CoV-2), which causes coronavirus disease 2019 (COVID-19), spread like wildfire across the entire world in the first exceptionally severe pandemic of the 21st century.[1] Humanity had last seen a comparable worldwide viral infection in the 20th century, with the 1918 influenza pandemic caused by an H1N1 virus that infected approximately one-third of the world's population; deaths were estimated at approximately 50 million people.[2,3]

In this century, the first cases of a "pneumonia of unknown cause" were reported in Wuhan, China in December 2019, with the first death reported on January 11, 2020.[4] A few days later, a dashboard showing COVID-19 cases in real time was started as a collaboration of several centers at Johns Hopkins University. The infection spread at such speed that the World Health Organization (WHO) declared it first to be a public health emergency and finally a pandemic on March 11, 2020, noting it was the first one caused by a coronavirus.[5]

At that point, the number of cases outside China had increased 13-fold and the number of countries reporting cases had tripled. Dr. Tedros A. Ghebreyesus, WHO Director-General, expressed being deeply concerned "both by the alarming levels of spread and severity, and by the alarming levels of inaction," and urged countries to take action immediately to contain the virus.[6] The WHO recommended that people with mild respiratory symptoms should isolate themselves, and social distancing was advised even for countries with no reported cases. On March 11, 2020, there were 118,000 cases globally (in 114 countries) with 4291 deaths (case fatality rate [CFR] of 3.6%), of which 1267 cases and 38 deaths (CFR 3%) were in the United States.[7]

Simultaneously, a review in *JAMA Insights* of the first published COVID-19 case studies from China reported that critical care would be "an integral component of the global response" to the infection.[8] Approximately two-thirds of patients had been reported to require intensive care for respiratory support, after progressing to acute respiratory distress syndrome (ARDS). ARDS is characterized by (1) loss of integrity of capillary endothelium, (2) inflammation with recruitment of resident tissue macrophages, and (3) immune activation. Left untreated, ARDS can lead to pulmonary edema and death from progressive respiratory failure. The time between symptom onset and admission to the intensive care unit (ICU) was estimated to be 9 to 10 days. The authors raised the concern that in some regions, the lack of intensive care infrastructure might lead to health systems being overwhelmed if mechanical ventilation capacity were to be exceeded.[8]

As patients with COVID-19 pneumonia were observed to develop ARDS, they were initially managed following widely accepted clinical practice guidelines, based on disease severity.[9] Therapeutic measures for patients with ARDS included conservative fluid strategies for patients without shock after initial resuscitation, antibiotics for potential bacterial pneumonia or secondary infections, and lung-protective ventilation strategies such as mechanical ventilation with lower tidal volumes and lower inspiratory pressures.[8] Proning for more than 12 hours per day was recommended for patients with severe ARDS, and disease management decisions were to be personalized for each patient. Modifications to the usual standard of care such as private rooms, distancing between patients, and exercising caution because of the risk for dispersion of aerosolized virus were implemented.

A case report of the clinical management of the first US COVID-19 case, diagnosed on January 20, 2020, was published in early March in the *New England Journal of Medicine*.[10] The patient's initial symptoms on admission were treated with antipyretics, fluid replacement, guaifenesin for cough, and antiemetics (ondansetron). As the disease progressed to pneumonia on day 9 of illness, the patient was treated with oxygen supplementation, antibiotics (vancomycin and cefepime), and compassionate use of an investigational antiviral therapy (intravenous remdesivir, an experimental antiviral).

Multiple therapies were tested during 2020 and 2021, in a desperate attempt to treat patients in a vacuum of definitive efficacy data. The US Food and Drug Administration (FDA) launched the Coronavirus Treatment Acceleration Program (CTAP), setting the regulatory stage for drug and biologicals manufacturers to develop products to meet this urgent need. As of May 12, 2021, excluding vaccines, there were more than 610 programs in planning stages, and more than 450 clinical trials had been reviewed by the FDA, resulting in nine COVID-19 treatments authorized for emergency use, and one treatment was approved (Fig. 16.1).[11]

In the face of the globally raging pandemic, the scientific community raced to unravel new antiviral therapies against COVID-19 disease. Meanwhile, they also, not surprisingly, explored the use of several existing antiviral, antimalarial, antiinflammatory, and even antibiotic agents for activity against the SAR-CoV-2 virus. One such repurposed drug is remdesivir, which was previously evaluated for treatment of Ebola virus disease and would become one of the most used tools in the COVID therapeutic armamentarium. A significant amount of research has been dedicated to remdesivir in COVID-19, as evidenced by the number of review articles published on this topic.[12–16] Its definitive efficacy was tested in a randomized clinical trial (RCT) setting within the Adaptive COVID-19 Treatment Trial (ACTT), launched by the National Institute of Allergy and Infectious Diseases (NIAID) to evaluate the safety and efficacy of investigational therapeutics for treatment of severe COVID-19 in hospitalized adults. Remdesivir was found to be superior to placebo in shortening the time to recovery in adults hospitalized with COVID-19 and lower respiratory tract infection.[17] Although hydroxychloroquine was the first repurposed medicine to receive an emergency use authorization (EUA) from the FDA, it was soon revoked because of lack of efficacy and potential safety concerns.[18,19] Remdesivir was the next to receive an EUA and the only therapy to date to have received full FDA approval (Fig. 16.2).

Similar to efforts in the United States, RCTs (SOLIDARITY and RECOVERY) were also initiated by the WHO and United Kingdom, respectively, to assess the efficacy and safety of a number of medicines previously approved for other uses.[19,20] Disappointingly, the SOLIDARITY trial reported little or no effect for

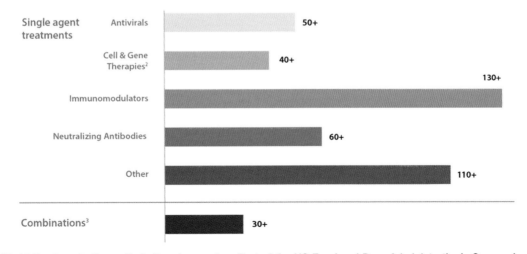

Type of COVID-19 Treatment Being Studied[1]

- Single agent treatments — Antivirals: 50+
- Cell & Gene Therapies[2]: 40+
- Immunomodulators: 130+
- Neutralizing Antibodies: 60+
- Other: 110+
- Combinations[3]: 30+

Fig. 16.1 COVID-19 Treatments Currently in Development as Part of the US Food and Drug Administration's Coronavirus Treatment Acceleration Program (CTAP). *1.* Corresponds to number of safe-to-proceed investigational new drugs (INDs). Excludes INDs related to vaccines. *2.* For additional information, see https://www.fda.gov/vaccines-blood-biologics/cellular-gene-therapy-products. *3.* Includes INDs with more than one product. (Reproduced from US Food and Drug Administration. Coronavirus Treatment Acceleration Program [CTAP]. June 2021. https://www.fda.gov/drugs/coronavirus-covid-19-drugs/coronavirus-treatment-acceleration-program-ctap).

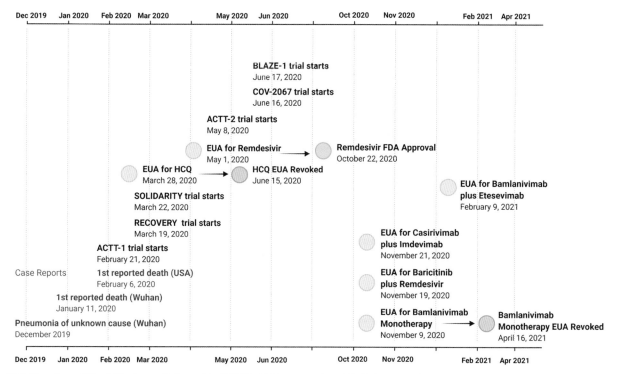

Fig. 16.2 Timeline of Key Milestones Relevant to COVID-19 Therapeutics. *ACTT,* Adaptive COVID-19 Treatment Trial; *EUA,* emergency use authorization; *HCQ,* hydroxychloroquine.

remdesivir, hydroxychloroquine, lopinavir, or interferon regimens on overall mortality, initiation of ventilation, or duration of hospital stay in hospitalized patients with COVID-19. The RECOVERY trial investigated whether treatment with lopinavir-ritonavir, hydroxychloroquine, corticosteroids, azithromycin, colchicine, intravenous immunoglobulin (children only), convalescent plasma, synthetic neutralizing antibodies (REGN-COV2), tocilizumab, aspirin, baricitinib, infliximab, or anakinra (in children only) prevented death in patients with COVID-19. In this trial, encouraging results were observed with dexamethasone, which lowered the 28-day mortality among those who were receiving either invasive mechanical ventilation or oxygen alone at randomization.[20] Also encouraging was the observation that tocilizumab, an interleukin-6 (IL-6) receptor monoclonal antibody, improved survival and other clinical outcomes in hospitalized COVID-19 patients with hypoxia and systemic inflammation, in addition to the benefits of systemic corticosteroids.[21]

The adaptive design of the ACTT platform allowed for the evaluation of additional therapies over time, such as baricitinib, a Janus kinase (JAK) inhibitor, in combination with remdesivir in ACTT-2,[22] and interferon-beta 1a (IFN-β1a) in combination with remdesivir, in ACTT-3.[23] Baricitinib given in combination with remdesivir showed a shorter recovery time relative to remdesivir alone and led to an EUA from the FDA.

In parallel, neutralizing monoclonal antibodies (mAbs) that bind directly to the receptor binding domain (RBD) of the SARS-CoV-2 S protein to compete with the cellular receptor angiotensin-converting enzyme-2 (ACE2) emerged as promising therapeutic approaches for the treatment of COVID-19. Bamlanivimab monotherapy was the first mAb to receive an EUA for the treatment of mild to moderate COVID-19 in adults and pediatric patients at high risk for progressing to severe COVID-19 and/or hospitalization. However, this EUA was later revoked because of the potential for increased risk for treatment failure as a result of the emergence of SARS-CoV-2 viral variants resistant to bamlanivimab alone. It was later combined with another mAb, etesevimab, which binds to another distinct, but overlapping, epitope within the RBD of the S protein of SARS-CoV-2. The combination received an EUA based on the results of the BLAZE-1 trial.[24] Another combination of RBD-binding mAbs, casirivimab and imdevimab, was also given an EUA based on the results of the COV-2067 trial.[25]

In the following section, the therapies will be discussed in further detail. Although not widely authorized for emergency use, there are numerous other repurposed or repositioned drugs that have been evaluated in RCTs and are being used in varying degrees worldwide and thus are discussed in a separate section. This section also includes a comprehensive list of investigational therapies (new and repurposed) currently in clinical trials to serve as a reference point. Finally, the evolving treatment guidelines for COVID-19 management at different phases of the disease are discussed.

Treatments Authorized for Emergency Use

As part of the mechanism to facilitate availability of treatments, vaccines, and other measures during public health emergencies, the US FDA issued EUAs to a number of medicines as of May 15, 2021. The initial date of EUA issuance, authorized use, and primary endpoint data from the pivotal trial supporting the respective EUAs are presented in Table 16.1.

Antiviral Monotherapy: Remdesivir

On May 1, 2020, the FDA issued an EUA for Veklury (remdesivir) for the treatment of hospitalized patients with severe COVID-19, defined as patients meeting one or more of the following four criteria—(1) oxygen saturation (SpO_2), (2) requiring supplemental oxygen, (3) requiring mechanical ventilation, and (4) requiring extracorporeal membrane oxygenation (ECMO). The EUA was based on a phase III, randomized double-blind trial, the ACTT-1, in which treatment with remdesivir was compared with placebo.[17] With supportive evidence from three randomized controlled clinical trials that included patients hospitalized with mild-to-severe COVID-19 (including ACTT), on October 22, 2020, a full approval was granted for the use of remdesivir (as Veklury) for the treatment of COVID-19 in adults and pediatric patients (12 years and older and weighing at least 40 kg), requiring hospitalization.[26] It was the first treatment to gain full FDA approval for COVID-19.

Pharmacological Properties

Remdesivir (GS-5734) is a phosphoramidate prodrug of a nucleoside analog, GS-443902, that directly inhibits viral replication of SARS-CoV-2.[27] It undergoes intracellular activation to form the pharmacologically active remdesivir triphosphate (RDV-TP), which competes with adenosine triphosphate (ATP) for incorporation into RNA-dependent RNA polymerase. This, in turn, leads to premature termination of viral RNA transcription and inhibition of subsequent RNA synthesis (Fig. 16.3).

In cellular assays, remdesivir demonstrated antiviral activity against a clinical isolate of SARS-CoV-2 in primary human airway epithelial cells with a 50% effective concentration (EC_{50}) of 9.9 nM after 48 hours of treatment. In other cell lines (Calu-3 and A549-hACE2), EC_{50} values were 115 nM and 280 nM after 48 and 72 hours, respectively.[26]

Whereas remdesivir (the prodrug) and its metabolites (GS-704277 and GS-441524) can be measured in plasma, the active moiety (triphosphate GS-443902) can only be detected intracellularly. Therefore activation to the triphosphate form was evaluated using peripheral blood mononuclear cells as clinical surrogates.[28] The pharmacokinetics of remdesivir and its metabolites (GS-704277 and GS-441524) was dose-proportional across the 3- to 225-mg dose range in healthy participants, after administration of single intravenous doses. Remdesivir was developed as an intravenous formulation because of its large first-pass hepatic extraction. After multiple once-daily doses of 150 mg remdesivir for 14 days, the major metabolite GS-441524 accumulated approximately 1.9-fold in plasma.[29]

Dosing and Indication

Single-dose vials of remdesivir are available in both solution and lyophilized injection formulations; the lyophilized formulation has a long shelf life and is stable at room temperature because of its better physiochemical stability.[28] The United States Prescribing Information (USPI) states that remdesivir is indicated for adults and pediatric patients (12 years of age and older and weighing at least 40 kg) for the treatment of COVID-19 requiring hospitalization, and that it should be administered only in a hospital or in a health care setting capable of providing acute care comparable to inpatient hospital care. The recommended dosage consists of a single intravenous loading dose of 200 mg remdesivir on day 1 followed by once-daily maintenance doses of 100 mg remdesivir starting on day 2. Before initiating remdesivir, estimated glomerular filtration rate (eGFR), prothrombin time, and liver function are assessed for any dosage adjustments. The recommended treatment duration is 5 days, which can be extended for up to 5 additional days (for a total treatment duration of up to 10 days) if no clinical improvement is observed.[26]

Clinical Efficacy

NIAID ACTT-1 (in Mild/Moderate and Severe COVID-19): Primary Evidence of Efficacy

In this pivotal phase III trial designated ACTT-1 (NCT04280705), 1062 hospitalized patients with COVID-19 received a 10-day course of remdesivir or placebo. The primary outcome was the time to recovery by day 29, on which a patient met the criteria for category 1 (not hospitalized and no limitations of activities), 2 (not hospitalized, with limitation of activities, home oxygen requirement, or both), or 3 (hospitalized, not requiring supplemental oxygen and no longer requiring ongoing medical care) on an 8-category ordinal scale. The time to recovery was shorter for patients who received remdesivir compared with those on placebo (see Table 16.1). In the severe disease stratum (N = 957), the median time to recovery was 11 days, relative to 18 days (rate ratio [RR] for recovery, 1.31; 95% confidence interval [CI], 1.12–1.52). Mortality by day 29 was numerically lower in the remdesivir group (11.4%) compared with placebo (15.2%), but the difference was not statistically significant (hazard ratio [HR] 0.73; 95% CI, 0.52–1.03]).[17]

Table 16.1 Emergency Use Authorizations Issued by the US Food and Drug Administration

Drug	Authorized for Emergency Use	Primary Endpoint
Remdesivir for certain hospitalized COVID-19 patients	Treatment of suspected or laboratory-confirmed COVID-19 in hospitalized pediatric patients weighing 3.5 kg to <40 kg or hospitalized pediatric patients younger than 12 years of age weighing at least 3.5 kg[a]	
Baricitinib in combination with remdesivir	Treatment of suspected or laboratory-confirmed COVID-19 in hospitalized adults and pediatric patients 2 years of age or older requiring supplemental oxygen, invasive mechanical ventilation, or extracorporeal membrane oxygenation (ECMO)	
Casirivimab and imdevimab	Treatment of mild to moderate COVID-19 in adults and pediatric patients (12 years of age and older weighing at least 40 kg) with positive results of direct SARS-CoV-2 viral testing, and who are at high risk for progressing to severe COVID-19 and/or hospitalization.	
Bamlanivimab and etesevimab	Treatment of mild to moderate COVID-19 in adult and pediatric patients with positive results of direct SARS-CoV-2 viral testing who are 12 years of age and older weighing at least 40 kg (about 88 lb), and who are at high risk for progressing to severe COVID-19 and/or hospitalization.	

[a]On October 22, 2020, the FDA approved remdesivir (Veklury) for use in adults and pediatric patients (12 years of age and older and weighing at least 40 kg) for the treatment of COVID-19 requiring hospitalization. The EUA continues to authorize Veklury for emergency use by licensed health care providers for the treatment of suspected or laboratory-confirmed COVID-19 in hospitalized pediatric patients weighing 3.5 kg to <40 kg or hospitalized pediatric patients younger than 12 years of age weighing ≥3.5 kg.

Data from Beigel JH, Tomashek KM, Dodd LE, et al. Remdesivir for the treatment of Covid-19: final report. *N Engl J Med.* 2020;383:1813-1826; Kalil AC, Patterson TF, Mehta AK, et al. Baricitinib plus remdesivir for hospitalized adults with Covid-19. *N Engl J Med.* 2021;384:795-807; US Food and Drug Administration. Casirivimab/imdevimab: fact sheet for health care providers—emergency use authorization (EUA) of casirivimab and imdevimab. https://www.fda.gov/media/145611/download; and US Food and Drug Administration. Bamlanivimab/etesevimab: fact sheet for health care providers—emergency use authorization (EUA) of bamlanivimab and etesevimab. https://www.fda.gov/media/145802/download.

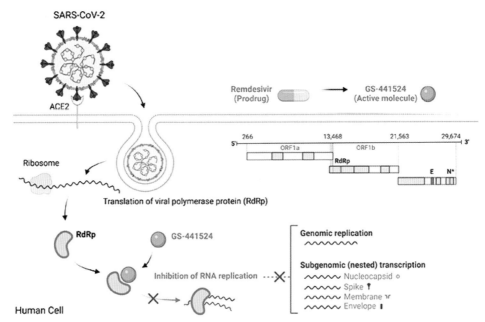

Fig. 16.3 Mechanism of Action of Remdesivir. Potential mechanism of action of remdesivir against coronavirus replication. As illustrated on the left, remdesivir undergoes intracellular activation to form the pharmacologically active remdesivir triphosphate (RDV-TP, GS-441524), which competes with adenosine triphosphate for incorporation into incorporation into RNA-dependent RNA polymerase (RdRp), leading to premature termination of viral RNA transcription and inhibition of subsequent RNA synthesis. ACE2, Angiotensin-converting enzyme-2. (Created using BioRender, based on the template Remdesivir: Potential Repurposed Drug Candidate for COVID-19.)

GS-US-540-5773 (in Severe COVID-19): Supportive Data

This randomized, open-label trial (NCT04292899) evaluated the safety and efficacy of 5 days versus 10 days of remdesivir in hospitalized patients with severe COVID-19.[30] The primary endpoint, clinical status on day 14, did not demonstrate a significant difference in efficacy between 5- and 10-day regimens of remdesivir. The absence of a standard-of-care alone arm limited the interpretability of the data. However, an external (synthetic) control arm based on retrospectively collected data from contemporaneously hospitalized patients with severe COVID-19 showed that by day 14, remdesivir was associated with 62% reduced odds of death (adjusted odds ratio [aOR], 0.38; 95% CI, 0.22–0.68, $P = .001$) versus standard-of-care treatment in patients with severe COVID-19.[31]

GS-US-540-5774 (in Moderate COVID-19): Supportive Data

The randomized, open-label trial NCT04292730 evaluated the safety and efficacy of 5 days versus 10 days of remdesivir compared with standard-of-care in hospitalized patients with moderate COVID-19. A statistically significant difference in the odds of improvement at day 11 favoring the 5-day (but not the 10-day) treatment group over standard of care was demonstrated. Notwithstanding the limitations of its open-label design, this trial provided supportive evidence for the efficacy of remdesivir in patients hospitalized with COVID-19 of moderate severity (i.e., patients hospitalized but not requiring supplemental oxygen).[32]

Clinical Safety

The safety profile of remdesivir was informed by data from three phase III studies in hospitalized adult patients with COVID-19 (N = 1313), four phase I studies in healthy adults (N = 131), and from patients with COVID-19 who received remdesivir under the EUA or a compassionate use program.[26] In the comparative ACTT-1 trial, the rates of severe (grade 3) or potentially life-threatening (grade 4) adverse events for remdesivir were comparable to placebo (8% vs. 9%), as were serious adverse events (0.4% vs. 0.6%) and adverse events leading to study drug discontinuation (2% vs. 3%). Adverse events of lower grade (1 or 2) were not collected. The most common adverse reactions ($\geq 5\%$, all grades) observed with remdesivir were nausea and elevations in liver transaminases. The overall efficacy and safety data support a flexible recommendation for 5- to 10-day treatment duration regimens to allow providers latitude in tailoring treatments per clinical response.

Key warnings and precautions include hypersensitivity reactions, which may be mitigated with slower infusion rates, and transaminase elevations requiring close laboratory testing and monitoring. Remdesivir is contraindicated in patients with a history of clinically significant hypersensitivity reactions, such as infusion-related and anaphylactic reactions. Coadministration of remdesivir with chloroquine or hydroxychloroquine is not recommended because of potential antagonistic effects on intracellular metabolic activation and the antiviral activity of remdesivir.

Immunomodulator and Antiviral Combination: Baricitinib and Remdesivir

On November 19, 2020 the FDA issued an EUA for the emergency use of baricitinib in combination with remdesivir for the treatment of COVID-19 (suspected or confirmed) in hospitalized adults and pediatric patients 2 years of age or older requiring supplemental oxygen, invasive mechanical ventilation, or ECMO. The EUA was based primarily on a phase III randomized double-blind trial, the ACTT-2, in which baricitinib improved the time to recovery when given in combination with remdesivir relative to remdesivir alone, in patients who required supplemental oxygen but not invasive mechanical ventilation.[22] The FDA review also included data for baricitinib from the approved indication of rheumatoid arthritis and from populations studied for other indications, including pediatric patients.

Pharmacological Properties

Baricitinib is an orally administered, selective inhibitor of JAK1 and JAK2 that is approved for the treatment of rheumatoid arthritis. As a JAK–STAT signaling inhibitor, baricitinib inhibits the intracellular signaling pathway of cytokines known to be elevated in severe COVID-19, including IL-2, IL-6, IL-10, interferon-gamma (IFN-γ), and granulocyte-macrophage colony-stimulating factor. In addition, through the use of artificial intelligence–inspired algorithms, it was identified as a potential therapeutic because of its high affinity (half-maximal inhibitory concentration [IC_{50}] of 34 nM) against AP2-associated protein kinase 1 (AAK1), which may lead to interrupted SARS-CoV-2 cellular entry and intracellular assembly of viral particles[33,34] (Fig. 16.4). The human pharmacokinetic (PK) profile of baricitinib is characterized by dose-proportional increases in systemic exposure and an elimination half-life of 12 hours.[35] After once-daily administration, the unbound peak

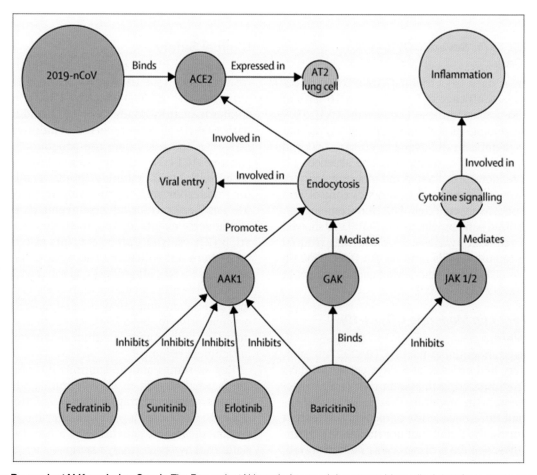

Fig. 16.4 The BenevolentAI Knowledge Graph. The BenevolentAI knowledge graph integrates biomedical data from structured and unstructured sources. It is queried by a fleet of algorithms to identify new relationships to suggest new ways of tackling disease. *2019-nCoV,* 2019 novel coronavirus; *AAK1,* AP2-associated protein kinase 1; *ACE2,* angiotensin-converting enzyme-2; *AT2,* •••; *GAK,* cyclin g-associated kinase; *JAK,* Janus kinase. (Reprinted with permission from Elsevier, Richardson et al. Baricitinib as potential treatment for 2019-nCoV acute respiratory disease, *Lancet.* 2020;395:e30–e31.)

concentration (103 nM) at a 10-mg daily dose was projected to exceed the IC_{50} for AAK1, further supporting evaluation in patients with COVID-19.[34]

Dosing and Indication

Baricitinib is available as oral tablets. In the EUA for baricitinib in combination with remdesivir, the recommended dosage in adults with an estimated glomerular filtration rate (eGFR) ≥ 60 mL/min/1.73 m^2 is 4 mg once daily for 14 days of total treatment or until hospital discharge, whichever is first. The authorization to use in pediatric patients comes from data in other indications, with a recommended dose of 4 mg once daily for patients ≥ 9 years, and 2 mg once daily for patients aged 2 through < 9 years, for 14 days or until hospital discharge. For both adults and pediatric patients, dosage adjustments are required for those with renal or hepatic impairment; the drug is not recommended for patients who are on dialysis, have end-stage renal disease, or have experienced acute kidney injury.[36]

Clinical Efficacy

The EUA was based on data from a randomized double-blind, placebo-controlled trial (ACTT-2) in which patients received either remdesivir and baricitinib (n = 515) or remdesivir and placebo (n = 518).[22] Randomization was stratified to trial site and disease severity at the time of enrollment. Remdesivir was administered by intravenous infusion as a 200-mg loading dose on day 1, then 100 mg daily from day 2 to day 10, or until hospital discharge or death. Baricitinib was administered as a 4-mg dose once daily for 14 days or until hospital discharge. Patients with an eGFR less than 60 mL per minute received baricitinib 2 mg once daily. Patients had to have laboratory-confirmed SARS-CoV-2 infection and at least one of the following to be enrolled in the trial: radiographic infiltrates by imaging, SpO$_2$ 94% or less on room air, a requirement for supplemental oxygen, or a requirement for mechanical ventilation or ECMO. Mean age was 55 years (with 30% of patients aged 65 or older); 63% of patients were male, 51% were Hispanic or Latino, 48% were White, 15% were Black or African American, and 10% were Asian; 14% did not require supplemental oxygen, 55% required supplemental oxygen, 21% required noninvasive ventilation or high-flow oxygen, and 11% required invasive mechanical ventilation or ECMO.

The primary endpoint was median time to recovery defined as discharged from hospital or hospitalized but not requiring supplemental oxygen or ongoing medical care. For the overall population, the median time to recovery was 7 days for baricitinib plus remdesivir *versus* 8 days for placebo plus remdesivir (RR for recovery, 1.16; 95% CI, 1.01–1.32; $P = .03$) (see Table 16.1). In secondary analyses, by day 29, fewer patients died or progressed to noninvasive ventilation/high-flow oxygen or invasive mechanical ventilation with baricitinib plus remdesivir (22.5%) compared

with remdesivir alone (28.4%) (RR, 0.77; 95% CI, 0.60–0.98). The Kaplan–Meier estimates of mortality at day 28 numerically favored the combination, with 5.1% (95% CI, 3.5–7.6) in the combination arm compared with 7.8% (95% CI, 5.7–10.6) with remdesivir alone, but the difference was not statistically significant (HR for death 0.65; 95% CI, 0.39–1.09). The upper bound of the confidence limit of the hazard ratio suggests that the combination was not likely to have an unacceptable increase in mortality. Additionally, the incidence of new use of oxygen was lower in the combination group than in the control group (22.9% vs. 40.3%; difference, -17.4 percentage points; 95% CI, -31.6 to -2.1), as was the incidence of new use of mechanical ventilation or ECMO (10.0% vs. 15.2%; difference, -5.2 percentage points; 95% CI, -9.5 to -0.9).[22]

Clinical Safety

Although higher than the FDA-approved dose of 2 mg for rheumatoid arthritis, the dosing period for baricitinib 4 mg once daily for the treatment of COVID-19 was limited to 14 days and substantial safety information from indications other than COVID-19 was available at the 4-mg dose to inform the safety profile. Safety data for the combination was available for 507 patients hospitalized with COVID-19. In the ACTT-2 trial, fewer patients experienced serious adverse events in the combination arm (15%) compared with remdesivir alone (20%), and a similar pattern was seen with treatment-emergent adverse events (41.3% vs. 47.5%). The rate of discontinuations because of adverse events was also lower in the combination arm (6.7%) compared with remdesivir alone (11.6%). On the other hand, an increase in thrombotic events was observed in the combination arm (4%) versus 3%, with 5 patients experiencing serious pulmonary embolism compared with 1 patient with remdesivir alone.[36] This is consistent with previous observations in patients with rheumatoid arthritis. Common nonserious adverse events were decreases in GFR and hypertension. There was no increase in the overall infections observed after 14 days of combination treatment compared with placebo. Overall, the safety profile observed in patients with COVID-19 in ACTT-2 was consistent with the established safety profile for baricitinib.[36]

There were no clinical data for baricitinib in pediatric patients with COVID-19. Instead, the dosing recommendations were derived from these available sources and insights: (1) PK data in pediatric patients with juvenile idiopathic arthritis, atopic dermatitis, and in diseases referred to as type I interferonopathies; (2) data from adults with COVID-19; (3) considerations that the disease in adults and pediatric patients is sufficiently similar once patients progress to require supplemental oxygen, invasive mechanical ventilation, or ECMO; and (4) that there are no known COVID-19–specific pathophysiological differences (pediatric vs. adult), which can significantly affect the PK profile of baricitinib.[36]

Neutralizing Antibody Combination: Casirivimab and Imdevimab

On November 21, 2020 the FDA issued an EUA for (REGEN-COV) casirivimab and imdevimab (administered together) for the treatment of mild to moderate COVID-19 in adults and pediatric patients (12 years of age and older weighing at least 40 kg) at high risk for progressing to severe COVID-19 and/or hospitalization.[25] The basis of approval stemmed from a randomized double-blind, placebo-controlled clinical trial in nonhospitalized adults with mild to moderate COVID-19 symptoms, which showed that the combination reduced COVID-19–related hospitalization or emergency department (ED) visits in patients at high risk for disease progression compared with placebo.

Of note, the product is not authorized for patients hospitalized for COVID-19 or who require oxygen therapy as a result of COVID-19 because a beneficial effect of casirivimab and imdevimab treatment has not been shown in patients hospitalized for COVID-19. Moreover, mAbs such as casirivimab and imdevimab may be associated with worse clinical outcomes when administered to hospitalized patients with COVID-19 requiring high-flow oxygen or mechanical ventilation.

Pharmacological Properties

Casirivimab and imdevimab (immunoglobulin G1λ [IgG1λ]) are recombinant human IgG1 mAbs, unmodified in the Fc regions. The mAbs are covalent heterotetramers consisting of two heavy and two light chains, produced by recombinant DNA technology in Chinese hamster ovary cell suspension cultures. They bind to nonoverlapping epitopes of the spike protein RBD of SARS-CoV-2 with an IC_{50} of 81.8 pM[25,37] (Fig. 16.5).

In a cell-based assay (Vero E6 cells), the combination neutralized SARS-CoV-2 with EC_{50} of 31.0 pM

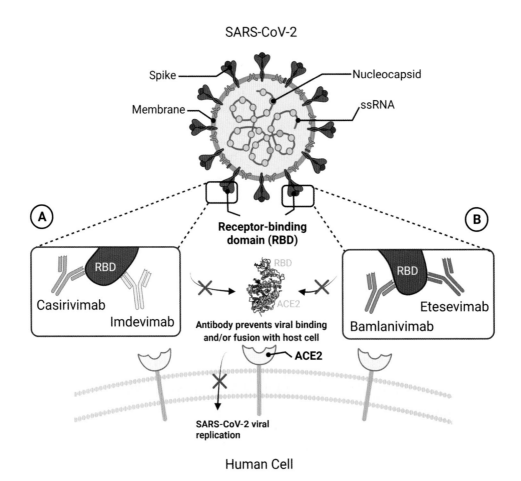

Fig. 16.5 Mechanism of Action of Monoclonal Antibodies With Emergency Use Authorization. Monoclonal antibodies (mAbs) are generated against the receptor binding domain *(RBD)* of the spike (S) protein of SARS-CoV-2. The anti-RBD mAbs prevent binding of the S protein to its cognate receptor, angiotensin-converting enzyme-2 *(ACE2),* on target host cells. The mAbs bind to distinct epitopes on the RBD. (Created using BioRender, based on Taylor PC, Adams AC, Hufford MM, et al. Neutralizing monoclonal antibodies for treatment of COVID-19. *Nat Rev Immunol.* 2021;21:382-393.)

(0.005 µg/mL). The combination was also shown to possibly mediate antibody-dependent cell-mediated cytotoxicity with natural killer cells and antibody-dependent cellular phagocytosis with macrophages. The human PK profiles of casirivimab and imdevimab are characterized by dose-proportional exposures (between 600- and 4000-mg) and mean estimated half-lives of 32 and 27 days, respectively.[25]

Dosing and Indication

The authorized dosage is 1200 mg of casirivimab and 1200 mg of imdevimab administered together as a single intravenous infusion as soon as possible after a positive viral test for SARS-CoV-2, and within 10 days of symptom onset. The drugs are available in a co-formulated vial (in a 1:1 ratio) and also as individual vials. The combination can be subcutaneously administered in the event intravenous infusion is not feasible and would delay treatment. The optimal dosing regimen for treatment of COVID-19 has not yet been established; the authorized dosing regimen may be updated with additional data from clinical trials.

As noted earlier, the EUA is for mild to moderate COVID-19 in adults and pediatric patients (12 years of age and older weighing at least 40 kg) who are at high risk for progressing to severe COVID-19 and/or hospitalization. Conditions that may place patients at higher risk for progression to severe COVID-19 include older age, obesity, diabetes, hypertension, chronic kidney disease, and others. The efficacy and safety of casirivimab with imdevimab have not been evaluated in hospitalized patients. Therefore the combination is not authorized for patients in these settings: (1) patients who are hospitalized, (2) patients who require oxygen therapy because of COVID-19, and (3) patients requiring an increase in baseline oxygen flow rate while on chronic oxygen therapy for non–COVID-19 conditions.

Clinical Efficacy

Mild to Moderate COVID-19 (R10933-10987-COV-2067)

The EUA was based on data from a phase I/II/III trial, COV-2067.[25] In the phase III trial, adults with at least one risk factor for severe COVID-19 received 600 mg each of casirivimab and imdevimab (n = 838), 1200 mg of each mAb (n = 1529), 4000 mg of each mAb (n = 700), or placebo (n = 1500) in a randomized design. Based on phase I/II efficacy results, the phase III portion of the protocol was amended to compare a 1200 mg dose of each mAb versus placebo, and 600 mg dose of each mAb versus placebo.

At baseline, the median age was 50 years (with 13% of subjects ages 65 years or older), 52% of the subjects were females, 84% were White, 36% were Hispanic or Latino, and 5% were Black or African American. Among patients with baseline symptom data, 42% had severe symptoms, 42% had moderate symptoms, 15% had mild symptoms, and 2% reported no symptoms. The median duration of symptoms was 3 days; mean viral load was 6.2 log10 copies per milliliter at baseline. Demographics and disease characteristics at baseline were well balanced across the treatment groups.[25]

The primary endpoint was the proportion of subjects with one or more COVID-19–related hospitalizations or all-cause death through day 29. The modified full analysis set was subjects with a positive reverse transcription polymerase chain reaction (RT-PCR) result and with at least one risk factor for severe COVID-19. As shown in Table 16.1, COVID-19–related hospitalization or death occurred in 7 (1.0%) patients in the casirivimab and imdevimab 600-mg group compared with 24 (3%) in the placebo group, corresponding to a 70% reduction ($P = .0024$). Similar results were observed for the higher dose, thus supporting the EUA of the 600-mg dose for both mAbs.[25]

Clinical Safety

The safety of 600 mg casirivimab plus 600 mg imdevimab is based on an analysis from ambulatory (nonhospitalized) subjects with COVID-19 from the COV-2067 trial. In the phase III portion of the trial, treatment-emergent adverse events were observed in 59 (7%) patients in the 600-mg dose group of each mAb (n = 827) compared with 189 (10%) in the placebo group (n = 1843). Fewer patients reported serious adverse events in the 600-mg dose group (1%–2%) compared with placebo (4%). Infusion-related reactions of grade 2 or higher severity were observed in 2 subjects in the 600-mg dose group compared with none in the placebo group.

Key warnings and precautions include serious hypersensitivity reactions such as anaphylaxis and potential for severe infusion-related reactions, which may be mitigated with slowing or stopping the infusion. Additionally, clinical worsening of COVID-19 after administration of REGEN-COV has been reported, although it is not known if these events were related to drug or disease progression. Thus the combination is not authorized for use in patients hospitalized for COVID-19 who require oxygen therapy for COVID-19 or who require an increase in baseline oxygen flow rate because of COVID-19 when receiving chronic oxygen therapy for comorbidity not related to COVID-19.[25]

Neutralizing Antibody Combination: Bamlanivimab and Etesevimab

On February 9, 2021 the FDA issued an EUA for emergency use of bamlanivimab and etesevimab administered together for the treatment of mild to moderate COVID-19 in adults and pediatric patients (12 years of age and older weighing at least 40 kg) with positive results of direct SARS-CoV-2 viral testing and who are at high risk for progressing to severe COVID-19 and/or hospitalization.[38] The EUA was based on the phase II/III

BLAZE-1 trial, a randomized double-blind, placebo-controlled clinical trial.[39]

Pharmacological Properties

Bamlanivimab and etesevimab are neutralizing IgG1 mAbs that bind to distinct but overlapping epitopes within the RBD of the spike protein of SARS-CoV-2.[38] The antibodies were derived from two patients who recovered from COVID-19 in North America and China.[40,41]

SARS-CoV-2 neutralizing antibody discovery efforts have focused on targeting the multidomain surface spike protein, a trimeric class I fusion protein that mediates viral entry. The viral entry depends on the interaction between the RBD and the ACE2 cellular receptor. Antibodies that bind the RBD and interfere with ACE2 binding can have potent neutralizing activity.[40] Bamlanivimab is a recombinant neutralizing human IgG1κ mAb to the spike protein of SARS-CoV-2, unmodified in the Fc region. Bamlanivimab binds the spike protein with a dissociation constant (KD) = 0.071 nM and blocks spike protein attachment to the human ACE2 receptor with an IC_{50} value of 0.17 nM (0.025 μg/mL). Etesevimab is a recombinant neutralizing human IgG1κ mAb to the spike protein of SARS-CoV-2, with amino acid substitutions in the Fc region (L234A, L235A) to reduce effector function. Etesevimab binds the spike protein with a dissociation constant KD = 6.45 nM and blocks spike protein attachment to the human ACE2 receptor with an IC_{50} value of 0.32 nM (0.046 μg/mL (see Fig. 16.5). The human PK profiles of bamlanivimab and etesevimab are dose proportional between 700- and 7000-mg doses, with half-lives of 18 days and 25 days, respectively.[24]

Dosing and Indication

The authorized dosages for the treatment of mild to moderate COVID-19 in adults and pediatric patients (12 years of age and older weighing at least 40 kg) is bamlanivimab 700 mg with etesevimab 1400 mg. The recommendation is to administer the antibodies as soon as possible after a positive viral test for SARS-CoV-2 and within 10 days of symptom onset. Under this EUA, bamlanivimab and etesevimab are diluted and administered together as a single intravenous infusion. Different dilutions are needed for patients weighing 50 kg or more versus patients weighing less than 50 kg.[24]

Clinical Efficacy

Mild to Moderate COVID-19 (BLAZE-1): Phase II Portion

The design of the phase II portion of BLAZE-1 included subjects receiving a single infusion of bamlanivimab 2800 mg and etesevimab 2800 mg (N = 112), bamlanivimab alone (at doses of 700 mg [N = 101], 2800 mg [N = 107], or 7000 mg [N = 101]) or placebo (N = 156).[39] The primary endpoint was the change in viral load from baseline to day 11. For the combination treatment, the differences in the change in log viral load at day 11 compared with placebo

were 0.09 (95% CI, –0.35 to 0.52; P = .69) for 700 mg, –0.27 (95% CI, –0.71 to 0.16; P = .21) for 2800 mg, 0.31 (95% CI, –0.13 to 0.76; P = .16) for 7000 mg, and –0.57 (95% CI, –1.00 to –0.14; P = .01).[39] The proportion of patients with COVID-19–related hospitalizations or ED visits was 5.8% (9 events) for placebo, 1.0% (1 event) for 700 mg, 1.9% (2 events) for 2800 mg, 2.0% (2 events) for 7000 mg, and 0.9% (1 event) for combination treatment, supporting the activity of these agents.[39]

Mild to Moderate COVID-19 (BLAZE-1): Phase III Portion

In the phase III portion, subjects received a single intravenous infusion of bamlanivimab 700 mg and etesevimab 1400 mg (N = 511) or placebo (N = 258).[24] The median age was 56 years (30% aged 65 years or older), 53% were females, 87% were White, 27% were Hispanic, and 8% were African American. Majority of the subjects had mild COVID-19 (76%) and the rest (24%) had moderate disease. The primary endpoint, proportion of subjects with COVID-19–related hospitalization (defined as ≥24 hours of acute care) or death by any cause by day 29, occurred in 6% of subjects in the placebo arm (15 subjects) compared with 0.8% (4 subjects) in the experimental arm, corresponding to an 87% reduction (P < .0001) (see Table 16.1). Counting just the 29-day mortality alone, there were 4 deaths in the placebo arm and no deaths in subjects treated with bamlanivimab 700 mg and etesevimab 1400 mg together (P = .01).[24]

Clinical Safety

The safety of bamlanivimab administered with etesevimab is primarily based on exposure of approximately 1400 ambulatory (nonhospitalized) subjects who received doses of bamlanivimab and etesevimab together, at the recommended dose of (bamlanivimab 700 mg, etesevimab 1400 mg) or higher. Safety data for the 700-mg bamlanivimab and 1400-mg etesevimab combination has not been reported at the time of writing this chapter. In the phase III trial, adverse events occurred in 13% of subjects who received 2800 mg of bamlanivimab plus 2800 mg of etesevimab and in 12% of placebo-treated subjects.[42] The combination is generally well tolerated. The most common treatment-emergent adverse events observed with bamlanivimab plus etesevimab have been nausea, dizziness, and pruritus, and none occurred in more than 1% of participants. Across ongoing, blinded clinical trials, a case of anaphylaxis and other cases of infusion-related reactions (n = 16, 1.1%) have been reported with the combination, which resolved upon stopping infusion and treatment (once with epinephrine).[24]

The key warnings and precautions to take with the combination are related to hypersensitivity reactions. Although clinical worsening of COVID-19 symptoms has been observed with the combination, it is not known whether it was related to the combination or disease progression. Thus the combination is not authorized for use in patients hospitalized for COVID-19, who require oxygen therapy for COVID-19, or who require an increase in baseline oxygen flow rate because of COVID-19 when receiving chronic oxygen therapy for comorbidity not related to COVID-19.

Repurposed Drugs and New Molecular Entities in Clinical Development

In addition to medicines authorized under an EUA program or that have full approval in at least one country (remdesivir), numerous organizations are involved in developing new molecular entities or in repositioning or repurposing medicines previously approved for other indications to address processes that drive the pathogenesis of COVID-19. These processes include the replication of SARS-CoV-2 early on during the disease process and the dysregulated immune and inflammatory response to SARS-CoV-2 that leads to tissue and organ damage[43] (Fig. 16.6).

One of the most successful repurposing efforts has been the use of corticosteroid therapy, including primarily dexamethasone (and to a lesser extent, methylprednisolone), to manage the severe complications associated with the immune and inflammatory response phase of COVID-19. Therefore this section begins with an overview of dexamethasone similar to that provided for drugs with EUA.

Dexamethasone

On September 2, 2020, the WHO issued a living guidance entitled "Corticosteroids for COVID-19."[44] The interim guideline suggests two recommendations regarding the use of corticosteroids according to COVID-19 disease severity, based on a prospective meta-analysis of randomized trials for corticosteroid therapy for COVID-19. For patients with severe and critical COVID-19, the WHO recommends the use of systemic (i.e., intravenous or oral) corticosteroids. For patients with nonsevere COVID-19, the WHO suggests not to use corticosteroids.

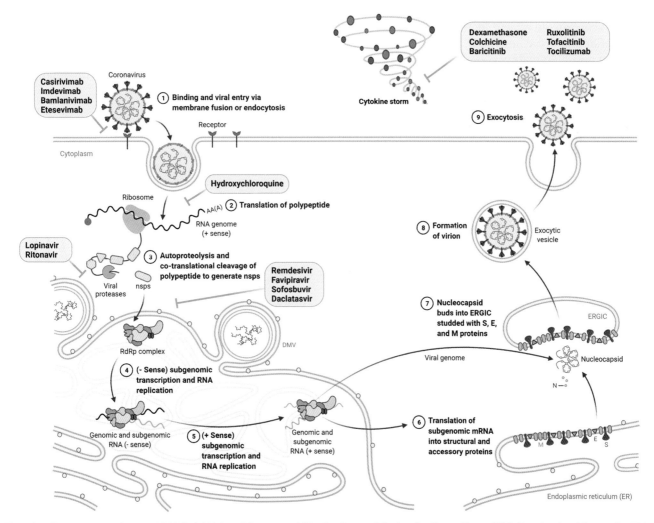

Fig. 16.6 The Infection Cycle of SARS-COV-2 and Suggested Mechanisms of Action for Some Drugs With Randomized Controlled Trial Data. *ERGIC*, Endoplasmic reticulum–Golgi intermediate compartment. (Created using BioRender based on Hartenian E, Nandakumar D, Lari A, et al. The molecular virology of coronaviruses. *J Bio Chem*. 2020;295:12910-12934.)

Research findings on dexamethasone, a corticosteroid, from the United Kingdom's national Randomised Evaluation of COVID-19 Therapy (RECOVERY) trial[20] was the main evidence initiating and supporting the WHO recommendations. The use of dexamethasone resulted in lower 28-day mortality among patients with COVID-19 who required invasive mechanical ventilation or oxygen therapy, but not among patients who did not receive respiratory support at randomization.

Pharmacological Properties

The general rationale for the use of dexamethasone for patients with severe COVID-19 is related to the pathogenesis of the disease. In the later disease phase, patients with COVID-19 suffer from organ tissue damage that is mainly driven by a dysregulated immune and inflammatory response (i.e., a hyperinflammatory state or cytokine storm) as a result of SARS-CoV-2 infection.[45,46] The use of corticosteroids for antiinflammatory and immunosuppressant effects may reduce organ tissue damage that can lead to long-term health problems (e.g., heart failure, long-term breathing problems, strokes, and even mortality.[47] Dexamethasone has potent glucocorticoid effects: increasing the production of antiinflammatory compounds, decreasing the production of proinflammatory compounds, and increasing apoptosis in inflammatory cells, by suppressing the

migration of neutrophils and decreasing lymphocyte proliferation[48,49] (Fig. 16.7).

Dexamethasone (9α-fluoro-16α-methylprednisolone) was synthesized in 1957 because of the need for a steroid with a longer duration of action.[46] The biological half-life of dexamethasone is 36 to 72 hours.[50] Oral doses of dexamethasone in the 1.5- to 6-mg dose range have a half-life of approximately 7 hours; a 20-mg oral tablet has a half-life of 4 hours, and a 4-mg intravenous dose has a half-life of 9 hours.[51,52] The absolute bioavailability of dexamethasone is 81% (95% CI, 54–121) in healthy subjects.[51]

Dosing and Indication

Dexamethasone is available in various formulations, including tablets with a range of 0.5 to 6 mg, an oral solution with a range of 0.5 mg/5 mL to 1 mg/mL, and injectable suspension with a range of 4 mg/mL to 20 mg/5 mL.[53] The glucocorticoid effect of 1 mg of dexamethasone is equivalent to that of 8 mg of prednisolone or 25 mg of hydrocortisone.[46] A general dosing recommendation for the treatment of inflammation for adults whose age is 18 years or older is to start with a dose of 0.75 mg daily and to increase to 9 mg daily, with doses divided two or four times daily.[54,55] For children ages 17 years or younger, 0.02 to 0.3 mg per kilogram of body weight per day is recommended, with dosing divided three or four times daily.[55] As with other drugs,

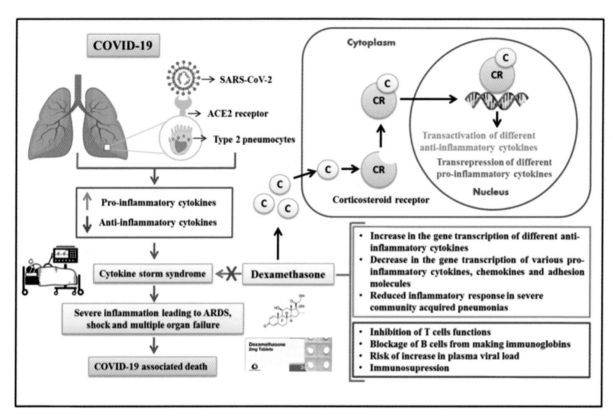

Fig. 16.7 Overview of Dexamethasone and Its Mode of Action in COVID-19 Patients. *ACE2,* Angiotensin-converting enzyme-2; *ARDS,* acute respiratory distress syndrome. (Reproduced from Patel SK, Saikumar G, Rana J, et al. Dexamethasone: a boon for critically ill COVID-19 patients? *Travel Med Infect Dis.* 2020;37:101844.)

a lower dose or less frequent dosing schedule would be needed for seniors, with consideration of their kidney and liver function. In addition, for a life-threatening condition, 10 mg of intravenous dexamethasone, followed by 4 mg of intramuscular administration given every 6 hours is recommended, with tapering over 7 days to discontinue the therapy.[56] Although the use of dexamethasone is recommended for patients with severe COVID-19, it remains unclear what the most appropriate dose would be in its treatment.[57]

Clinical Efficacy

The RECOVERY trial[20] is a multicenter, randomized, open-label study assessing 28-day mortality as the primary outcome among 6425 hospitalized patients with COVID-19. The use of dexamethasone (6 mg once daily for up to 10 days) reduced the 28-day mortality most significantly for patients who required invasive mechanical ventilation at randomization (28-day mortality: 29.3% in dexamethasone arm vs. 41.4% in control arm; rate ratio, 0.64; 95% CI, 0.51–0.81). Some extent of the survival benefit was also observed among patients who received oxygen therapy but did not require invasive mechanical ventilation (28-day mortality: 23.3% in dexamethasone arm vs. 26.2% in control arm; rate ratio, 0.82; 95% CI, 0.72–0.94). However, the use of dexamethasone did not reduce the 28-day mortality rate among patients who did not require any respiratory support at randomization (28-day mortality: 17.8% in dexamethasone arm vs. 14.0% in control arm; RR, 1.19; 95% CI, 0.92–1.55).

Other corticosteroids have been investigated for COVID-19 and compared with the effectiveness of dexamethasone. Recently, a finding from a prospective triple-blinded randomized controlled trial was published, which demonstrated methylprednisolone (2 mg/kg/day) showed significantly better clinical outcomes compared with dexamethasone (6 mg/day) among a total of 86 patients who were hospitalized for COVID-19.[57] The study used a 9-point WHO ordinal scale from 0 (uninfected) to 8 (death), with the lower the score, the better. The methylprednisolone group showed significantly lower values at day 5 (4.02 in methylprednisolone arm vs. 5.21 in the dexamethasone arm, $P = .002$) and day 10 (2.90 in methylprednisolone arm vs. 4.71 in dexamethasone arm, $P = .001$) of admission. The mean length of hospital stay (7.43 ± 3.64 days in the methylprednisolone arm vs. 10.52 ± 5.47 days in the dexamethasone arm, $P = .015$) and the need of a ventilator (18.2% in the methylprednisolone arm vs. 38.1% in the dexamethasone arm, $P = .040$) also supported the conclusion.

Clinical Safety

Adverse Events

Dexamethasone is generally tolerated.[49,53,58] Its short-term use is not associated with any serious adverse drug effects or allergic reactions. The most common reported adverse drug effect is insomnia (sleep disorder), along with agitation, depression, acne, increased appetite, indigestion, nausea, and vomiting. However, its long-term use (i.e., >2 weeks) may be associated with psychological problems (e.g., irritation, mood swings, and memory issues), vision problems (e.g., glaucoma and cataract), bone and joint pain (i.e., increasing risk for osteoporosis), signs of infections (e.g., fever and sore throat), or symptoms of intestinal bleeding (e.g., abdominal pain and dark stools). In particular, dexamethasone is not recommended for patients who have a history of infectious diseases, such as tuberculosis, fungal infections, and parasite infections, because it may hide and worsen the harmful effects of certain infections.

Drug–Drug Interactions

Antibiotics (e.g., erythromycin) and antifungal drugs (e.g., ketoconazole, itraconazole, posaconazole, and voriconazole) can increase the plasma concentration of dexamethasone, leading to higher risk for adverse drug reactions of dexamethasone.[58] In contrast, the use of dexamethasone can decrease the concentration of anticoagulants (e.g., apixaban and rivaroxaban), leading to higher risk for a blood clot or stroke. Dexamethasone can also decrease the efficacy of human immunodeficiency (HIV) drugs (e.g., protease inhibitors such as ritonavir and nonnucleoside reverse transcriptase inhibitors such as etravirine) and tuberculosis drugs (e.g., isoniazid).[58]

Special Populations

Dexamethasone may delay a child's growth.[58] For pregnant or breastfeeding women, adverse drug reactions of dexamethasone have not been studied enough, but animal research showed a risk for side effects to the fetus.[55]

Other Repurposed Medicines With Randomized Controlled Trial Data

A useful framework was proposed by Khani et al.[59] for COVID-19 therapeutics by adapting the classification system recommended by the American College of Cardiology/American Heart Association based on strength of recommendation (Class I = strong benefit, Class IIa = moderate benefit, Class IIb = weak benefit, and Class III = no benefit or harmful) and quality of evidence (A = high-quality RCT, B-R = moderate-quality RCT, B-NR = moderate-quality non-RCT, C-LD = limited data, and C-EO = expert opinion).[60] Based on this classification and considering that a number of investigational therapeutics besides those that have received EUA or approval have been evaluated in an RCT, a summary of the outcomes is provided in Table 16.2, modified from the review by Khani et al.[59] Agents with non-RCT data have not been considered, given the high potential to yield biased or misleading results.

Table 16.2 Investigational Therapeutics With Randomized Controlled Trial Data in Patients With COVID-19

Drug (Alphabetical)	Author	N	Trial Description	Outcomes
Colchicine	Deftereos et al/Greece [61]	105	Prospective, open-label, RCT in 105 patients hospitalized with COVID-19; randomized 1:1 from April 3 to April 27, 2020, to standard medical treatment or colchicine plus standard medical treatment	Primary endpoint (baseline to clinical deterioration, defined as a 2-grade increase on an ordinal clinical scale) occurred in 7 patients (14.0%) in the control group and in 1 patient (1.8%) in the colchicine group (OR, 0.11; 95% CI, 0.01–0.96; $P = .02$). Mean event-free survival time was 18.6 days for control vs. 20.7 days for colchicine ($P = .03$)
	Tardif/USA COLCORONA [62]	4488	Randomized, double-blind trial in nonhospitalized patients with COVID-19; assigned to colchicine (0.5 mg twice daily for 3 days, once daily thereafter) or placebo for 30 days	Primary endpoint not met. Composite of death or hospitalization for COVID-19 occurred in 4.7% in the colchicine group vs. 5.8% on placebo (OR, 0.79; 95.1% (CI, 0.61–1.03; $P = .08$)
Favipiravir, baloxavir marboxil	Lou et al/China [63]	29	Randomized trial of 3 arms in hospitalized adult patients with COVID-19 assigned in a 1:1:1 ratio to baloxavir marboxil, favipiravir, or control	14-day treatment resulted in viral negative status in 70% (baloxavir marboxil), 77% (favipiravir), and 100% (control) of patients. No statistically significant benefit shown with addition of baloxavir marboxil or favipiravir
	Chen et al/China [64]	240	Prospective, randomized controlled, open-label multicenter trial involving adult patients with COVID-19; randomly assigned to conventional therapy plus umifenovir (Arbidol) or favipiravir (1600 mg × 2/first day followed by 600 mg × 2/day) for 10 days	Clinical recovery rate of day 7 not significantly different between treatment arms (favipiravir (71/116) vs. arbidol (62/120) ($P = .1396$). Favipiravir significantly improved latency to relief for pyrexia and cough
Hydroxychloroquine	WHO SOLIDARITY trial/multiple countries [19]	1853	Randomized trial of remdesivir, hydroxychloroquine, lopinavir, and interferon-beta 1a in patients hospitalized with COVID-19	Death occurred in 104/947 patients receiving hydroxychloroquine and in 84/906 receiving its control (RR, 1.19; 95% CI, 0.89–1.59; $P = .23$). No benefits observed with initiation of ventilation or duration of hospital stay
	RECOVERY/United Kingdom [18]	4716	Randomized controlled, open-label platform trial in patients hospitalized with COVID-19 and randomly assigned to hydroxychloroquine vs. usual care	Enrollment closed after interim analysis showing lack of efficacy. Death within 28 days occurred in 421 patients (27.0%) in the hydroxychloroquine group and in 790 (25.0%) in the usual-care group (RR, 1.09; 95% CI, 0.97–1.23; $P = .15$)
Interferon-beta 1a (IFN-β1a)	Davoudi-Monfared et al/Iran [65]	81	Randomized trial of IFN-β1a in patients with severe COVID-19 comparing IFN-β1a plus national protocol medications (NPCs) (hydroxychloroquine + lopinavir-ritonavir or atazanavir-ritonavir) vs. NPC as control group	Time to clinical response not significantly different (IFN 9.7 ± 5.8 vs. control 8.3 ± 4.9 days, $P = .95$). However, 28-day overall mortality lower for IFN (19%) vs. NPC (43.6%) and day 14 discharge rate higher for IFN (66.7%) vs. NPC (43.6%)
	WHO SOLIDARITY trial/multiple countries [19]	4100	Randomized trial of remdesivir, hydroxychloroquine, lopinavir, and IFN-β1a in patients hospitalized with COVID-19	Death occurred in 243/2050 patients receiving IFN and in 216/2050 receiving its control (RR, 1.16; 95% CI, 0.96–1.39; $P = .11$). No benefits observed with initiation of ventilation or duration of hospital stay

Drug (Alphabetical)	Author	N	Trial Description	Outcomes
Ivermectin	Ahmed et al/Bangladesh[66]	72	Randomized trial of oral ivermectin alone (12 mg once daily for 5 days), oral ivermectin plus doxycycline (12 mg ivermectin single dose and 200 mg doxycycline on day 1, followed by 100 mg every 12 h for the next 4 days), and a placebo control group	Virological clearance was earlier in the 5-day ivermectin treatment arm vs. placebo (9.7 vs. 12.7 days; $P = .02$), but not for ivermectin + doxycycline arm (11.5 days; $P = .27$)
	López-Medina/Columbia[67]	476	Double-blind, randomized trial conducted at a single site in Cali, Colombia in which patients were randomized to ivermectin, 300 mcg/kg of body weight/day for 5 days (n = 238) or placebo (n = 238)	Median time to resolution of symptoms was 10 days (IQR, 9–13) in the ivermectin group compared with 12 days (IQR, 9–13) in the placebo group (HR for resolution of symptoms, 1.07 [95% CI, 0.87–1.32]; $P = .53$ by log-rank test)
Lopinavir/ritonavir	Cao et al/China[27]	199	Randomized controlled, open-label trial in patients assigned in a 1:1 ratio to lopinavir-ritonavir twice daily for 14 days plus standard care vs. standard care alone (control)	Primary endpoint (time to clinical improvement) not significantly different (HR, 1.31; 95% CI 0.95–1.80). Mortality at 28 days was similar (19.2% vs. 25%) as was percentage of patients with detectable viral RNA
	WHO SOLIDARITY trial/multiple countries[19]	2771	Randomized trial of remdesivir, hydroxychloroquine, lopinavir, and IFN-β1a in patients hospitalized with COVID-19	Death occurred in 148/1399 patients receiving lopinavir and in 146/1372 receiving its control (RR, 1.00; 95% CI, 0.79–1.25; $P = .97$). No benefits observed with initiation of ventilation or duration of hospital stay
	RECOVERY Collaborative Group/United Kingdom[68]	5040	Investigator-initiated, individually randomized, open-label, platform trial to evaluate the effects of potential treatments in patients admitted to hospital with COVID-19	No significant difference in the proportion of patients who met the primary outcome of 28-day mortality between the two randomized groups (374 [23%] patients for lopinavir-ritonavir vs. 767 [22%] patients for usual-care group (RR, 1.03; 95% CI, 0.91–1.17; $P = .60$)
Ruxolitinib	Cao et al/China[69]	43	Prospective, multicenter, single-blind, randomized controlled phase II trial in patients with severe COVID-19	No significant clinical improvement in ruxolitinib recipients vs. control group (primary endpoint). Among secondary endpoints, ruxolitinib recipients had significantly faster improvement in chest CT at day 14 compared with the control group (18 [90%] vs. 13 [61.9%]; $P = .0495$) and no deaths (vs. 14.3% in control group)
Sofosbuvir/daclatasvir	Sadeghi et al/Iran[70]	66	Open-label, multicenter, RCT in adults with moderate or severe COVID-19 randomized to sofosbuvir and daclatasvir plus standard care or control (standard care alone)	Clinical recovery within 14 days achieved by 29/33 (88%) in the treatment arm and 22/33 (67%) in the control arm ($P = .076$); shorter median duration of hospitalization (6 days [IQR, 4–8]) vs. 8 days [IQR, 5–13] for control)
Sofosbuvir/daclatasvir v. ribavirin	Eslami et al/Iran[71]	62	Patients severe COVID-19 divided into two arms (ribavirin vs. sofosbuvir/daclatasvir)	Median duration of stay 5 days for sofosbuvir/daclatasvir vs. 9 days for ribavirin. Mortality in the sofosbuvir/daclatasvir group was 2/35 (6%) and 9/27 (33%) for ribavirin, (relative risk, 0.17; 95% CI, 0.04–0.73; $P = .02$)
Sofosbuvir/daclatasvir/ribavirin	Abbaspour Kasgari et al/Iran[72]	48	Single-center RCT in adults with moderate COVID-19 randomly assigned to 400 mg sofosbuvir, 60 mg daclatasvir, and 1200 mg ribavirin (intervention group) or to standard care (control group)	Median duration of hospital stay was 6 days in both groups ($P = .398$). Trends observed in favor of the sofosbuvir/daclatasvir/ribavirin arm for recovery and lower death rates, but trial was too small to draw conclusions

(Continued)

Table 16.2 Investigational Therapeutics With Randomized Controlled Trial Data in Patients With COVID-19 (continued)

Drug (Alphabetical)	Author	N	Trial Description	Outcomes
Tocilizumab (TCZ)	Salvarani et al/Italy[73]	126	Prospective, open-label, RCT that randomized patients hospitalized with COVID-19 pneumonia to receive tocilizumab or standard of care in 24 hospitals in Italy	Trial prematurely interrupted after an interim analysis for futility. No benefit on disease progression was observed compared with standard care
	Hermine et al/France[74]	131	Cohort-embedded, investigator-initiated, multicenter, open-label, bayesian RCT assigned to receive TCZ, 8 mg/kg, IV plus usual care on day 1 and on day 3 if clinically indicated (TCZ group) or to receive usual care alone	TCZ did not reduce WHO-CPS scores lower than 5 at day 4 but might have reduced the risk for noninvasive ventilation (NIV), mechanical ventilation (MV), or death by day 14. No difference on day 28 mortality
	Stone et al/USA[75]	243	Randomized, double-blind, placebo-controlled trial in patients with confirmed severe ARS, assigned in a 2:1 ratio to standard care plus single dose of either tocilizumab (8 mg/kg) or placebo	HR (TCZ vs. placebo) for intubation or death 0.83 (95% CI, 0.38–1.81); HR for disease worsening 1.11 (0.59–2.10). Not effective for preventing intubation or death in moderately ill hospitalized patients
	RECOVERY Collaborative Group/United Kingdom[21]	4116	Randomized, controlled, open-label, platform trial in patients with hypoxia (oxygen saturation <92% on air or requiring oxygen therapy) and evidence of systemic inflammation (C-reactive protein ≥75 mg/L)	Patients allocated to TCZ were more likely to be discharged from hospital within 28 days (57% vs. 50%; RR, 1.22; 1.12–1.33; $P < .0001$)

Modified from Khani E, Khiali S, Entezari-Maleki T. Potential COVID-19 therapeutic agents and vaccines: an evidence based review. J Clin Pharmacol. 2021;61(4):429-460; updated with newer data.
CPS, Clinical Progression Scale; CT, computed tomography; HR, hazard ratio; IQR, interquartile range; OR, odds ratio; RCT, randomized controlled trial; RR, rate ratio; WHO, World Health Organization.

Colchicine

Colchicine is an antiinflammatory medication used to treat gout, pericarditis, and coronary disease. Results from an initial RCT in 105 patients suggested it had the potential to be an important option in COVID-19,[61] triggering a 4000+ patient RCT named COLCO-RONA.[62] However, the primary endpoint (composite of death or hospitalization for COVID-19) was not met. Although secondary endpoints appeared to suggest a trend, the efficacy of colchicine was not conclusively established.

Favipiravir

Favipiravir is an antiviral drug that selectively inhibits RNA polymerase, which is necessary for viral replication. Although published RCT data have not been as clear in demonstrating efficacy, favipiravir is approved in Russia for the treatment of COVID-19 based on the interim results of an RCT showing SARS-CoV-2 viral clearance in 62.5% (25/40) of patients within 4 days versus 30% (6/20) in the standard of care arm.[76] A literature review/meta-analysis of 11 studies also suggests that favipiravir induces viral clearance by 7 days and contributes to clinical improvement within 14 days.[77] Additional studies are needed for a definitive conclusion. A phase III trial, PRESECO (Preventing Severe COVID Disease), is currently investigating favipiravir in the United States in patients with mild to moderate symptoms to prevent disease progression and hospitalization.[78]

Baloxavir Marboxil

Baloxavir marboxil is an antiviral drug currently approved by FDA for the treatment of influenza. It was tested in an RCT based on in vitro data suggesting potential in COVID-19, given its effects on endonuclease function, which results in inhibition of mRNA transcription. However, the results showed no benefit relative to standard antiviral therapy.[63]

Hydroxychloroquine

On June 15, 2020, the FDA revoked the EUA for hydroxychloroquine and chloroquine. Definitive evidence of its lack of efficacy came from the WHO SOLIDARITY and the UK RECOVERY trials, which showed no significant difference in 28-day mortality, longer duration of hospitalization, and lower likelihood of discharge compared with those in the usual-care group.[18,19]

Interferon-Beta 1a

Based on laboratory studies suggesting that type 1 IFN can inhibit SARS-CoV-2 and two closely related viruses, SARS-CoV and Middle East respiratory syndrome coronavirus (MERS-CoV), RCTs were triggered to assess its clinical potential, including the WHO SOLIDARITY trial. The results showed no benefits with respect to mortality rate, ventilation, or duration of hospital stay.[19] However, it is being further evaluated in combination with remdesivir in the NIAID's ACTT-3 compared with remdesivir plus placebo in 969 patients.[23]

Ivermectin

Based on in vitro data showing ivermectin, an antiparasitic drug approved by the FDA, to inhibit SAR-COV-2 in cell cultures and its activity in RNA viruses (influenza and West Nile virus), RCTs were initiated across several regions, although it was not clear that systemic inhibitory SARS-CoV-2 concentrations could be achieved even at doses exceeding currently approved doses. RCT data indicated earlier virological clearance (9.7 vs 12.7 days for placebo; $P = .02$), suggesting potential in COVID-19.[66] However, in a large RCT performed at a single site in Colombia in 476 adults with mild COVID-19 disease and symptoms for 7 days or fewer (at home or hospitalized), a 5-day course of once-daily 300 mcg/kg ivermectin did not significantly improve the time to resolution of symptoms compared with placebo.[67]

Lopinavir and Ritonavir

Lopinavir and ritonavir are protease inhibitors approved for the management of HIV infection, with strong in vitro data in SARS-CoV and MERS-CoV. However, data from three RCTs in patients with COVID-19 did not demonstrate efficacy for the combination on overall mortality, initiation of ventilation, or duration of hospital stay.[19,27,68] The collective in vitro and clinical data suggest that the typical doses used in HIV result in concentrations below what would be required to have an impact on SARS-CoV-2 replication.

Ruxolitinib

Ruxolitinib is a potent JAK1 and JAK2 inhibitor approved for the treatment of polycythemia vera and myelofibrosis. Because patients with severe COVID-19 experience excessive levels of proinflammatory cytokines (cytokine storm), which signal through JAK1 and JAK2, inhibition of these pathways with ruxolitinib was evaluated in clinical trials. In a prospective RCT in 41 patients with severe COVID-19, no significant clinical improvement was observed.[69] However, ruxolitinib recipients showed improvement based on follow-up chest CT scans and earlier recovery from lymphopenia, triggering phase III trials (DEVENT and RUXCOVID) in patients with severe COVID-19. However, neither trial met their primary endpoints of death, respiratory failure requiring mechanical ventilation, or admission to the ICU.[79,80]

Sofosbuvir and Daclatasvir

Anti–hepatitis C virus nucleotide analogs, such as sofosbuvir, daclatasvir, and ribavirin were hypothesized to be active in COVID-19, based on molecular docking and polymerase extension experiments showing inhibitory effects against SARS-CoV-2 RNA-dependent RNA polymerase (RdRp). In a small RCT in adults with moderate or severe COVID-19, sofosbuvir and daclatasvir significantly reduced the duration of hospital stay compared with standard care alone and showed a numerical trend toward fewer deaths. This was verified by an individual patient data meta-analysis suggesting improved survival and clinical recovery in patients with moderate to severe COVID-19. In another RCT, sofosbuvir and daclatasvir were more effective than ribavirin in improving clinical symptoms, duration of hospitalization, and death compared with ribavirin. The data collectively support future evaluations in larger RCTs.[70-72]

Tocilizumab

Because SARS-CoV-2 infection is often associated with excessive production of IL-6 from bronchial cells, tocilizumab, a recombinant humanized anti–human IL-6 receptor mAb was considered a promising candidate, particularly in critically ill patients with lung injury and high levels of IL-6.[60] Multiple RCTs have evaluated clinical outcomes in moderately to severely ill patients who were hospitalized with an inflammatory response.[21,73–75] Of the four RCTs, three failed to show any significant improvements in clinical symptoms, prevention of intubation, or overall mortality relative to the control group. However, the RECOVERY trial showed improvement in survival and other clinical outcomes with tocilizumab in hospitalized COVID-19 patients with hypoxia and systemic inflammation, which were additional to the benefits of systemic corticosteroids.[21]

Investigational Treatments in Clinical Trials for COVID-19: A Reference List

As previously discussed, various therapeutic modalities in clinical development have been designed to deliver primarily single-agent treatments for COVID-19. More recently, combination approaches are being increasingly evaluated to address the rapid evolution and emergence of variants. Regulatory authorities have strongly emphasized that individual mAb products be developed with the expectation that they will be combined with one or more mAb products that bind to different epitopes to minimize the risk for losing activity against emergent variants.[81]

Besides the CTAP website, several organizations are actively monitoring the development of new treatments and vaccines, including FasterCures, a center of the Milken Institute, which has developed an online tracking system based on publicly available information.[82] A list of investigational antiviral agents, antibodies, cell-based therapies, RNA-based therapies, and other medicines in development for the holistic management of patients with COVID-19 is provided later. As vast amounts of clinical data are being generated rapidly across the globe, it is not possible to provide a comprehensive clinical data summary of all of the agents in development. The following list is intended to serve as a reference point from which emerging clinical trial information could be accessed.

Therapeutic Management: Current Guidelines and Unmet Needs

To account for the rapid evolution as well as to help clarify the therapeutic tactics employed for COVID-19 across the globe, Siddiqi and Mehra[83] proposed a useful framework of clinical phenotyping to distinguish the phase where the viral pathogenicity is dominant versus the phase when the

---

List of Investigational Therapies in Clinical Trials for COVID-19

ANTIVIRALS

- PF-07321332 (SARS-CoV2-3CL protease inhibitor)
- Emetine hydrochloride
- DAS181, recombinant sialidase (nebulized)
- Ganovo (danoprevir), hepatitis C virus (HCV) NS3 protease inhibitor;
- Ritonavir
- Interferon (IFN), approved in China to treat hepatitis C (HCV)
- ASC09, HIV protease inhibitor

- BTL-TML
- Galidesivir
- Levovir (clevudine)
- Favilavir/ Favipiravir/ T-705/ Avigan, licensed in Japan to treat influenza
- Remdesivir, nucleotide analog
- Lopinavir/ritonavir, HIV-1 protease inhibitor
- Virazole (ribavirin for inhalation solution)
- AT-527, oral purine nucleotide prodrug

- Selzentry (maraviroc), a CCR5 coreceptor antagonist
- Sofusbuvir
- Arbidol (umifenovir), licensed in Russia and China for treatment of respiratory viral infections
- Prezcobix (darunavir, HIV-1 protease inhibitor/cobicistat, CYP3A inhibitor)
- Hyperimmune immunoglobulin (hIVIG) + remdesivir
- Neurosivir (NA-831)

- PF-07304814 (intravenous protease inhibitor)
- Truvada (emtricitabine and tenofovir, both HIV-1 nucleoside analog reverse transcriptase inhibitors)
- EIDD-2801, oral ribonucleoside analog
- Tamiflu (oseltamivir), neuraminidase inhibitor
- Atazanavir, protease inhibitor
- Daklinza (daclatasvir), HCV NS5A inhibitor

List of Investigational Therapies in Clinical Trials for COVID-19

ANTIBODIES

- CPI-006
- Ultomiris (ravulizumab-cwvz), complement inhibitor
- Soliris (eculizumab), complement inhibitor
- MEDI3506, monoclonal antibody (mAb) targeting interleukin (IL)-33
- Itolizumab, anti-CD6 immunoglobulin G1 (IgG1) mAb Abatacept (Orencia)
- CT-P59; antibodies from recovered COVID-19 patients
- Remsima (infliximab), anti–tumor necrosis factor (TNF) antibody
- CERC-002, anti-LIGHT mAbs
- SAB-185, polyclonal hyperimmune globulin (H-IG)
- COVID-19 immunoglobulin, plasma derived
- Avastin (bevacizumab), vascular endothelial growth factor inhibitor

- Leronlimab (PRO 140), a CCR5 antagonist
- EB05, nonsteroidal antiinflammatory molecule (sPLA2 inhibitor)
- LY3127804, anti–angiopoietin 2 antibody
- LY-CoV555 antibody from recovered patients
- LY-CoV1404 antibody from a convalescent COVID-19 patient
- Polyclonal hyperimmune globulin (H-IG)
- Sylvant (siltuximab), IL-6 targeted monoclonal
- GC5131A, plasma-derived therapy
- Nonviral gene therapy to produce mAbs
- Polyclonal hyperimmune globulin (H-IG)
- Gamunex-C, contains anti-SARS-CoV-2 polyclonal antibodies from recovered plasma donors
- Otilimab, anti– GM-CSF antibody
- Antibody 47D11
- Actemra (tocilizumab), IL-6 receptor antagonist

- Lenzilumab, anti–granulocyte-macrophage colony-stimulating factor (GM-CSF) antibody
- TJM2 (TJ003234), anti–GM-CSF antibody
- IC14, recombinant chimeric anti-CD14 mAbs
- IFX-1, anti-C5a antibody
- JS016 antibody candidate (LY-CoV016 + LY-CoV555)
- Antibodies from recovered COVID-19 patients
- Mavrilimumab, anti–GM-CSF factor receptor-alpha mAb
- Convalescent plasma (blood plasma from recovered patients)
- Octagam; intravenous immunoglobulin (IVIG)
- Ilaris (canakinumab), IL-1 beta-blocker
- PD-1 blocking antibody; thymosin

- Antibody combination REGN-COV2 (REGN10933+REGN10987) against the spike protein
- Gimsilumab, anti–GM-CSF factor mAb
- COVI-SHIELD/COVI-TRACE/COVI-GUARD antibody cocktail that binds to three different epitopes
- BDB-001, monoclonal anti-C5a antibody
- Gamifant (emapalumab), anti-IFN-γ antibody
- Meplazumab, anti-CD147 antibody
- BRII-196 and BRII-198, antibodies from recovered COVID-19 patients
- TY027, mAb targeting SARS-CoV-2
- Opdivo (nivolumab), PD-1 blocking antibody
- Combo of two antibodies (AZD7442)
- Prolastin, alpha-1 antitrypsin antibody
- VIR-7831 and VIR-7832, antibodies from recovered SARS patients

CELL-BASED THERAPIES

- AgenT-797, allogeneic invariant natural killer (NK) T cells
- Allogeneic T-cell therapies
- ACT-20, allogeneic cell preparation of mesenchymal stem cells from umbilical cord tissue
- MultiStem, bone marrow stem cells
- CLBS119, autologous peripheral blood-derived CD34+ cell therapy
- AmnioBoost, concentrated allogeneic MSCs and cytokines derived from amniotic fluid
- AlloRx stem cells, umbilical cord mesenchymal stem cell therapy

- CAP-1002, allogenic cardiosphere-derived cells
- CK0802, allogeneic cell therapy containing T-regulatory cells from umbilical cord blood processed to express lung homing markers on the cell surface
- Autologous adipose-tissue derived mesenchymal stem cells (ADMSCs) and allogeneic MSCs
- CYNK-001, allogeneic, NK cell therapy
- Ryoncil (remestemcel-L), allogenic mesenchymal stem cells

- CYP-001 (Cymerus MSC), mesenchymal stem cells
- DWP710, DW-MSC, a mesenchymal stem cell therapy
- Chimeric antigen receptors (CAR)/T-cell receptors (TCR)-T-cell therapy
- Allocetra, early apoptotic cells
- Allogenic, adipose-derived mesenchymal stem cells (HB-adMSCs)
- Bone marrow–derived allogenic mesenchymal stem cells (BM-Allo-MSC)
- Umbilical cord–derived mesenchymal stem cells

- Astrostem-V, allogenic, adipose-derived mesenchymal stem cells (HB-adMSCs)
- Mesenchymal stem cells
- PLX cell product, placenta-based cell therapy
- MSV allo, allogenic mesenchymal stem cells
- SBI-101, biological/device combo product with allogeneic mesenchymal stem cells and a phasmapheresis device
- StemVacs, universal donor NK cell–based therapy

(Continued)

List of Investigational Therapies in Clinical Trials for COVID-19

RNA-BASED THERAPIES

- Ampligen; (rintatolimod)
- OT-101, a transforming growth factor-beta (TGF-β) antisense drug candidate

OTHERS

- Firazyr (bradykinin B2 antagonist)
- MRx-4DP0004 (strain of *Bifidobacterium breve*)
- Senicapoc
- ABX464
- Zilucoplan, synthetic macrocyclic peptide inhibitor of terminal complement protein C5
- Risankizumab mAb and remdesivir + lenzilumab
- LAM-002A (apilimod dimesylate), PIKfyve kinase inhibitor
- ADX-1612, HSP 90 inhibitor
- ADX-629, orally available reactive aldehyde species (RASP) inhibitor
- Cerocal (ifenprodil), NP-120, an NDMA receptor glutamate receptor antagonist targeting Glu2NB
- Vascepa (icosapent ethyl), a form of eicosapentaenoic acid
- Otezla (apremilast), inhibitor of phosphodiesterase 4 (PDE4)
- Solnatide (synthetic molecule with a structure based on the lectin-like domain of human TNF-alpha)
- Dutasteride, antiandrogen
- AT-001, aldose reductase inhibitor
- Metablok (LSALT peptide), selective dipeptidase-1 antagonist
- ARMS-1
- Calquence (acalabrutinib), Bruton's tyrosine kinase (BTK) inhibitor
- Farxiga (dapagliflozin), sodium-glucose cotransporter 2 (SGLTs) inhibitor
- ATYR1923, fusion protein (immunomodulatory domain of histidyl tRNA synthetase fused to the Fc region of a human antibody) modulator of neuropilin-2
- Bemcentinib, selective AXL kinase inhibitor
- Activase (alteplase), tissue plasminogen activator (tPA)

- Fadraciclib (CYC065), cyclin-dependent kinase (CDK)2/9 inhibitor
- Raloxifene (Evista), an estrogen agonist/antagonist
- Ryanodex (dantrolene sodium), skeletal muscle relaxant
- Peginterferon lambda
- Eritoran, TLR-4 antagonist
- EDP1815, oral single strain of microbe
- Gleevac (imatinib), kinase inhibitor
- Traumakine (INF-β1a)
- Pepcid (famotidine), histamine-2 (H₂) receptor antagonist
- FSD-201 (ultramicronized palmitoylethanolamide)
- Losmapimod, oral selective p38 mitogen-activated protein kinase inhibitor
- MSTT1041A (anti-ST2, the receptor for IL-33)
- UTTR1147A (IL-22-Fc)
- CIGB-258, immunoregulatory peptide, Jusvinza
- TD139, specific inhibitor of galectin-3, inhalation powder
- Tricor (fenofibrate), peroxisome proliferator–activated receptor (PPAR) alpha agonist
- Cinvanti (aprepitant), a substance P/neurokinin-1 receptor antagonist
- Razuprotafib, Tie 2–activating compound (AKB-9778)
- Cenicriviroc, chemokine receptor 2 and 5 dual antagonist
- IMU-838, selective oral dihydroorotate dehydrogenase (DHODH) inhibitor
- N-803, IL-15 superagonist (nogapendekin alfa inbakicept)
- Brilacidin, a defensin mimetic
- Nangibotide

- Ivermectin
- M5049, small molecule that block the activation of Toll-like receptor (TLR)7 and TLR8
- Cozaar (losartan), angiotensin-2 receptor blocker (ARB)
- Diovan (valsartan), ARB
- Camostat mesylate, transmembrane protease serine 2 (TMPRSS2) inhibitor, approved in Japan to treat multiple conditions, including pancreatitis
- Nafamostat, approved in Japan to treat pancreatitis and other diseases
- Heparin; low molecular weight heparin (enoxaparin), anticoagulant
- Adaptive COVID-19 Treatment Trial 3 (ACTT-3), remdesivir + INF-β1a
- Olumiant (baricitinib), Janus kinase (JAK) inhibitor
- NT-I7 (efineptakin alfa), long-acting human IL-7
- Aviptadil, synthetic form of vasoactive intestinal polypeptide (RLF-100)
- Apixaban (Eliquis) blood thinner, direct oral anticoagulant
- Jakafi/jakavi (ruxolitinib)
- ST266, cell-free biological made from antiinflammatory proteins secreted by placental cells
- Veyonda (idronoxil)
- Recombinant human IFN-α1b
- Colchicine
- Dipyridamole (Persantine), anticoagulant
- Chloroquine/ hydroxychloroquine, antimalarial
- Methylprednisolone/ ciclesonide (Alvesco)/ hydrocortisone/ corticosteroids
- VentaProst, inhaled epoprostenol delivered by a dedicated delivery system

- PTC299, oral small molecule inhibitor of dihydroorotate dehydrogenase (DHODH)
- PUL-042 inhalation solution
- Azithromycin, antibiotic
- Yeliva (opaganib, ABC294640), oral sphingosine kinase-2 (SK2) selective inhibitor
- RHB-107 (upamostat, WX-671), serine protease inhibitor
- Levaquin (levofloxacin), a fluoroquinolone antibacterial
- Ceftriaxone, broad-spectrum cephalosporin antibiotic
- Apabetalone (RVX-208), selective BET (bromodomain and extraterminal) inhibitor
- Bucillamine, a cysteine derivative thiol-based drug
- Nitazoxanide, antiprotozoal
- ST-001 nanoFenretinide (fenretinide)
- Silmitasertib, small molecule drug, targets CK2 and CK2-inhibitor
- AQCH, plant-derived (phytopharmaceutical) drug
- Kineret (anakinra), IL-1 receptor antagonist
- SNG001, inhaled formulation of IFN-β1a
- UNI9011 (Union Therapeutics), FW-1022 (First Wave Bio), DWRX2003 (Daewoong) niclosamide
- Lysteda/Cyklokapron/ LB1148 (tranexamic acid), an antifibrinolytic
- APN01; recombinant soluble human angiotensin-converting enzyme-2 (ACE2)
- Micardis (telmisartan)

List of Investigational Therapies in Clinical Trials for COVID-19

- Recombinant human plasma gelsolin (rhu-pGSN)
- Vazegepant, CGRP receptor antagonist
- BIO-11006, inhaled peptide
- BLD-2660, synthetic small molecule inhibitor of calpain (CAPN) 1, 2, and 9
- Auxora (CM4620-IE), calcium release–activated calcium (CRAC) channel inhibitor
- Piclidenoson, A3 adenosine receptor agonist
- Entresto (sacubitril, a neprilysin inhibitor, and valsartan, an ARB)
- DSTAT (dociparstat sodium), glycosaminoglycan derivative of heparin
- Pacritinib, oral kinase inhibitor with specificity for JAK2, IRAK1, and CSFIR
- Roscovitine seliciclib, cyclin-dependent kinase (CDK)2/9 inhibitor

- Brensocatib, oral, reversible inhibitor of dipeptidyl peptidase 1 (DPP1)
- Rebif (INF-β1a)
- Xpovio (selinexor), oral, selective inhibitor of nuclear export (SINE) compound
- EPAspire, oral formulation of highly purified eicosapentaenoic acid free fatty acid (EPA-FFA) in gastroresistant capsules
- Flarin (lipid ibuprofen)
- Proxalutamide (GT0918), antiandrogen
- LAU-7b (fenretinide)
- Nitric oxide
- MN-166 (ibudilast), orally bioavailable, small molecule macrophage migration inhibitory factor (MIF) inhibitor and phosphodiesterase (PDE) 4 and 10 inhibitor

- CD24Fc, biological immuno-modulator (nonpolymorphic regions of CD24 attached to the Fc region of human IgG1)
- Organicell Flow, acellular product derived from amniotic fluid
- OP-101, dendrimer-based therapy
- PP-001
- Leukine (sargramostim, rhu–GM-CSF factor)
- Xeljanz (tofacitinib), Janus kinase (JAK) inhibitor
- Aplidin (plitidepsin), approved in Australia to treat multiple myeloma
- Ruconest (recombinant human C1 esterase inhibitor)
- PB1046, long-acting, sustained-release human vasoactive intestinal peptide (VIP) analog

- Tradipitant, a neurokinin-1 receptor antagonist
- Aldactone (spironolactone), aldosterone antagonist
- Almitrine
- Leflunomide, pyrimidine synthesis inhibitor; dihydroorotate dehydrogenase inhibitor (DHODH- Brequinar)
- Pulmozyme (nebulized dornase alfa), a recombinant DNase enzyme
- VP01, C21, angiotensin-2 type 2 receptor activator
- merimepodib, IMPDH inhibitor
- Luvox (fluvoxamine), a selective serotonin reuptake inhibitor
- Interferon/peginterferon alpha-2b, PegIntron, Sylatron, IntronA, Pegihep
- Desidustat, a hypoxia-inducible factor prolyl hydroxylase inhibitor

Prepared from Milken Institute's COVID-19 Treatment and Vaccine Tracker Spreadsheet[82]; not exhaustive; as of Apr 30, 2021.

host inflammatory response overtakes the pathological condition. Overlaid on this framework are the National Institutes of Health treatment recommendations for FDA EUA/approved therapies for managing patients with varying severities of disease[84] (Fig. 16.8).

It should be acknowledged that this is a simplified depiction of a complex disease progression that is unpredictable and, in many cases, deadly. Two key aspects that inform therapeutic intervention are the nature/order of appearance of symptoms and the timing of the progression of events. Useful insights were reported by Larsen et al.,[85] who modeled the order of symptom occurrence to help patients and medical professionals more quickly distinguish COVID-19 from other respiratory diseases. They applied a Markov process to an ordered set of clinical observations and constructed transition probabilities based on patient data collected from various literature reports on the frequencies of symptoms in COVID-19, influenza, MERS, and SARS. The analysis revealed that whereas influenza typically started with cough, COVID-19 and other coronavirus-related diseases (SARS and MERS) commenced with fever. Further, whereas fever and cough were the first and second symptoms for COVID-19, SARS, and MERS, the upper gastrointestinal tract (i.e., nausea/vomiting)

seemed to be affected before the lower gastrointestinal tract (diarrhea) in COVID-19, and MERS and SARS typically had the opposite sequence. Although this type of insight around the initial symptomatology may not be as critical as a diagnostic test as the authors themselves point out, it is invaluable to use such information to initiate testing, because the ultimate goal is to stop further spread of the disease.[85]

A more challenging aspect of disease and therapy management appears to be the timing, that is, the large interindividual variability in disease progression and associated symptoms. In general terms, symptoms typically begin with a fever (day 1), followed by or in conjunction with dry cough and other symptoms (e.g., headache, fatigue, loss of taste/smell), many of which last for a week or two. However, during this period, patients begin to either recover from the disease (~80%–90%) or take a turn for the worse (10%–20%) attributable to cytokine excess, progress toward ARDS, and tissue/organ damage. From a therapeutic interventional standpoint, the key seems to be predicting or identifying promptly the time point at which that turn for the worse occurs so that corticosteroids, other immune-modulators, and anticoagulants could be administered to reverse the clinical deterioration. The

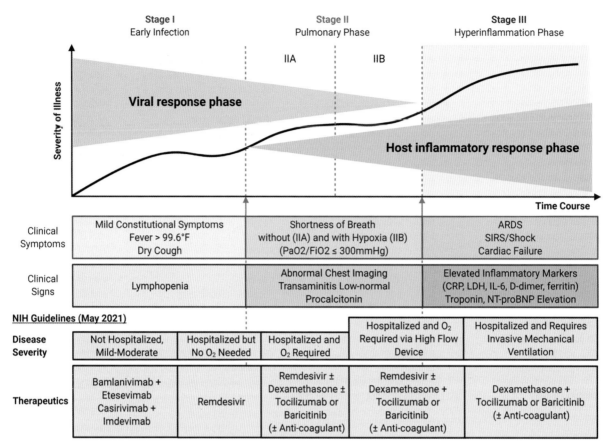

Fig. 16.8 Classification of COVID-19 Disease States and Therapeutic Strategy Based on National Institutes of Health (NIH) Treatment Guidelines for Therapies With US Food and Drug Administration Emergency Use Authorization and Approval. Three escalating phases of COVID-19 disease progression, with associated signs and symptoms. The *bottom rows* (disease severity and therapeutics) have been added to reflect the NIH Panel's recommendations for managing patients with varying severities of disease with the potential addition of anticoagulation, which has emerged as a core component of treatment management during cytokine excess. For details, refer to Therapeutic Management, COVID-19 Treatment Guidelines (nih.gov). *ARDS*, Acute respiratory distress syndrome; *CRP*, C-reactive protein; *LDH*, lactate dehydrogenase; *NTproBNP*, N-terminal pro-brain natriuretic peptide; *SIRS*, severe inflammatory response syndrome. (Modified from Siddiqi HK, Mehra MR. COVID-19 illness in native and immunosuppressed states: a clinical–therapeutic staging proposal. *J Heart Lung Transplant.* 2020;39[5]:405–407.)

complicated safety profile of these agents, however, further underscores the need for highly efficacious novel antiviral therapies that can be given within the first 3 to 5 days of onset of symptoms. Across the globe, a variety of protocols are being used to manage patients and the guidelines and protocols continue to evolve based on empiric experience. Combining empiric evidence and modeling the approaches described previously will enable us to plan therapeutic interventions in a more optimal and timely manner.

Conclusion

Despite the remarkable innovations and progress with vaccines around the world, much of the world's population will remain unvaccinated well into 2022 and likely even beyond. With the rapid and widespread appearance of variants of concern, one or more such variants could invariably find a way to escape the vaccines. Given this scenario, it is vitally important to also have new treatment strategies to tackle the various manifestations and devastating effects of COVID-19.

Significant strides have been made over the past year by the global scientific community to parse out and repurpose older medicines and in parallel to design and develop new antiviral molecules, mAbs, and other medications to manage the clinical manifestations of COVID-19. Yet, there continues to be a high unmet global need for targeted medicines with proven efficacy using objective clinical endpoints and excellent safety that can be easily delivered to very large numbers of patients to slow disease progression, prevent symptoms from becoming serious and life threatening, and enable quick recovery. Thanks to the rapid and ever-deepening understanding of SARS-CoV-2 human protein–protein interactions, new molecular entities are being developed and authorized at an unprecedented pace (e.g., at the time of finalizing this chapter, the FDA issued new or updated EUAs for sotrovimab,[86] tocilizumab,[87] and baricitinib,[88] and new RCT data have been reported, such as for tofacitinib,[89] demonstrating lower risk for death or respiratory failure). The quick development and approval of new molecular entities combined with effective vaccines hold great promise in containing the pandemic.

Disclosures

Sriram Krishnaswami and Sujatha Menon are employees and stockholders of Pfizer; Amparo de la Peña is an employee and minor stockholder at Cognigen, a division of Simulations Plus; Sarah Kim declares no conflicts of interest.

REFERENCES

1. Carvalho T, Krammer F, Iwasaki A. The first 12 months of COVID-19: A timeline of immunological insights. *Nature Reviews Immunology*. 2021;21:245–256.
2. Center for Disease Control and Prevention. 1918-Influenza, ": 1918 Pandemic (H1N1 virus)," 20 Mar 2019. [Online]. Available: https://www.cdc.gov/flu/pandemic-resources/1918-pandemic-h1n1.html.
3. Taubenberger JK, Morens DM. 1918 Influenza: the Mother of All Pandemics. *Emerg Inf Dis*. 2006;12(1):15–22.
4. Taylor DB, "A Timeline of the Coronavirus Pandemic," NY Times, 17 Mar 2021. Online]. Available: https://www.nytimes.com/article/coronavirus-timeline.html.
5. Cucinotta D, Vanelli M. WHO Declares COVID-19 a Pandemic. *Acta Biomed*. 2020;91(1):157–160.
6. World Health Organization, "Director-General's opening remarks at the media briefing on COVID-19," 11 Mar 2020. [Online]. Available: https://www.who.int/director-general/speeches/detail/who-director-general-s-opening-remarks-at-the-media-briefing-on-covid-19—11-march-2020.
7. Johns Hopkins University, "Coronavirus Resource Center," 11 Mar 2020. [Online]. Available: https://coronavirus.jhu.edu/.
8. Murthy S, Gomersall CD, RA Fowler. Care for Critically Ill Patients With COVID-19. *JAMA Insights*. 2020;323(15):1499–1500.
9. Fan E, Del Sorbo L, Goligher EC, et al. An Official American Thoracic Society/European Society of Intensive Care Medicine/Society of Critical Care Medicine Clinical Practice Guideline: Mechanical Ventilation in Adult Patients with Acute Respiratory Distress Syndrome. *American J Resp Crit Care Med*. 2017;195(9):1253–1263.
10. Holshue ML, DeBolt C, Lindquist S, et al. First case of 2019 novel coronavirus in the United States. *N Engl J Med*. 2020;382:929–936.
11. US Food and Drug Administration. CTAP, "Coronavirus Treatment Acceleration Program (CTAP)," June 2021. [Online]. Available: https://www.fda.gov/drugs/coronavirus-covid-19-drugs/coronavirus-treatment-acceleration-program-ctap.
12. Frediansyah A, Nainu F, Dhama K, et al. Remdesivir and its antiviral activity against COVID-19: a systematic review. *Clinical Epidemiology and Global Health*. 2020;2021(9):123–127.
13. Okoli GN, Rabbani R, Copstein L, et al. Remdesivir for coronavirus disease 2019 (COVID-19): a systematic review with meta-analysis and trial sequential analysis of randomized controlled trials. *Infectious Diseases (2021)*. 2021:1–9.
14. Jorgensen SCJ, Kebriaei R, Dresser LD. Remdesivir: review of pharmacology, pre-clinical data, and emerging clinical experience for COVID-19. *Pharmacotherapy: The Journal of Human Pharmacology and Drug Therapy*. 2020;40(7):659–671.
15. Eastman RT, Roth JS, Brimacombe KR, et al. Remdesivir: a review of its discovery and development leading to emergency use authorization for treatment of COVID-19. *ACS central Science 6*. 2020;5:672–683.
16. Singh AK, Singh A, Singh R, Misra A. Remdesivir in COVID-19: a critical review of pharmacology, pre-clinical and clinical studies. *Diabetes & Metabolic Syndrome: Clinical Research & Reviews*. 2020;14(4):641–648.
17. Beigel JH, Tomashek KM, Dodd LE, et al. Remdesivir for the Treatment of Covid-19 — Final Report. *N Engl J Med*. 2020;383:1813–1826.
18. Horby P, Mafham M, Linsell L, et al. RECOVERY Collaborative Group. Effect of hydroxychloroquine in hospitalized patients with Covid-19. *N Engl J Med*. 2020;383(21):2030–2040.
19. Pan H, Peto R, HenaoRestrepo A-M, et al. Repurposed antiviral drugs for COVID-19: interim WHO Solidarity Trial results. *N Engl J Med*. 2021;384(6):497–511.
20. Horby P, Lim WS, Emberson JR, et al. Dexamethasone in hospitalized patients with COVID-19. *N Engl J Med*. 25 February 2021;384(8):693–704.
21. Ayujayeb A, Vatish M, Tavoukjian V, et al. Tocilizumab in patients admitted to hospital with COVID-19 (RECOVERY): preliminary results of a randomised, controlled, open-label, platform trial. *The Lancet*. 2021;397(10285):1637–1645.
22. Kalil AC, Patterson TF, Mehta AK, et al. Baricitinib plus remdesivir for hospitalized adults with COVID-19. *N Engl J Med*. 2021;384:795–807.
23. National Institutes of Health. ACTT-3, "NCT04492475: Adaptive COVID-19 Treatment Trial 3," [Online]. Available: https://clinicaltrials.gov/ct2/show/NCT04492475.
24. US Food and Drug Administration. Bamlanivimab/Etesevimab, "Fact sheet for health care providers: Emergency Use Authorization (EUA) of Bamlanivimab and Etesevimab," [Online]. Available: https://www.fda.gov/media/145802/download.
25. US Food and Drug Administration. Casirivimab/Imdevimab, "Fact sheet for health care providers: Emergency Use Authorization (EUA) of Casirivimab and Imdevimab," [Online]. Available: https://www.fda.gov/media/145611/download.
26. Gilead Sciences. Veklury, "United State Package Insert," Gilead Sciences, Inc., Oct 2020. [Online]. Available: https://www.gilead.com/-/media/files/pdfs/medicines/covid-19/veklury/veklury_pi.pdf.
27. Cao B, Wang Y, Wen D, et al. A trial of lopinavir-ritonavir in adults hospitalized with severe Covid-19. *N Engl J Med*. 2020;382(19):1787–1799.
28. Humeniuk R, Mathias A, Kirby BJ, et al. Pharmacokinetic, pharmacodynamic, and drug-interaction profile of remdesivir, a SARS-CoV-2 replication inhibitor. *Clin Pharmacokint*. 2021;60:569–583.
29. Humeniuk R, Mathias A, Cao H, et al. Safety, tolerability, and pharmacokinetics of remdesivir, an antiviral for treatment of COVID-19, in healthy subjects. *Clin Tran Sci*. 2020;13(5):896–906.
30. Goldman JD, Lye DCB, Hui DS, et al. Remdesivir for 5 or 10 days in patients with severe Covid-19. *N Eng J Med*. 2020;383(19):1827–1837.
31. Olender SA, Perez KK, Go AS, et al. Remdesivir for severe COVID-19 versus a cohort receiving standard of care. *Clinical Infectious Diseases (2020)*. 2020;73(11):e4166–e4174.

32. Spinner CD, Gottlieb RL, Criner GJ, et al. Effect of remdesivir vs standard care on clinical status at 11 days in patients with moderate COVID-19: a randomized clinical trial. *JAMA*. 2020;324(11):1048–1057.

33. Richardson P, Griffin I, Tucker C, et al. Baricitinib as potential treatment for 2019-nCoV acute respiratory disease. *Lancet*. 2020;395:e30–e31.

34. Stebbing J, Phelan A, Griffin I, et al. COVID-19: combining antiviral and anti-inflammatory. *Lancet*. 2020;20:400–401.

35. Eli Lilly and Company. Olumiant, "Baricitinib: United States Package Insert," 7 July 2020. [Online]. Available: https://uspl.lilly.com/olumiant/olumiant.html#pi.

36. US Food and Drug Administration. FDA-Review, "Emergency Use Authorization of Baricitinib for the treatment of COVID-19," 12 December 2020. [Online]. Available: https://www.fda.gov/media/144473/download.

37. Taylor PC, Adams AC, Hufford MM, et al. Neutralizing monoclonal antibodies for treatment of COVID-19. *Nature Reviews Immunology*. 2021;21:382–393.

38. US Food and Drug Administration Bamlanivimab/Etesevimab, "FDA Emergency Use Authorization," 25 February 2021. [Online]. Available: https://www.fda.gov/media/145801/download.

39. Gottlieb RL, Nirula A, Chen P, et al. Effect of bamlanivimab as monotherapy or in combination with etesevimab on viral load in patients with mild to moderate COVID-19. *JAMA*. 2021;325(7):632–644.

40. Jones BE, Brown-Augsburger PL, Corbett KS, et al. The neutralizing antibody, LY-CoV555, protects against SARS-CoV-2 infection in non-human primates. *Science Translational Medicine*. 05 Apr 2021;13(593):1--17.

41. Shi R, Shan C, Duan X, et al. A human neutralizing antibody targets the receptor-binding site of SARS-CoV-2. *Nature*. 2020;584:120–124.

42. US Food and Drug Administration. CDER_Review, "FDA CDER Review of Bamlanivimab 700 mg and Etesevimab 1400 mg for Emergency Use Authorization," 9 Feb 2021. [Online]. Available: https://www.fda.gov/media/146255/download.

43. Hartenian E, Nandakumar D, Lari A, et al. The molecular virology of coronaviruses. *J Bio Chem*. 2020;295(37):12910–12934.

44. World Health Organization, 2 September 2020. [Online]. Available: https://www.who.int/publications/i/item/WHO-2019-nCoV-Corticosteroids-2020.1.

45. National Institutes of Health, "COVID-19 Treatment Guidelines," 21 April 2021. [Online]. Available: https://www.covid19treatmentguidelines.nih.gov/therapeutic-management/.

46. Ferner RE, DeVito N, Aronson JK, et al, "Drug vignettes: Dexamethasone," Centre for Evidence-Based Medicine, Nuffield Department of Primary Care Health Sciences, University of Oxford, 26 June 2020. [Online]. Available: https://www.cebm.net/covid-19/dexamethasone/. [Accessed 11 May 2021].

47. Mayo Clinic, "COVID-19 (coronavirus): Long-term effects," 13 April 2021. [Online]. Available: https://www.mayoclinic.org/diseases-conditions/coronavirus/in-depth/coronavirus-long-term-effects/art-20490351.

48. Patel SK, Saikumar G, Rana J, et al. Dexamethasone: A boon for critically ill COVID-19 patients? *Travel Medicine and Infectious Disease*. 2020;37:101844.

49. Johnson DB, Lopez MJ, and Kelley B, "Dexamethasone," StatPearls Publishing, 5 Sept 2020. [Online]. Available: https://www.ncbi.nlm.nih.gov/books/NBK482130/.

50. Schimmer BP, Parker KL. Goodman and Gilman's The Pharmacological Basis of Therapeutics. In: Brunton L, ed. *In Adrenocorticotropic hormone; adrenocortical steroids and their synthetic analogues; inhibitors of the syntheses and actions of adrenocortical hormones*. 11th edition Columbus, Ohio: The McGraw-Hill Companies, Inc; 2006

51. Spoorenberg SMC, Deneer VHM, Grutters JC, et al. Pharmacokinetics of oral vs. intravenous dexamethasone in patients hospitalized with community-acquired pneumonia, *Br J Clin Pharmacol*, July 2014;78(1):78-83.

52. Dexcel Pharma Technologies. Hemady, "Dexamethasone Oral Tablets: United States Package Insert," 10 2019. [Online]. Available: https://www.accessdata.fda.gov/drugsatfda_docs/label/2019/211379s000lbl.pdf.

53. World Health Organization, "Coronavirus disease (COVID-19): Dexamethasone," 25 June 2020. [Online]. Available: https://www.who.int/news-room/q-a-detail/coronavirus-disease-covid-19-dexamethasone.

54. Matheson EC, Thomas H, Case M, et al. Glucocorticoids and selumetinib are highly synergistic in RAS pathway-mutated childhood acute lymphoblastic leukemia through upregulation of BIM. *Haematologica*. 2019;104(9):1804–1811.

55. "Dexamethasone, Oral Tablet (Medically reviewed by Victor Nguyen, PharmD, MBA - Written by University of Illinois-Chicago, Drug Information Group)," Medical News Today, 23 July 2020. [Online]. Available: https://www.medicalnewstoday.com/articles/322409. [Accessed 23 May 2021].

56. Orton S, Censani M. Iatrogenic Cushing's syndrome due to intranasal usage of ophthalmic dexamethasone: a case report. *Pediatrics*. 2016;137(5):e20153845.

57. Ranjbar K, Moghadami M, Mirahmadizadeh A, et al. Methylprednisolone or dexamethasone, which one is superior corticosteroid in the treatment of hospitalized COVID-19 patients: a triple-blinded randomized controlled trial. *BMC Infectious Diseases*. 2021;21(1):337.

58. "Dexamethasone Oral," WebMD, [Online]. Available: https://www.webmd.com/drugs/2/drug-1027-5021/dexamethasone-oral/dexamethasone-oral/details. [Accessed 23 May 2021].

59. Khani E, Khiali S, Entezari-Maleki T. Potential COVID-19 therapeutic agents and vaccines: an evidence based review. *J Clin Pharmacol*. 2021;61(4):429–460.

60. Halperin JL, Levine GN, Al-Khatib SM, et al. Further evolution of the ACC/AHA Clinical Practice Guideline Recommendation Classification System: a report of the American College of Cardiology/American Heart Association Task Force on Clinical Practice Guidelines. *J Am Coll Cardiol*. 2016;67(13):1572–1574.

61. Deftereos SG, Giannopoulos G, Vrachatis DA, et al. Effect of colchicine vs standard care on cardiac and inflammatory biomarkers and clinical outcomes in patients hospitalized with coronavirus disease. *JAMA Netw Open*. 2020;3(6):e2013136.

62. Tardiff JC, Bouabdallaoui N, L'Allier PL, et al, "Efficacy of Colchicine in Non-Hospitalized Patients with COVID-19," 27 Jan 2021. [Online]. Available: https://www.medrxiv.org/content/10.1101/2021.01.26.21250494v1.

63. Lou Y, Liu L, Yao H, et al. Clinical outcomes and plasma concentrations of baloxavir marboxil and favipiravir in COVID-19 patients: an exploratory randomized, controlled trial. *Eur J Pharm Sci.* 2020;157:105631.

64. Chen C, Zhang Y, Huang J, et al, "Medrxiv," 15 Apr 2020. [Online]. Available: https://www.medrxiv.org/content/10.1101/2020.03.17.20037432v4. [Accessed 5 June 2021].

65. Davoudi-Monfared F, Rahmani H, Khalili H, et al. A randomized clinical trial of the efficacy and safety of interferon β-1a in treatment of severe COVID-19. *Antimicrob Agents Chemother.* 2020;64(9) e01061–e01020.

66. Ahmed S, Karim MM, Ross AG, et al. A five-day course of ivermectin for the treatment of COVID-19 may reduce the duration of illness. *Int J Infect Dis.* 2020;103:214–216.

67. López-Medina E, López P, Hurtado IC, et al. Effect of ivermectin on time to resolution of symptoms among adults with mild COVID-19: a randomized clinical trial. *JAMA.* 2021;325(14):1426–1435.

68. RECOVERY Collaborative Group. Lopinavir–ritonavir in patients admitted to hospital with COVID-19 (RECOVERY): a randomised, controlled, open-label, platform trial. *The Lancet.* 2020;396:1345–1352.

69. Cao Y, Wei J, Zou L, et al. Ruxolitinib in treatment of severe coronavirus disease 2019 (COVID-19): a multicenter, single-blind, randomized controlled trial. *J Allergy Clin Immunol.* 2020;146(1):137–146.

70. Sadeghi A, Asgari AA, Norouzi A, et al. Sofosbuvir and daclatasvir compared with standard of care in the treatment of patients admitted to hospital with moderate or severe coronavirus infection (COVID-19): a randomized controlled trial. *J Antimicrob Chemother.* 2020;75(11):3379–3385.

71. Eslami G, Mousaviasl S, Radmanesh E, et al. The impact of sofosbuvir/daclatasvir or ribavirin in patients with severe COVID-19. *J Antimicrob Chemother.* 2020;75(11):3366–3372.

72. Abbaspour-Kasgari HA, Moradi S, Shabani AM, et al. Evaluation of the efficacy of sofosbuvir plus daclatasvir in combination with ribavirin for hospitalized COVID-19 patients with moderate disease compared with standard care: a single-centre, randomized controlled trial. *J Antimicrob Chemother.* 2020;75(11):3373–3378.

73. Salvarani C, Dolci G, Massari M, et al. Effect of tocilizumab vs standard care on clinical worsening in patients hospitalized with COVID-19 pneumonia: a randomized clinical trial. *JAMA Intern. Med.* 2021;181(1):24–31.

74. Hermine O, Mariette X, Tharaux PL, et al. Effect of tocilizumab vs usual care in adults hospitalized with COVID-19 and moderate or severe pneumonia: a randomized clinical trial. *JAMA Intern. Med.* 2021;181(2):32–40.

75. Stone JH, Frigault MJ, Serling-Boyd NJ, et al. Efficacy of tocilizumab in patients hospitalized with Covid-19. *N Engl J Med.* 2020;383(24):2333–2344.

76. Ivashchenko AA, Dmitriev KA, Vostokova NV, et al, "Medxriv," 4 August 2020. [Online]. Available: https://www.medrxiv.org/content/10.1101/2020.07.26.20154724v1.full.pdf. [Accessed 5 June 2021].

77. Manabe T, Kambayashi D, Akatsu H, Kudo K. Favipiravir for the treatment of patients with COVID-19: a systematic review and meta-analysis. *BMC Infect Dis.* 2021;21:489.

78. ClinicalTrials.gov. T. P. S. C.-1. (. Study 25 Mar 2021. [Online]. Available: https://clinicaltrials.gov/ct2/show/NCT04600895.

79. ClinicalTrials.gov. RUXCOVID_DEVENT, ": Assessment of Efficacy and Safety of Ruxolitinib in Participants With COVID-19-Associated ARDS Who Require Mechanical Ventilation (RUXCOVID-DEVENT)," 15 Mar 2021. [Online]. Available: https://clinicaltrials.gov/ct2/show/study/NCT04377620?term=DEVENT&draw=2&rank=2.

80. ClinialTrials.gov. RUXCOVID, ": Study to Assess the Efficacy and Safety of Ruxolitinib in Patients With COVID-19 Associated Cytokine Storm (RUXCOVID)," 2 Jun 2021. [Online]. Available: https://clinicaltrials.gov/ct2/show/NCT04362137.

81. US Food and Drug Administration. Guidance, "Development of Monoclonal Antibody Products Targeting SARS CoV-2, Including Addressing the Impact of Emerging Variants, During the COVID-19 Public Health Emergency," Feb 2021. [Online]. Available: https://www.fda.gov/media/146173/download.

82. Milken Institute, "COVID-19 Treatment and Vaccine Tracker," 30 April 2021. [Online]. Available: https://covid-19tracker.milkeninstitute.org/#treatment_antibodies.

83. Siddiqi HK, Mehra MR. COVID-19 illness in native and immunosuppressed states: A clinical–therapeutic staging proposal. *The Journal of Heart and Lung Transplantation.* 2020;39(5):405–407.

84. National Institutes of Health. Treatment-Guideline, "Therapeutic Management of Adults With COVID-19," 24 May 2021. [Online]. Available: https://www.covid19treatmentguidelines.nih.gov/therapeutic-management/.

85. Larsen JR, Martin MR, Martin JD, et al. Modeling the Onset of Symptoms of COVID-19. *Front. Public Health.* 2020;8.

86. US Food and Drug Administration. Sotorovimab, "Fact Sheet Emergency Use Authorization (EUA) of Sotroviamb," FDA, May 2021. [Online]. Available: https://www.fda.gov/media/149534/download.

87. US Food and Drug Administration. Tocilizumab, "Fact sheet for healthcare providers: Emergency Use Authorization (EUA) for ACTEMRA (tocilizumab)," 2021 June 2021. [Online]. Available: https://www.fda.gov/media/150321/download.

88. US Food and Drug Administration. Baricitinib Monotherapy, "Fact sheet for healthcare providers: Emergency Use Authorization (EUA) for Baricitinib," 28 July 2021. [Online]. Available: https://www.fda.gov/media/143823/download.

89. Guimarães PO, Quirk D, Furtado RH, et al. Tofacitinib in patients hospitalized with COVID-19 pneumonia. *N Eng J Med.* 2021;385:406–415.

CHAPTER

17 Novel Therapeutic Targets for SARS-CoV-2 and COVID-19

Srinivasan Krishnaswami, PhD, and Ben Geoffrey A.S., PhD

Factors That Affect Therapy for Treatment of COVID-19

Symptoms

Symptoms of COVID-19 are many[1,2]; some of them are as mild as those of normal influenza and others quite severe. Treatment provided to a patient with mild COVID-19 symptoms may be different from given to one with more serious symptoms such as difficulty of breathing. COVID-19 may lead to a few other manifestations such as cardiac problems in critically ill patients.

Most patients experience mild to moderate respiratory illness among other symptoms and recover quickly without requiring any special treatment. Aged patients and those with prior medical issues such as cardiovascular disease, diabetes, chronic respiratory disease, and cancer are at risk for developing serious complications and other manifestations. Several chapters in this book deal with varied manifestations, indicating that COVID-19 treatment is about not only respiratory illness but also potentially other severe symptoms, including tissue damage.

Disease Progression and Severity

In the time course of COVID-19, there are three stages: (1) early infection phase, (2) pulmonary phase, and (3) hyperinflammation phase.[3,4] It is important to note that some patients have only mild symptoms associated with an upper respiratory tract infection, or stage 1, whereas others progress to more advanced stages. The medication varies across stages. Pneumonia sets in at the pulmonary phase. Stage 3, or the hyperinflammation phase, leads to organ failures. Avoiding a cytokine storm remains a critical challenge in the progression of the disease.

Prevention and Control of Infection

To slow transmission of severe acute respiratory syndrome coronavirus 2 (SARS-CoV-2) one needs to know about the virus, the disease itself, and how it could spread. Social distancing and washing hands or using an alcohol-based rub frequently go a long way to avoid spread of the virus. SARS-CoV-2 spreads primarily through droplets of saliva or discharge from the nose when an infected person coughs or sneezes, which is why wearing face masks and social distancing have been shown to be effective against the spread of the virus. The transmission of SARS-CoV-2 also can be airborne.[5]

In addition to the previously mentioned basic protective measures, when infection is suspected, identification of certain biomarkers becomes necessary for COVID-19 treatment. To form a therapeutic strategy, it is important to classify severity based on identified immune-related biomarkers so that appropriate treatment would be provided. A list of such biomarkers includes the following types:

1. Hematological (lymphocyte count, neutrophil count, neutrophil-to-lymphocyte ratio [NLR])
2. C-reactive protein (CRP)
3. Erythrocyte sedimentation rate (ESR)
4. Procalcitonin (PCT)
5. Interleukin-6 (IL-6)
6. Biochemical (D-dimer, troponin, creatine kinase [CK], aspartate aminotransferase [AST]), especially those related to coagulation cascades in disseminated intravascular coagulation (DIC) and acute respiratory distress syndrome (ARDS)[6]

Emerging Therapeutic Treatments of the Disease

Among the emerging therapeutic treatments for COVID-19, vaccines play an important part in preventing infection, but they are discussed elsewhere in a separate chapter in this book.

Among the many drug discovery efforts for COVID-19, drug repurposing has taken central stage thus far in the small molecule space wherein attempts have been made to repurpose drugs approved for other diseases into drugs for COVID-19. Some of these drugs have been accorded emergency use authorization and the repurpose drug remdesivir has been granted approval by the US Food and Drug Administration (FDA). A list of emerging treatments for COVID-19 includes use of various repurpose drugs, neutralizing monoclonal antibodies (mAbs), and cell and gene therapy covering convalescent plasma and stem cells. Most of these treatments are of tentative nature, some having greater promise than others.[7] Further investigations continue in search of newer and more promising treatments for COVID-19. Countless journal articles, clinical practice guidelines, and other scientific reports on COVID-19 treatment have appeared in the last 18 months. Many clinical trials to evaluate promising repurpose drugs are also progressing. Given that mortaltiy of severe COVID-19 in unvaccinated persons remains high despite current treatment options, identification of newer targets and newer therapies for treatment of COVID-19 continues to be an important challenge in medical science.

Brief Description of Structure and Parts of SARS-CoV-2

Information on virus genome, structure, entry, replication, and transmission is covered in detail in Chapter 2. SARS-CoV-2 is an RNA virus, and, once sequenced, the protein products of the viral genome can be determined.[8,9] The proteins are encoded through codons of three nucleotides. Each codon encodes for a particular amino acid, and the resulting amino acids are polymerized together to form a protein. The start and stop codons decide the beginning and termination of the polymerization process of the protein. From the genome, one can obtain the encoded protein products. The functions and structure of these proteins can be determined using bioinformatics approaches, which are discussed in a subsequent section.

The structural and functional details of a druggable proteome of SARS-CoV-2 have been determined through various bioinformatics and experimental approaches, and a detailed description is given elsewhere.[9] Approximately two-thirds of the viral RNA genome of SARS-CoV-2 is translated into what are known as nonstructural proteins (NSPs). Besides this, the proteome encoded by the viral genome involves accessory proteins and four essential structural proteins that contribute to the stability and assembly of the virus, and they are the spike (S) receptor binding glycoprotein, which is the protein responsible for binding with the host angiotensin-converting enzyme-2 (ACE2) receptor and consequently plays a key role in the viral entry. For this discussion the nucleocapsid protein will be referred to with the symbol (N); the membrane protein will be referred to with the symbol (M), which is a transmembrane protein involved in the interaction with N, which will be referred to with the symbol (TM); and a small envelope protein that plays a vital role in assembly and stability of the virus will be referred to with the symbol (E). The functionality of SARS-CoV-2 can be broadly summarized as follows. The nonstructural proteins are predominantly involved in the viral replication process inside the human cell. The structural proteins referred to as M, N, S, and E proteins participate in viral assembly and stability. Other proteins known as accessory proteins interact with the host in functions such as shutting down host functions to redirect resources to viral replication, avoiding immune responses, and inducing pathogenicity. One of the compelling therapeutic strategies against COVID-19 is to inhibit the function of these proteins essential to the viral cycle of SARS-CoV-2 to stop both entry and replication of the virus, as described in the following sections.

Therapeutic Targets for the Treatment of COVID-19

The strategy for a therapeutic attack is twofold: virus-targeted antiviral therapy and host-directed antiviral therapy (Fig. 17.1).

In virus targeted antiviral therapies, the targets are certain virus domains to block entry of virus into the human cell and the viral enzymes produced by the virus to hijack the host machinery for its survival and the replication of the virus.

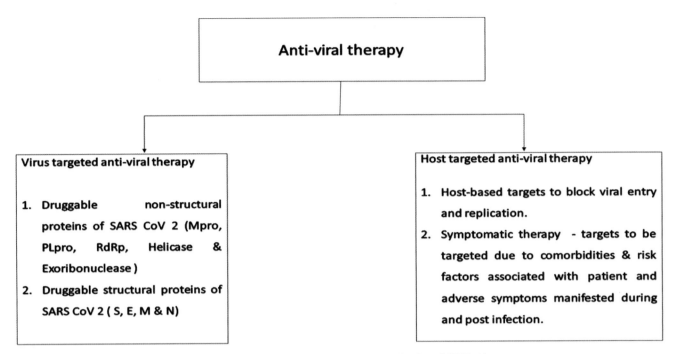

Fig. 17.1 Broad Areas of Antiviral Therapy Against COVID-19.

Table 17.1 Simplified View of Virus and Host Targeted Therapies and Disease Progression

Stage of Disease Progression	Virus-Targeted Therapy	Host-Targeted Therapy
Stage 1: Early viral infection	1. To prevent viral entry into cell: *Example:* Specific monoclonal antibodies 2. To prevent viral replication: Antivirals *Example:* Remdesivir or Favipiravir	None
Stage 2: Pulmonary infection—susceptibility to develop pneumonia	Antiviral to lessen viral replication.	Immunomodulator (*example:* dexamethasone) + anticoagulants
Stage 3: Hyperinflammation—acute respiratory syndrome (ARDS), sepsis, organ failures etc.	—	Immunomodulators + anticoagulants + other standard care

In host-targeted antiviral therapy, the targets are receptors and proteins in the host whose function is critical for the virus to enter and hijack the host machinery for its replication and drug targets specific to different adverse symptoms caused by COVID-19.[10–12] The adverse symptoms of COVID-19 are caused primarily by the unregulated immune response of the body.

Elements of both virus-targeted and host-targeted therapies are important for the treatment of COVID-19. The two types of therapies in the context of disease progression are shown in Table 17.1. No immunosuppressants are used in stage 1 as the body's natural resistance to the virus would be affected at that stage. No antivirals are used in stage 3. Immunomodulators or suppressants are required at both stages 2 and 3.

Human genetic diversity introduces much more complexity to the COVID-19 disease progression and treatment than what is depicted in Table 17.1. Many repurpose drugs are being used as part of either virus-targeted therapy or host-targeted therapy (Tables 17.3 and 17.4).

The following is a brief discussion on what drug targets are and current approaches being followed to identify them. Most drug targets are proteins. Proteins are involved in many essential functions in living beings. Noted German researcher Paul Ehrlich once said, "drugs will not act unless they are bound" to protein targets. Drug targets are those proteins whose function or non-function and/or their overexpression or underexpression are causing the disease. Small or large therapeutic molecules can bind to binding cavities of these proteins and induce conformational changes within the proteins. Such changes could inhibit or activate the function of protein to restore normalcy of function from the disease condition of the body. The molecules that inhibit the function of proteins are called inhibitors or antagonists; the molecules that activate the function are called agonists. A sound understanding of the molecular-level mechanism of the disease leads to effective identification of the proteins involved in the molecular pathways and mechanisms of the disease and proteins with binding cavities that can qualify as drug targets.

Experimental Studies to Identify Druggable Targets

A target is called "druggable" if its activity (or function) can be modulated by a therapeutic drug. Proteins and nucleic acids are both examples of biological targets. A potential drug target should have druggability, have an acceptable toxicity profile, and be assayable in addition to the fact that its three-dimensional (3D) structure is known. There are two classes of methods for identification of targets, target deconvolution and target discovery. A gamut of experimental methods to identify targets are known both in vitro and in vivo and described in a seminal reference.[13] The experimental methods include various affinity methods and genetic methods. Affinity chromatography is one of the most used methods for target deconvolution. Target deconvolution means looking for a target for an active compound. This results in screening of many molecules. In the target discovery method, the search is for a new target for which there is not yet a drug compound. Various biological assays and bioinformatics approaches are used for target discovery and target-based drug discovery.

Biological Assays

To understand the molecular mechanisms of disease, scientists perform experiments, specifically *assays. In vitro* assays are cell-based models, and *in vivo* assays are carried out inside living systems. Many different assays are used for drug target identification and validation; a few of them are mentioned here as examples. One major class of assays used in target identification and validation is *functional assays,* which are experiments designed to determine the role or function of a protein in a biological process or pathway.

As an example, to determine the activity of the target RNA-dependent RNA polymerase (RdRp) (NSP12), typical assays include the following[14]:
1. Polymerase elongation template element (PETE)
2. Fluorescence-based alkaline phosphatase–coupled polymerase assay (FAPA)
3. Fluorometric RdRp activity assay
4. Scintillation proximity assay
5. Cell-based assays

When these assays are carried out in the presence of an antagonist, a decrease in the replication activity may be observed. To find the efficacy of the drug remdesivir, which has been approved by FDA for treatment of COVID-19, such assays were used to determine its inhibitory activity against RdRp.[14]

Bioinformatics Approaches

Traditionally, in bioinformatics approaches, algorithms such as BLAST are used, to compute similarity of a given protein against proteins with a known structure and function present in bioinformatics databases.[15–18] Through this process, one can predict the structure and function of a given protein by comparing its similarity with known targets. In every drug discovery project, one is also able to leverage and capitalize on the data available from experiments carried out previously, aided by bioinformatics, which is being further enhanced by advanced data-driven techniques.[19] In the case of SARS-CoV-2, much of the knowledge from other virus systems such as SARS-CoV, Ebola, and Middle East respiratory syndrome coronavirus (MERS-CoV) led to recognition of similar target types for SARS-CoV-2.

Bioinformatics not only provides historical experimental data on structure, activity, and other properties of biomolecules but also gives insights from analysis of the data. Further, it provides many approaches not only for identification of targets but also for drug discovery. Current trends in bioinformatics encompass an approach that integrates many factors such as predicting disease-relevant genes, constructing gene networks, protein–protein interaction networks, biological pathway analysis, etc.

In silico or computational techniques, including molecular modeling techniques, can provide information on a variety of factors, such as:
1. Binding orientation of small molecule inhibitors with protein structures in 3D space through molecular docking techniques
2. Information on functional groups such as amino acid residues and other moieties that bind to the drug
3. Stability and properties of ligand–protein complexes using molecular dynamics simulation

A combination of these techniques as part of an integrated approach guide the researcher in discovering new drug molecules and new drug targets. A summary of methods of target and drug discovery is given in Box 17.1.

The literature published in the last 18 months reveals the extensive use of various bioinformatics approaches related to COVID-19.[17,18] Bioinformatics enables scientists to reduce the number of experiments and quicken the target discovery, drug discovery, or drug repurposing process. Drug repurposing is particularly attractive because the knowledge of the drug safety is already available, which saves time and reduces cost.

In addition to the previous description, it is important to point out that bioinformatics approaches are enhanced by integration of various data. Genomics, transcriptomic, and metabolomic data are integrated with proteomics (proteins) data through data science techniques to make predictions about protein biomarkers of a disease. The predictive modeling method helps narrow the search space of druggable protein targets from a list of proteins involved in the disease pathway. The druggable proteins identified should be unique to the disease to avoid off-target effects.

■ **Box 17.1** Key steps in Target and Drug Discovery

Step 1: Identify differentially expressed proteins in the disease.
Step 2: Use bioinformatics and AI[a] approaches to identify structure and function of those proteins.
Step 3: Druggability analysis of the proteins.
Step 4: Functional assays to experimentally validate the druggable protein target.
Step 5: Select an experimentally validated target for drug discovery.
Step 6: Learn binding pocket information from crystal structures of protein-ligand complex.
Step 7: Use molecular modelling and AI approaches to screen hits (either repurpose drugs or NCE[b]s) by molecular docking of drug molecules in the binding pocket.
Step 8: Prioritize top hits using calculated docking scores or binding energies.
Step 9: In Vitro/In Vivo evaluation of safety and efficacy to identify lead molecules.
Step 10: Clinical trials of the drug lead candidates to identify active drug molecule.

---

[a]AI stands for "artificial intelligence" approaches, where using trained mathematical models, structure and properties are predicted;

[b]NCE stands for "new chemical entity" which means new drug molecule.

To identify the differential expression of genes and their protein products in the diseased and the normal case, various forms of high-throughput expression profiling is carried out and data are deposited in many public research databases, such as the National Center for Biotechnology Information Expression Atlas.[20,21] Various forms of data analysis–based machine learning algorithms are used to identify the differentially expressed genes, which are then mapped to their respective protein products.[22] The protein products that are identified with druggable pockets and unique differential expression with respect to the disease are proposed as possible therapeutic targets.[22]

Further, functional assays are carried out to validate a proposed target. If target protein inhibition is proposed as a therapeutic strategy to overcome the overexpression of the target protein in the disease, gene knockout experiments are performed, in which the gene corresponding to the target is knocked out and thus the target protein is not expressed; if an attempt to induce the disease fails in such a case, the target can be considered and experimentally validated.[23] Although experimental methods are still required to validate proposed targets, the machine learning and bioinformatics approaches are useful to carry out the data analysis required to identify perturbed molecular pathways in a disease, which leads to identifying novel therapeutic targets. A dedicated resource of COVID-19–related differential gene expression data is available at CovidExpress for the leveraging of bioinformatics and machine learning approaches in identifying novel therapeutic targets.[24]

A recent example of identifying a drug target and repurposing a known drug molecule for COVID-19 is related to

baricitinib, a known immunomodulator. Baricitinib is an oral Janus kinase (JAK)1/JAK2 inhibitor approved for the treatment of rheumatoid arthritis. Based on a large repository of structured medical information extracted from the scientific literature using machine learning, scientists identified JAK1/JAK2 and AP2-associated protein kinase 1 (AAK1) proteins as potential targets for treatment of COVID-19.[25,26] AAK1 is known to regulate endocytosis. Further, it was predicted through modeling studies that baricitinib would bind to the AAK1 protein as well, which would inhibit virus entry. A combination of baricitinib with an antiviral drug (remdesivir) is in clinical testing. Thus a multifaceted approach comprising experimental, theoretical, computational, and data science–based techniques is used to identify drug targets and drug molecules for COVID-19.

The host genetic diversity that determines susceptibility to SARS-CoV-2 and disease severity makes a case for the use of precision medicine methodology in COVID-19 therapeutics. One of the challenging problems in COVID-19 treatment, for example, is the knowledge gap of predicting which patients have a genetic predilection for a cytokine storm and thus would benefit most from immunosuppressive medication such as corticosteroids. To deal with this challenge, Lam C. et al.[27] used a precision medicine–based artificial intelligence (AI)[a] model to make recommendations on the use of corticosteroids for COVID-19.[27]

Virus-Targeted Antiviral Therapy: Druggable Nonstructural Proteins

In this section, the functions of the nonstructural proteins of SARS-CoV-2 are briefly described to indicate why some of these proteins are targets to treat COVID-19. Table 17.2 provides a summary of the various NSPs and their functions. The idea has been to inhibit functions of these NSPs by binding them with small molecules of appropriate structure. The function of NSP11 is yet not understood.

Papain-Like Protease

Papain-like protease (PLpro) is a named subdomain of NSP3. Viral proteins also act on the host to shut down the immune system to enable their proliferation and growth. The human body has the capacity to sense antigens or foreign agents such as viruses and bacteria. It signals the immune machinery of the body to destroy them. PLpro has been identified with the function of interfering with the immune signaling proteins in the human body and consequently shutting down the host's innate immune response. Targeting PLpro with drug molecules to inhibit its function can be one of the therapeutic strategies in SARS-CoV-2. There purposing approach based on small molecules has not used this strategy in any significant way. However, there have been reports on efforts to

---

[a]AI stands for artificial intelligence approaches, in which by the use of trained mathematical models, structure and properties are predicted.

Table 17.2 Various Nonstructured Proteins and Their Functions

Target NSP	Target Function
NSP1	Degrades host mRNA, inhibits IFN signaling
NSP2	Degrades host mRNA, inhibits IFN signaling
NSP 3 (PLpro)	Degrades host mRNA, inhibits IFN signaling, cleaves polyprotein
NSP$_4$	Required for replication, DMV morphology formation with NSP3
NSPp5 (Mpro)	Cleaves polyprotein
NSP6	DMV morphology formation with NSP3 and NSP4
NSP7 (RdRp)	Forms hexadecameric complex, processivity clamp RdRp and Primase complex
NSP8 (RdRp)	Forms hexadecameric complex, processivity clamp RdRp and primase complex
NSP9	RNA binding
NSP10	Stimulates activity of NSP14 and NSP16
NSP12 (RdRp)	RdRp, virus replication and transcription
NSP13	Virus mRNA capping, RNA helicase, 5′-triphosphatase
NSP14	Virus mRNA capping and proofreading: 3′5′-exoribonuclease
NSP15	Endoribonuclease, favors cleavage of RNA
NSP16	Virus mRNA capping

DMV, Double-membrane vesicles; *IFN*, interferon; *Mpro*, main protease; *NSP*, nonstructured protein; *PLpro*, papain-like protease; *RdRp*, RNA-dependent RNA polymerase.
Naqvi AAT, Kisa F, Mohammad T et al. Insights into SARS CoV-2 genome, structure, evolution, pathogenesis and therapies: structural genomics approach. *Biochim Biophys Acta Mol Basis of Dis.* 2020;1866(10):165878. doi:10.1016/j.bbadis.2020.165878; and Arya R, Kumari S, Pandey B, et al. Structural insights into SARS-CoV-2 proteins. *J Mol Biol.* 2021;433(2):166725. doi: 10.1016/j.jmb.2020.11.024.

develop new drug molecules to inhibit PLpro.[28] A few molecules, including large peptides, have been found to bind to PLpro, as pictorially represented in Fig. 17.2.

Main Protease

The main protease (Mpro, also known as 3CLpro), which is a named subdomain part of the NSP5, is involved in the function of cleaving the polyproteins into functional proteins in the viral cycle and thus lends itself to being a therapeutic target. An inhibitor bound in the active site is shown in Fig. 17.3.

RNA Polymerase (NSP12-NSP7-NSP8)

In the viral replication of coronaviruses, RdRp plays a key role, and it is formed by a complex of NSP12-NSP7-NSP8 and thus it lends itself to be a therapeutic target for a drug molecule. It is notable that remdesivir, a drug designed for the Ebola virus, through repurposing strategies has received a great deal of attention as an RdRp inhibitor and potential treatment for COVID-19. RdRp with a bound inhibitor is shown in Fig. 17.4.

The binding pose and interaction of remdesivir with the target, which is an approved drug for this target, is shown in Fig. 17.5.

Remdesivir is a prodrug. The active form of remdesivir is shown in Fig. 17.5. The figure shows the binding conformation of the active form of remdesivir and the RdRp target in the background.

Fig. 17.6 shows the types of interactions between active form of remdesivir and the RdRp target and the interacting residues of RdRp. Most of the interactions are either H-bonding or van der Waals interactions.

Helicase (NSP13)

Helicase is a named part of NSP13 that plays a key role in catalyzing the unwinding in the 5′ to 3′ direction of double-stranded RNA (dsRNA) or structured RNA into single strands. Although it is known to possess a zinc-binding domain, this can be targeted with metal chelators. Helicase with bound inhibitor is shown in Fig. 17.7.

Exoribonuclease/Guanine-N7 Methyltransferase (NSP14-NSP10 Complex)

The protein exoribonuclease (ExoN) is involved in the proofreading of viral genome synthesis. It is being proposed that in addition to RdRp inhibitors, exoribonuclease inhibitors could be an additional therapeutic strategy of attack against SARS-CoV-2 viruses. Exoribonuclease with a bound inhibitor in the active site is shown in Fig. 17.8

The binding site of S-adenosyl-L-methionine is (SAM) is an attractive target to develop inhibitors using small molecules that could impede SAM or guanosine-P3-adenosine-5′,5′-triphosphate (GpppA) binding, thus suppressing the N7-methyltransferase (MTase) activity of NSP14 and thereby affecting replication.

Other nonstructural proteins (NSPs) involved in essential function of the viral cycle that can be targeted by drug molecules are (1) RNA nucleotide-2′O-methyltransferase complex (NSP16-NSP10), (2) RNA uridylate–specific

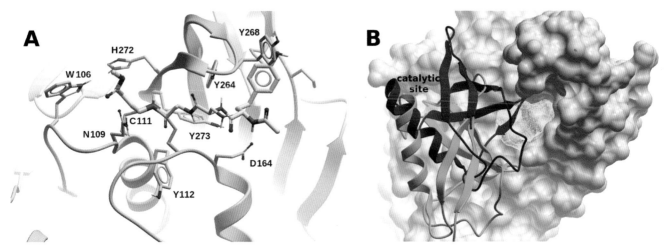

Fig. 17.2 (A) The complex of papain-like protease (PLpro) and a peptide inhibitor VIR251 covalently bound to the active site (PDB ID 6XW4). (B) Catalytic binding site indicated by the *yellow mesh;* ubiquitin, a human protein, is depicted in *red;* and ISG15 is depicted in *green ribbon.* The N-terminus of these two proteins is inserted within the catalytic site. Ubiquitin and ISG15 regulate immune response. It is proposed that PLpro hinders their role as immune regulators and a small molecule might inhibit the interaction of these two proteins with PLpro. (From Cavasotto CN, Sánchez Lamas M, Maggini J. Functional and druggability analysis of the SARS CoV-2 proteome. *Eur J Pharmacol.* 2021;890[2021]:17370. https://doi.org/10.1016/j.ejphar.2020.173705.)

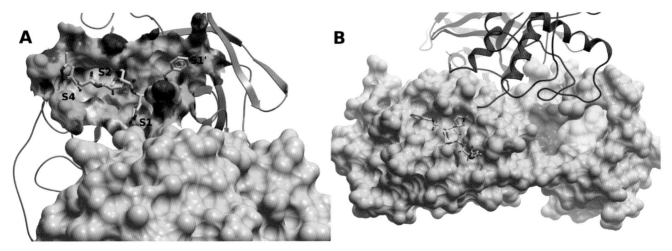

Fig. 17.3 The Main Protease of SARS-CoV-2 Along With Its Binding Site in Complex With Peptide Inhibitor N3 (PDB 6LU7). (A) Protein subsites S1, S2, S4, and S1′ are labeled and featured in different colors. Main protease (Mpro) is dimeric and has two protomers. The molecular surface of the one protomer is shown in *light green.* (B) A potential active site *(brown)* on Mpro with a catalytic site nearby lined by amino acid residues T199, Y237, Y239, L271, L272, G275, M276, and A285-L287 *(yellow surface)* is shown. Mpro is represented by a *green* molecular surface. N3 is also displayed within the catalytic site *(light yellow).* The other protomer is represented in the *magenta ribbon.* It is proposed that a small molecule binding to this potential site might interfere with homodimerization and inhibit the replication of the virus by interfering with its viral cycle. (From Cavasotto CN, Sánchez Lamas M, Maggini J. Functional and druggability analysis of the SARS CoV-2 proteome. *Eur J Pharmacol.* 2021;890[2021]:17370. https://doi.org/10.1016/j.ejphar.2020.173705.)

endoribonuclease (NSP15), (3) nonstructural protein 9 (NSP9), (4) adenosine diphosphate (ADP)-ribose-phosphatase (NSP3 domain), (5) ubiquitin-like 1 domain (NSP3), (6) SARS-unique domain (NSP3 domain), and (7) nucleic acid–binding region (NAB, NSP3 domain). Examples of use of these targets for drug therapy are not available.

Potential Inhibitors of Virus Replication

Blocking of virus replication in host cells is attempted by inhibition of either selected polymerases such as

RdRp or selected proteases such as 3CLpro proteins or PLpro proteins.[28,29] Considerable literature exists on studies of inhibition of both of these targets. Inhibition of RdRp has been a more successful approach based on the FDA approval status for remdesivir than inhibition of proteases such as 3CLpro, although the latter has received greater attention from medicinal scientists, as indicated by the voluminous literature available thus far. Among the repurpose drugs, protease inhibitors such as

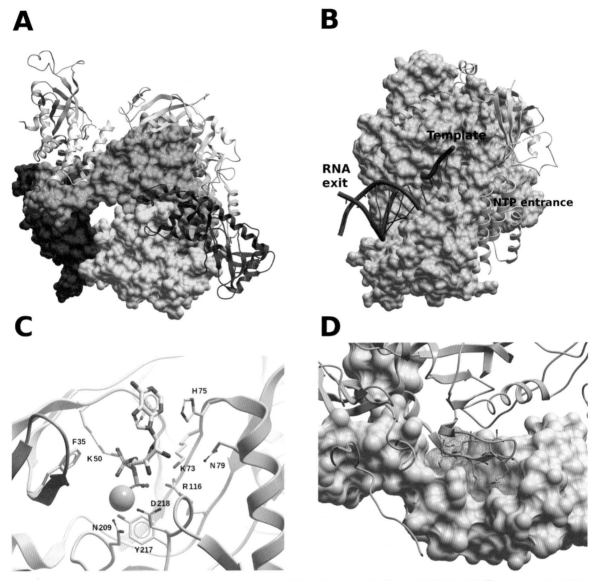

Fig. 17.4 A Ligand Bound in the Active Site of the RNA-Dependent RNA polymerase (RdRp) of SARS-CoV-2. The color code of (A) which represents different parts of the complex is as follows, NSP7: *white ribbon;* NSP8-2: *light blue ribbon*; NSP8-1: *yellow ribbon.* The RNA polymerase is characterized by three subdomains called palm, fingers, and thumb. The colour code representing the NSP12 domains are as follows: palm, *yellow;* fingers, *tans;* thumb, *red;* interface, *pale green ribbon;* nucleotidyl transferase domain (NiRAN), *magenta ribbon.* (B) RdRp complex bound to RNA. NSP12 is displayed as a *green surface.* Primer RNA, *blue;* template RNA, *red;* NSP7, *yellow ribbon;* NSP8-1, *gray ribbon.* (C) A molecule of ADP-Mg²⁺ within the NiRAN domain of NSP12. Interacting residues are shown, in what may constitute a druggable binding site. (D) Target site in NSP8 *(light yellow surface).* The predicted binding site is represented using a *blue mesh* representation, and NSP12 is shown as gray ribbon. *NTP,* Nucleoside triphosphate. (From Cavasotto CN, Sánchez Lamas M, Maggini J. Functional and druggability analysis of the SARS CoV-2 proteome. *Eur J Pharmacol.* 2021;890[2021]:17370. https://doi.org/10.1016/j.ejphar.2020.173705.)

boceprevir have not been found as promising as polymerase inhibitors such as nucleoside analogs (remdesivir). Various trials are underway with newer candidates for both classes of inhibitors to block SARS-CoV-2 replication.

Apart from remdesivir, another antiviral drug, favipiravir, originally indicated for influenza is now being widely used prominently against COVID-19. Molnupiravir is an investigational drug currently undergoing clinical trials. These three drugs are repurposed compounds belonging to the class of nucleosides.

Virus-Targeted Antiviral Therapy: Druggable Structural Proteins

Structural proteins S, E, M, and N are the viral proteins whose function is essential in the viral cycle and by way of their involvement in the assembly and stability of the virus. They could also be attractive targets for drug molecules, as described in later in this section.

Spike Protein

The spike-protein of SARS-CoV-2 is a large homotrimeric multidomain glycoprotein.[30] Many glycosylated S

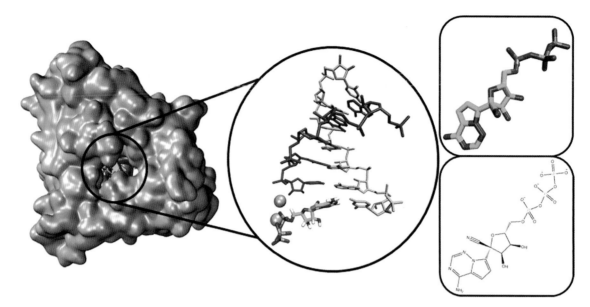

Fig. 17.5 Graphic Depiction of the Binding Pose of the Active Form Derived From Remdesivir With RNA-Dependent RNA Polymerase. (From Arba M, Wahyudi ST, Brunt DJ, et al. Mechanistic insight on the remdesivir binding to RNA-dependent RNA polymerase (RdRp) of SARS CoV-2. *Comput Biol Med.* 2021;129:104156. doi:10.1016/j.compbiomed.2020.104156.)

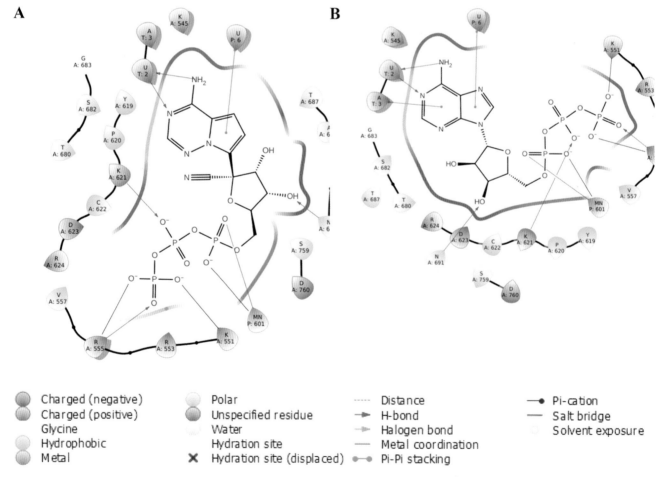

Fig. 17.6 Interacting Residues of RNA-Dependent RNA Polymerase With the Active Form Derived From Drug Remdesivir. (From Arba M, Wahyudi ST, Brunt DJ, et al. Mechanistic insight on the remdesivir binding to RNA-dependent RNA polymerase (RdRp) of SARS CoV-2. *Comput Biol Med.* 2021;129:104156. doi:10.1016/j.compbiomed.2020.104156.)

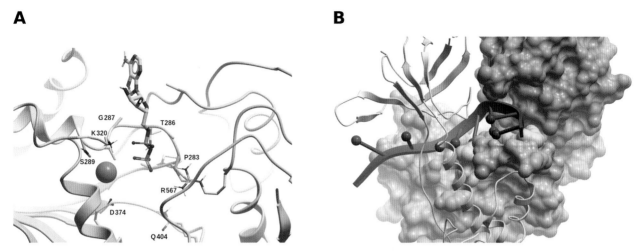

Fig. 17.7 Ligand Bound in the Active Site of Helicase, a Nonstructural Druggable Protein of SARS-CoV-2. (A) Adenosine diphosphate–Mg^{2+} bound within NSP13. This site has been identified as being involved in nucleoside triphosphate hydrolysis in SARS-CoV and could constitute a druggable site. (B) Two potential borderline druggable binding sites identified in NSP13. NSP13 is represented as a *green ribbon,* but NSP13 domains 1A and 2A are displayed as *gray* and *tan* molecular surfaces, respectively. NSP13 is represented as a *green ribbon,* but NSP13 domains 1A and 2A are displayed as *gray* and *tan* molecular surfaces, respectively, with the structure of RNA in *blue.* Small molecules binding to these sites might interfere with RNA binding, thereby inhibiting the replication. (From Cavasotto CN, Sánchez Lamas M, Maggini J. Functional and druggability analysis of the SARS CoV-2 proteome. *Eur J Pharmacol.* 2021;890[2021]:17370. https://doi.org/10.1016/j.ejphar.2020.173705.)

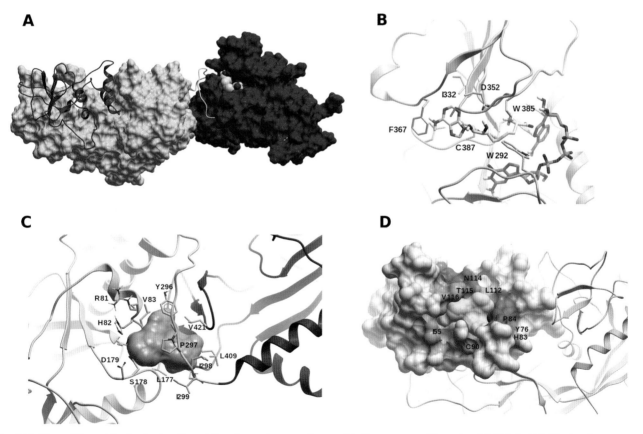

Fig. 17.8 Ligand Bound in the Active Site of Exoribonuclease, a Druggable Nonstructural Protein of SARS-CoV-2. The binding site and structure of ExoN/MTase (NSP14-NSPp10) complex is shown in Fig. 17.8. (A) ExoN NSP14 domain (in green) and the methyltransferase (MTase) domain (in red) are connected by the hinge loop F286-G300 *(yellow).* NSP10 is shown in *dark gray ribbon,* and a S-adenosyl-L-methionine (SAM) molecule *(light yellow carbons)* is displayed within the catalytic site. (B) Model of SAM *(light yellow carbons)* within the catalytic site of the MTase domain of SARS-CoV-2 NSP14 with a proposed small molecule inhibitor guanosine-P3-adenosine-5′,5′-triphosphate (GpppA) *(green carbons).* (C) Potential druggable (allosteric) binding site in the vicinity of the hinge region F286-G300 (in *yellow*), including Y296 and P297. The linked NSP14 domains ExoN and MTase are displayed in *green* and *magenta,* respectively. (D) Druggable site *(yellow* surface) within a potential active site on NSP10 *(lighter or darker brown).* The ExoN domain of NSP14 is shown as *green ribbon.* (From Cavasotto CN, Sánchez Lamas M, Maggini J. Functional and druggability analysis of the SARS CoV-2 proteome. *Eur J Pharmacol.* 2021;890[2021]:17370. https://doi.org/10.1016/j.ejphar.2020.173705.)

proteins cover the surface of SARS-CoV-2 and bind to the host cell receptor ACE2, mediating viral cell entry.[31] When the S protein binds to the receptor, TM protease serine 2 (TMPRSS2), a type 2 TM serine protease located on the host cell membrane, promotes virus entry into the cell by activating the S protein. Once the virus enters the cell, the virus hijacks the replication mechanism of the host and replicates itself.

With a size of 180 to 200 kDa, the S protein consists of an extracellular N-terminus, a TM domain anchored in the viral membrane, and a short intracellular C-terminal segment. S normally exists in a metastable, prefusion conformation; once the virus interacts with the host cell, extensive structural rearrangement of the S protein occurs, allowing the virus to fuse with the host cell membrane. The spikes are coated with polysaccharide molecules to camouflage them, evading surveillance of the host immune system during entry. The total length of SARS-CoV-2 spike is 1273 amino acids and consists of a signal peptide (amino acids 1–13) located at the N-terminus S1 subunit (14–685 residues), and the S2 subunit (686–1273 residues); the last two regions are responsible for receptor binding and membrane fusion, respectively.

S1 Subunit

In the S1 subunit, there are two binding domains: the N-terminal domain (14–305 residues) and the RBD (319–541 residues).

S2 Subunit

The fusion peptide (FP) (788–806 residues), heptapeptide repeat sequence 1 (HR1) (912–984 residues), HR2 (1163–1213 residues), TM domain (1213–1237 residues), and cytoplasm domain (1237–1273 residues) make up the S2 subunit.

During viral infection, target cell proteases activate the S protein by cleaving it into S1 and S2 subunits, which is necessary for activating the membrane fusion domain after viral entry into target cells.

The host RBD of the spike is situated in the S1 subunit, which binds to the cell receptor ACE2 in the region of aminopeptidase N of the receptor. Mutations (e.g., from SARS-CoV to SARS-CoV-2) of key residues play an important role in enhancing the interaction with ACE2. F486 in SARS-CoV-2, compared with I472 in SARS-CoV RBD, forms strong aromatic–aromatic interactions with ACE2 Y83; E484 in SARS-CoV-2 (C terminal domain [CTD]), compared with P470 in SARS RBD, forms ionic interactions with K31, which leads to higher affinity for receptor binding for SARS-CoV-2. For the spike to qualify as an attractive therapeutic target, the RBD should be a conserved region among the many mutations of SARS-CoV-2; whether this is the case is unclear.

The S2 subunit comprises successively an FP, heptapeptide repeat 1 (HR1), HR2, TM domain, and cytoplasmic domain (CD) and is responsible for viral fusion and entry. FP is a short segment of 15 to 20 conserved amino acids of the viral family, composed mainly of hydrophobic residues, such as glycine (G) or alanine (A), which anchor to the target membrane when the S protein adopts the pre-hairpin conformation. Research has shown that FP plays an essential role in mediating membrane fusion by disrupting and connecting lipid bilayers of the host cell membrane. HR1 and HR2 are composed of a repetitive heptapeptide: HPPHCPC, in which H is a hydrophobic or traditionally bulky residue, P is a polar or hydrophilic residue, and C is another charged residue. HR1 and HR2 form the six-helical bundle (6-HB), which is essential for the viral fusion and entry function of the S2 subunit. HR1 is located at the C-terminus of a hydrophobic FP, and HR2 is located at the N-terminus of the TM domain. The downstream TM domain anchors the S protein to the viral membrane, and the S2 subunit ends in a CT.

RBD binds to ACE2, and S2 changes conformation by inserting FP into the target cell membrane, exposing the pre-hairpin coiled-coil of the HR1 domain and triggering interaction between the HR2 domain and HR1 trimer to form 6-HB, thus bringing the viral envelope and cell membrane into proximity for viral fusion and entry. HR1 forms a homotrimeric assembly in which three highly conserved hydrophobic grooves on the surface that bind to HR2 are exposed. The HR2 domain forms both a rigid helix and a flexible loop to interact with the HR1 domain. In the postfusion hairpin conformation, there are many strong interactions between the HR1 and HR2 domains inside the helical region, which is designated the fusion core region–HR1 core and HR2 core regions. Targeting the heptad repeat (HR) has attracted much attention.

In summary, the spike has at least three sites to be targeted: (1) the RBD, which can be targeted to prevent viral entry; (2) the HR1, which can be targeted to prevent viral fusion into the cell membrane; and (3) the serine protease inhibitor of TMPRSS2, which can prevent the cleavage of the spike protein at the S1/S2 and S2 sites, which is required for viral entry.

Envelope Protein

Structural protein E of SARS-CoV-2 is a small homopentameric membrane protein (75 amino acids per protomer) that has been shown to possess the essential function of being involved in the viral particle assembly in SARS-CoV-2. The N-terminal region of the structural protein E spans the lipid bilayer twice, and the C-terminal is exposed to the interior of the SARS-CoV-2 virus. In infectious bronchitis virus and SARS-CoV virus, the E protein interacts with the viral M protein through an undefined region. It also interacts with host protein associated with Lin Seven 1, a factor associated with pathogenesis through its C-terminus. In many coronaviruses, the E protein works as an ion-channeling viroporin, which affects the production of inflammatory mediators such as cytokines, consequently affecting the immune response. No binding sites of E are known for small molecule binding.

Membrane and Nucleocapsid Proteins

Structural protein M of SARS-CoV-2 is a membrane homodimeric glycoprotein that forms part of the virion. In SARS-CoV, the structural proteins M and N interact and act as a nexus between virus membrane formation and RNA association in the virion. They are also known to interfere with the immune signaling and immune response of the host by way of inhibiting interferon (IFN) signaling in the case of SARS-CoV and MERS-related diseases.

For a more detailed functional description of the druggable proteome of SARS-CoV-2, crystal structure to access the protein structure of these known drug targets of SARS-CoV-2, analysis of the binding sites and details of compounds active (in vitro) against these targets, the 2021 review by Cavasotto et al.[9] may be accessed.

Potential Inhibitors of Viral Entry

1. For the RBD as the target, monoclonal neutralizing antibodies are the potential inhibitors. A few promising therapeutic solutions based on mAbs are known and being used: cocktail of bamlanivimab and etesevimab, cocktail of casirivimab and imdevimab, and sotrovimab.
2. For the HR1 domain as the target, generally, peptides are chosen as the fusion inhibitor. Some of the peptides are SARS-CoV-2 HR2P (1168–1203) residues or a lipopeptide EK1C4. A non–peptide inhibitor, nelfinavir mesylate, is also known.
3. For the spike protein cleavage site at the S1/S2 as the target, protease inhibitors are used. Examples are camostat mesylate, a potent serine protease inhibitor of TMPRSS2, and E64d, a potent cysteine protease inhibitor of cathepsin L.

Another class of drug called ivermectin has been found effective in some trials for decreasing replication of SARS-CoV-2. Ivermectin is an antiparasitic drug. The mechanism proposed for its alleged effectiveness against SARS-CoV-2 is as follows. Ivermectin complexes with transport factors called importin alpha and importin beta and prevents them from transporting the SARS-CoV-2 virus into the cell,[32] thus preventing virus entry. However, among all virus entry inhibitors, mAbs appear to be receiving greater attention owing to their perceived better performance in actual use.

Host-Targeted Antiviral Therapy

Besides targeting the viral proteome that comes under the category of direct viral-targeted antiviral therapy, druggable proteins in the host that are involved in viral entry and viral hijacking of host mechanisms for replication also could be targeted. Viruses causing respiratory illnesses such as influenza, parainfluenza, and coronaviruses rely on host-human proteases for the activation of their entry factors that facilitate membrane fusion and entry into airway epithelial cells. The transmembrane protease serine 2 (TMPRSS2) plays a crucial role in both the cleavage and activation of both hemagglutinin (HA) of human influenza viruses and the spike (S) protein of SARS-causing coronaviruses. Although TMPRSS2 plays an indispensable role for host development and homeostasis, attempts have been made to target TMPRSS2 to block viral entry as one of the strategies in host-targeted antiviral therapy against COVID-19. Currently, camostat, which is a serine protease inhibitor and currently under clinical trials, can block viral entry of SARS-CoV-2 and influenza viruses through the mechanism mentioned previously, and this will constitute for the design of inhibitors with a broad spectrum of antiviral activity against respiratory viruses. However, such targets are not without limitations, as was the case with camostat. Although camostat inhibited SARS-CoV-2 entry and replication, it did not eliminate viral replication, which indicates the presence of other means for entry of the spike.

Another alternative strategy for host-directed antiviral therapies that is being explored is the depletion of intracellular nucleotide pools necessary to viral replication. However, this approach is not without challenges, as reflected by the general fact that among approved antiviral drug therapies for many diseases, only about 10% of them constitute host-directed antiviral therapy.[33]

Targets to Improve Immune Response Against the SARS-CoV-2 Virus

SARS-CoV-2 affects the immune system and avoids being eliminated in early stages. The human immune system lags in its response, but when it eventually responds it might result in uncontrolled secretion of inflammatory cytokines, thus creating critical conditions that lead to pulmonary tissue damage, functional impairment, reduced lung capacity, and multiorgan failure. At the same time, insufficiency of immunity would increase viral replication and tissue damage. Thus a balanced host immune response against SARS-CoV-2 is necessary to control infection.

A few host-targeted therapies have shown potential against COVID-19 and are in use:
1. Tocilizumab (TCZ) is a recombinant humanized anti–IL-6R monoclonal antibody. It inhibits both the soluble and membrane-bound forms of the IL-6 receptor and has been tried in cases of serious infections.[34] Sarilumab is another recombinant monoclonal antibody targeting IL-6R, which has been found effective.
2. INFs have been proposed as a potential treatment for COVID-19 because of their antiviral properties. INFs (α, β) are cytokines with antiviral properties.

Some of the viral proteins are known to shut down the human immune system, and therefore reactivation of the human immune system to fight the virus forms a therapeutic strategy against COVID-19. Because the INFs trigger cytokine release, early administration of IFN-β in combination with antiviral drugs could be a promising therapeutic strategy against COVID-19.[35] Results of many clinical trials are unknown.

Many antiinflammatory molecules are under preclinical trials.[36]

Targets and Emerging Therapeutic Strategies Addressing Morbidity Caused by COVID-19 During and After Infection

In studies carried out to analyze the genomic data of mild, moderate, and severe COVID-19 infection, it was found that persons with a genetic make-up corresponding to an elevated immune response and cytokine storm are likely candidates for severe COVID-19 infection.[37-40] Cytokines are cell-signaling proteins that mediate immune response and inflammation, and immunomodulatory therapies are being adopted as therapeutic strategy against COVID-19.[41] In developing immunomodulatory therapies against COVID-19, strategies include inhibition of specific cytokines or signaling molecules and nonspecific immune suppression with corticosteroids such as dexamethasone. Inhibitors of cytokines such as IL-1 and IL-6 include anakinra, tocilizumab, sarilumab, and siltuximab; of anti–tumor necrosis factor-α, adalimumab, and infliximab; and of JAK, baricitinib, and ruxolitinib. Immune modulatory therapy increases the risk for other microbial infections, and antimicrobial therapies are sometimes used for prevention.

Another complication caused by COVID-19 is blood clotting, which is treated with blood thinners or anticoagulants.[10] Having comorbidities also puts one at increased risk for COVID-19–related severity and fatality. According to early reports, preexisting respiratory diseases, diabetes, and hypertension have been identified as leading risk factors for severe and fatal COVID-19.[11] As data on comorbidities associated with poor outcome of COVID-19 are emerging, consensus on specific therapeutic strategies is evolving. Another emerging area for new treatment strategies is long-COVID.[12] Consensus on treatments in these areas is expected to develop with time as our knowledge improves.

Interaction Between Virus and Human Proteins (Protein–Protein Interaction)

Quite a few research efforts have been made in identifying interactions between the virus and human proteins.[42,43] New targets have been identified and repurpose drugs have been proposed based on cell-line data. A brief description on the process followed to identify protein–protein interactions is as follows:

1. Collection of literature experimental data or create database on physical interaction between human protein and SARS-CoV-2 based on experiments

2. Use bioinformatics tool to map the protein–protein interactions
3. Analysis of interactome

In addition, data on host–drug interactions are retrieved from literature. Subsequently, an analysis of interactome leads to identification of new targets and therapeutic leads, which is then subjected to experimental validation. Such an exhaustive procedure has been followed in their work on identifying new targets for repurposing known drugs by Gordon et al.[43] From the analysis of interactome, ideas are derived for new targets and therapeutic solutions, followed by experimental validation. Initially, these researchers[43] identified human proteins that physically associated with each of the SARS-CoV-2 proteins using affinity-purification mass spectrometry, which led to a list of 332 high-confidence protein–protein interactions between SARS-CoV-2 and human proteins. Of the protein–protein interactions, 66 were identified as druggable human proteins or host factors targeted by 69 approved or investigational compounds. After screening a subset of multiple viral assays, the researchers found two sets of compounds that displayed antiviral activity: inhibitors of mRNA translation and predicted regulators of the sigma-1 and sigma-2 receptors.

In another example of protein–protein interaction analysis, researchers found that one of the drugs chlorpromazine (CPZ), an antipsychotic drug, showed an in vitro activity in the cell-line in terms of half maximum inhibitory concentration of 8.2 μM against SARS-CoV-2.[44] Subsequently it was put to phase III clinical trial. Drugs such as CPZ target many proteins in the host. It was observed from data that host protein calmodulin (CALM1) interacts with ORF3 protein from porcine epidemic diarrhea virus having Coronaviridae genome. CALM1 has a controlling effect on Ca^{2+}/calmodulin-dependent protein kinase II (CAMKII proteins), which are targeted by coronaviruses, as well. Indeed, CAMK2D and CAMK2G interact with NSP3 of SARS-CoV and NSP2 of mouse hepatitis virus, respectively. CPZ also interacts with CALM1. The interactions with CALM1 could account for the inhibition of coronaviruses, including SARS-CoV-2 by CPZ.[42,44]

The researchers manually curated the literature to assemble a unique dataset of 1311 coronavirus-host protein–protein interactions.[42] A technique called network analysis revealed coronavirus connections to RNA processing and translation, DNA damage and pathogen sensing, IFN production, and metabolic pathways. This led to renewed focus on protein–protein interactions with translation modulators (GIGYF2-EIF4E2), components of the nuclear pore, proteins involved in mitochondria homeostasis (PHB, PHB2, STOML2), and methylation pathways (MAT2A/B).

In other reports,[45,46] researchers describe the factors on how SARS-CoV-2 disrupts the immune response of the host through specific protein–protein interactions. NSP16 binds mRNA recognition domains of U1/U2 small nuclear RNA (snRNA) and disrupts mRNA splicing. NSP1 binds in the mRNA entry channel of the ribosome to disrupt protein translation. NSP8 and NSP9 bind the signal recognition particle and disrupt protein trafficking. These disruptions of protein production suppress the IFN response to infection.

Analysis of protein–protein interactions followed by experimentation for validation has the potential to lead to new targets and new antiviral therapies for COVID-19, particularly by repurposing known drugs.

Overview of Therapies Based on Repurpose Drugs and Corresponding Targets

Antiviral therapies (virus-targeted therapies) have the greatest effect early in the course of the disease, whereas immunosuppressive/antiinflammatory therapies (host-targeted therapies) are more beneficial in the later stages of COVID-19. Hence, combination of both therapies is being explored for COVID-19. Tables 17.3 and 17.4 provide a list of therapies based on repurpose drugs, some of which are currently used in many regions of the world and some are yet to be proven. There are many clinical trials underway with repurpose drug candidates.[47]

A combination of both therapies is employed at different stages of the disease progression, as discussed in Table 17.1. There are numerous repurpose molecules and drugs that have been studied for treatment of COVID-19. Many of them are in clinical trials.[48] Some of the molecules show promise during preclinical trials but do not pass clinical trials. A few of the drugs mentioned in Tables 17.3 and 17.4 have already been employed in therapies to save millions of lives

Table 17.3 Selected Examples of Virus-Targeted Therapies

Function	Repurpose Drug	Target/Action Related to COVID-19
Antiviral	Favipiravir[a]: Active form is derived from nucleoside metabolite	RdRp polymerase inhibitor
Antiviral	Remdesivir: Prodrug of active form has nucleoside structure	RdRp polymerase inhibitor
Antiviral	Sofosbuvir/daclatasvir: Sofosbuvir—synthetic nucleoside drug Daclatasvir—nonnucleoside drug	Sofosbuvir: RdRp inhibitor. In HCV treatment, daclatasvir binds to NSP5A and prevents replication. In COVID-19, the mechanisms are expected to be similar[b]
Antiviral	Ribavirin: Synthetic nucleoside drug	Mechanism not established. Could be by RdRp polymerase inhibition
Antiviral	Molnupiravir: Synthetic nucleoside	RdRp polymerase inhibitor.[c] Drug under investigation
Antiviral	Oseltamivir	Neuraminidase inhibitor. Not considered effective against SARS-CoV-2[a]
Antiviral	Darunavir	3CLpro protease inhibitor. Not effective against SARS-CoV-2[a]
Antiviral	Lopinavir/ritonavir	3CLpro protease inhibitor. Not effective against SARS-CoV-2[a]
Antiviral	Nelfinavir	3CLpro protease inhibitor. Effective in vitro. More studies underway. Combination drug with virus entry inhibitor, cepharanthine[d]
Prevention of viral entry	Neutralizing monoclonal antibodies: (not repurposed) cocktail of (1) casirivimab and imdevimab and (2) sotrovimab	Binds to RBD of spike protein
Prevention of viral entry	Cepharanthine, an experimental alkaloid having macrocyclic structure	Predicted to bind to RBD domain of spike protein[e]

HCV, Hepatitis C; RBD, receptor binding domain; RdRp, RNA-dependent RNA polymerase.
Among the virus targeted therapies, RdRp polymerase, 3CLpro protease, PLpro protease and receptor binding domains of the S1 portion of spike protein of the virus are the targets that have received a lot of attention. In host-targeted therapy, many antiinflammatory drugs and immune modulators are under trial. Popular targets in this are interleukin-6 receptors and Janus kinase-1 (JAK1) and JAK2 proteins.[a]Parastoo T, Eftekhari S, Chizari M, et al. A review of potential suggested drugs for coronavirus disease (COVID-19) treatment. Eur J Pharmacol. 2021;895:173890. https://doi.org/10.1016/j.ejphar.2021.173890.
[b]Sacramento CQ, Fintelman-Rodrigues N, Temerozo JR, et al. In vitro antiviral activity of the anti-HCV drugs daclatasvir and sofosbuvir against SARS-CoV-2, the aetiological agent of COVID-19. J Antimicrob Chemother. 2021;76(7):1874-1885. https://doi.org/10.1093/jac/dkab072.
[c]Kabinger F, Stiller C, Schmitzova J, et al. Mechanism of molnupiravir-induced SARS CoV-2 mutagenesis. bioRxiv 2021.05.11.443555. doi: 10.1101/2021.05.11.443555.
[d]Ohashi H, Watashi K, Saso W, et al. Potential anti-COVID-19 agents, cepharanthine and nelfinavir, and their usage for combination treatment. iScience 2021;24(4):102367. https://doi.org/10.1016/j.isci.2021.102367.
[e]Rogosnitzky M, Okediji P, Koman, I. Cepharanthine: a review of the antiviral potential of a Japanese-approved alopecia drug in COVID-19. Pharmacol Rep. 2020;72:1509-1516. https://doi.org/10.1007/s43440-020-00132-z.

Table 17.4 Selected Examples of Host-Targeted Therapies

Function	Repurpose Drug	Target/Action Related to COVID-19
Antiviral and immune modulation[d]	IFN-β1a	Activates proteins that degrade RNA; clinical trials in combination with antivirals also under study
Antiinflammatory	Tocilizumab	Blocks IL-6 receptors
Antiinflammatory	Sarilumab	Binds to IL-6 receptors
Antiinflammatory	Anakinra	Binds to the IL-1 type I receptor (IL-1RI), thereby inhibiting the action of elevated levels IL-1. Not promising. Ongoing clinical trials
Antiinflammatory and immunosuppressant	Corticosteroids: Dexamethasone	Inhibits the enzyme phospholipase A2 and blocks the synthesis of the inflammatory mediators
Antiinflammatory	Colchicine	Decreases cytokine production by inhibiting activation of the NLRP3 inflammasome.[b] Minimal clinical data
Antiinflammatory and immunosuppressant	Ruxolitinib	JAK1 and JAK2 inhibitor. Not found greatly promising in COVID-19 treatment
Immunomodulator	Baricitinib	JAK1 and JAK2 inhibitor. Promising in combination with remdesivir
Immune response modulators	Tofacitinib	An orally administered selective inhibitor of JAK1 and JAK3, with functional selectivity for JAK2; promising results
Prevents viral entry	Nafamostat mesilate or camostat	TMPRSS2 receptor inhibitor. No large clinical trial results[c,d]
Prevents viral entry	Teicoplanin	Proposed to block cathepsin-L receptor[e]
Prevents viral entry (originally indicated as antiparasitic)	Ivermectin	Binds to transport factors importin alpha and Importin beta. Not considered promising. Many clinical trials are underway.
Obstructing viral entry	Hydroxychloroquine or chloroquine	Many targets are proposed. One of the targets is gangliosides and sialic acids.[f] Not considered effective
Treatment of thromboembolism	Anticoagulants[g]	Direct thrombin inhibitors such as dabigatran and direct factor Xa inhibitors such as apixaban, edoxaban, and rivaroxaban
Antiinflammatory action and interaction with viral proteins	2-Deoxy-D-glucose	Not specific to single target.[d] Efficacy is unclear, and clinical trials results data are not yet available. It was originally meant for cancer treatment. But the product has been launched as treatment for COVID-19[h]

[a]Lin FC, Young HA. Interferons: success in anti-viral immunotherapy. *Cytokine Growth Factor Rev.* 2014;25(4):369–376. doi:10.1016/j.cytogfr.2014.07.015.

[b]Reyes AZ, Hu KA, Teperman J, et al. Anti-inflammatory therapy for COVID-19 infection: the case for colchicine. *Ann Rheum Dis.* 2021;80:550–557. https://ard.bmj.com/content/80/5/550

[c]Chitalia VC, Munawar AH. A painful lesson from the COVID-19 pandemic: the need for broad-spectrum, host-directed antivirals. *J Transl Med.* 2020;18(1):1–6. doi:10.1186/s12967-020-02476-9.

[d]Verma A, Adhikary A, Woloschak G, et al. A combinatorial approach of a polypharmacological adjuvant 2-deoxy-D-glucose with low dose radiation therapy to quell the cytokine storm in COVID-19 management. *Int J Radiat Biol.* 2020;96(11):1323–1328. doi:10.1080/09553002.2020.1818865.

[e]Ceccarelli G, Alessandri F, d'Ettorre G, et al. Is teicoplanin a complementary treatment option for COVID-19? The question remains. *Int J Antimicrob Agents.* 2020;56(2):106029. doi:10.1016/j.ijantimicag.2020.106029.*IL,* Interleukin; *JAK,* Janus kinase.

[f]Saghir SAM, AlGabri NA, Alagawany MM, et al. Chloroquine and hydroxychloroquine for the prevention and treatment of COVID-19: a fiction, hope or hype? An updated review. *Ther Clin Risk Manag.* 2021;17:371–387 doi:10.2147/TCRM.S301817

[g]Chandra A, Chakraborty U, Ghosh S, Dasgupta S. Anticoagulation in COVID-19: current concepts and controversies. *Postgrad Med J.* https://pmj.bmj.com/content/postgradmedj/early/2021/04/12/postgradmedj-2021-139923.full.pdf.

[h]Dr. Reddy's announces commercial launch of 2-DG. The Hindu. https://www.thehindu.com/business/Industry/dr-reddys-announces-commercial-launch-of-2-dg/article35011071.ece.

throughout the world against COVID-19. The lessons have been immense, and new candidates for repurposing are emerging every day thanks to docking studies of computational bioinformatics. Owing to the damages caused by severity of disease through cytokine storm, many of the investigations have centered around control of immune response and inflammation in the patient. Preventing the virus entry into human cells has been partially successful through use of mAbs from the initial reports, but whether they stand the test of rigor and time, particularly against virus variants is still under investigation.

Viral Mutations and Selection of Drug Targets

Although we have a list of potential targets, drug target prioritization is a process not based on a single criterion but optimized based on multiple criteria. For example, if the virus is mutating rapidly, identifying conserved regions in the viral genome becomes an important criterion. In 2021, Almubaid et al.[49] identified NSP13 to be the conserved region among 1200 genome samples of SARS-CoV-2 across the first

7 months of 2020. In another study, genetic variance studies among SARS-CoV-2 and SARS-CoV reported conserved drug proteins.[50] It was found that Mpro, PLpro, and RdRp are conserved largely between SARS-CoV-2 and SARS-CoV.

Observed Mutations of SARS-CoV-2

In 2020, three of every four residents of Manaus, Brazil had been infected with SARS-CoV-2.[51] Yet, the virus caused a second wave of illness and death in late 2020 and early 2021. The reason was several mutations resulting in a variant called P.1.[51] Researchers sequenced SARS-CoV-2 genomes from 184 patient samples collected in Manaus. The research project was focused on viral genomics and epidemiology for public health. Genomic data revealed the P.1 variant had acquired 17 new mutations. Of these, 10 were in the spike protein to make it easier for the P.1 spike to bind to the human ACE2 receptor.

The first P.1 variant case was detected by genomic surveillance on December 6, 2020, after which it spread rapidly. When the researchers developed a mathematical model that integrated the genomic data with mortality data, they found that P.1 may be 1.7 to 2.4 times more transmissible than earlier variants.

All viruses mutate, some faster than others. SARS-CoV-2 mutates much slower than, for example, HIV. Yet, hundreds of mutations of SARS-CoV-2 have already occurred. Some of the mutations elicit a concern with respect to infectivity and transmissibility. Three classifications of mutations of SARS-CoV-2 were defined by a US government interagency group.[52] The three classes of variants are:
1. Variant of interest
2. Variant of concern
3. Variant of high consequence

Currently, there is no variant classified as a variant of high consequence. However, a few of the variants have been classified as variants of concern.

Rapid genome sequencing characterizes various mutations. Typically, the mutation is reflected in one or more substitutions of key amino acid residues in the proteins.

The list of variants of concern are given in the Table 17.5.[53] The mutations in the variants of concern, as given in Table 17.5, have occurred in the RBD of the spike protein. Amino acid substitutions related to these variants are:
- L452R is present in B.1.526.1, B.1.427 (epsilon), and B.1.429 (epsilon) lineages, as well as the B.1.617 (kappa, delta) lineages and sublineages.
- E484K is present in B.1.525 (eta), P.2 (zeta), P.1 (gamma), and B.1.351 (beta), but only some strains of B.1.526 (iota) and B.1.1.7 (alpha).
- The combination of K417N, E484K, and N501Y substitutions is present in B.1.351 (beta).
- The combination of K417T, E484K, and N501Y substitutions is present in P.1 (gamma).

These substitutions in the variants of concern category are thought to result in evasion of antibodies and higher infectivity.[54] It is not clear whether monoclonal antibody cocktail therapy would be effective against some of the mutations of spike protein.[55] The variants will necessitate newer therapies and consequently newer antibodies. If the mutations occur on other parts of the virus, such as NSPs, the resulting impact could be envisaged[56]; now, however, mutations of spike proteins are causing the concern. Quite a few mutations are covered under the category variants of interest, the details of which are available.[52]

Conclusion

Development of therapeutic solutions for COVID-19 treatment is happening at a rapid pace. The understanding of disease progression, disease mechanisms, and nuances of therapeutic treatment for COVID-19 has advanced significantly in the recent past, with a promise of therapeutic solutions of high potential for the near future. Both virus-targeted therapy and host-targeted therapy are likely to provide novel therapeutic solutions. Effective host-targeted therapy, for example, use of a corticosteroid as an antiinflammatory and immunosuppressant to avoid cytokine storm in the treatment of COVID-19, will continue to be important. Identification of new targets through analysis of protein–protein interactions between virus and host is poised to shape superior understanding of mechanisms and lead to novel treatments. Need for accuracy of analysis and predictions of targets and therapies by bioinformatics methods will increase further. SARS-CoV-2 variants that could cause higher infectiveness and/or transmissivity pose a challenge for drug therapy.

Table 17.5 Key SARS-CoV-2 Mutation Variants of Concern

Name	Lineage
Alpha from Britain	B.1.1.7
Beta from South Africa	B.1.351
Gamma from Brazil	P.1
Delta from India	B.1.617.2
Epsilon from the United States	B.1.427
Epsilon from the United States	B.1.429

REFERENCES
1. Tsai P-H, Lai W-Y, Lin Y-Y, et al. Clinical manifestation and disease progression in Covid-19 infection. J Chin Med Assoc. 2021;84(1):3–8. https://journals.lww.com/jcma/Fulltext/2021/01000/Clinical_manifestation_and_disease_progression_in.2.aspx. Accessed on 20/6/2021.
2. World Health Organization. Coronavirus disease (COVID-19). https://www.who.int/health-topics/coronavirus#tab=tab_1, Accessed on 20/6/2021.

3. National Institutes of Health. Clinical spectrum of SARS-CoV-2 Infection. October 19, 2021. https://www.covid19treatmentguidelines.nih.gov/overview/clinical-spectrum/, Accessed on July 1, 2021.

4. MED Mastery. Symptom onset. https://www.medmastery.com/guide/covid-19-clinical-guide/covid-19-disease-progression.

5. World Health Organization. Modes of transmission of virus causing COVID-19: implications for IPC precautions recommendations. https://www.who.int/news-room/commentaries/detail/modes-of-transmission-of-virus-causing-covid-19-implications-for-ipc-precaution-recommendations. Accessed on July 1, 2021.

6. Ponti G, Maccaferri M, Ruini C, Tomasi A, Ozben T. Biomarkers associated with COVID-19 disease progression. *Crit Rev Clin Lab Sci.* 2020;57(6):389–399. doi:10.1080/10408363.2020.1770685.

7. Zimmer C, Wu KJ, Corum J, Kristofferson M. Coronavirus drug and treatment tracker. NY Times. https://www.nytimes.com/interactive/2020/science/coronavirus-drugs-treatments.html, Accessed on July 1, 2021.

8. Kumar BK, Sekhar KVGC, Kunjiappan S, Jamalis J, Balaña-Fouce R, Tekwani BL, & Sankaranarayanan M. Druggable targets of SARS-CoV-2 and treatment opportunities for COVID-19. *Bioorganic chemistry.* 2020;104:104269. doi:10.1016/j.bioorg.2020.104269.

9. Cavasotto CN, Sánchez Lamas M, Maggini J. Functional and druggability analysis of the SARS CoV-2 proteome. *European journal of pharmacology.* 2021;890:17370. doi:10.1016/j.ejphar.2020.173705.

10. Hadid T, Kafri Z, Al-Katib A. Coagulation and anticoagulation in COVID19. *Blood Reviews.* 2021;47:10076. doi:10.1016/j.blre.2020.100761.

11. Sanyaolu A, Okorie C, Marinkovic A, et al. Comorbidity and its Impact on Patients with COVID-19. *SN comprehensive clinical medicine.* 2020:1–8. doi:10.1007/s42399-020-00363-4.

12. Nalbandian A, Sehgal K, Gupta A, et al. Post-acute COVID-19 syndrome. *Nature medicine.* 2021:1–15. doi:10.1038/s41591-021-01283-z.

13. Van den Broeck MM. Drug Targets, Target Identification, Validation, and Screening. In: Wermuth CG, Aldous D, Raboisson P, Rognan D, eds. *The Practice of Medicinal Chemistry.* 4th ed. London: Academic Press; 2015.

14. Wei Zhu W, Chen CZ, Gorshkov K, et al. RNA-dependent RNA polymerase as a target for COVID-19 drug discovery. *SLAS Discovery.* 2020;25(10):1141–1151. doi:10.1177/2472555220942123.

15. Ray M, Sable NM, Sarkar S, Hallur V. Essential interpretations of bioinformatics in COVID-19 pandemic. *Meta Gene.* 2021:100844. doi:10.1016/j.mgene.2020.100844.16.

16. Jiang Z, Zhou Y. Using bioinformatics for drug target identification from the genome. *Am J Pharmacogenomics.* 2005;5:387–396. doi:10.2165/00129785-200505060-00005.

17. Whittaker PA. The role of bioinformatics in target validation. *Drug Discov Today Technol.* 2004 Oct;1(2):125–133. doi:10.1016/j.ddtec.2004.08.002.

18. Chen YP, Chen F. Identifying targets for drug discovery using bioinformatics. *Expert Opin Ther Targets.* 2008 Apr;12(4):383–389. doi:10.1517/14728222.12.4.383.

19. Auwul R, Rahman R, Gov E, et al. Bioinformatics and machine learning approach identifies potential drug targets and pathways in COVID-19. *Briefings in Bioinformatics.* 2021:bbab120. doi:10.1093/bib/bbab120.

20. Barrett T, Suzek TO, Troup DB, et al. NCBI GEO: mining millions of expression profiles—database and tools. *Nucleic acids research.* 2005;33(suppl_1):D562–D566. doi:10.1093/nar/gki022.

21. Papatheodorou I, Fonseca NA, Keays M, et al. Expression Atlas: gene and protein expression across multiple studies and organisms. *Nucleic acids research.* 2018;46(D1):D246–D251. doi:10.1093/nar/gkx1158.

22. Caruso FP, Scala G, Cerulo L, Ceccarelli M. A review of COVID-19 biomarkers and drug targets: resources and tools. *Briefings in bioinformatics.* 2021;22(2):701–713. doi:10.1093/bib/bbaa328.

23. Walke DW, Han C, Shaw J, et al. In vivo drug target discovery: identifying the best targets from the genome. *Current opinion in biotechnology.* 2001;12(6):626–631. doi:10.1016/s0958-1669(01)00271-3.

24. Djekidel MN, Rosikiewicz W, Peng JC, et al. "CovidExpress: an interactive portal for intuitive investigation on SARS-CoV-2 related transcriptomes." bioRxiv (2021) 2021.05.14.444026, doi: 10.1101/2021.05.14.444026.

25. Richardson P, Griffin I, Tucker T et al. "Baricitinib as potential treatment for 2019-nCoV acute respiratory disease" *Lancet*, February 15, 2020;39(10223):E30–E31. 10.1016/S0140-6736(20)30304-4.

26. Stebbing J, Krishnan V, de Bono S, et al. Mechanism of baricitinib supports artificial intelligence-predicted testing in COVID-19 patients. *EMBO Mol Med.* 2020 Aug 7;12(8):e12697. doi:10.15252/emmm.202012697.

27. Lam C, Siefkas A, Zelin NS, et al. Machine learning as a precision-medicine approach to prescribing COVID-19 pharmacotherapy with remdesivir or corticosteroids. *Clin Ther.* 2021. doi:10.1016/j.clinthera.2021.03.016 2021 Mar 29 S0149-2918(21)00128-4.

28. Amin SA, Banerjee S, Gayen S, Jha T. Protease targeted COVID-19 drug discovery: What we have learned from the past SARS-CoV inhibitors?. *Eur J Med Chem.* 2021 Apr 5;215:113294. doi:10.1016/j.ejmech.2021.113294.

29. Fu L, Ye F, Feng Y, et al. Both Boceprevir and GC376 efficaciously inhibit SARS CoV-2 by targeting its main protease. *Nat Commun.* 2020;11:4417. doi:10.1038/s41467-020-18233-x.

30. Yuan H, Yang C, Xu X-F, et al. Structural and functional properties of SARS CoV-2 spike protein: potential antivirus drug development for COVID-19. *Acta Pharmacologica Sinica.* 2020;41(9):1141–1149. doi:10.1038/s41401-020-0485-4.

31. Naqvi AAT, Kisa F, Mohammad T, et al. Insights into SARS CoV-2 genome, structure, evolution, pathogenesis and therapies: Structural genomics approach. *Biochimica et Biophysica Acta (BBA)-Molecular Basis of Disease.* 2020;1866(10):165878. doi:10.1016/j.bbadis.2020.165878.

32. Caly L, Druce JD, Catton MG, et al. The FDA-approved drug ivermectin inhibits the replication of SARS CoV-2 in vitro. *Antiviral Research.* 2020;178:104787. doi:10.1016/j.antiviral.2020.104787.

33. Chitalia VC, Munawar AH. A painful lesson from the COVID-19 pandemic: the need for broad-spectrum, host-directed antivirals. *Journal of Translational Medicine.* 2020;18(1):1–6. doi:10.1186/s12967-020-02476-9.

34. Samaee H, Mohsenzadegan M, Ala S, Maroufi SS, Moradimajd P. Tocilizumab for treatment patients with COVID-19: Recommended medication for novel disease. *Int Immunopharmacol.* 2020;89(Pt A):107018. doi:10.1016/j.intimp.2020.107018.

35. Nakhlband A, Fakhari A, Azizi H. Interferon-beta offers promising avenues to COVID-19 treatment: a systematic review and meta-analysis of clinical trial studies. *Naunyn Schmiedebergs Arch Pharmacol.* 2021;394(5):829–838. doi:10.1007/s00210-021-02061-x.

36. Guo H, Zhou L, Ma Z, Tian Z, Zhou F. Promising Immunotherapies against COVID-19. *Adv. Therap.* 2021:2100044. doi:10.1002/adtp.202100044.

37. Jain R, Ramaswamy S, Harilal D, et al. Host transcriptomic profiling of COVID-19 patients with mild, moderate, and severe clinical outcomes. *Computational and Structural Biotechnology Journal.* 2021;19:153–216. doi:10.1016/j.csbj.2020.12.016.

38. Wang F, Huang S, Gao R, et al. Initial whole-genome sequencing and analysis of the host genetic contribution to COVID-19 severity and susceptibility. *Cell Discovery.* 2020;6(1):1–16. doi:10.1038/s41421-020-00231-4.

39. Debnath M, Banerjee M, Berk M. Genetic gateways to COVID-19 infection: Implications for risk, severity, and outcomes. *The FASEB Journal.* 2020;34(7):8787–8795. doi:10.1096/fj.202001115R.

40. COVID-19 Host Genetics Initiative. The COVID-19 Host Genetics Initiative, a global initiative to elucidate the role of host genetic factors in susceptibility and severity of the SARS CoV-2 virus pandemic. *European Journal of Human Genetics.* 2020;28(6):715. doi:10.1038/s41431-020-0636-6.

41. Rizk JG, Kalantar-Zadeh K, Mehra MR, et al. Pharmaco-immunomodulatory therapy in COVID19. *Drugs.* 2020:1–2. doi:10.1007/s40265-020-01367-z.

42. Perrin-Cocon L, Diaz O, Jacquemin C, et al. The current landscape of coronavirus-host protein–protein interactions. *J Transl Med.* 2020;18(1):319. doi:10.1186/s12967-020-02480-z.

43. Gordon DE, Jang GM, Bouhaddou M, et al. A SARS CoV-2 protein interaction map reveals targets for drug repurposing. *Nature.* 2020;583:459–468. doi:10.1038/s41586-020-2286-9.

44. Plaze M, Attali D, Prot M, et al. Inhibition of the replication of SARS CoV-2 in human cells by the FDA-approved drug chlorpromazine. *International Journal of Antimicrobial Agents.* 2021;57(3):106274. doi:10.1016/j.ijantimicag.2020.106274.

45. Abhik K, Banerjee MR, Blanco EA, et al. SARS CoV-2 disrupts splicing, translation, and protein trafficking to suppress host defenses. *Cell.* 2020;183(5):1325–1339. doi:10.1016/j.cell.2020.10.004.

46. Schubert K, Karousis ED, Jomaa A, et al. SARS CoV 2 Nsp1 binds the ribosomal mRNA channel to inhibit translation. *Nat Struct Mol Biol.* 2020;27:959–966. doi:10.1038/s41594-020-0511-8.

47. Robinson J. Everything you need to know about the COVID-19 therapy trials,. Pharmaceutical J. March 18, 2022 https://pharmaceutical-journal.com/article/feature/everything-you-need-to-know-about-the-covid-19-therapy-trials. Accessed on June 30, 2021.

48. Milken Institute," COVID-19 Treatment and Vaccine Tracker," [Online]. Available: https://covid-19tracker.milkeninstitute.org/#treatment_antibodies Accessed July 1, 2021.

49. Almubaid Z, Al-Mubaid H. Analysis and comparison of genetic variants and mutations of the novel coronavirus SARS CoV-2. *Gene Reports.* 2021;23:101064. doi:10.1016/j.genrep.2021.101064.

50. Wu C, Liu Y, Yang Y, et al. Analysis of therapeutic targets for SARS CoV-2 and discovery of potential drugs by computational methods. *Acta Pharmaceutica Sinica B.* 2020;10(5):766–788. doi:10.1016/j.apsb.2020.02.008.

51. Tracking the Evolution of a 'Variant of Concern' in Brazil, https://directorsblog.nih.gov/tag/spike-protein/, Accessed on July 1, 2021.

52. Centers for Disease Control and Prevention. SARS-CoV-19 Variant Classifications and Definitions. https://www.cdc.gov/coronavirus/2019-ncov/variants/variant-info.html. Accessed on July 1, 2021.

53. https://www.news-medical.net/health/Viral-Clades-of-SARS-CoV-2.aspx, Accessed on July 1, 2021.

54. Jiahui C, Gao K, Want R, Wei G-W. Prediction and mitigation of mutation threats to COVID-19 vaccines and antibody therapies. *Chem Sci.* 2021;12:6129–6948. doi:10.1039/D1SC01203G.

55. Planas D, Veyer D, Baidaliuk A, et al. Reduced sensitivity of SARS-CoV-2 variant Delta to antibody neutralization. *Nature.* 2021;596:276–280. doi:10.1038/s41586-021-03777-9.

56. Banoun H. Evolution of SARS CoV-2: review of mutations, role of the host immune system. *Nephron.* 2021. doi:10.1159/000515417.

Vaccine Basics and the Development and Rollout of COVID-19 Vaccines

Subramani Mani, MBBS, PhD, and Daniel Griffin, MD, PhD

OUTLINE

Historical Introduction to Vaccines

At the end of 2019, a novel human pathogen was first identified in China and resulted in a pandemic that posed the greatest infectious threat that humans had encountered in modern times. The virus responsible for the pandemic, severe acute respiratory syndrome coronavirus 2 (SARS-CoV-2), soon infected hundreds of millions of people, resulting in millions of deaths worldwide. To develop a critical understanding of the coronavirus disease 2019 (COVID-19) and its causative agent SARS-CoV-2, to study the evolution of the pandemic over time in different parts of the world, and eventually to control the pandemic, it is necessary to examine the challenges various viral infections posed over the centuries and the role of vaccines in containing them.

Smallpox became a scourge in the Indian subcontinent more than two millennia ago and gradually spread to other parts of the world. Although a vaccine was developed for the disease by Edward Jenner in the later part of the 18th century, the concept of *virus* evolved during the last decades of the 19th century and crystallized only in the early years of the 20th century. As nicely put by William Summers, viruses are a conceptualization of scientists. The "virus" described by Jenner in 1778 during smallpox vaccination, the view provided by Pasteur at the time of his rabies vaccine in 1885, and the "virus" concept provided by Stanley in 1935 when he crystallized the poliovirus are naturally different.[1] The first human virus to be discovered was the yellow fever virus in 1901, and the first to be visualized was the tobacco mosaic virus in 1939 using an electron microscope.[2] The first approach to combating viruses was by vaccination. Throughout the 19th and first half of the 20th century, all the vaccines were developed using viruses grown in animals and chicken egg embryos. This was the methodology for the development of vaccines for smallpox, rabies, yellow fever, and influenza. Polio represented an advance in our options for how we could manipulate and ultimately combat viruses; the successful growth of the poliovirus in cell cultures led to the development of the polio vaccine in the early 1950s of the 20th century using a cell culture approach.[2]

Emerging viruses are defined as those causing new human infections that had never been encountered earlier, and reemerging viruses are defined as those causing opportunistic infections after lying quiescent for many years or even decades. Most emerging viruses are zoonotic, jumping to humans from wildlife reservoirs or through an intermediate domestic animal host. Human immunodeficiency virus (HIV), avian influenza viruses, Nipah virus (NiV), severe acute respiratory syndrome coronavirus (SARS-CoV), Middle East respiratory syndrome coronavirus (MERS-CoV), Lassa mammarenavirus, Zika virus, and the more recent severe acute respiratory syndrome coronavirus 2 (SARS-CoV-2) are prominent emerging viruses. The Ebolaviruses (Bundibugyo virus, Sudan virus, Tai Forest virus, and Ebola virus [formerly Zaire Ebola virus]) reemerged in the 1990s after the first well-recognized outbreak of the 1970s.

Viral evolution plays a significant role in the viral agent's survival. By their mechanisms of mutation and recombination, the survival of many viruses is ensured, as variants arise that can evade the host immune responses. A classic case in point is the influenza A virus, which has not been eliminated even in the presence of effective vaccines and antiviral drugs with some efficacy such as amantadine and oseltamivir.[2]

Viruses also have been found to be causative agents for many tumors. In 1911, Peyton Rous first demonstrated the transmission of sarcoma in chickens through cell-free filtrates. Since then, over the course of a century, many viruses, including human papillomaviruses (HPV), Epstein Barr virus, Kaposi sarcoma herpesvirus, human T-cell leukemia virus-1 and human T-cell leukemia virus-2, hepatitis B virus (HBV), and hepatitis C virus (HCV), have been implicated in various types of cancers, together causing a significant percentage of human cancer deaths.[3] Vaccines also have been developed to prevent infection against some of these viruses, for example HPV and HBV.[4]

Working with the fowl cholera bacterium, Louis Pasteur developed a method of growing and weakening the microbe in culture. He discovered that these weakened or attenuated bacteria caused a mild form of the disease and protected the chickens when exposed to the virulent form. Pasteur gave the name *vaccine* to this attenuated strain based on the Latin *vacca* which means cow. He was honoring Dr. Jenner and his work using cowpox inoculation to prevent smallpox.[5]

The rest of the chapter is organized as follows. The chapter begins with a discussion of the science of vaccinology incorporating the basic concepts of the various types of immunity, and the different stages of the vaccine development process to ascertain safety and efficacy. The discussion then proceeds to describe the promising SARS-CoV-2 vaccines under various stages of development, with a focus on those undergoing phase III clinical trials, including those that have been accorded emergency use authorization (EUA) or approval by different regulatory agencies. Finally, the chapter provides a summary of the vaccine rollout under way in the developed and developing countries and the challenges posed by emerging SARS-CoV-2 variants for acquiring population immunity.

Vaccines and Vaccinology

The science of vaccinology is founded on the basic principles of immunology, which are outlined in the following section.

Innate and Adaptive Immunity

The human body fights infections using two basic immune mechanisms called *innate* and *adaptive* immunity. Innate immunity is the body's first line of defense

and is activated immediately within minutes to a few hours of the entry of pathogens. Macrophages and neutrophils are recruited to quickly engulf and destroy extracellular pathogens by phagocytosis. Pathogen recognition is achieved in an antigen-specific manner using related molecular structures called pathogen-associated molecular patterns (PAMPs). PAMPs are broad patterns made up of essential polysaccharides and polynucleotides found in various pathogens, but these are absent in the host receptors. In innate immunity there is no memory trigger of past exposures. "Natural antibodies," which are evolutionarily selected immunoglobulins based mostly on germline sequences, also play a role in innate immune mechanisms.

Adaptive immunity is a tailored, precise, and specific response to pathogen entry. The body mounts an initial adaptive immune response over a period of a few days to weeks. The pathogen is recognized precisely by receptors that are generated by a random process of differentiation of B and T lymphocytes. Clones of highly specific T lymphocytes that can discriminate between even very small differences in the molecular structure of pathogen epitopes are generated and recruited for the adaptive immune response. The pathogen epitopes are made of polypeptides or polysaccharides and represent the uniqueness of a pathogen. A primary adaptive B-cell response takes about a week to be detected, but the memory of the event is retained and a secondary response typically has a shorter lag phase of 3 or 4 days. Moreover, in the primary response, low-affinity immunoglobulin M (IgM) antibodies predominate initially followed by the development of higher affinity IgG antibodies. High-affinity IgG antibodies dominate the secondary response. The kinetics of the initiation of an adaptive T-cell response follows a similar time course with the ability to detect expansion of T cells, with a T-cell receptor repertoire being first detectable 3 to 4 days after pathogen challenge. Fig. 18.1 presents a depiction of the primary and secondary immune response curves. Fig. 18.2 shows the interaction of innate and adaptive immune systems. The dendritic cells act as intermediaries between the innate and adaptive immune systems. The interested reader is referred to publications by Punt et al.[5] and Virella[6] for further details.

Population Immunity

In vaccinology, the concept of population immunity, also referred to as herd immunity,[a] plays a significant role. When a community attains population immunity, it can be expected to be protected from the onslaught of a specific pathogenic infection. One way to obtain this type of immunity is by the natural course of disease

---

[a]Because *herd* pertains to nonhuman primates and animals, we prefer to use *population* immunity.

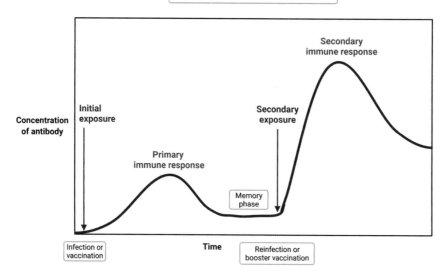

Fig. 18.1 Primary and Secondary Immune Response Curves. The primary response curve solely the result of innate immunity initially has a slow rise. The adaptive response kicks in after a time delay. The primary response then mostly subsides and enters a memory phase that retains the ability to initiate a vigorous response if the same or a very similar pathogen is encountered subsequently, triggering the steeper, larger and more sustained secondary response. (Created using Biorender.)

Interaction of Innate and Adaptive Immunity

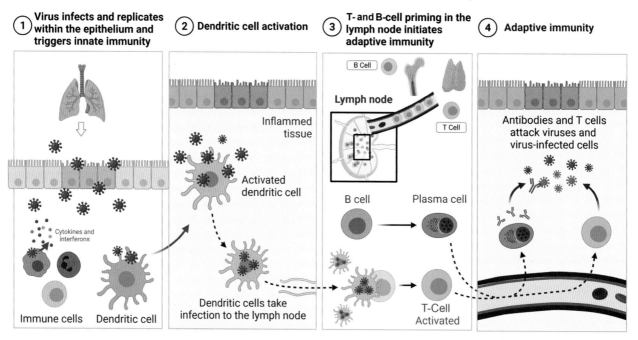

Fig. 18.2 Interaction of innate and Adaptive Immunity. The development of the immune response after exposure to pathogen is shown in four steps. First the immune cells engage the invading pathogen with the release of cytokines and interferons. The dendritic cells then get activated carrying the pathogen to the lymph nodes, where a more specific adaptive immune response is generated (step 3). In the germinal center of the lymph node B and T cells get activated. B cells get transformed into plasma cells and generate highly specific antibodies. Activated T cells and plasma cells enter the circulation and reach the site of infection to engage the pathogen (step 4). (Created using Biorender.)

transmission when a significant proportion (60%–95%) of individuals in a community are exposed and subsequently get infected by the pathogen. However, this can impose a high burden of mortality and morbidity on

the population. A much more desirable approach to attain population immunity is through vaccination or immunization. However, the proportion of a population in a community or geographic region who must be

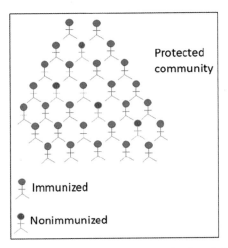

Fig. 18.3 Population Immunity in a Community. Population immunity is acquired when a sufficiently large proportion of a population becomes immune to a specific pathogen. Population immunity confers a direct protective effect for the immunized and indirectly protects the nonimmunized members of a community by shielding them from becoming infected by breaking the transmission chain.

immunized with a vaccine for a specific infectious disease depends on the transmissibility of the pathogen in question. For example, measles is a highly contagious disease, and for effective protection, 95% coverage is needed. This is to ensure that the entire population is shielded from the pathogen. Population immunity confers a direct protective effect on the immunized, but it also provides indirect protection for the nonimmunized individuals by disabling the transmission chain, as shown in Fig. 18.3.

History of Vaccines

From a functional perspective there are two predominant categories of vaccines: prophylactic and therapeutic. Prophylactic vaccines are typically administered as part of a preventive strategy before a person is exposed to a pathogen or develops the disease. Therapeutic vaccines are administered as a treatment strategy for an existing disease or clinical condition.

Edward Jenner is credited with developing an approach to smallpox vaccination in 1796 using anecdotal evidence and previous observations that milkmaids who developed cowpox lesions were protected from smallpox. Although Jenner is properly credited for his investigations, publications, and prolific correspondence that championed vaccination, Benjamin Jesty, a farmer, had also become aware of the protection from smallpox that an earlier cowpox infection provided. Based on this knowledge, Jesty inoculated his wife and two sons with fluid from a cowpox lesion on one of his cows in 1774.[7] This ultimately turned out to be a safer approach than the Turkish variolation method that involved introducing a small quantity of infective smallpox material into a skin incision, with a resultant 2% mortality. The credit for sheep anthrax vaccine goes

to Louis Pasteur, who made a public demonstration of his anthrax vaccination methodology in 1881 by inoculating 25 sheep, with another 25 sheep retained as controls. When challenged with anthrax spores, 24 of the 25 vaccinated sheep survived compared with only 2 of 25 survivors in the control group. However, Pasteur did not give credit to Henri Toussaint, who developed the method to inactivate anthrax bacteria using phenol.[7] Later, Pasteur developed a killed vaccine for rabies from air-dried spinal cords of infected rabbits. He successfully vaccinated a 9-year-old boy, Joseph Meister, bitten by a rabid dog in 1885, and Meister survived. This was the first therapeutic vaccination, because Meister was vaccinated after exposure to rabies.

Starting with serendipity and observation in the late 1700s, vaccine methodologies evolved into empiric approaches involving isolation, inactivation, and the use of killed microbes in the late 19th and first half of the 20th centuries. For diphtheria and tetanus, toxins were identified as the cause of the disease, and antiserum made against toxins in horses was used in passive vaccination. From 1880 to 1950, vaccines were developed successfully to tackle rabies, diphtheria, tetanus, and polio. The bacillus Calmette-Guérin (BCG) vaccine for tuberculosis was also developed during this period.

The second half of the 20th century saw two new successful vaccine development approaches: recombinant DNA technology and glycoconjugation or polysaccharide-protein conjugation. By 1980, the recombinant method yielded two effective vaccines, one for HBV and the other for HPV. By 1990, the polysaccharide-protein conjugation method enabled the development of the meningococcal ACWY (MenACWY), *Haemophilus influenzae* type b (Hib), and pneumonia vaccines. These newer vaccines are also referred to as subunit vaccines because they contain only parts of the pathogen but are capable of generating an adequate immune response after vaccination. In the first decade of the 21st century, genome-derived reverse vaccinology approaches using bioinformatics methods were employed to develop the meningococcal B (MenB) vaccine. Fig. 18.4 illustrates the vaccination milestones.

Public Health Impact of Vaccines

The 20th century saw the development of new and effective vaccines for many infectious diseases, resulting in a dramatic reduction in mortality and morbidity from the onslaught of these diseases. Just in the 20th century alone, smallpox killed more than 500 million people before the worldwide eradication strategy of the disease succeeded, and smallpox was eliminated as a disease in 1980. Although effective vaccines have been developed for influenza, approximately 30,000 people on average succumb to the complications resulting from influenza in the United States alone each year. This translates to approximately half a million deaths globally every year

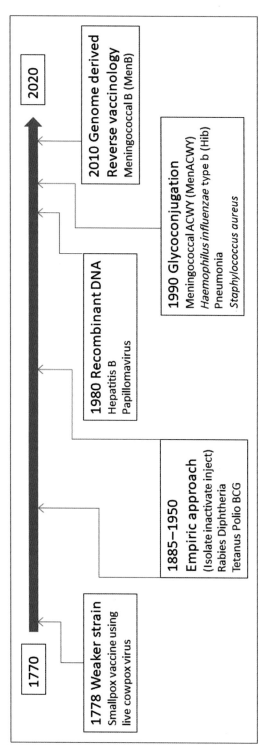

Fig. 18.4 Vaccination Milestones. Serendipity to empiric approaches to epitope prediction and reverse vaccinology. Starting with weaker pathogen strains in the late 18th century to genome-derived vaccination approaches of the 21st century, vaccinology has traveled a long way. *BCG*, Bacillus Calmette-Guérin.

Table 18.1 Annual Morbidity From Common Vaccine-Preventable Diseases Recommended for Universal Vaccine Use in US Children Before 1990

Disease	20th-Century Morbidity[a]	1998 Morbidity[b]	Percent Decrease
Smallpox	48,164	0	100
Diphtheria	175,885	1	99.99
Pertussis	147,271	6279	95.7
Tetanus	1314	34	97.4
Polio (paralytic)	16,316	0	100
Measles	503,282	89	99.99
Mumps	152,209	606	99.6
Rubella	47,745	345	99.3

[a]Average annual number of cases before universal vaccine use recommended. Smallpox, 1900–1904; diphtheria, 1920–1922; pertussis, 1922–1925; tetanus, 1922–1926; polio, 1951–1954; measles, 1958–1962; mumps, 1968; rubella, 1966–1968.
[b]Number of cases reported for each disease in 1998.
Modified from the Centers for Disease Control and Prevention. Ten great public health achievements—United States, 1900–1999. *MMWR Morb Mortal Wkly Rep*. 1999;48(12):241–243.

from influenza. Measles causes more than 100,000 deaths worldwide in spite of the availability of an effective vaccine from the 1960s. The reasons for the failure to control outbreaks of diseases in many countries of the world, even when effective vaccines are available, can be traced to economic disparities, widespread ignorance among the populace, lack of political will in the countries' leadership, and inadequate allocation of resources for public health. However, a substantial increase in the life expectancy of children and by extension in the whole populace was observed globally in the second half of the 20th century as a result of the impact of vaccination and immunization campaigns led by the World Health Organization (WHO) and the respective public health authorities of various countries.

The dramatic reduction in mortality and morbidity of various infectious diseases observed in the last century in the United States clearly illustrates the significant impact of vaccines in the prevention and control of various infectious diseases. By the end of the 20th century, the percentage reduction in morbidity for smallpox, diphtheria, pertussis, tetanus, paralytic polio, measles, mumps, and rubella varied between 99.3% and 100% (see Table 18.1 for additional details). Paralytic polio is on the verge of global eradication, having been eliminated from the developed world and most developing countries. However, there were isolated reports of paralytic polio during a period of 19 months (January 2019 to July 2020) in 5 countries of Asia (Afghanistan, China, Myanmar, Pakistan, Philippines) and 14 countries of Africa.[8] Among these countries, only Afghanistan and Pakistan have documented paralytic polio caused by wild-type poliovirus. Paralytic polio cases in the other countries are oral polio vaccine–associated paralytic poliomyelitis resulting from circulating vaccine-derived poliovirus.

Types of Vaccines

As noted earlier, the field of vaccinology started with live attenuated and inactivated vaccines. During the last part of the 20th century, and more so in this century, the focus has shifted to subunit vaccines particularly for tackling emergent viral diseases. These subunit vaccines typically consist of surface proteins that can induce a significant immune response, and they could also be conjugated with polysaccharides. Subunit vaccines also can be engineered with DNA or RNA segments that encode for the immunogenic proteins. These vaccines are also referred to as recombinant vaccines. Because the recombinant vaccines consist of specific immunogens, they typically elicit a better immune response than inactivated vaccines. Recombinant vaccines are also considered safe when compared with live attenuated vaccines because there is no danger of virulence. The vaccine types are illustrated in Fig. 18.5.

Nucleic Acid Vaccines

These vaccines use antigen-encoding plasmid DNA or RNA. In this case the vaccine does not possess the genome to make the microbe but just the genetic material necessary to make the required immunogens needed for protective immunity. The DNA has to be delivered inside cells and into the nucleus so that it can be transcribed first to messenger RNA (mRNA) and then translated into the relevant immunogenic proteins, making use of the cell machinery. The cells subsequently secrete the immunogens or they get attached to the surface. If mRNA is used, it need only enter the cytoplasm of cells, where it is directly translated into proteins using the host cellular machinery. Because mRNAs can be directly translated into proteins using the cellular ribosomal apparatus, they have a superior protein (antigen) expression profile. Moreover, antigen-specific targeting is facilitated by the expression of specific antigens in

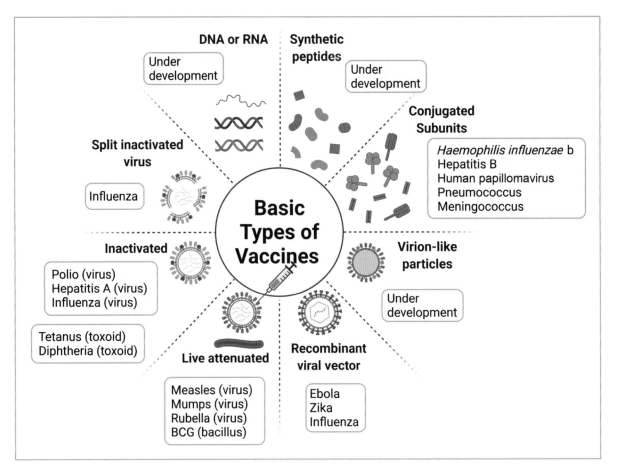

Fig. 18.5 Basic Types of Vaccines. The figure illustrates the traditional approaches (inactivated and live attenuated), methods successfully pioneered in late 20th century (conjugated subunits) and the recent approaches (split inactivated virus and recombinant viral vector) and newer paradigms, including some under development (DNA/RNA, synthetic peptides, and virion-like particles). *BCG,* Bacillus Calmette-Guérin. (Created using Biorender.)

antigen-presenting cells (APCs). The body's own cells are responsible for manufacturing the vaccine using their own cellular architecture and components, resulting in protective immunity. Both humoral and cell-mediated immune responses are generated by this method.[9]

There are a few additional advantages for nucleic acid vaccines. These vaccines are cell-free. No handling of live virus is needed, so a biosafety level 2 (BSL2) laboratory is not needed for vaccine development. Moreover, production can be speeded up because manufacturing is synthetic. The disadvantage is that mRNA is fragile and cold storage is needed to prevent degradation.

Therapeutic Vaccines

Therapeutic vaccination involves the administration of a vaccine to manage or treat a preexisting disease or clinical condition. The general goal here is to target noninfectious diseases such as cancer, Parkinson disease, Alzheimer disease, multiple sclerosis, arthritis, or conditions such as obesity, high blood pressure, and drug addictions. The challenge here is to critically understand the disease pathogenesis and pathological conditions and come up with suitable targets for vaccination. Note that in the case of noninfectious diseases, we are

dealing with host proteins as opposed to pathogen-derived proteins as targets, and this can cause problems with immune targeting. The recognition of specific conformational forms in the pathological processes associated with the disease is a key step in the development of effective therapeutic vaccines.[10,11] Identification of circulating cytotoxic T cells specific to tumor antigens indicates that induction of an immunogenic response to mutated tumor host proteins is feasible.

Therapeutic vaccines are broadly categorized into cancer vaccines and noninfectious noncancer (NINC) vaccines. Current cancer vaccines include personalized tumor immunotherapy, prostate cancer vaccine, and the use of BCG vaccine for bladder cancer. NINC vaccines are an area of intense investigation, with vaccines for addiction, high blood pressure, and obesity, currently in exploratory stages (see Fig. 18.6 for more details.)

The first use of therapeutic vaccination was to address the infectious disease rabies. The vaccine is still in use effectively to this day for this purpose with excellent efficacy as long as it is used early enough after infection. There may be a role for therapeutic vaccination in patients with COVID-19 who continue to have symptoms past the initial 4 weeks of illness.

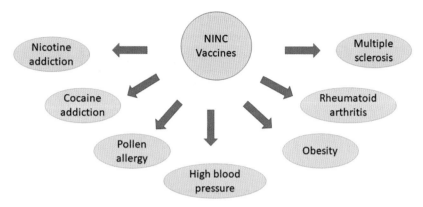

Fig. 18.6 Noninfectious Noncancer *(NINC)* Vaccines. Because these vaccines target human host proteins there are many underlying challenges in the development of these types of therapeutic vaccines. (Modified from Giese M. *Introduction to molecular vaccinology.* New York; 2016.)

Vaccines, Immunity, and Age

Age exerts a significant influence on the immune system. Generating immunological response by vaccination is easier in the young, whereas immune protection is quite challenging in older people. Low efficacy of seasonal influenza vaccine in the elderly has been well documented.[12,13] Immune competence decreases with increasing age, which is termed immunosenescence.[14] This can result from changes at multiple levels of the immune system over time, such as reduced lymphopoiesis in the bone marrow and thymus atrophy. These in turn result in a lower output of native T lymphocytes. Likewise, T-cell receptors and B-cell receptors are also negatively affected by aging. This implies that a conventional vaccine based on young adult responses may not be highly effective in older adults.[14,15] Supplementation of vaccination with immunotherapy by an infusion of neutralizing monoclonal antibodies might be needed in the elderly for enhanced protection.

Vaccine Protection Mechanisms

It is critical to understand what vaccines can and cannot do. Vaccines do not prevent pathogen entry or transient pathogen growth. Stimulating the host immune response by activating innate and adaptive immune mechanisms, vaccines can block pathogens from establishing a firm foothold by inhibiting the growth, development, and unchecked replication of these organisms. They can prevent the occurrence of clinical manifestations of disease or reduce the severity and complications resulting from infections. The goal of vaccination is to induce adaptive immunity that is specific for vaccine antigens. This facilitates the development of persistent antibodies, and memory B-cell and T-cell responses. This cascade of events protects the vaccinated individual during later contact with the virulent pathogen. The vaccine components engage the innate immune mechanism to induce protective adaptive immune responses.

Vaccine Development Process

Creating an effective and safe vaccine involves the successful completion of five critical stages: exploratory, preclinical, clinical trials, US Food and Drug Administration (FDA) review and approval, and, finally, manufacturing the required number of doses. These stages are usually sequential, and successful completion of a specific stage is necessary to move forward to the next stage. The COVID-19 pandemic has seen some changes to this paradigm with production often occurring before FDA review or approval. The exploratory stage incorporates in silico medicinal chemistry and biological experimentation, which leads to the preclinical stage, which typically involves testing for safety and efficacy on laboratory animals and possibility even primates. Successful completion of these two stages moves the process forward to the most important stage, the clinical trials stage, which will be discussed in some detail. Fig. 18.7 illustrates these five stages of the vaccine development process. The figure also shows the accelerated timeline with overlapping stages (stages 3, 4, and 5) for possible emergency use authorization in the case of pandemics.

Clinical Trials

A candidate vaccine advances to the clinical trials stage to evaluate the safety and efficacy of the vaccine in a rigorous and transparent manner. This task is accomplished by progressively larger complex human trials that are conducted in three sequential phases: phases I, II, and III. Safety of the candidate vaccine is assessed using healthy volunteers in phase I. In phase II, preliminary efficacy, dosage protocol, and additional safety determinations are made. The phase III clinical trial is the most critical, complex, and challenging step of the vaccine development process. Typically, it is a large randomized, placebo-controlled, double-blinded clinical trial involving the enrollment of thousands or even tens of thousands of subjects based on strict inclusion and exclusion criteria. It is clearly an expensive and

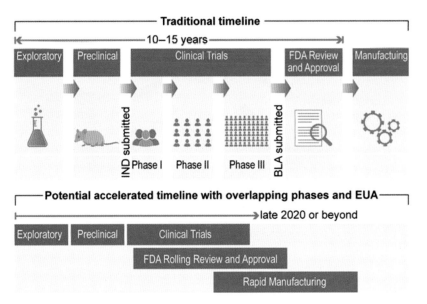

Fig. 18.7 Five Stages of the Vaccine Development Process. The cascade of five stages starting with exploratory work, preclinical (animal experiments), clinical trials in humans, US Food and Drug Administration (*FDA*)/regulatory agency approval, and ending with manufacturing stage are illustrated. To successfully complete all these stages typically takes one to two decades, and most vaccine prospects fail in the early stages. *BLA*, Biological license application; *EUA*, emergency use authorization; *IND*, investigational new drug. (Data from GAO-20-215SP, FDA, and US Department of Health and Human Services.)

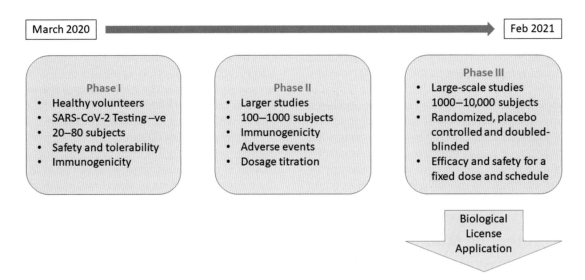

Fig. 18.8 Major Phases of a COVID-19 Candidate Vaccine Clinical Trial: Phase I, Phase II, and Phase III. This is a warp-speed and highly compressed timeline that many SARS-CoV-2 candidate vaccines successfully followed. The trial complexity increases as the development process moves from phase I to phase II and to phase III. −ve denotes negative.

resource-intensive undertaking. Successful completion of this important phase is mandatory for regulatory review and approval; the vaccine then moves on to the manufacturing stage. Fig. 18.8 presents additional details of the different phases of the clinical trials stage for a COVID-19 candidate vaccine.

Vaccine Development Timeline

The vaccine development process involves five sequential stages, including a three-phase clinical trial stage; it usually takes many years to decades to develop a successful vaccine. For example, development of the

meningococcal B vaccine, including licensing, took almost 15 years (Fig. 18.9). The shortest recorded time was for the live attenuated Jeryl Lynn mumps vaccine, developed by Maurice Hilleman at Merck laboratories in a span of about 5 years.[16]

Vaccine Development Failures

Even when the causative pathogen is isolated and sequenced, a safe and effective vaccine may not materialize in spite of persistent efforts. For example, there are no licensed effective vaccines currently in the

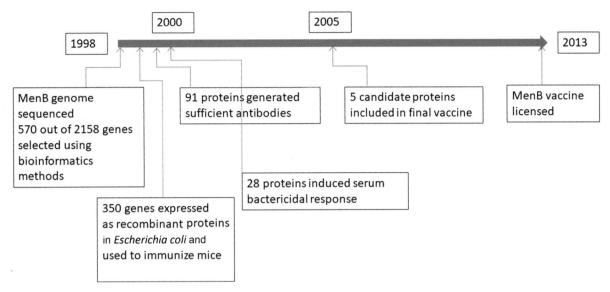

Fig. 18.9 Reverse Vaccinology Framework and Timeline for Meningococcal B Vaccine Development. Starting in 1998 when the Meningococcus B was sequenced, it took 15 years for the development pipeline to be completed, and the license was granted in 2013. (Modified from Modjarrad K, Koff W. *Human Vaccines: Emerging Technologies in Design and Development*. San Diego, CA: Academic Press; 2017.)

market for HIV, HCV, and malaria. HIV mutates continuously in the human host, which poses significant challenges for vaccine development. HCV shows enormous diversity, and animal models for testing potential vaccines are limited. Moreover, our understanding of protective immune responses against HCV are still evolving.[17] In general, developing vaccines against parasites is problematic because of their larger genomes. The malarial parasite genome has more than 5000 genes, which provide hundreds of potential targets and a plethora of vaccine candidates over the different stages of the parasitic life cycle. We need a better understanding of the mechanisms and key targets of immunity to develop a successful and durable vaccine for malaria.[18]

COVID-19 Vaccine Development

COVID-19 emerged as the biggest public health challenge mankind has faced over the last 100 years. To combat the disease and bring the pandemic under control, various teams, spread over many countries, are engaged in developing successful vaccines against SARS-CoV-2.

Vaccine Candidate Mechanisms

Apart from the more traditional approaches of using an attenuated and inactivated virus, many of the leading candidate vaccines use one of these three methods: mRNA coding a SARS-CoV-2 gene, recombinant SARS-CoV-2 surface protein, and viral vector packaging SARS-CoV-2 gene, as the key mechanism to induce an effective antibody response in the vaccinated host. These approaches are illustrated in Fig. 18.10. The live attenuated, mRNA, recombinant surface protein and viral vector incorporating SARS-CoV-2 gene(s) approaches

induce both humoral and cellular immunity–like natural infections. However, the inactivated pathogen-based vaccines can initiate only a humoral immune response.

mRNA Vaccines

Because mRNA vaccines are novel and have generated considerable interest and curiosity in recent years, the discussion now turns to the mRNA vaccine paradigm in additional detail.

The mRNA nanoparticle vaccine framework has brought a revolutionary transformation in the field of vaccinology,[19] offering many advantages over conventional approaches to trigger an immune response by the injection of attenuated or fully inactivated pathogens. The mRNA vaccines consist of bare mRNA strands transcribed in vitro and packaged in a lipid nanoparticle (LNP) bubble. They do not have any protein components or viral particles. Fig. 18.11, *panel A*, shows mRNA strands packaged in an LNP.

mRNA Preparation and Target Selection

The in vitro transcribed (IVT) mRNA undergoes some modifications and purifications that confer significant benefits. The removal of double-stranded RNA (dsRNA) contaminants enables IVT mRNA to avoid degradation through innate immunity.[20] A key modification involving the substitution of N1-methyl-pseudouridine base for uridine enhances translation by a factor of 10 and prevents the immune trigger associated with PAMP sensors such as Toll-like receptors (TLRs) or the retinoic acid–inducible gene I (RIG-I).[21–23] This in turn protects from excessive inflammatory reactions, thereby minimizing vaccine side effects.[23]

All of the candidate mRNA vaccines target the spike protein S and incorporate the whole sequence of the

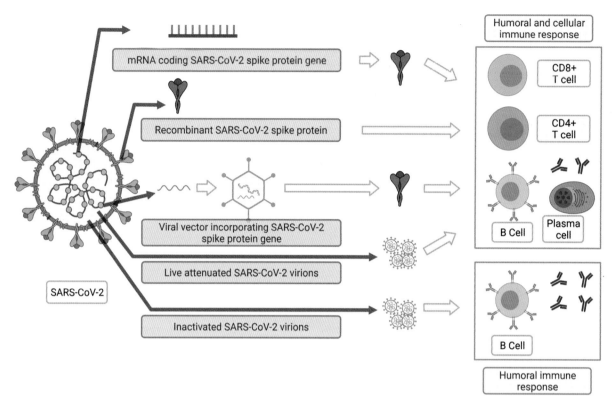

Fig. 18.10 Key Mechanisms Used in SARS-CoV-2 Vaccines. All the leading COVID-19 vaccines use one of these five key mechanisms to generate an adequate immune response in the vaccinated individual. The first four—mRNA coding SARS-CoV-2 spike protein gene, recombinant SARS-CoV-2 spike protein, recombinant viral vector, and live attenuated SARS-CoV-2 virions—induce both humoral and cellular responses, and the fifth, inactivated SARS-CoV-2 virions, generates only a humoral response. (Created using Biorender.)

mRNA code for the S protein. Although the receptor binding domain (RBD) segment of the S protein might suffice for the generation of SARS-CoV-2 neutralization antibodies, targeting the whole spike protein facilitates a broader immune response involving B cells and T cells.[23] Likewise, targeting the whole S protein would confer protection against many variants.[24]

mRNA Delivery and Mechanism of Action

Translation of mRNA and protein expression is directly related to the quantity of mRNA that is able to enter the cytoplasm of cells. The efficient delivery of IVT mRNA strands is accomplished by encapsulating the mRNA inside an LNP bubble. Once injected into the muscle, the mRNA-LNP complex is internalized and routed through the endolysosomal compartment, and the LNPs enable the mRNA to ultimately reach the myocyte cytoplasm from the endosomes.[19] The mRNA strands and the locally translated antigen are transported by the APCs in the skeletal muscle to the local draining lymph nodes, thereby generating vaccine-specific T-cell and B-cell responses.[25] Fig. 18.11, panels B, C, and D (mRNA vaccine immune response), illustrate this mRNA journey and initiation of both innate and adaptive immune responses. The mRNA vaccines predominantly trigger B cells to induce neutralizing antibodies but CD8 + and CD4 + T-cell responses are also generated in varying degrees.[19] In the germinal centers

of lymph node, antigen-activated B cells generate high-affinity neutralizing antibodies. Through a natural selection process mimicking evolution, some of these B cells are transformed into long-lived plasma cells and memory B cells.[23,26] The long-lived plasma cells typically survive for many years, retaining the capacity to secrete antibodies without the necessity of a fresh antigen stimulus, and the memory B cells are activated during subsequent episodes of pathogen exposure.[23,26]

Advantages and Disadvantages

The mRNA vaccines have considerable advantages. One critical feature of the mRNA framework is that the viral antigens are created in the host cell using its cellular machinery and the injected mRNA as the template for creating the protein antigen, thereby mimicking the natural pathogenesis of a viral infection.[19] This ensures the same posttranslational modifications, protein folding, and conformational changes enabling incorporation of the antigen in the membrane of APCs in the prefusion conformation.[19] This in turn will favor the development of specific antibodies tailored to the pathogen antigen.[27] There are also other desirable properties such as (1) not needing a vector for delivery of the antigen, thereby avoiding problems resulting from the possibility of preexisting antivector immunity[28]; and (2) the mRNA strands forming the core of the vaccine can be easily tailored to eliminate side effects or to address

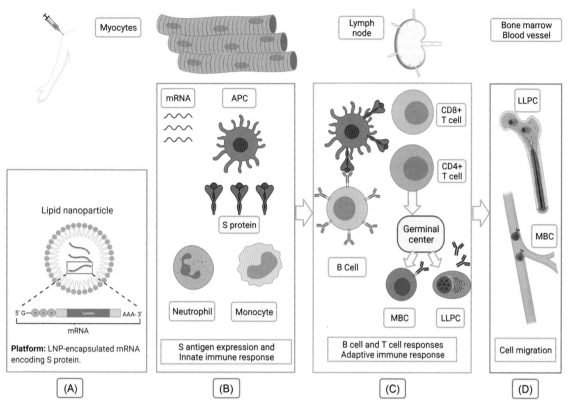

Fig. 18.11 mRNA Vaccine Immune Response. Once injected into the muscle, the lipid nanoparticle (LNP) complex containing the in vitro transcribed mRNA *(panel A)* is internalized and reaches the cytoplasm of the myocyte via the endosomes. The local translation of the mRNA generates spike proteins, which trigger an innate immune response *(panel B)*. The antigen-presenting cells *(APCs)* in the muscle transport the expressed spike protein to the lymph nodes, where specific B- and T-cell responses are triggered *(panel C)*. Some of the B cells get transformed into long-lived plasma cells *(LLPCs)* and memory B cells *(MBCs)* and migrate *(panel D)*. (Created using Biorender.)

mutations and related genetic drift, resulting in variants causing antigenic changes.[29] Moreover, unlike DNA vaccines, which need to be delivered directly into cell nuclei by electroporation, an mRNA vaccine can be administered by a routine intramuscular injection as antigen translation occurs in the cell cytoplasm.[27]

There are also some notable disadvantages for the mRNA formulations. Cold chain and storage restrictions in general are a concern. The BNT162b2 needs to be stored at –70°C for prolonged periods but will remain stable undiluted for about 2 weeks at –25°C. The BNT162b2 has been approved for storage at normal refrigerator temperatures for up to a month, and future modifications may allow for longer periods. The mRNA-1273 remains stable at –20°C for up to 6 months and at refrigerated conditions for up to 30 days. The CVnCoV (CureVac) remains stable for 3 months at 5°C. Fig. 18.12 summarizes the many advantages and disadvantages of the mRNA vaccine paradigm.

Recombinant Protein Vaccines

Although the mRNA and viral vector vaccines secured an early lead in the SRAS-CoV-2 vaccine race, recombinant protein subunit vaccines are also likely to play a significant role in the COVID-19 vaccine landscape.[30–34] The spike protein emerged as the dominant antigen target for most COVID-19 vaccines and that holds firm for the protein subunit vaccine framework also. There are three types based on the target antigen candidate— (1) full-length S-protein, (2) RBD of the S protein, and (3) multiple-epitope based, which uses segments of the RBD, S2 unit, and many other SARS-CoV-2 proteins.[30]

The protein subunit vaccines confer some significant advantages and strengths. They have a commendable track record of safety and efficacy based on the development of an effective acellular pertussis vaccine, HBV vaccine and the Shingrix subunit vaccine for herpes zoster.[35] Compared with mRNA vaccines, which typically require a cold chain for maintaining their potency, the subunit vaccines need only simple refrigeration. Whereas viral vector platforms can compromise the robustness of immune response with booster doses because of antivector immunity,[36] the protein subunit vaccines are well suited for primary vaccinations followed by subsequent boosters.[30] The Novavax protein subunit vaccine is a leading contender in this class of COVID-19 vaccines.

Candidate Vaccines

As of September 10, 2021, there were 114 candidate vaccines undergoing clinical evaluation, that is, in phase I, phase II, phase I/II (combined), phase II/III (combined),

mRNA Vaccines: Advantages and Disadvantages

Fig. 18.12 **mRNA Vaccine Advantages and Disadvantages.** From an efficacy perspective there are three main advantages: (1) the proteins expressed by the host cells resemble the viral proteins from a natural infection leading to (2) precise and specific immunity, and (3) the vaccines are easily modifiable to tackle variants by "editing" the mRNA strands as needed to create booster doses. *IVT*, In vitro transcription; *LNP*, lipid nanoparticle. (Data from Bettini E, Locci M. SARS-CoV-2 mRNA vaccines: immunological mechanism and beyond. *Vaccines.* 2021;9[2]:147; Kowalzik F, Schreiner D, Jensen C, et al. mRNA-based vaccines. *Vaccines.* 2021;9[4]:390; and Kim J, Eygeris Y, Gupta M, Sahay G. Self-assembled mRNA vaccines. *Adv Drug Deliv Rev.* 2021;170:83-112.)

phase III trials, or phase IV long-term clinical studies (postapproval). Another 206 candidate vaccines were in the preclinical stages of development.[37] Table 18.2 provides additional details about these candidate vaccines.

Next, this discussion will consider a few of the leading candidate vaccines undergoing phase III trials in more detail.

University of Oxford/AstraZenica (UOAZ) ChAdOx1 Viral Vector Vaccine

ChAdOx1 nCoV-19 (AZD1222) is a replication-deficient vaccine that incorporates the full-length SARS-CoV-2 spike glycoprotein gene and uses a chimpanzee adenovirus as vector to express the specific antigen.[38]

The UOAZ vaccine is undergoing two phase III trials, one in the United States and the other in the United Kingdom. The US phase III trial recruited more than 32,000 adults 18 years or older and studied the safety and efficacy of the vaccine (see Fig. 18.13 for additional details).

The UK trial combined phases II and III with the stated goal of determining the efficacy, safety, and immunogenicity of the candidate vaccine in adults (18 years and older) and children (2–11 years). The protocol called for the assessment of humoral and cellular immunogenicity on days 0, 7, 14, 28, 42, 56, 182, and 364. The trial is enrolling 60 children (2–11 years), 12,030 adults (18–64 years), and 240 older subjects (65 years and older). It is a double-blind placebo-controlled trial.

A pooled interim analysis reported an efficacy of 70.4% (95% confidence interval [CI], 54.8–80.6) for symptomatic COVID-19 and projected an acceptable safety profile.[39]

Moderna/NIAID mRNA-1273 Vaccine

The Moderna/NIAID candidate vaccine underwent a phase III trial to assess its safety, efficacy, and immunogenicity in adults 18 years and older. It was a double-blind, placebo-controlled trial. Fig. 18.14 provides additional details of the clinical trial. Moderna has completed phase I[40] and phase II[41] studies successfully, establishing and confirming the safety and immunogenicity for a two-dose regimen of the vaccine,[41] and the phase III study is ongoing. This mRNA vaccine encodes the prefusion stabilized full-length spike glycoprotein of SARS-CoV-2 and is encased in an LPN bubble.[42]

Based on symptomatic COVID-19 as the endpoint the reported efficacy for the vaccine was 94.1% (95% CI, 89.3–96.8) without any significant safety concerns apart from local reactions and flu-like symptoms in a small subset of trial participants.[42] Based on the phase III study results, the FDA granted an EUA for this vaccine in December 2020 Subsequently, FDA gave regular approval for this vaccine on January 31, 2022.

BioNTech/Pfizer BNT162b2 mRNA Vaccine

The BNT162b2 candidate vaccine underwent a randomized placebo-controlled, multisite phase III trial to assess its efficacy and safety. The vaccine moved to phase III after successfully completing a combined phase I/II study. It is a LPN-formulated, nucleoside-modified mRNA vaccine that encodes the prefusion stabilized SARS-CoV-2 full-length spike glycoprotein.[43] In the phase I/II study

Table 18.2 Number of Prospective COVID-19 Vaccines in Clinical and Preclinical Phases as of September 10, 2021

Platform	Preclinical	Clinical Phases						
		All Phases	Phase I	Phase I/II	Phase II	Phase II/III	Phase III	Phase IV
Protein subunit (PS)	71	39	10	12	3	1	13	0
Viral vector (nonrepli-cating) (VVnr)	21	17	7	4	0	2	1	3
DNA	16	11	4	4	0	2	1	0
Inactivated virus (IV)	9	16	4	2	0	1	7	2
RNA	25	19	8	2	2	2	2	3
Viral vector (replicating) (VVr)	19	2	0	0	1	1	0	0
Virus-like particle (VLP)	18	5	1	2	1	1	0	0
VVr + antigen-presenting cell (VVr + APC)		2	1	0	1	0	0	0
Live attenuated virus (LAV)	2	2	2	0	0	0	0	0
VVnr + antigen-presenting cell (VVnr + APC)	21	1	0	1	0	0	0	0
Live-attenuated bacterial vector (LABV)	2							
Bacterial vector (replicating) (BVr)	1							
Cellular-based vaccine (cell)	1							
Total	**206**	**114**	**37**	**27**	**8**	**10**	**24**	**8**

Data from the World Health Organization: COVID-19 vaccine tracker and landscape. https://wwwwhoint/publications/m/item/draft-landscape-of-covid-19-candidate-vaccines.

University of Oxford/AstraZeneca Viral Vector Vaccine
(Start: August 2020; Completion: February 2023; Trial registered in United States)

- Timeline
  - Start: August 2020
  - Completion: February 2023
- Randomized double-blind placebo-controlled
- Phase 3; 32,459 participants
- Vaccine type: nonreplicating viral vector vaccine
- Outcome measures
  - Primary
    - PCR positive symptomatic COVID-19 over 12 months
    - Safety and tolerability of two IM doses compared to placebo
  - Secondary
    - Prevention of SARS-CoV-2 asymptomatic infection over 12 months
    - Periodic immunogenicity study

- Study protocol
  - Adults ≥18 years
  - 2 IM doses of AZD1222 or placebo given 4 weeks apart
  - Follow up visits at day 28, 80, 182, and 364
  - Test for COVID-19 if symptoms develop

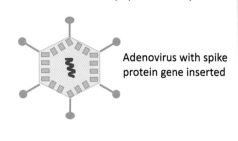

Adenovirus with spike protein gene inserted

Abstracted from https://clinicaltrials.gov/ct2/show/record/NCT04516746; accessed September 13, 2021.

Fig. 18.13 University of Oxford/AstraZeneca Viral Vector Candidate Vaccine. It is a nonreplicating viral vector vaccine. The figure provides the timeline, outcome measures, and other phase III study protocol details. *IM*, Intramuscular; *PCR*, polymerase chain reaction.

Moderna/NIAID mRNA Vaccine
(Start: July 2020; Completion: October 2022)

- Timeline
  - Start: July 2020
  - Completion: October 2022
- Randomized double-blind, placebo-controlled
- Phase 3; 30,420 participants
- Vaccine type: mRNA
- Outcome measures
  - Safety
    - Local and systemic adverse reactions
  - Efficacy
    - Immunogenicity of mRNA by titer of SARS-CoV-2–specific binding antibody
    - Through 2 years after final dose

- Dose
  - Vaccine arm will receive 1 IM injection of 100 microgram of mRNA Day 1 and Day 29
  - Placebo arm will receive 1 IM injection of matching placebo (normal saline) on Day 1 and Day 29
- Study population
  - Adults ≥18 years

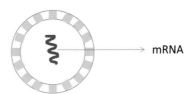

Abstracted from https://clinicaltrials.gov/ct2/show/record/NCT04470427; accessed September 14, 2021.

Fig. 18.14 Moderna/National Institute of Allergy and Infectious Diseases *(NIAID)* mRNA Vaccine. Timeline, outcome measures, and other phase III study protocol details. mRNA strand coding for spike protein is shown surrounded by a lipid envelope. *IM*, Intramuscular.

BioNTech/Pfizer mRNA Vaccine
(Start: April 2020; Completion: May 2023)

- Timeline
  - Start: April 2020
  - Completion: May 2023
- Randomized placebo-controlled, blinded trial
- mRNA vaccine
  - Lipid nanoparticle–formulated
  - Nuceloside-modified
  - Encodes trimerized SARS-COV-2 full-length spike glycoprotein
- Outcome measures
  - Primary
    - Safety
    - Adverse reactions
  - Secondary
    - Periodic immunogenicity study
    - Confirmed COVID-19 incidence

- Multisite
  - Phase II/III
  - 43,998 participants
- Study protocol
  - 3 age groups
    - Adults 18–55 years
    - Adults 56–85 years
    - Children/adolescents 12–17 years
  - Two-dose IM injection 21 days apart

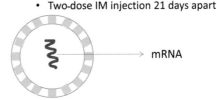

Abstracted from https://clinicaltrials.gov/ct2/show/study/NCT04368728; accessed September 14, 2021.

Fig. 18.15 BioNTech/Pfizer mRNA Vaccine. Timeline, outcome measures, and other phase II/III study protocol details. mRNA strand coding for spike protein is shown, surrounded by a lipid envelope. *IM*, Intramuscular.

using 45 healthy adult volunteers, the investigators observed 1.9 to 4.6 times neutralizing antibody titer levels when compared with convalescent human serum.[44]

Using the primary endpoint of symptomatic COVID-19, BNT162b2 had an efficacy of 95% (95% CI, 90%–97.9%) with a good safety profile.[43] Based on the phase III study result the FDA granted an EUA for this vaccine in December 2020. Subsequently, in August 2021, the FDA approved the vaccine for individuals 16 years and older and granted EUA for use in children and adolescents 5 through 15 years.[45] Fig. 18.15 presents additional details of the study.

Janssen Ad26-COV2-S Vaccine

The Janssen Ad26-COV2-S vaccine makes use of a recombinant, nonreplicating human adenovirus type 26 vectors and encodes the full-length SARS-CoV-2 spike glycoprotein in a prefusion-stabilized conformation.[46] The vaccine successfully completed phase I and phase II studies[47] before embarking on the phase III clinical trial.

Based on the primary endpoint of moderate to severe-critical COVID-19 manifesting at least 28 days after the administration of a single dose, Ad26-COV2-S vaccine had an efficacy of 66.3% (95% CI, 59.9–71.8) with a good safety profile comparable to those of other COVID-19 vaccines in phase III trials.[46] Based on the phase III study result the FDA granted an EUA for this single-dose vaccine in February 2021.[48] The phase III trial of the vaccine is ongoing.

Gam-Covid-Vac rAd26-rAd5 Vaccine

The Gam-Covid-Vac, also referred to as the Sputnik V vaccine, makes use of two adenovirus vectors (rAd26 and rAd5), with both vectors carrying the gene for the full-length SARS-CoV-2 spike glycoprotein.[49] The vaccine is administered as a two-dose regimen, 21 days apart. The phase I/II studies of the rAd26-rAd5 vaccine demonstrated a good safety profile and induced strong humoral and cellular immune responses in trial participants.[50]

Based on the primary endpoint of reverse transcription polymerase chain reaction (RT-PCR)-confirmed COVID-19 manifesting from day 21 after the administration of the first dose, rAd26-rAd5 vaccine had an efficacy of 91.6% (95% CI, 85.6–95.2) with a good safety profile.[49] The phase III trial of the vaccine is ongoing.

Sinovac (CoronaVac) Vaccine

The Sinovac candidate vaccine underwent a randomized placebo-controlled, blinded trial in two sites: Brazil and Indonesia. It is an inactivated vaccine. The phase I/II studies were successful from safety and immunogenicity perspectives; the vaccine was well tolerated by the participants and induced humoral responses against SARS-CoV-2.[51]

The details of the phase III study are shown in Fig. 18.16, and the virus inactivation process to create the Sinovac vaccine is illustrated in Fig. 18.17.

Novavax Protein Subunit Vaccine

The Novavax vaccine labeled NVX-CoV2372 uses the full-length S protein with mutations in the S1/S2 cleavage sites, making it protease resistant, and additional substitutions in the S2 subunit to stabilize it at the prefusion conformation.[33] This recombinant SARS-CoV-2 termed rSARS-CoV-2 was optimized in the baculovirus insect cell expression system.[52] The vaccine is mixed with the Matrix-M adjuvant, consisting of two nanosized particles, before use to augment the T helper 1 (Th1) and Th2 type immune responses.[30,33]

The Novavax protein subunit vaccine completed a phase I study and moved to phase II and phase III studies. It is a double-blinded, randomized controlled study, which uses a recombinant spike protein nanoparticle configuration. Additional details of the vaccine and the protocol of the ongoing phase III studies are shown in Fig. 18.18. The generation of the spike protein nanoparticle based on the baculovirus insect cell system used in the development of the Novavax vaccine is illustrated in Fig. 18.19.

Phase I study participants were split randomly into three groups: 83 study subjects were administered vaccine with adjuvant, 25 were given the vaccine without adjuvant, and 23 received the placebo. The first group (vaccine with adjuvant) elicited immune responses that exceeded neutralizing antibody titers

Sinovac Vaccine
(Start: July 2020; Completion: April 2023)

- **Phase III timeline**
  - Indonesia: 1620 participants
    - Start: July 2020
    - Completion: August 2021
  - Turkey: 13,000 participants
    - Start: September 2020
    - Completion: April 2022
  - Chile: 2300 participants
    - Start: November 2020
    - Completion: March 2022
  - Global: 14,000 participants
    - Start: August 2021
    - Completion: April 2023
- **Randomized placebo-controlled, blinded trial**
- **Adsorbed COVID-19–inactivated vaccine**

- **Outcome measures**
  - Primary
    - Safety
    - Adverse reactions
  - Secondary
    - Periodic immunogenicity study
    - Confirmed COVID-19 incidence
- **Study protocol**
  - 3 age groups
    - Adults 18–59 years (Indonesia, Turkey, Chile)
    - Adults ≥60 years (Chile)
    - Children/adolescents (6 months–17 years)
  - Two-dose IM injection 14 days apart in adults 18 years or more
  - Two-dose IM injection 28 days apart in the 6 months through 17 years age group

Abstracted from https://clinicaltrials.gov/ct2/show/NCT04508075; https://clinicaltrials.gov/ct2/show/study/NCT04582344; https://www.clinicaltrials.gov/ct2/show/NCT04651790; https://clinicaltrials.gov/ct2/show/NCT04992260; accessed September 14, 2021.

Fig. 18.16 Sinovac Vaccine Phase III Study. Timeline, outcome measures, and other phase III study protocol details. *IM,* Intramuscular.

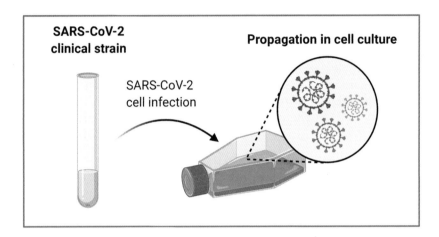

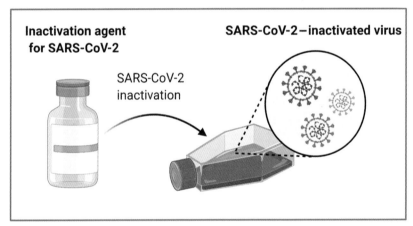

Platform: Inactivated virus vaccine produced from viral propagation in cells infected with a SARS-CoV-2 clinical strain.

Fig. 18.17 Sinovac Vaccine and Virus Inactivation. Cell culture propagation and inactivation steps in the development of the Sinovac inactivated virus vaccine. (Created using Biorender.)

observed in COVID-19 convalescent serum. The vaccine with adjuvant combination also elicited CD4+ T-cell responses with a predominant Th1 phenotype.[33]

A phase II study of the Novavax vaccine with a target of 4400 participants was started in late August 2020, and a phase III study with a plan to enroll 48,000 participants in multiple countries commenced in November 2020. The interim results of the phase III study[53] are included in Table 18.3.

A Critical Look at SARS-CoV-2 Vaccine Phase III Trials

This section will examine the efficacy of different vaccines based on the results of phase III trials. Table 18.3 summarizes efficacy measures of mRNA-1273 (Moderna), BNT162b2 (BioNTech-Pfizer), ChAdOx1 (Oxford-AstraZeneca), Ad26-COV2-S (Janssen), rAd26-rAd5 (Sputnik V), and NVX-CoV2373 (Novavax) vaccines. All except Novavax have been given EUA or approval by one or more regulatory agencies. The reported efficacy ranges vary from 66.3% for the Janssen vaccine to 95% for the BioNTech-Pfizer vaccine.

The safety profiles of these vaccines based on phase III trials have been encouraging and reassuring. Localized symptoms such as pain and swelling at the injection site and some systemic manifestations resembling a mild version of flu with fever, headache, and nausea in a subset of trial participants receiving the vaccine have been documented. However, no serious adverse events have been causally linked to these vaccines during the phase III trials.

For evaluation of vaccine efficacy, the primary outcome was development of symptomatic COVID-19. However, from a transmission and population immunity perspective it is important to determine if these vaccines prevent the development of asymptomatic disease or

Novavax Protein Subunit Vaccine
(Start: November 2020; Completion: June 2023)

- Timeline
  - United Kingdom
    - Start: November 2020
    - Completion: January 2022
  - Mexico, Puerto Rico, and United States
    - Start: December 2020
    - Completion: June 2023
- Randomized blinded, placebo-controlled study
- Recombinant spike protein nanoparticle vaccine
- Phase III
  - United Kingdom
    - 15,000 participants
  - Mexico, Puerto Rico, United States
    - 33,000 participants

- Outcome measures
  - Primary
    - Symptomatic mild, moderate, or severe COVID-19 (Day 28–Day 750)
    - Adverse reactions
  - Secondary
    - Immunogenicity study
- Study protocol
  - Mexico, Puerto Rico, and United States
    - Adults 18 years and older
    - Adolescents 12 through 17 years
  - United Kingdom
    - Adults 18 through 84 years
  - Two IM injections Day 0 and Day 21

Abstracted from https://clinicaltrials.gov/ct2/show/record/NCT04611802; https://clinicaltrials.gov/ct2/show/NCT04583995; accessed September 14, 2021.

Fig. 18.18 Novavax Protein Subunit Vaccine Study Protocol. Timeline, outcome measures, and other phase III study protocol details. *IM,* Intramuscular.

prevent a person from getting infected with SARS-CoV-2 and transmitting the virus to susceptible individuals. We have efficacy measures for asymptomatic infections as part of phase III trial only for two vaccines: an efficacy of 27.3% for the ChAdOx1[39] and an efficacy of 66% for the Ad-26-COV2-S.[46] Mehrotra et al.[54] caution that vaccine protection against COVID-19 based on efficacy for the prevention of symptomatic COVID-19 could result in a larger proportion of asymptomatic SARS-CoV-2 infections.[54] This is an untoward but plausible outcome if the administered vaccines are unable to confer sterilizing immunity.[54,55]

Note that efficacy assessments with symptomatic COVID-19 as the primary endpoint could be problematic. A vaccine that suppresses COVID-19 symptoms, thereby transforming symptomatic infections to asymptomatic ones without reducing viral load and transmission characteristics, could lead to more infections in the community because asymptomatic individuals are less likely to undergo testing and isolation.[54] However, if vaccine coverage is high and approaches population immunity in the community, the increase in the number of asymptomatic infections and the resulting excess transmission would be directed increasingly more toward the vaccinated, who are already protected from symptomatic disease.[54]

Promises, Pitfalls, and Challenges of Vaccine Development During Pandemic Times

Based on the progress made so far, it is evident that vaccine development is proceeding at an accelerated pace compared with historical vaccine development

efforts. There is the pressure of the pandemic that is infecting large numbers of people daily and causing significant fatalities on a daily basis worldwide.[56] As we already noted, over the duration of the pandemic, SARS-CoV-2 has infected hundreds of millions of people worldwide, with total fatalities in multimillions. These are the people who tested positive for the virus. Assuming the magnitude of infection to be 10-fold would still leave out a large majority of the world's population as potential targets of the virus. For the pandemic to resolve there needs to be about 75% population immunity, which could be acquired through infection or vaccination. Assuming current mortality rates, achieving population immunity globally through spread of infection would result in additional deaths of tens of millions of people. Thus developing and deploying safe and effective vaccines globally is a much more desirable option for population immunity acquisition. However, releasing a vaccine to sections of the general population, before completing a successful phase III trial, and establishing the safety and efficacy of the candidate vaccine, is also a very risky proposition.

Although neutralizing antibodies have been demonstrated in persons recovering from an infection with SARS-CoV-2, it is not clear if the infection confers long-lasting immunity; a number of cases of reinfection were reported and documented even before the first year of the pandemic had passed.

Vaccines for measles, mumps, rubella, polio, smallpox and influenza have a long history of safe use, and they were all developed with stringent regulatory requirements and scientific rigor. It is notable that the SARS-CoV-1 vaccine generated worrisome immune

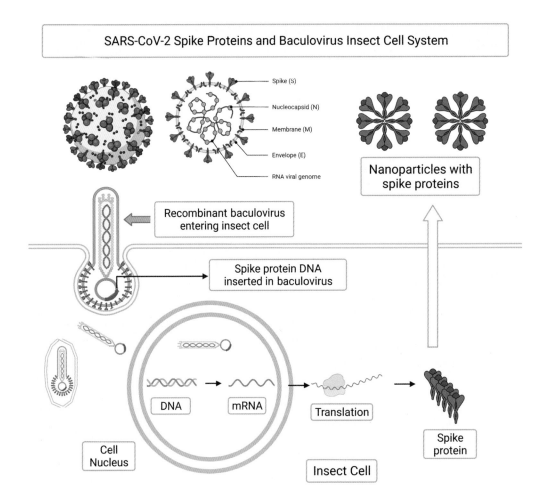

Fig. 18.19 SARS-CoV-2 Spike Proteins and the Baculovirus Insect Cell System. Creation of the nanoparticles studded with SARS-CoV-2 spike proteins using the baculovirus insect cell system. The baculovirus carrying the modified spike protein gene enters the insect cell by endocytosis. Subsequently, the nucleocapsid is released into the cytoplasm, which then migrates to the insect cell nucleus. The expression of viral DNA occurs inside the nucleus. In the nucleus of the cell the recombinant spike protein gene is transcribed into mRNA, which then enters the translation process, resulting in the formation of spike proteins. These are harvested from the insect cell to create the nanoparticles studded with the spike proteins. This is the process followed in the development of the Novavax vaccine. (Modified from Fabre ML, Arrías PN, Masson T, et al. Baculovirus-derived vectors for immunization and therapeutic applications. In: *Emerging and Reemerging Viral Pathogens.* San Diego, CA: Academic Press; 2020:197-224; and Corum J, Zimmer C. How the Novavax vaccine works. *New York Times.* New York: Times Inc.; 2021. Created using Biorender.)

Table 18.3 Efficacy of mRNA-1273, BNT162b2-mRNA, ChAdOx1 Ad26-COV2-S, rAd26-rAd5, and NVX-CoV2373 Vaccines

Vaccine	Number of Doses	Symptomatic COVID-19 Cases			Vaccine-Placebo Ratio	Efficacy (%)	95% Confidence Interval
		Total	Vaccine Arm	Placebo Arm			
mRNA-1273	2	196	11	185	1:1	94.1	89.3–96.8
BNT162b2	2	170	8	162	1:1	95	90–97.9
ChAdOx1	2	131	30	101	1:1	70.4	54.8–80.6
Ad26-COV2-S	1	682	173	509	1:1	66.3	59.9–71.8
rAd26-rAd5	2	78	16	62	3:1	91.6	85.6–95.2
NVX-CoV2373	2	106	10	96	1:1	89.7	80.2–94.6

Data from Baden LR, El Sahly HM, Essink B, et al. Efficacy and safety of the mRNA-1273 SARS-CoV-2 vaccine. *N Engl J Med.* 2021;384(5):403–416; Polack FP, Thomas SJ, Kitchin N, et al. Safety and efficacy of the BNT162b2 mRNA Covid-19 vaccine. *N Engl J Med.* 2020;383(27):2603–2615; Voysey M, Clemens SAC, Madhi SA, et al. Safety and efficacy of the ChAdOx1 nCoV-19 vaccine (AZD1222) against SARS-CoV-2: an interim analysis of four randomised controlled trials in Brazil, South Africa, and the UK. *Lancet.* 2021;397(10269):99–111; Sadoff J, Gray G, Vandebosch A, et al. Safety and efficacy of single-dose Ad26.COV2.S vaccine against COVID-19. *N Engl J Med.* 2021;384(23):2187–2201; Logunov DY, Dolzhikova IV, Shcheblyakov DV, et al. Safety and efficacy of an rAd26 and rAd5 vector-based heterologous prime-boost COVID-19 vaccine: an interim analysis of a randomised controlled phase 3 trial in Russia. *Lancet* 2021;397(10275):671–681; and Heath PT, Galiza EP, Baxter DN, et al. Safety and efficacy of NVX-CoV2373 Covid-19 vaccine. *N Engl J Med.* 2021;385(13):1172–1183.

responses in ferrets and monkeys, whereas mice were reportedly safe.[57] Anti–SARS-CoV-1 spike protein antibodies generated by a vaccinia vector worsened lung injury in Chinese macaques after being administered a challenge dose of the virus; this was the result of infection and proinflammatory reprogramming of macrophages.[58] In general, vaccine-associated disease enhancement remains a distinct possibility. Lax regulation by the FDA in 2020 resulted in the marketing of many SARS-CoV-2 antibody tests with questionable sensitivity and specificity. That is a cautionary tale.

The WHO has provided preferred target characteristics for a safe and effective SARS-CoV-2 vaccine.[59] Table 18.4 summarizes the desired properties for a COVID-19 vaccine.

COVID-19 Vaccine Rollout

Immunity After Vaccination

The first COVID-19 vaccine to be evaluated by the FDA was the mRNA-based vaccine produced by Pfizer-BioNTech. On November 18, 2020, Pfizer and BioNTech announced the results of their phase III efficacy study. They reported a vaccine efficacy of 95% ($P < .0001$) that was consistent across age, sex, race, and ethnicity. They reported no severe cases of COVID-19 in their vaccinated individuals and no safety issues. This announcement was soon followed by Moderna reporting the results of their Coronavirus Efficacy and Safety Study (COVE). Moderna reported that this trial demonstrated that their mRNA vaccine had 94.1% efficacy and a similar 100% efficacy against severe disease. Moderna also reported no safety concerns for their vaccine.

December 10, the FDA independent scientific advisory committee on vaccines reviewed the Pfizer-BioNTech application for EUA, and on December 17 this committee reviewed Moderna's application. Both times the committee recommended for EUA for these

vaccines, and in December 2020 the first doses of these vaccines began to be administered in the United States.

Along with efficacy data, additional data were presented on the ability of these vaccines to generate robust B-cell responses that generated high levels of neutralizing antibodies and robust T-cell responses. This information formed the basis for the initial EUA, but as time passes ongoing studies would confirm that at 6 months antibody levels remained high and protection was still durable for both vaccines. Based on these data, expectations were that protection would last at a minimum for 1 year.

Meanwhile, outside the United States, the results of the AstraZeneca AZD1222 ChAdOx vaccine interim analysis were released. This vaccine used replication-incompetent adenoviral vector technology. The data released were a bit more complicated because of a manufacturing issue, but the report was of a 62% vaccine efficacy overall but a similar 100% protection against hospitalization or death from COVID-19. After release, safety concerns would arise regarding rare but increased rates of clots in vaccine recipients.

It was several months later that the data became available on the next vaccine that would be given EUA in the United States, the Johnson and Johnson (J&J) vaccine produced by the Janssen division. This vaccine used replication-incompetent adenoviral vector technology, much like the AstraZeneca vaccine, but in this case was a one-dose vaccine using human adenovirus instead of a chimpanzee adenovirus. The J&J Ad26-COV2-S vaccine trial was the largest and fastest enrolled vaccine trial up to this point in history, with almost 40,000 participants included from multiple sites in multiple countries. As early as 14 days after the single-dose vaccination, an efficacy of 67% was reported, and by 28 days 100% protection against hospitalization or death from COVID-19. This was one of the first primary trials that also produced efficacy against asymptomatic infection that would be presented to the FDA. After 29 days and out to day 71 a 74% reduction in

Table 18.4 Preferred Characteristics of a SARS-CoV-2 Vaccine Based on World Health Organization Guidelines	
Vaccine Feature	**What Is Preferred**
Indication	Active immunization to prevent COVID-19
Contraindication	None
Target population	All ages
Safety and reactogenicity	High benefit-to-risk profile
Efficacy	Minimum 70% efficacy
	Onset of protection within 2 weeks of administration of vaccine
Dose regimen	Single dose plus annual booster if needed
Duration of protection	At least 1 year
Route of administration	Nonparenteral preferred
Stability and storage	Shelf life of 6 to 12 months at room temperature
Accessibility	Capability to quickly scale up production

asymptomatic COVID-19 was reported. Although initial safety reports suggested no concerns a short time after its widespread administration, its use in the United States would pause because of concerns about clots associated with low platelet levels in younger women. The vaccine administration would then resume in the United States but going forward would carry a warning.

Breakthrough Infections

The massive vaccination campaign throughout the world and in the United States served as a source of information on the rate and characteristics of breakthrough infections in fully vaccinated individuals. Although initially the Centers for Disease Control and Prevention (CDC) started by tracking all breakthrough infections after COVID-19 vaccination on May 14, they transitioned to only reporting cases that required hospitalization or resulted in death. The CDC established a vaccine breakthrough case definition of a person who has SARS-CoV-2 RNA or antigen detected on a respiratory specimen collected 14 days or more after completing the primary series of an FDA-authorized COVID-19 vaccine. The data collected by the CDC did support the effectiveness found in the vaccine trials with evidence that breakthrough infections were rare and evidence that vaccination may make illness less severe.[60]

Several studies looked at breakthrough infections in fully vaccinated individuals and suggested that this was much in line with rates suggested from the initial studies that supported vaccine EUA.[61] This was followed by publications describing vaccine breakthrough infections with SARS-CoV-2 variants.[62]

Vaccine Challenges Posed by SARS-CoV-2 Variants

Although SARS-CoV-2 variants of concern quickly affected the efficacy of some of our monoclonal antibody therapy, the significance for vaccine efficacy was initially a different matter. The mRNA vaccines were tested in locations and times with a low frequency of variants of concern; however, real-world data soon emerged on the efficacy of these vaccines in areas of the world with rising numbers of infections because of these variants of concern. In May 2020, a letter to the editor was published in the *New England Journal of Medicine* describing the success of the mass vaccination program in Qatar. In Qatar there had been a B.1.1.7 wave followed by a rapid expansion of B.1.351, with viral genome sequencing suggesting that 50% of the infections were caused by B.1.351 and 45% were caused by B.1.1.7. They estimated that the effectiveness of the vaccine against the B.1.1.7 variant and the B.1.351 variants were 89.5% and 75%, respectively.[63] Other vaccines were also tested against variants of concern. Moderna reported positive initial booster data against

SARS-CoV-2 variants of concern.[64] In a phase IIa-b trial the Novavax NVX-CoV2373 vaccine was reported to have achieved an efficacy of 60% with 93% of the sequenced isolates being the B.1.351 variant.[65] Many vaccine producers anticipate second-generation vaccines with improved efficacy against variants of concern.

The Road Ahead

Although many considered vaccines to be the definitive solution for ending this pandemic, many questions remained in terms of the vaccine distribution process and the impact of variants of concern on vaccine efficacy. After initially peaking in the United States with over 3.5 million vaccine doses being administered per day, by early May the number of doses per day had dropped below 2 million. Vaccines were quickly administered in certain countries such as Israel, the United Kingdom, and the United States; however, many countries had limited access to vaccines and saw tremendous increases in infection rates as countries with high vaccination rates saw decreases. The catastrophes in Brazil and India are warnings to the world of what happens when nonpharmaceutical interventions such as masking, physical distancing, and shutdowns were eased before widespread vaccination. The impact of the high numbers of infections and the impact of viral variants will take many years to be fully appreciated.

Conclusion

The rapidity with which COVID-19 vaccines were developed, produced, and distributed is without historical precedent. Although many questions remain regarding duration of protection, requirement for boosters, and adjusted vaccines to protect against variants, it did not take long to see that countries that achieved rapid widespread vaccination of their populations experienced rapid reduction in cases, hospitalizations, and deaths.

REFERENCES

1. Summers W. Historical roots: The family tree of viral pathogenesis. In: Katze M, Korth M, Law L, Nathanson N, eds. *Viral Pathogenesis*. 3rd edn; 2016.
2. Enquist L, Racaniello V. Virology: From contagium fluidum to virome. In: Knipe D, Howley P, eds. *Field's virology*. 6th edn. Philadelphia: Wolters Kluwer; 2013.
3. DiMaio D, Fan H. Viruses, cell transformation, and cancer. In: Knipe D, Howley P, eds. *Field's virology*. 6th edn. Philadelphia: Wolters Kluwer; 2013.
4. Wallace N, Galloway D. Viral oncogenesis. In: Katze M, Korth M, Law L, Nathanson N, eds. *Viral Pathogenesis*. 3rd edn; 2016.
5. Punt J, Stranford S, Jones P, Owen J: Kuby immunology: W. H. Freeman; 2018.
6. Virella G. *Medical immunology*. 7th edn: CRC Press; 2020.
7. Giese M. *Introduction to molecular vaccinology*: Springer; 2016.

8. Polio this week as of August, 2020 [http://polioeradication.org/polio-today/polio-now/this-week/]

9. Barrett A. Licensed vaccines for humans. In: Milligan G, Barrett A, eds. *Vaccinology, an essential guide*: Wiley Blackwell; 2015.

10. Hu Z, Ott PA, Wu CJ. Towards personalized, tumour-specific, therapeutic vaccines for cancer. *Nature Reviews Immunology*. 2018;18(3):168.

11. Guo C, Manjili MH, Subjeck JR, Sarkar D, Fisher PB, Wang X-Y. Therapeutic cancer vaccines: past, present, and futureAdvances in cancer research119: Elsevier; 2013:421–475.

12. Domnich A, Arata L, Amicizia D, Puig-Barberà J, Gasparini R, Panatto D. Effectiveness of MF59-adjuvanted seasonal influenza vaccine in the elderly: a systematic review and meta-analysis. *Vaccine*. 2017;35(4):513–520.

13. DiazGranados CA, Denis M, Plotkin S. Seasonal influenza vaccine efficacy and its determinants in children and non-elderly adults: a systematic review with meta-analyses of controlled trials. *Vaccine*. 2012;31(1):49–57.

14. Pera A, Campos C, López N, Hassouneh F, Alonso C, Tarazona R, Solana R. Immunosenescence: implications for response to infection and vaccination in older people. *Maturitas*. 2015;82(1):50–55.

15. Allen JC, Toapanta FR, Chen W, Tennant SM. Understanding immunosenescence and its impact on vaccination of older adults. *Vaccine*. 2020;38(52):8264–8272.

16. Hilleman M. The development of live attenuated mumps virus vaccine in historic perspective and its role in the evolution of combined measles-mumps-rubella. In: Plotkin S, ed. *History of vaccine development*: Springer; 2011:207–215.

17. Bailey JR, Barnes E, Cox AL. Approaches, progress, and challenges to hepatitis C vaccine development. *Gastroenterology*. 2019;156(2):418–430.

18. Beeson JG, Kurtovic L, Dobaño C, Opi DH, Chan J-A, Feng G, Good MF, Reiling L, Boyle MJ. Challenges and strategies for developing efficacious and long-lasting malaria vaccines. *Science Translational Medicine*. 2019;11(474).

19. Verbeke R, Lentacker I, De Smedt SC, Dewitte H. The dawn of mRNA vaccines: The COVID-19 case. *Journal of Controlled Release*. 2021.

20. Baiersdörfer M, Boros G, Muramatsu H, Mahiny A, Vlatkovic I, Sahin U, Karikó K. A facile method for the removal of dsRNA contaminant from in vitro-transcribed mRNA. *Molecular Therapy-Nucleic Acids*. 2019;15:26–35.

21. Karikó K, Muramatsu H, Welsh FA, Ludwig J, Kato H, Akira S, Weissman D. Incorporation of pseudouridine into mRNA yields superior nonimmunogenic vector with increased translational capacity and biological stability. *Molecular therapy*. 2008;16(11):1833–1840.

22. Pardi N, Hogan MJ, Porter FW. Weissman D: mRNA vaccines—a new era in vaccinology. *Nature reviews Drug discovery*. 2018;17(4):261.

23. Bettini E, Locci M. SARS-CoV-2 mRNA vaccines: immunological mechanism and beyond. *Vaccines*. 2021;9(2):147.

24. Liu L, Wang P, Nair MS, Yu J, Rapp M, Wang Q, Luo Y, Chan JF-W, Sahi V, Figueroa A. Potent neutralizing antibodies against multiple epitopes on SARS-CoV-2 spike. *Nature*. 2020;584(7821):450–456.

25. Liang F, Lindgren G, Lin A, Thompson EA, Ols S, Röhss J, John S, Hassett K, Yuzhakov O, Bahl K. Efficient targeting and activation of antigen-presenting cells in vivo after modified mRNA vaccine administration in rhesus macaques. *Molecular Therapy*. 2017;25(12):2635–2647.

26. Sallusto F, Lanzavecchia A, Araki K, Ahmed R. From vaccines to memory and back. *Immunity*. 2010;33(4):451–463.

27. Cagigi A, Loré K. Immune Responses Induced by MRNA Vaccination in Mice, Monkeys and Humans. *Vaccines*. 2021;9(1):61.

28. Xu Y, Li X, Zhu B, Liang H, Fang C, Gong Y, Guo Q, Sun X, Zhao D, Shen J. Characteristics of pediatric SARS-CoV-2 infection and potential evidence for persistent fecal viral shedding. *Nature medicine*. 2020;26(4):502–505.

29. Kowalzik F, Schreiner D, Jensen C, Teschner D, Gehring S, Zepp F. mRNA-Based Vaccines. *Vaccines*. 2021;9(4):390.

30. Pollet J, Chen W-H, Strych U. Recombinant protein vaccines, a proven approach against coronavirus pandemics. *Advanced Drug Delivery Reviews*. 2021.

31. Wu Y, Huang X, Yuan L, Wang S, Zhang Y, Xiong H, Chen R, Ma J, Qi R, Nie M. A recombinant spike protein subunit vaccine confers protective immunity against SARS-CoV-2 infection and transmission in hamsters. *Science Translational Medicine*. 2021;13(606):eabg1143.

32. Dai L, Zheng T, Xu K, Han Y, Xu L, Huang E, An Y, Cheng Y, Li S, Liu M. A universal design of betacoronavirus vaccines against COVID-19, MERS, and SARS. *Cell*. 2020;182(3):722–733.e711.

33. Keech C, Albert G, Cho I, Robertson A, Reed P, Neal S, Plested JS, Zhu M, Cloney-Clark S, Zhou H, et al. Phase 1–2 Trial of a SARS-CoV-2 Recombinant Spike Protein Nanoparticle Vaccine. *New England Journal of Medicine*. 2020;383(24):2320–2332.

34. Tian J-H, Patel N, Haupt R, Zhou H, Weston S, Hammond H, Logue J, Portnoff AD, Norton J, Guebre-Xabier M. SARS-CoV-2 spike glycoprotein vaccine candidate NVX-CoV2373 immunogenicity in baboons and protection in mice. *Nature communications*. 2021;12(1):1–14.

35. Vetter V, Denizer G, Friedland LR, Krishnan J, Shapiro M. Understanding modern-day vaccines: what you need to know. *Annals of medicine*. 2018;50(2):110–120.

36. Ura T, Okuda K, Shimada M. Developments in viral vector-based vaccines. *Vaccines*. 2014;2(3):624–641.

37. World Health Organization: COVID-19 vaccine tracker and landscape. In: Available on-line: https://wwwwhoint/publications/m/item/draft-landscape-of-covid-19-candidate-vaccines. 2021.

38. Ramasamy MN, Minassian AM, Ewer KJ, Flaxman AL, Folegatti PM, Owens DR, Voysey M, Aley PK, Angus B, Babbage G. Safety and immunogenicity of ChAdOx1 nCoV-19 vaccine administered in a prime-boost regimen in young and old adults (COV002): a single-blind, randomised, controlled, phase 2/3 trial.*The Lancet*. 2020;396:1979–1993.

39. Voysey M, Clemens SAC, Madhi SA, Weckx LY, Folegatti PM, Aley PK, Angus B, Baillie VL, Barnabas SL, Bhorat QE. Safety and efficacy of the ChAdOx1 nCoV-19 vaccine (AZD1222) against SARS-CoV-2: an interim analysis of four randomised controlled trials in Brazil, South Africa, and the UK. *The Lancet*. 2021;397(10269):99–111.

40. Jackson LA, Anderson EJ, Rouphael NG, Roberts PC, Makhene M, Coler RN, McCullough MP, Chappell JD, Denison MR, Stevens LJ. An mRNA vaccine against SARS-CoV-2—preliminary report. *New England Journal of Medicine*. 2020;383:1920–1931.

41. Chu L, McPhee R, Huang W, Bennett H, Pajon R, Nestorova B, Leav B. Group m-S: A preliminary report of a randomized controlled phase 2 trial of the safety and immunogenicity of mRNA-1273 SARS-CoV-2 vaccine. *Vaccine.* 2021;39(20):2791–2799.

42. Baden LR, El Sahly HM, Essink B, Kotloff K, Frey S, Novak R, Diemert D, Spector SA, Rouphael N, Creech CB. Efficacy and safety of the mRNA-1273 SARS-CoV-2 vaccine. *New England Journal of Medicine.* 2021;384(5):403–416.

43. Polack FP, Thomas SJ, Kitchin N, Absalon J, Gurtman A, Lockhart S, Perez JL, Pérez Marc G, Moreira ED, Zerbini C, et al. Safety and Efficacy of the BNT162b2 mRNA Covid-19 Vaccine. *New England Journal of Medicine.* 2020;383(27):2603–2615.

44. Mulligan MJ, Lyke KE, Kitchin N, Absalon J, Gurtman A, Lockhart S, Neuzil K, Raabe V, Bailey R, Swanson KA. Phase 1/2 study of COVID-19 RNA vaccine BNT162b1 in adults. *Nature.* 2020:1–8.

45. US. Food and Drug Administration. *FDA approves first Covid-19 vaccine.* Washington DC: FDA; 2021.

46. Sadoff J, Gray G, Vandebosch A, Cárdenas V, Shukarev G, Grinsztejn B, Goepfert PA, Truyers C, Fennema H, Spiessens B. Safety and efficacy of single-dose Ad26. COV2. S vaccine against COVID-19. *New England Journal of Medicine.* 2021;384(23):2187–2201.

47. Sadoff J, Le Gars M, Shukarev G, Heerwegh D, Truyers C, de Groot AM, Stoop J, Tete S, Van Damme W, Leroux-Roels I. Interim Results of a Phase 1–2a Trial of Ad26. COV2. S Covid-19 Vaccine. *New England Journal of Medicine.* 2021;384(19):1824–1835.

48. US Food and Drug Administration. *Janssen Covid-19 vaccine.* Washington DC: FDA; 2021.

49. Logunov DY, Dolzhikova IV, Shcheblyakov DV, Tukhvatulin AI, Zubkova OV, Dzharullaeva AS, Kovyrshina AV, Lubenets NL, Grousova DM, Erokhova AS. Safety and efficacy of an rAd26 and rAd5 vector-based heterologous prime-boost COVID-19 vaccine: an interim analysis of a randomised controlled phase 3 trial in Russia. *The Lancet.* 2021;397(10275):671–681.

50. Logunov DY, Dolzhikova IV, Zubkova OV, Tukhvatullin AI, Shcheblyakov DV, Dzharullaeva AS, Grousova DM, Erokhova AS, Kovyrshina AV, Botikov AG. Safety and immunogenicity of an rAd26 and rAd5 vector-based heterologous prime-boost COVID-19 vaccine in two formulations: two open, non-randomised phase 1/2 studies from Russia. *The Lancet.* 2020;396(10255):887–897.

51. Zhang Y, Zeng G, Pan H, Li C, Hu Y, Chu K, Han W, Chen Z, Tang R, Yin W. Safety, tolerability, and immunogenicity of an inactivated SARS-CoV-2 vaccine in healthy adults aged 18–59 years: a randomised, double-blind, placebo-controlled, phase 1/2 clinical trial. *The Lancet Infect Dis.* 2021;21(2):181–192.

52. Fabre ML, Arrías PN, Masson T, Pidre ML, Romanowski V. *Baculovirus-derived vectors for immunization and therapeutic applications. In: Emerging and Reemerging Viral Pathogens.* San Diego: Academic Press; 2020:197–224.

53. Heath PT, Galiza EP, Baxter DN, Boffito M, Browne D, Burns F, Chadwick DR, Clark R, Cosgrove C, Galloway J. Safety and efficacy of NVX-CoV2373 COVID-19 vaccine. *New Engl J Med.* 2021;385(13):1172–1183.

54. Mehrotra DV, Janes HE, Fleming TR, Annunziato PW, Neuzil KM, Carpp LN, Benkeser D, Brown ER, Carone M, Cho I. Clinical endpoints for evaluating efficacy in COVID-19 vaccine trials. *Ann Int Med.* 2020;174(2):221–228.

55. Leshem E, Lopman BA. Population immunity and vaccine protection against infection. *Lancet (London, England).* 2021;397(10286):1685–1687.

56. Worldometers.info: COVID-19 Coronavirus Pandemic. 2021.

57. Mao L, Wang M, Chen S, He Q, Chang J, Hong C, Zhou Y, Wang D, Miao X, Hu Y. Neurological manifestations of hospitalized patients with COVID-19 in Wuhan, China: a retrospective case series study. *JAMA Neurol.* 2020;77(6):683–690.

58. Graepel KW, Kochhar S, Clayton EW, Edwards KE. Balancing expediency and scientific rigor in severe acute respiratory syndrome coronavirus 2 vaccine development. *J Infect Dis.* 2020;222(2):180–182.

59. World Health Organization: WHO target product profiles for Covid-19 vaccines. 2020.

60. COVID-19 Vaccine Breakthrough Case Investigation and Reporting [https://www.cdc.gov/vaccines/covid-19/health-departments/breakthrough-cases.html]

61. Keehner J, Horton LE, Pfeffer MA, Longhurst CA, Schooley RT, Currier JS, Abeles SR, Torriani FJ. SARS-CoV-2 infection after vaccination in health care workers in California. *New England Journal of Medicine.* 2021;384:1774–1775.

62. Hacisuleyman E, Hale C, Saito Y, Blachere NE, Bergh M, Conlon EG, Schaefer-Babajew DJ, DaSilva J, Muecksch F, Gaebler C. Vaccine Breakthrough Infections with SARS-CoV-2 Variants. *New England Journal of Medicine.* 2021;384(23):2212–2218.

63. Abu-Raddad LJ, Chemaitelly H, Butt AA. Effectiveness of the BNT162b2 Covid-19 Vaccine against the B. 1.1. 7 and B. 1.351 Variants. *New England Journal of Medicine.* 2021;385(2):187–189.

64. Hussey C, Talukdar L. *Moderna Announces Positive Initial Booster Data Against SARS-CoV-2 Variants of Concern.* Cambridge, MA: Business wire; 2021.

65. Shinde V, Bhikha S, Hoosain Z, Archary M, Bhorat Q, Fairlie L, Lalloo U, Masilela MS, Moodley D, Hanley S. Efficacy of NVX-CoV2373 covid-19 vaccine against the b. 1.351 variant. *New England Journal of Medicine.* 2021;384(20):1899–1909.

Glossary

Acroparesthesia A sensation of burning pain, tingling, and numbness in the upper and lower limbs, mainly affecting the fingers and toes.

ACTT-1 Adaptive COVID-19 Treatment Trial is the pivotal, randomized trial that established the efficacy of remdesivir in patients hospitalized with COVID-19.

ACTT-2 Adaptive COVID-19 Treatment Trial is the pivotal, randomized trial that established the efficacy of baricitinib plus remdesivir in patients hospitalized with COVID-19.

Acute coronary syndrome (ACS) The term refers to a set of conditions such as acute myocardial infarction and unstable angina (acute myocardial ischemia) that are acute manifestations of coronary artery disease. The cause of ACS is a sudden interruption in blood flow to the cardiac muscle.

Acute hemorrhagic stroke A sudden loss of neurological function caused by bleeding into the brain parenchyma (tissue) or in the subarachnoid spaces surrounding the brain as a result of the rupture of a blood vessel. In general, intracerebral hemorrhage relates to smaller blood vessels that bleed into the brain parenchyma whereas subarachnoid hemorrhage relates to the bleeding of larger vessels into the subarachnoid space.

Acute ischemic stroke A sudden loss of neurological function caused by neuronal death that occurs when blood flow to an area of the brain is acutely blocked. Most often, this is secondary to a blood clot that is either thrombotic or embolic in nature.

Acute kidney injury (AKI) An abrupt decrease in kidney function as measured by increases in serum creatinine and/or decreases in urine output that occur over hours to days.

Acute motor and sensory axonal neuropathy A subtype of Guillain-Barré syndrome characterized by acute onset of distal weakness, loss of deep tendon reflexes, and sensory symptoms characterized by its affinity to affect sensory nerves and roots in addition to only motor nerves, as in acute motor axonal neuropathy. Pathological findings show severe axonal degeneration of motor and sensory nerve fibers with little demyelination.

Acute respiratory distress syndrome (ARDS) Condition in which fluid accumulates in the lung air sacs leading to hypoxemia, that is, reduced oxygen saturation of the blood.

Acute tubular necrosis (ATN) A subtype of acute kidney injury (AKI) characterized on light microscopy by kidney tubule cell injury. It is the most common cause of AKI in kidney biopsy studies in the setting of a COVID-19 infection.

Adaptive immunity Parts of the immune system that undergo gene rearrangement and clonal expansion to mount a specific response to infection. It is divided into humoral (antibody) and T-cell components.

Advanced maternal age Pregnant patients aged 35 and older.

Aerosol-generating procedure (AGP) Any medical procedure that can induce the production of aerosols of various sizes, including particles as small as less than 5 μm.

Ageusia Ageusia is the loss of taste functions of the tongue, particularly the inability to detect sweetness, sourness, bitterness, saltiness, and savory taste.

Agonist An agonist is a compound that can bind to and cause activation of a receptor and mimics the activity of the substrate that binds to the receptor.

Albuminocytological dissociation Albuminocytological dissociation of the cerebrospinal fluid (CSF) is defined as an increase in total protein concentration with normal total nucleated cell count. It is suspected to occur in diseases that alter the blood–brain barrier, increase the production of protein, or obstruct the flow of CSF, such as acute inflammatory demyelinating polyneuropathy.

Angiotensin-converting enzyme-2 (ACE2) receptor The ACE2 receptor is a protein on the surface of many different cell types throughout the nasopharynx, lungs, brain, vasculature, heart, liver, and gastrointestinal tract that plays a role in regulating blood pressure, wound healing, and inflammation through the renin-angiotensin-aldosterone pathway. The SARS-CoV-2 virus spike protein binds to the ACE2 receptor to gain entrance into human cells. The SARS-CoV-2 spike protein is also known to damage the epithelium via downregulation of ACE2.

Angiotensin-converting enzyme type 2 (ACE2) A protein on the surface of cells that the virus binds to in order to gain entry into the host cell.

Anosmia A loss of the sense of smell generally related to a blocked nose or infection, but can be due to damage of the olfactory receptor neurons in the nose or brain areas that process smell.

Antagonist An antagonist is a compound that can bind to a receptor and block the binding of the substrate to the receptor, thus producing inhibition.

Antibody-dependent enhancement (ADE) The worsening of the manifestations of a new infection by preexisting antibodies. This can occur as a result of prior infection (e.g., in individuals with a prior dengue virus infection newly infected with a different strain) or vaccination (e.g., in persons immunized with a formalin-inactivated vaccine against respiratory syncytial virus [RSV]).

Antiviral medications against SARS-CoV-2 Drugs inhibiting replication or transcription of SARS-CoV-2 that can be given either orally or parenterally.

Anxiety An experience of abnormal or overwhelming sense of apprehension, fear, distress, or uneasiness often with physical signs (rapid heart rate, sweating, muscle tension).

Aphthous ulcer Aphthous ulcers or canker sores are painful round or oval soft tissue lesions in the mouth with a white or yellow center and a red border. They can be found on or under the tongue, inside cheeks or lips, at the base of the gums, or on the soft palate. Typically, they heal without scarring in 1 to 2 weeks.

Aqueous humor The clear fluid filling the space in the front of the eyeball between the lens and the cornea.

ARDS Acute respiratory distress syndrome. Lung injury resulting in hypoxia (low blood oxygen saturation). A hallmark of pulmonary manifestation of SARS-CoV-2 infection.

Assay An experimental procedure.

Assayable drug target A target for which high-throughput experimental screening against many compounds is possible.

Bacteriophage A virus that attaches itself to a susceptible bacterium and infects the host cells as well as forces the bacterium cells to produce viral components instead of bacterial components.

Bioinformatics The application of tools of computation and analysis to the capture and interpretation of biological data.

Biomarker A biological molecule found in blood, other body fluids, or tissues that is a sign of a normal or abnormal process or of a condition or disease.

BLAST A bioinformatics algorithm to compare the sequence similarity of proteins.

Blepharitis Inflammation of the eyelids.

Blood–brain barrier A highly selective border of endothelial cells within the blood vessels that vascularize the central nervous system (CNS) that prevents solutes in the blood from nonselectively crossing into the extracellular fluid of the CNS, where neurons reside. This barrier tightly regulates the movement of ions, molecules, and cells between the blood and the brain and can protect the brain from toxins and pathogens. Alteration of this barrier is an important component of the pathological processes and progression of several neurological diseases.

Breakthrough infection An infection resulting from the same pathogen occurring in an individual who has been fully vaccinated against the pathogen is referred to as a breakthrough infection. The term denotes a breach of the immunity cover conferred by the vaccine.

Budding For enveloped viruses, the acquisition of a lipid membrane envelope occurs through a process called "budding" that can occur at any cellular membrane, such as the endoplasmic reticulum, Golgi, endoplasmic reticulum–Golgi intermediate compartment, or plasma membrane. The viral nucleocapsid comes into the close proximity of S, E, and M proteins inserted into a cellular membrane. Interactions between the nucleocapsid and the cytoplasmic tails of the other viral structural proteins induce local curvature of the cellular membrane, resulting in the formation of a bud-like structure. The bud is then pinched off by membrane scission to release the enveloped virus.

Catatonia A psychomotor disturbance and potentially life-threatening state that may include muscle rigidity, stupor, mutism, purposeless movements, negativism (refusing to follow an instruction or doing the opposite of the request), echolalia (repeatedly echoing words spoken by another individual), echopraxia (repeating movements made by another individual), and inappropriate posturing and is associated with medical and psychiatric conditions.

Chemokine A subset of cytokines specifically involved in recruitment of immune cells to the site of infection.

Chemosis Swelling of the conjunctiva.

Compliance Refers to the capacity of the lung parenchyma to expand/contract, that is, inflate/deflate or increase/decrease in volume as a function of the transpulmonary pressure. It is a measure of change in lung volume (LV) over transpulmonary pressure (TPP), that is, LV/TPP.

Congenital infections A maternal infection with the potential for mother-to-child transmission.

Conjunctiva Loose connective tissue that covers the surface of the eyeball and folds back on itself to form the inner layer of the eyelid.

Cornea The transparent part of the eye that covers the iris, pupil, and anterior chamber.

COVAN COVID-19–associated nephropathy, which is a form of collapsing focal segmental glomerulosclerosis.

COVID-19 Disease manifestations of SARS-CoV-2 infection, including one or more of the following: fever, respiratory symptoms, gastrointestinal symptoms, headache, myalgias, fatigue, respiratory failure, and death.

COVID-19–associated coagulopathy (CAC) CAC is a coagulation disorder resulting from SARS-CoV-2 infection. The pathophysiological processes of CAC are multifactorial. Direct invasion of the vascular endothelium by SARS-CoV-2, inflammatory cytokines, and coagulation factors, including factor VIII, play a role in thrombus formation in COVID-19.

COVID-19 post–intensive care syndrome New or worsening physical, mental, and neurocognitive symptoms that adversely affect daily functioning and quality of life for survivors of COVID-19.

COVID-19 vaccination A portion of SARS-CoV-2 (mRNA, protein subunit, or vector vaccines) is injected into an individual to elicit a T- and B-cell immune response to the virus to reduce infection and/or severity of illness.

Coronavirus Treatment Acceleration Program (CTAP) CTAP is a special emergency program for possible coronavirus therapies created by the US Food and Drug Administration to move new treatments to patients as quickly as possible, while at the same time finding out whether they are helpful or harmful.

Cytokine A number of substances, such as interferons, interleukins, and growth factors, secreted by certain cells of the immune system, that have proinflammatory or antiinflammatory effects on other cells.

Cytokine storm Severe immune reaction in which too many cytokines are quickly released into the blood, with signs and symptoms including fever, inflammation, severe fatigue, and nausea; may be life threatening and lead to multiple organ failure.

Damage-associated molecular pattern (DAMP) DAMPs are molecules released by dying cells or by cells that are damaged, infected, or under stress. DAMPs can be recognized by immune sensors and trigger inflammatory and immune responses. DAMPs activate pattern recognition receptors in the immune cells setting in motion an inflammatory reaction with the release of cytokines and other inflammatory mediators. Examples of DAMPs include adenosine triphosphate, nuclear DNA, mitochondrial DNA, and histones.

D-Dimer Metabolic product of blood clot breakdown and fibrin degradation. D domains are components of fibrin monomers that coalesce by end-to-end alignment of D domains forming fibrin. Plasmin degrades fibrin, releasing the D-dimer antigen. D-Dimers also play a role in platelet bonding and aggregation. D-Dimer values 500 ng/mL or less are considered normal. D-Dimer is elevated in disseminated intravascular coagulation, DIC, COVID-19–associated coagulopathy, and other thrombotic disorders.

Deep vein thrombosis (DVT) A condition that occurs when blood clot forms in the deep veins, mostly in the lower extremities. Patients present with leg pain and swelling.

Delayed cord clamping Practice of delaying the cutting or clamping of the umbilical cord for a prespecified interval, often 60 to 120 seconds, after birth.

Delirium A cognitive disturbance characterized by confused thinking and disrupted attention; disordered speech and hallucinations may be present; and resulting from an underlying medical or psychiatric condition.

Delta variant Variant of SARS-CoV-2 that appears more transmissible than the SARS-CoV-2 strains that circulated earlier in the pandemic.

Depression An affective/mood state in which a patient has low mood or withdrawal/apathy combined with many of the following symptoms: disrupted sleep, change in appetite, low energy, feelings of guilt/worthlessness/hopelessness, impaired concentration, slowed movements or lack of motivation, and suicidal ideation.

Differentially expressed gene A gene is declared differentially expressed if a difference or change observed in read counts or expression levels/index between two experimental conditions is statistically significant.

Disseminated intravascular coagulation (DIC) A serious coagulation disorder and a recognized complication in various conditions such as sepsis, some malignancies, and many other inflammatory disorders. Excessive clotting results in a depletion of platelets with consequent bleeding in various tissues and organs. DIC can lead to shock, heart attack, stroke, and acute respiratory distress syndrome.

Drug target A molecule in the body, usually a protein, that is intrinsically associated with a particular disease process and that could be addressed by a drug to produce a desired therapeutic effect.

Druggable genome A set of genes encoding proteins whose activity can be modulated using small molecule compounds.

Dysbiosis The disruption of healthy microbiome homeostasis as a result of imbalance in the microflora, a shift in the local distribution, or changes in the functional composition and metabolic activities, often of the bacterial communities in the normal flora.

Dysgeusia A condition in which a person's perception of taste is altered; everything seems sweet, sour, bitter, or metallic.

Eclampsia The convulsive manifestation of the hypertensive disorders of pregnancy, defined by new-onset tonic-clonic, focal, or multifocal seizures in the absence of other causative conditions such as epilepsy, cerebral arterial ischemia and infarction, intracranial hemorrhage, or drug use.

Elastance The elastic resistance offered by lung parenchyma to inflation. It is a function of the pressure required to inflate the lungs. Elastance is inversely related to (reciprocal of) compliance.

Electroporation Application of high-voltage electrical pulses to living cells to enable membrane permeability. DNA vaccines use this methodology to deliver genetic material into the nucleus of cells. DNA delivery by electroporation can be accomplished by intramuscular and intradermal routes.

Emergency medicine services (EMS) A system of emergency services that provides prehospital treatment and stabilization for serious illness and injuries and transport to definitive care facilities.

Encephalopathy A broad term for any disease or damage to the brain that can cause an alteration in brain function or structure. This disease or damage can be related to an infectious agent, a metabolic or mitochondrial dysfunction, vascular disorder, trauma, hypoxia, or any neurotoxin.

End-stage kidney disease (ESKD) A condition in which a patient's kidneys have failed to the point of needing dialysis therapy or a kidney transplant to maintain life.

Epidemic curve A histogram that shows the course of a disease outbreak or epidemic by plotting the number of cases by time of onset.

Emergency use authorization (EUA) A mechanism to facilitate the availability and use of medical countermeasures, including vaccines, during public health emergencies, such as the current COVID-19 pandemic. EUAs still require rigorous testing, monitoring and reporting, but proceed at a faster pace.

Extracorporeal membrane oxygenation (ECMO) A process by which a machine pumps and oxygenates a patient's blood outside the body, allowing the heart and lungs to rest.

Functional assay An experimental procedure carried out to identify the function of a protein.

Furin A serine endoprotease that proteolytically activates many substrates ranging from pathogenic agents to growth factors, receptors, and extracellular matrix proteins.

Ganglioside A molecule most commonly found on the cell membrane of neurons that plays an important role in the action of ion channels and in intracellular communication. The loss of function of gangliosides leads to severe neurodegenerative disorders that may or may not be reversible.

Gestational hypertension Defined as a systolic blood pressure of 140 mm Hg or more or a diastolic blood pressure of 90 mm Hg or more, or both, on two occasions at least 4 hours apart after 20 weeks of gestation, in a woman with a previously normal blood pressure.

Glomerulonephritis A group of kidney disorders represented by inflammation and damage to the glomeruli. There are many causes, including infection, autoimmune processes, and genetic conditions.

Ground-glass opacity (GGO) Radiological patterns of attenuation in the lung manifested in chest computed tomography images and chest x-ray films. These hazy diffuse patterns are peripherally distributed in SARS-CoV-2 infection. GGOs have a broad range of causes, resulting from conditions such as partial collapse of alveoli, interstitial thickening, or fibrosis.

Guillain-Barré syndrome Also known as acute inflammatory demyelinating polyneuropathy, is a rare autoimmune disorder in which the body's immune system begins to attack and damage nerves, causing sensory symptoms generally followed by weakness and paralysis. Symptoms generally progress over hours to days and peak within the first 2 weeks after symptoms appear.

Hemolysis, elevated liver enzymes, and low platelets (HELLP) syndrome The clinical manifestation of hemolysis, elevated liver enzymes, and low platelet count (HELLP) syndrome is one of the more severe forms of preeclampsia and has the following criteria to make the diagnosis: lactate dehydrogenase (LDH) elevated to 600 IU/L or more, aspartate aminotransferase (AST) and alanine aminotransferase (ALT) elevated more than twice the upper limit of normal, and the platelets count less than $100,000 \times 10\ 9/L$.

Herpetiform ulcers Herpetiform ulcers are crops of 10 to 100 pinpoint lesions that eventually fuse together and form large, irregularly shaped ulcers. They are so called because of their similarity in appearance to herpes; however, herpetiform ulceration is not caused by the herpes simplex virus.

Host-targeted antiviral therapy Therapy that targets the host proteins to disrupt the viral life cycle.

Human leukocyte antigen DR isotype (HLA-DR) A class 2 major histocompatibility complex antigen expressed on cell surfaces originally defined as mediating graft-versus-host disease. The expression of these molecules may be increased in response to signaling during infection.

Hypertensive disorders of pregnancy A spectrum of conditions that occur in pregnancy or in the immediate postpartum period, including gestational hypertension, preeclampsia, eclampsia, and HELLP syndrome.

Hyposalivation A noticeable and measurable decrease of the amount of saliva in a person's mouth. A person may experience dryness of mouth (xerostomia) without actually having decrease in saliva.

Hypoxia A medical condition in which tissues in the body are deprived of oxygen.

Hypoxic-ischemic brain injury A condition that is caused by a lack of blood flow to the whole brain to meet its metabolic demand resulting from to limited oxygen supply. This is commonly seen in cases of cardiac arrest, but can be seen in several systemic disease processes that limit oxygen delivery to the brain.

Immunocompromise Primary or secondary (acquired) deficits in cellular and/or humoral immunity that predispose to severe infection.

Immunoglobulin isotypes The main immunoglobulin (Ig) isotypes are M, G, A, and E. IgM, a pentamer, is typically the first produced by the host in response to a novel pathogen. Switching to other isotypes requires help by CD4+ T cells. IgG antibodies are further divided into subclasses with distinct regulatory properties. IgA is the main form secreted onto mucous membranes, where it serves to block infection. IgE is mainly involved in allergic responses.

Immunomodulators Drugs that can support the immune function by modifying, in a beneficial way, the immune system's response to a threat.

Immunosenescence The ability of the human body to mount an adequate immune response to pathogens diminishes with age. This phenomenon is referred to as immunosenescence.

Incubation period The duration from the time of exposure to the pathogen to the manifestation of symptoms of the disease.

Infectivity Viral infectivity is defined as the capacity of a virus to efficiently enter host cells and use its resources to replicate and produce infectious viral particles that can further perpetuate infection and disease within the host. In the context of SARS-CoV-2 variants, various changes in the characteristics of the virus, ranging from increased angiotensin-converting enzyme-2 binding affinity that may promote more efficient host cell entry to increased replicative potential of the virus, which may be reflected by higher viral loads in patients, may all contribute to the enhancement of viral infectivity.

Inflammasome An inflammasome is a cytosolic multiprotein complex that is formed when immune sensors detect pathogens or danger signals. Inflammasomes are an essential part of the innate immune system. When activated, they can induce inflammation and recruit immune cells to the sites of infection or cell damage.

Innate immunity Parts of the immune system that are invariant, that is, do not undergo rearrangement of receptor genes or undergo clonal expansion in response to a specific infection.

Interferon (IFN) A family of signaling molecules produced by both innate and adaptive immune cells and so named for their ability to block viral replication.

Interferon response Playing an integral role in the innate immune response, interferons (IFNs) are cytokines that are secreted by cells in response to viral infection and interfere with viral replication. The activation of IFN receptor complexes by IFNs result in the induction of a large number of IFN-stimulated genes that act concertedly to effectively contain the infection.

Interferon-stimulated genes (ISG) Genes specifically induced by interferon as part of the innate response to infection.

Isogenic recombinant viruses To perform a comparative study that more closely mimics the native condition, a full-length genomic sequence of the virus that is capable of producing infectious viral particles and expresses the same proteins as the original virus can be engineered in vitro. Mutations in spike can be introduced into the sequence before the full-length viral RNA is transcribed and the virus is produced. By producing both a mutant form and a wild type form of the virus, a direct comparison can be made between them to study any changes in the behavior or characteristics of the virus resulting from the presence of the mutation.

Keratitis Inflammation of the cornea.

Kidney replacement therapy A generic term for therapy that replaces the normal blood filtering functions of the kidneys when they have failed. This includes therapies such as hemodialysis, peritoneal dialysis, continuous kidney replacement therapy, prolonged intermittent kidney replacement therapy, and kidney transplant.

Kidney transplant recipient A patient who has undergone a kidney transplant to reverse kidney failure.

Lipid nanoparticle (LNP) Nonviral delivery system originally approved by the US Food and Drug Administration for delivery of small interfering RNA and currently adapted for mRNA delivery. LNP is composed of many lipid components such as amine lipid, phospholipid, and cholesterol.

Long-COVID Long-COVID, also termed the *long-hauler syndrome*, refers to the persistence of symptoms of COVID-19 beyond 8 to 12 weeks.

Long-lived plasma cell (LLPC) In the germinal centers of lymph nodes, activated B cells get transformed into long-lived plasma cells through a process of evolutionary selection. LLPCs survive for a number of years, retaining their ability to secrete specific antibodies without the need for a fresh trigger.

Major histocompatibility complex (MHC) Proteins encoded by highly polymorphic genes that are essential for adaptive immunity. MHC proteins present antigenic peptides for cellular recognition. Human leukocyte antigen (HLA)-A, B, and C are members of MHC class I, and mainly present antigenic peptides to cytotoxic CD8+ T cells, whereas HLA-D (class II) mainly presents antigenic peptides to CD4+ T cells.

Mania An affective/mood state often consisting of increased energy, insomnia, rapid speech, feelings of euphoria or grandiosity.

Mechanical ventilation barotrauma Invasive mechanical ventilation or oxygen therapy causes damage to the alveolar sacs resulting in air leak to the pleural cavity and surrounding structures, including the heart and subcutaneous tissues.

Meibomian orifices Openings of the meibomian glands, which are oil glands that line the rims of the eyelids and produce an oil that protects the surface of the eye.

Microaspiration Microaspiration is aspiration of small volumes of oropharyngeal secretions or gastric fluid into their lungs.

Middle East respiratory syndrome (MERS) CoV (MERS-CoV) A viral respiratory illness caused by the coronavirus MERS-CoV, it first emerged in 2012 in Saudi Arabia and spread to many countries in the region. By 2018, MERS-CoV had infected more than 2000 people, causing 803 deaths.

Miscarriage Miscarriage, or early pregnancy loss, is defined as a nonviable, intrauterine pregnancy with either an empty gestational sac or a gestational sac containing an embryo or fetus without fetal heart activity within the first 12 6/7 weeks of gestation.

Molecular mimicry A leading mechanism by which infectious or chemical agents may induce autoimmunity. It occurs when similarities between foreign and self-peptides favor an activation of autoreactive T or B cells by a foreign-derived antigen in a susceptible individual.

Monoclonal antibodies against SARS-CoV-2 Laboratory-produced antibodies given as parenteral infusions that recognize the SARS-CoV-2 spike protein to block viral entry and reduce the severity of COVID-19.

Morbidity Any departure, subjective or objective, from a state of physiological or psychological well-being.

Mortality rate A measure of the frequency of occurrence of death in a defined population during a specified interval of time.

Mucormycosis A significant fungal infection in humans caused by mucormycetes molds. The infection can become widespread and can be fatal. Diabetes and steroid therapy are predisposing factors.

Multisystem inflammatory syndrome in children (MIS-C) A rare but serious consequence of SARS-CoV-2 infection that appears to be a delayed immunologic response to the virus and involves systemic inflammation and multiorgan involvement.

Mutation notations Gene mutations are most often annotated as AnnnB, where A is the one-letter abbreviation for the amino acid usually found at position nnn in the gene of interest, and B is amino acid found in the mutant.

Myocarditis Inflammation of the heart muscle. The predominant cause of myocarditis is a viral infection. Severe forms of myocarditis can lead to heart failure and cardiac arrhythmias.

Natural killer (NK) cells Also called large granular lymphocytes, these cells are part of the innate immune system. They exert cytotoxicity activity directed at cells expressing certain tumor antigens or cells with certain intracellular infections.

Neonatal death Defined as the death of a live-born infant, regardless of gestational age at birth, within the first 28 completed days of life.

Neutralizing antibody Antibody that prevents cellular infection by a virus, usually by binding to a viral protein involved in cell entry. Antibodies recognizing other viral surface proteins may bind without preventing cellular infection.

Non–ST-segment elevation myocardial infarction (NSTEMI) Part of the spectrum of acute coronary syndrome and a manifestation of coronary artery disease resulting in increased morbidity and mortality. NSTEMI is caused by a partial or near-complete thrombotic occlusion of a major coronary artery and less severe compared to STEMI. NSTEMI is a consequence of cardiac ischemia involving part of the cardiac muscle or myocardium.

Opportunistic infections Opportunistic infections are defined as infections by bacteria, fungi, viruses, or parasites that normally do not cause disease, but become pathogenic when the body's defense system is impaired.

Oral microbiome The term *microbiome* describes the ecological community of symbiotic, commensal, and pathogenic microorganisms in and on our body. Oral microbiome, oral microbiota, or oral microflora refers to the microorganisms found in the human oral cavity.

Oral virome Collection of all viruses found in the oral cavity of humans that include both eukaryotic and prokaryotic viruses.

Orbit The bony cavity in the skill that houses the eyeballs, the muscles that move the eyes, the tear glands, and the nerves and vessels that supply these structures.

Organizing pneumonia A rare lung condition, a nonspecific inflammatory pulmonary process formerly called bronchiolitis obliterans. Infection is the most common cause of organizing pneumonia, which usually manifests with fever, nonproductive cough, anorexia, and weight loss. Corticosteroids are the mainstay of treatment.

Pandemic An epidemic (the occurrence of more cases of disease than expected in a given area or among a specific group of people over a particular period of time) occurring over a very wide area (several countries or continents) and usually affecting a large proportion of the population.

PAPR A powered air-purifying respirator that uses a blower to force the ambient air through air-purifying elements to the inlet covering.

Pathogen-associated molecular pattern (PAMP) PAMPs are pathogen-derived stimuli that can activate immune sensors, consequently driving immune responses and inflammation. Examples of PAMPs include viral double-stranded RNA, bacterial cell wall components such as lipopolysaccharide and peptidoglycans, and flagellin from bacterial flagella.

Pathogenicity Pathogenicity denotes the ability of a pathogen to induce disease.

Pattern recognition receptor (PRR) Receptors detecting specific ligands to detect infection or cell damage, located on the membranes or in the cytoplasm of immune cells and other cell types.

Periconception The time preceding, including, and immediately after human conception.

Personal protective equipment (PPE) Equipment worn to minimize exposure to hazards that cause serious workplace injuries and illnesses. These injuries and illnesses may result from contact with chemical, radiological, physical, electrical, mechanical, or other workplace hazards. Personal protective equipment may include items such as gloves, safety glasses and shoes, earplugs or muffs, hard hats, respirators, or coveralls, vests, and full body suits.

Plateau pressure (P$_{plat}$) The maximum pressure that the alveoli of the lung can be subjected to during mechanical ventilation. P$_{plat}$ is typically maintained below 30 cm H$_2$O to minimize barotrauma.

Pneumothorax Air leak from the alveolar sac causing air accumulation between the chest wall and lungs resulting in compression of lungs and collapse of the lungs.

Polyethylene glycol (PEG) A large otherwise inert molecule that if covalently bound to another biologically active molecule (e.g., a monoclonal antibody or cytokine) can reduce its renal elimination and increase its plasma half-life.

Population immunity A community (population) in a geographic region is said to acquire population immunity when unvaccinated individuals who form a small minority are protected from infection by a pathogen because the rest of the members of the community have been fully vaccinated. Population immunity confers a direct protective effect on the immunized, but it also provides indirect protection for the nonimmunized individuals by disabling the transmission chain.

Positive end-expiratory pressure (PEEP) Setting on a mechanical ventilator that aids in distending the alveoli and enhances oxygen delivery to the body. Normal setting ranges from 5 to 10 cm H$_2$O.

Posterior reversible encephalopathy syndrome A syndrome characterized by headaches, seizures, and/or encephalopathy and the radiological finding of white matter vasogenic edema affecting predominantly the posterior occipital and parietal lobes of the brain. The syndrome is recognized most commonly through the constellation of symptoms with associated computed tomography or magnetic resonance imaging findings.

Postpartum period The postpartum period, also known as the puerperium and the "fourth trimester," refers to the time after delivery when maternal physiological changes related to pregnancy return to the nonpregnant state.

Posttraumatic stress disorder/symptoms A psychological reaction triggered by the experience of a highly stressful and potentially life-threatening event and characterized by flashbacks, recurrent nightmares, avoidance of the event, severe anxiety, and low mood.

Preeclampsia A disorder of pregnancy associated with new-onset hypertension, which occurs most often after 20 weeks of gestation and frequently near term.

Premature rupture of membranes Membrane rupture before labor that occurs before 37 weeks of gestation.

Preterm birth Defined as a delivery occurring at or after 20 0/7 weeks of gestation and before 37 0/7 weeks of gestation.

Programmed ribosomal frameshifting (PRF) PRF is a key event during the translation of SARS-CoV-2 ORF1ab to generate the polyprotein pp1ab. It refers to the controlled slippage of the ribosome during translation, which is mediated by the formation of a knot-like structure by the RNA and followed by a "slippery" sequence, causing the ribosome to pause and slide back, resulting in the rest of the mRNA sequence being translated in an alternative minus 1 (−1) frame. PRF is conserved in coronaviruses and facilitates the use of a single mRNA to generate two proteins with distinct C-terminal sequences, allowing for more efficient use of the small genome.

Proning The process of turning a patient with precise, safe motions from their back onto their abdomen (stomach) so the individual is lying face down. This helps promote aeration of the dorsal regions of the lung facing alveolar collapse from the gravitational effect of the supine position and also improves perfusion.

Proteome A proteome is the complete set of proteins expressed by an organism.

Pseudotyped viruses Pseudotyped viruses, also called pseudoviruses, are replication-defective, presenting relatively harmless and useful tools for laboratory research on viruses. Pseudoviruses can be engineered to express SARS-CoV-2 spike protein on their surfaces, which can be used to study certain aspects of viral behavior, such as the impact of sequence changes in spike on angiotensin-converting enzyme-2 binding and host cell entry, or neutralization by antibodies.

Psychosis May be an acute or chronic state in which a patient develops fixed delusions and/or hallucinations.

Pulmonary embolism (PE) Embolism is the lodging of a blood clot in an artery and causing obstruction to the blood flow. Pulmonary embolism is a condition with a blockage of the pulmonary artery, which supplies blood to the lungs.

Pulmonary fibrosis A lung disease characterized by chronic and progressive scarring of the lungs with inflammation and fibrosis. Patients have a worsening cough, shortness of breath, and declining lung function. Patients with pulmonary fibrosis have a poor prognosis with or without treatment.

Pulmonary hypertension Condition in which the mean pulmonary arterial pressure is greater than 25 mm Hg.

Pyroptosis A form of proinflammatory programmed cell death as opposed to apoptosis, which is a noninflammatory cell death protocol. Gasdermins, various caspases, and granzymes play a role in engineering cell death by forming pores in the cell membrane and consequent release of inflammatory molecules when the host is subjected to exogenous and endogenous stimuli. Pyroptosis is observed in cancer and various infectious, neurological, cardiovascular, and autoimmune diseases.

Quarantine A state, period, or place of isolation in which people (or animals) that have arrived from elsewhere or been exposed to infectious or contagious disease are placed.

Receptor binding domain A fragment from a virus that binds to a specific receptor, for example, host angiotensin-converting enzyme-2 in the case of SARS-CoV-2, to gain entry into host cells.

RECOVERY Trial RECOVERY is a large-enrollment clinical trial of potential treatments for people in the United Kingdom and South East Asia who are hospitalized with COVID-19.

Relative illness ratio A comparison of the rate of illness between two groups.

Renin-angiotensin system (RAS) RAS plays a critical role in cardiovascular homeostasis and blood pressure maintenance. To accomplish this, RAS regulates blood volume and systemic vascular resistance. Apart from the heart and blood vessels, RAS involves the kidneys, lungs, and the brain.

Reproductive number (R_0) The number of new cases an existing case is likely to generate on average. The R_0 of COVID-19 is estimated to be 2.2.

Repurposed drug Repurposing or repositioning is a way of identifying new uses for approved or investigational medicines that are outside the scope of the original medical indication.

Retina The layer of tissue in the back of the eye that sense light and sends images to the brain.

Rhabdomyolysis A condition in which skeletal muscle breaks down rapidly, releasing their intracellular components, including myoglobin. Myoglobin can precipitate in the renal tubules to form intratubular casts obstructing the tubule and leading to acute tubular damage and acute kidney injury.

Ribavirin An oral small molecule inhibitor of viral replication that acts by interfering with RNA synthesis and capping, licensed for treatment of hepatitis C virus and viral hemorrhagic fevers.

Risk factor An aspect of personal behavior or lifestyle, an environmental exposure, or an inborn or inherited characteristic that is associated with an increased occurrence of disease or other health-related event or condition.

RNA-dependent RNA polymerase (RdRp) An enzyme that coronaviruses use to carry out replication and transcription of their RNA genome. Drugs such as remdesivir inhibit RdRp.

Salivary diagnostics The ability to analyze molecules in saliva for detecting and monitoring oral and systemic diseases.

SARS-CoV The first severe acute respiratory syndrome coronavirus, which emerged in 2002 to 2003; also referred to as SARS-CoV-1 after the appearance of SARS-CoV-2.

SARS-CoV-2 Coronavirus that causes COVID-19.

SARS-CoV-2 monoclonal antibodies Laboratory-made proteins that are typically directed against the spike protein of SARS-CoV-2 and designed to block the viral attachment and entry into human cells.

Scotoma A blind spot or partial loss of vision in an otherwise normal visual field.

Severe acute respiratory syndrome (SARS) A viral respiratory illness caused by a coronavirus (SARS-CoV) first reported in Asia in February 2003. The illness spread to more than two dozen countries in North America, South America, Europe, and Asia before the outbreak was contained.

Severe maternal morbidity Generally refers to health-affecting and life-threatening events that occur during hospitalization for childbirth.

Sialadenitis Inflammation of a salivary gland and/or salivary ducts.

Small for gestational age (SGA) Infants with a birth weight below the 10th percentile for gestational age.

SOLIDARITY Trial SOLIDARITY is an international clinical trial to help find an effective treatment for COVID-19, launched by the World Health Organization, enrolling 12,000 patients in 500 hospital sites in over 30 countries.

Spike protein A surface protein of SARS-CoV-2 that facilitates cell entry by binding with angiotensin-converting enzyme-2.

Stillbirth The delivery of a fetus showing no signs of life as indicated by the absence of breathing, heartbeats, pulsation of the umbilical cord, or definite movements of voluntary muscles at 20 weeks or longer of gestation (if the gestational age is known), or a weight of 350 g or greater if the gestational age is not known.

ST-segment elevation myocardial infarction (STEMI) Most acute and serious manifestation of coronary artery disease that is characterized by significant morbidity and mortality. STEMI is caused by a complete thrombotic occlusion of a major coronary artery. STEMI is a consequence of cardiac ischemia involving the full thickness of the cardiac muscle or myocardium.

Synaptosome-associated protein of 25 kDa (SNAP-25) A kinesin heavy-chain (uKHC)-interacting protein involved in membrane fusion and synaptic function. SNAP-25 immunoreactivity in taste cells possessing synapses suggests that these cells may be gustatory receptor cells.

Taste 1 receptor member 3 (TASR13) The protein encoded by this gene is a G protein–coupled receptor involved in taste responses.

T-cell receptor (TCR) A protein present on the surface of T cells recognizing specific antigens presented by class I or II major histocompatibility complex proteins. Triggering the TCR results in cellular activation, cytokine expression, and clonal expansion, and may trigger cytotoxicity.

Telemedicine Telemedicine is the practice of medicine using technology to deliver care at a distance. A caregiver such as a physician, advanced practice provider, or nurse in one location uses a telecommunications infrastructure to deliver care to a patient at a distant site.

Teratogenicity Has the capability of producing fetal malformation.

Therapeutic vaccines Vaccines administered with the goal of managing or treating a preexisting disease or clinical condition. Cancer vaccines and noninfectious noncancer vaccines that are under development are examples.

Thrombocytopenia A reduction in the number of platelets or thrombocytes in blood. Normal platelet count range is 150,000 to 450,000 per microliter of blood.

Thromboembolism Formation of blood clots within blood vessels that can then get detached, leading to obstruction of arteries (embolus). Embolization results in loss of blood supply and organ damage.

Thrombotic microangiopathy A group of clinical syndromes characterized by hemolytic anemia, low platelets, and end organ damage. It is secondary to the formation of thrombi in capillaries and arterioles as a result of endothelial cell damage.

Toll-like receptors (TLRs) A class of pattern recognition receptors that initiate innate immune response by sensing conserved molecular patterns shared by group of microorganisms. They are triggered by microbial ligands.

Tracheostomy A surgical procedure of making an incision through the neck into the trachea for airway protection. It is used in patients on prolonged mechanical ventilatory support with acute respiratory failure.

Transcolonization Bacterial migration from one anatomical area to another area that is often observed in respiratory pathological conditions.

Transmembrane protease serine-2 (TMPRSS-2) A transmembrane protein that participates in many physiological and pathological processes. It is also involved in the entry and spread of coronaviruses, including severe acute respiratory syndrome coronavirus 2 (SARS-CoV-2).

Transneuronal spread Spread of a virus or pathogen from one area to another using a neuron's axonal transport to transfer. Transneuronal spread from the sensory olfactory neurons to the olfactory bulb, then to numerous areas of the brain, is a proposed mechanism of SARS-CoV-2 brain proliferation.

Troponins Troponins are proteins located in cardiac and skeletal myocytes. Troponins are of three types—troponin C, troponin T, and troponin I. Troponin C, found in the heart and skeletal muscle, is basically the same while there are different forms of troponin T and troponin I for the heart and skeletal muscle. Cardiac injury can be diagnosed by measuring the level of heart-specific troponin T and troponin I. These specific troponin tests are routinely employed for the detection of acute coronary syndromes, including acute myocardial infarction.

Validated drug target A protein's role in causing the disease has been experimentally confirmed.

Variant of interest (VOI) VOIs are variant strains of SARS-CoV-2 that can be distinguished by their genetic changes and are either predicted to or known to affect characteristics such as transmissibility, disease severity, immune escape, efficacy of treatments, or diagnostic capability. Additionally, VOIs must be associated with significant community transmission with increasing relative prevalence, increasing case numbers, or other apparent changes that suggest an emerging risk to public health.

Variants of concern Viruses constantly change through mutation A variant has one or more mutations that differentiate it from other variants in circulation. SARS-CoV-2 variants are being closely monitored for evidence of an increase in transmissibility, more severe disease, significant reduction in neutralization by antibodies generated during previous infection or vaccination, reduced effectiveness of treatments or vaccines, or diagnostic detection failures. A variant that shows any such changes are a variant of concern.

Venovenous extracorporeal membrane oxygenation (VV ECMO) Taking the blood from a large vein such as the inferior vena cava and returning to another large vein such as the superior vena cava through a membrane oxygenator that aids in oxygenating the blood.

Ventilator-associated pneumonia (VAP) VAP is a condition in which pneumonia occurs after 48 hours of patients being intubated and on the ventilator.

Vertical transmission Passage of a disease-causing agent (pathogen) from mother to fetus during pregnancy.

Vesiculobullous lesions Lesions characterized by fluid-filled vesicles and bullae that appear as blisters in the oral cavity mucosa. People affected with SARS-CoV-2 infection could present with vesiculobullous lesions in the oral cavity.

Viral cycle Viral life cycle typically involves the process of the virus infecting the host and replicating itself, and this includes attachment, entry, uncoating, replication, maturation, and release.

Viral egress The process by which a progeny virion exits the cell after replication and assembly. In the case of SARS-CoV-2, budding at the ERGIC membrane is followed by transportation in a secretory vesicle that fuses with the plasma membrane to release the virion from the cell.

Virion Infectious viral particles that are either located outside the host cell or ready to exit the host cell after assembly. For an enveloped virus, a complete viral particle consists of an RNA or a DNA core that is protected from environmental damage by the outer viral envelope that contains structural proteins that are essential to convey it to the next host (cell or organism) and permit successful infection.

Virulence Virulence is determined by the severity of the disease manifestation after the occurrence of infection.

Virus-targeted antiviral therapy Virus-targeting antiviral therapy targets the viral proteins to disrupt the viral life cycle.

Xerostomia Xerostomia refers to the sensation of having a dry mouth.

Zoonosis Zoonosis is an infectious disease caused by a pathogen that has jumped from a nonhuman animal to humans. Zoonotic pathogens may be bacterial, viral, or parasitic and can spread to humans through direct contact or through food, water, or the environment.

Zoonotic spillover A zoonotic spillover occurs when the virus from an infected animal host enters a human host, either directly from the natural reservoir (animal species that serve as the original hosts of the virus) or through an intermediate species that carries the virus from its source.

Acronyms

+ssRNA: Positive-sense, single-stranded RNA
3CLpro: 3-Chymotrypsin-like protease
6MWT: 6-Minute walk test
AAK-1: AP2-associated protein kinase 1
AAP: American Academy of Pediatrics
ACE: Angiotensin-converting enzyme
ACE2: Angiotensin-converting enzyme-2
ACE2 receptor: Angiotensin-converting enzyme-2 receptor
ACEI: Angiotensin-converting enzyme inhibitor
ACIP: Advisory Committee on Immunization Practices
ACOG: American College of Obstetricians and Gynecologists
ACS: Acute coronary syndrome
ACTT: Adaptive COVID-19 Treatment Trial
AD: Atopic dermatitis
ADAM17: A disintegrin and metallopeptidase domain 17
ADCC: Antibody-dependent cell-mediated cytotoxicity
ADCP: Antibody-dependent cellular phagocytosis
ADE: Antibody-dependent enhancement
AF: Atrial fibrillation
AGP: Aerosol-generating procedure
aHR: Adjusted hazard ratio
AIDP: Acute inflammatory demyelinating polyneuropathy
AKI: Acute kidney injury
ALI: Acute lung injury
ALT: Alanine transaminase
AMAN: Acute motor axonal neuropathy
AMI: Acute myocardial infarction
AMS: Altered mental status
AMSAN: Acute motor and sensory axonal neuropathy
Ang: Angiotensin
Ang-2: Angiopoietin-2
Anti-GBM: Anti–glomerular basement membrane
AOGEN: Angiotensinogen
APC: Antigen-presenting cell
APOL1: Apolipoprotein L1
aPTT: Activated partial thromboplastin time
ARB: Angiotensin receptor blocker
ARDS: Acute respiratory distress syndrome
AST: Aspartate transaminase
AT1R: Angiotensin type 1 receptor
AT2R: Angiotensin type 2 receptor
ATI: Acute tubular injury
ATS: American Thoracic Society
BALF: Bronchoalveolar lavage fluid

BBB: Blood–brain barrier
BCG: Bacillus Calmette-Guérin
BCR: B-cell receptor
BDBV: Bundibugyo virus
BKV: BK virus
BLAZE-1: Blocking Viral Attachment and Cell Entry with SARS-CoV-2 Neutralizing Antibodies trial
BMI: Body mass index
BPAP: Bilevel positive airway pressure
BSL2: Biosafety level 2
BVr: Bacterial vector replicating
C3: Complement component 3
C4: Complement component 4
CAC: COVID-19–associated coagulopathy
CAD: Coronary artery disease
Canadian ISTH: Subcommittee for Women's Health Issues in Thrombosis and Hemostasis
CAPR: Controlled air-purifying respirator
CAR: Chimeric antigen receptor
CARD: Caspase activation and recruitment domain
CARDS: Coronavirus disease–associated acute respiratory distress syndrome
CBb: Complement factor B catalytic subunit Bb
CCTA: Coronary computed tomography angiography
CD: Crohn's disease
CDC: Centers for Disease Control and Prevention
CFR: Case fatality rate
CHD: Coronary heart disease
CHF: Congestive heart failure
CI: Confidence interval
CIA: Chemiluminescent immunoassay
CK: Creatinine kinase
CLD: Chronic liver disease
CLEIA: Chemiluminescent enzyme immunoassay
CLIF-OF/CLIF-C: European Foundation for the Study of Chronic Liver Failure, Organ Failure and Cirrhosis
CMR: Cardiac magnetic resonance
CNS: Central nervous system
COPD: Chronic obstructive pulmonary disease
CoV: Coronavirus
COVAN: COVID-19–associated nephropathy
COVAX: COVID-19 Vaccines Global Access
COVE: Coronavirus Efficacy and Safety Study
COVID-19: Coronavirus disease 2019
CP: Convalescent plasma
CPAP: Continuous positive airway pressure
CRP: C-reactive protein
CRRT: Continuous renal replacement therapy
CRS: Cytokine-release syndrome

CSF: Cerebrospinal fluid
CSS: Cytokine storm syndrome
CT: Computed tomography
CT: Connecticut
CT: Cycle threshold or cytoplasmic domain fusion
CTA: CT angiography
CTAP: Coronavirus Treatment Acceleration Program
CTD: C-terminal domain
CTP: Child-Turcotte-Pugh
CTPA: Computed tomography pulmonary angiogram
CVA16: Coxsackievirus A16
CVD: Cardiovascular disease
CVL: Central venous line
CXR: Chest x-ray
DAD: Diffuse alveolar damage
DAMP: Damage-associated molecular pattern
DC: Dendritic cell
DECT: Dual-energy computed tomography
DIC: Disseminated intravascular coagulation
DLCO: Diffusing capacity for carbon monoxide
DOAC: Direct oral anticoagulant
dsRNA: Double-stranded RNA
DVT: Deep vein thrombosis
E: Envelope protein
EBOV: Ebola virus
EBV: Epstein Barr virus
EC50: Concentration producing 50% of maximum effect
ECMO: Extracorporeal membrane oxygenation
ED: Emergency department
EEG: Electroencephalography
eGFR: Estimated glomerular filtration rate
ELISA: enzyme-linked immunosorbent assay
EMB: Endomyocardial biopsy
EMS: Emergency medical services
ENT: Ear, nose, and throat
EPAP: Expiratory positive airway pressure
ER: Endoplasmic reticulum
ERA-EDTA: European Renal Association–European Dialysis and Transplant Association
ERGIC: Endoplasmic reticulum–Golgi intermediate compartment
ESICM: European Society of Intensive Care Medicine
ESKD: End-stage kidney disease
ESR: Erythrocyte sedimentation rate
EUA: Emergency Use Authorization by US Food and Drug Administration
EV71: Enterovirus 71
FACTT: Fluid and Catheter Treatment Trial
FBG: Fasting blood glucose
FD: Functional dyspepsia
FDA: US Food and Drug Administration
FiO$_2$: Fraction of inspired oxygen
FMT: Fecal microbiota transplantation
FP: Fusion peptide
FSGS: Focal segmental glomerulosclerosis
GAF: g-interferon activation factor

GAS: g-interferon activation site
GBS: Guillain-Barré syndrome
GC: Germinal center
GCSF: Granulocyte colony-stimulating factor
GFR: Glomerular filtration rate
GGO: Ground-glass opacity
GI: Gastrointestinal
GP: Glycoprotein
GPCR: G protein–coupled receptor
GWAS: Genome-wide association study
H$_2$RA: Histamine-2 receptor antagonists
HAPE: High-altitude pulmonary edema
HBP: High blood pressure
HBV: Hepatitis B virus
HCoV: Human coronavirus
HCV: Hepatitis C virus
HD: Hemodialysis
HF: Heart failure
HFMD: Hand, foot, and mouth disease
HFNC: High-flow nasal cannula
HHV: Human herpes virus
HIT: Heparin-induced thrombocytopenia
HIV: Human immunodeficiency virus
HLA: Human leukocyte antigen
HLA-DR: Human leukocyte antigen–DR isotype
HPV: Human papillomavirus
HPV: Hypoxic pulmonary vasoconstriction
HR: Hazard ratio
HR: Heptapeptide repeat
HRCT: High-resolution computed tomography
HSV-1: Herpes simplex virus-1
HTLV-1: Human T-cell leukemia virus-1
HTLV-2: Human T-cell leukemia virus-2
IBD: Inflammatory bowel disease
IBS: Irritable bowel syndrome
IBV: Infectious bronchitis virus
IC50: Inhibitory concentration producing 50% of maximum effect
ICA: Immunochromatographic assay
ICU: Intensive care unit
IDSA: Infectious Diseases Society of America
IDVI: Infectious Disease Vulnerability Index
IFN: Interferon
IFN-γ: Interferon gamma
IFN-I: Type I interferon
IFN-III: type III interferon
Ig: Immunoglobulin
IgG: Immunoglobulin G
IgG1: Immunoglobulin G subclass 1
iHD: Intermittent hemodialysis
IKK: Inhibitor of NF-κB kinase
IL: Interleukin
IL-1: Interleukin-1
IL-2: Interleukin 2
IL-4: Interleukin 4
IL-6: Interleukin 6
IL-6R: Interleukin-6 receptor

IL-8: Interleukin-8
IL-10: Interleukin 10
IL-12: Interleukin 12
IL-21: Interleukin 21
IL-23: Interleukin 23
IL-27: Interleukin 27
IPAP: Inspiratory positive airway pressure
IRF: Interferon regulatory factor
ISG: Interferon stimulated gene
ISGF: Interferon-stimulated gene factor
ISGF3: Interferon-stimulated gene factor 3
ISRE: Interferon-stimulated response element
ITSH: International Society of Thrombosis and Hemostasis
IV: Inactivated virus
IV: Intravenous
IVIG: Intravenous immunoglobulin
IVT: In vitro transcribed
JAK: Janus kinase
JAK-STAT: Janus kinase-signal transducer and activator of transcription
JH PACT: Johns Hopkins Postacute COVID-19 Team
JIA: Juvenile idiopathic arthritis
kb: Kilobase to describe genome length (1000 bases in length)
KDIGO: Kidney Disease: Improving Global Outcomes Guidelines
KM: Kaplan-Meier
KSHV: Kaposi sarcoma herpesvirus
LABV: Live attenuated bacterial vector
LAV: Live attenuated virus
LDH: Lactate dehydrogenase
LGP2: Laboratory of genetics and physiology 2
LLPC: Long-lived plasma cell
LMW: Low molecular weight
LNP: Lipid nanoparticle
LPS: Lipopolysaccharide
LV: Left ventricle
M: Membrane protein
mAb: Monoclonal antibody
MAD: Mean arteries diameter
MAP: Mean arterial pressure
MAS: Macrophage activation syndrome
MasR: Mas receptor
MAVS: Mitochondrial antiviral signaling protein
MBC: Memory B cell
MCP-1: Monocyte chemoattractant protein-1
MDA5: Melanoma differentiation–associated protein 5
MDI: Metered-dose inhaler
MELD: Model of end-stage liver disease
MenACWY: Meningococcal ACWY
MenB: Meningococcal B
MERS: Middle East respiratory syndrome
MERS-CoV: Middle East respiratory syndrome coronavirus
MFMU: The Maternal-Fetal Medicine Unit Network
MHC: Major histocompatibility complex

MHC-I: Major histocompatibility complex class I
MHC-II: Major histocompatibility complex class II
MIS-A: Multisystem inflammatory syndrome in adults
MIS-C: Multisystem inflammatory syndrome in children
ML: Machine learning
Mpro: Main protease, the same as 3CLpro
mRNA: Messenger ribonucleic acid
Mtb: *Mycobacterium tuberculosis*
mtDNA: Mitochondrial DNA
mTOR: Mammalian target of rapamycin
MV: Mechanical ventilation
MVD: Mean veins diameter
N: Nucleocapsid protein
NAAT: Nucleic acid amplification test
NAB: Nucleic-acid binding region
NAD$^+$: Nicotinamide adenine dinucleotide
NCBI: National Center for Biotechnology Information
NCD: Noncommunicable disease
NCE: New chemical entity
NCIP: Novel coronavirus infected pneumonia
nCoV-19: Novel coronavirus 2019
NETs: Neutrophil extracellular traps
NF-κB: Nuclear factor-kappa light-chain enhancer of activated B cells
NIAID: National Institute of Allergy and Infectious Diseases
NICE: National Institute for Health and Care Excellence
NIH: National institutes of health
NINC: Noninfectious noncancer vaccines
NIPPV: Noninvasive positive pressure ventilation
NiV: Nipah virus
NIV: Noninvasive ventilation
NJ: New Jersey
NK: Natural killer (cell)
NLRP3: NOD-, LRR-, and pyrin domain–containing protein 3
nM: Nanomolar
NO: Nitric oxide
NO$_2$: Nitrogen dioxide
NSAID: Nonsteroidal antiinflammatory drug
NSP: Nonstructural proteins
NST: NanoString transcriptomic
NSTEMI: Non–ST-segment elevation myocardial infarction
NTD: N-terminal domain
NT-proBNP: N-terminal pro-brain natriuretic peptide
NY: New York
OGD: Olfactory or gustatory dysfunction
OP: Organizing pneumonia
OR: Odds ratio
ORF: Open reading frame
P/F ratio: PaO$_2$/FiO$_2$ ratio
PaCO$_2$: Partial pressure of carbon dioxide
PAHO: Pan American Health Organization
PAMP: Pathogen-associated molecular pattern
PaO$_2$: Partial pressure of arterial oxygen

PaO$_2$/FiO$_2$ ratio: Partial pressure of oxygen in arterial blood/fraction of inspired oxygen concentration ratio
PAPR: Powered air-purifying respirator
PASC: Postacute sequelae of SARS-CoV-2 infection
PBMC: Peripheral blood mononuclear cell
PBW: Predicted body weight
PCI: Percutaneous coronary intervention
PCPF: Post–COVID-19 pulmonary fibrosis
PCP-III: Protein biomarker procollagen peptide
PCR: Polymerase chain reaction
PD: Peritoneal dialysis
PDB ID: Protein data bank identifier
PE: Pulmonary embolism
PEDV: Porcine epidemic diarrhea virus
PEEP: Positive end-expiratory pressure
PEG: Polyethylene glycol
PI-IBS: Postinfectious irritable bowel syndrome
PIRRT: Prolonged intermittent renal replacement therapy
PK: Pharmacokinetic
PLpro: Papain-like protease
PM: Particulate matter
PMM: Pneumomediastinum
Poly(A): Poly-adenylation
POOR: Permeability-originated obstruction response
PP: Polyprotein
PPE: Personal protective equipment
PPI: Protein-protein interaction
PPI: Proton pump inhibitor
Pplat: Plateau pressure
PRES: Posterior reversible encephalopathy
PRESECO: Preventing Severe COVID Disease Trial
PRR: Pattern recognition receptor
PS: Protein subunit
P-SILI: Patient self-inflicted lung injury
PSP: Primary spontaneous pneumothorax
PT: Prothrombin time
PTSD: Posttraumatic stress disorder
PTT: Partial thromboplastin time
PTX: Pneumothorax
PUI: Patient under investigation
R$_0$: Reproductive number
R/I: Recruitment-to-inflation ratio
RA: Renin-angiotensin
RALE: Radiographic assessment of lung edema
RAS: Renin-angiotensin system
RBD: Receptor binding domain
RCA: Right coronary artery
RCOG: Royal College of Obstetrician and Gynaecologists
RCT: Randomized controlled trial
RdRp: RNA-dependent RNA polymerase
RDV-TP: Remdesivir triphosphate
RECOVERY: Randomised Evaluation of COVID-19 Therapy
RIG: Retinoic acid–inducible gene

RIG-I: Retinoic acid–inducible gene 1
RIRs: Relative illness ratios
RNA: Ribonucleic acid
ROS: Reactive oxygen species
RR: Relative risk
RR: Respiratory rate
RRT: Renal replacement therapy
rRT-PCR: Real-time reverse transcriptase polymerase chain reaction
RSV: Respiratory syncytial virus
RTC: Replication and transcription complex
RT-LAMP: Reverse transcription loop-mediated isothermal amplification
RT-PCR: Reverse transcriptase polymerase chain reaction
RT-qPCR: Reverse transcription quantitative polymerase chain reaction
S: Spike protein
S1P: Sphingosine-1-phosphate
sACE2: Soluble ACE2
SAM: S-adenosyl-L-methionine
SARS: Severe acute respiratory syndrome
SARS-CoV: Severe acute respiratory syndrome–associated coronavirus
SARS-CoV-2: Severe acute respiratory syndrome coronavirus-2
SBECD: Sulfobutylether-B-cyclodextrin
SC5b-9: Soluble complement components 5b-9 (also known as terminal complement complex)
SCCM: Society of Critical Care Medicine
SCFAs: Short-chain fatty acids
SES: Socioeconomic status
SLE: Systemic lupus erythematosus
SLED: Sustained low-efficiency dialysis
SMFM: The Society of Maternal-Fetal Medicine
SP-D: Surfactant protein-D
SPM: Spontaneous pneumomediastinum
SpO$_2$: Peripheral capillary oxygen saturation
sRAGE: Soluble receptor for advanced glycation end products
SSRI: Selective serotonin reuptake inhibitor
STAT: Signal transducer and activator of transcription
STEMI: ST-segment elevation myocardial infarction
SUD: SARS-unique domain
SUDV: Sudan virus
SVI: Social Vulnerability Index
T2D: Type 2 diabetes
TACE: TNF-α–converting enzyme
TAFV: Tai forest virus
TAT: Turnaround time
TBK1: TANK-binding kinase 1
TCR: T-cell receptor
TEE: Transesophageal echocardiogram
Tfh: T follicular helper cells
TGF-β: Transforming growth factor-beta
Th: T-helper

Th1: Type 1 T helper cells
Th2: Type 2 T helper cells
Th9: Type 17 T helper cells
Th17: Type 17 T helper cells
TLR: Toll-like receptor
TLR3: Toll-like receptor 3
TM: Transmembrane
TMA: Thrombotic microangiopathy
TMPRSS: Transmembrane protease serine
TMPRSS2: transmembrane protease serine 2
TNF: Tumor necrosis factor
TNF-α: Tumor necrosis factor-alpha
TOM70: Translocase of outer membrane 70
Tr1: Type 1 regulatory T cells
TRAF: TNF receptor–associated factor
TRAIL: TNF-related apoptosis–inducing ligand
Treg: Regulatory T cells
Trm: Resident memory T cells
UC: Ulcerative colitis
UK: United Kingdom
UKILD: UK Interstitial Lung Disease Consortium
US: United States

USPI: United States Package Insert
V/Q: Ventilation/perfusion
VAP: Ventilator-associated pneumonia
VE: Vaccine effectiveness
VEGF: Vascular endothelial growth factor
VILI: Ventilator-induced lung injury
VLP: Virus-like particle
VOC: Variant of concern
VOHC: Variant of high consequence
VOI: Variant of interest
vRNP: Viral ribonucleoprotein
VSV: Vesicular stomatitis virus
VTE: Venous thromboembolism
VV ECMO: Venovenous extracorporeal membrane oxygenation
VVnr: Viral vector nonreplicating
VVr: Viral vector replicating
VWF: von Willebrand factor
VZ: Varicella zoster
WHO: World Health Organization
WOB: Work of breathing
WR: Waiting room

Index

Note: Page numbers followed by *f* indicate figures, *t* indicate tables, and *b* indicate boxes.